Attachment in Adulthood

Attachment in Adulthood

Structure, Dynamics, and Change

MARIO MIKULINCER

PHILLIP R. SHAVER

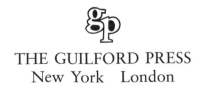

THE GUILFORD PRESS
New York   London

© 2007 The Guilford Press
A Division of Guilford Publications, Inc.
72 Spring Street, New York, NY 10012
www.guilford.com

Paperback edition 2010

Printed in the United States of America

This book is printed on acid-free paper.

Last digit is print number: 9   8   7   6   5   4

Library of Congress Cataloging-in-Publication Data

Mikulincer, Mario.
    Attachment in adulthood : structure, dynamics, and change /
Mario Mikulincer, Phillip R. Shaver.
      p. cm.
    Includes bibliographical references and index.
    ISBN-13: 978-1-59385-457-7 (cloth : alk. paper)
    ISBN-13: 978-1-60623-610-9 (paperback : alk. paper)
    1. Attachment behavior. I. Shaver, Phillip R. II. Title.
    BF575.A86M55 2007
    155.6—dc

                                          222006102548

To Salomon and Teresa Mikulincer, Deby Engel Mikulincer,
and Dan and Alon Mikulincer
—M. M.

To Robert and Frances Shaver, Gail Goodman,
and Danielle and Lauren Goodman-Shaver
—P. R. S.

About the Authors

Mario Mikulincer, PhD, received his doctorate in psychology from Bar-Ilan University, Ramat Gan, Israel, in 1985, and was Professor of Psychology there until 1992. In 2007, he established the Interdisciplinary Center (IDC) in Herzliya, Israel, and now serves as Dean of the New School of Psychology. He has published more than 220 articles and book chapters and two books, *Human Learned Helplessness: A Coping Perspective* (1994) and *Prosocial Motives, Emotions, and Behavior: The Better Angels of Our Nature* (2009) coauthored with Phillip R. Shaver. Dr. Mikulincer's research interests include attachment styles in adulthood, terror management theory, personality processes in interpersonal relationships, evolutionary psychology, and trauma and posttraumatic processes. He currently serves on the editorial boards of several academic journals and as associate editor of *Personal Relationships* and the *Journal of Personality and Social Psychology*. In 2004 he received the EMET Prize in Social Science, sponsored by the A. M. N. Foundation for the Advancement of Science, Art, and Culture in Israel, awarded by Prime Minister Ariel Sharon, for Dr. Mikulincer's contribution to psychology.

Phillip R. Shaver, PhD, received his doctorate in psychology from the University of Michigan, and is currently Distinguished Professor of Psychology at the University of California, Davis. He has served on the faculties of Columbia University, New York University, the University of Denver, and University at Buffalo, State University of New York. Dr. Shaver is associate editor of *Attachment and Human Development* and a member of the editorial boards of *Personal Relationships*, the *Journal of Personality and Social Psychology*, and *Emotion*. He has published several books, including *Measures of Personality and Social Psychological Attitudes* (1991) and *Handbook of Attachment: Theory, Research, and Clinical Applications*, 2nd edition (2008), as well as more than 175 scholarly articles and book chapters. Dr. Shaver's research focuses on emotions, close relationships, and personality development, viewed from the perspective of attachment theory. He has made notable contributions to the literatures on human emotions, close relationships, and psychology of religion. In 2002 Dr. Shaver received a Distinguished Career Award from the International Association for Relationship Research and in 2006 was elected President of that organization.

Preface

In this book we summarize, organize, and evaluate the large literature that has grown up around the concepts of "adult attachment" and "attachment style," as these were first conceptualized in the late 1980s in papers by Hazan and Shaver (1987) and Shaver, Hazan, and Bradshaw (1988). We organize the major research findings around a model of the attachment behavioral system in adulthood. The book provides a launching pad for anyone wishing to understand, contribute to, or clinically apply the large and still expanding literature on adult attachment.

Until now, students and researchers who wished to tap into the stream of research on adult attachment had to skim Bowlby's (1969/1982, 1973, 1980, 1988) weighty theoretical volumes, make their way through Ainsworth's important psychometric and empirical work (especially as summarized by Ainsworth, Blehar, Waters, & Wall, 1978), understand something about the Adult Attachment Interview (which is well described by Hesse, 1999), and ponder the various self-report measures of adult attachment, beginning with Hazan and Shaver's (1987) single-item measure of "romantic attachment" and running through a host of dimensional measures created by Collins and Read (1990), Simpson (1990), J. A. Feeney, Noller, and Hanrahan (1994), Brennan, Clark, and Shaver (1998), and Klohnen and John (1998), among others.

While involved in the process of self-education, interested researchers and clinicians were often perplexed by concepts such as behavioral system, hyperactivating and deactivating strategies, working model, safe haven and secure base, attachment–exploration balance, attachment styles, and segregated mental systems, and they were likely to be confused by the proliferation of adult attachment measures.

The interested reader's task was made easier in 1996, with the publication of J. A. Feeney and Noller's brief textbook, *Adult Attachment*, and in 1999, with the publication of the *Handbook of Attachment* (Cassidy & Shaver, 1999). But the former volume is already out of date given the rapid expansion of the research literature, and the latter volume is heavy on attachment in infancy and childhood and light on the large literature summarized here. In the *Handbook*, the kinds of research we discuss here were condensed into two chapters by Feeney (1999c) and Crowell, Fraley, and Shaver (1999), the latter dealing almost exclusively with measurement. Although there are interesting and excellent volumes dealing with the kinds of research we discuss here (e.g., Bartholomew & Perlman, 1994; Mikulincer & Goodman, 2006; Rholes & Simpson, 2004; Simpson & Rholes, 1998; Sperling & Berman, 1994), they are all collections of chapters by independent authors, so a reader has to do all of the integrative work.

The field has lacked a systematic, comprehensive overview of evolving theory, of the vast empirical literature, and of alternative measures and research methods. Here, we provide the comprehensive overview that has been missing, creating a foundation for future theorizing, research, and applications. In writing the book, we have benefited greatly from the edited volumes just mentioned and from excerpts of our own previously published work. We certainly do not wish to discourage anyone from beginning with Bowlby and reading all the way to the present in original sources (we have provided all the necessary references for those brave souls), but for many researchers and students this book will provide a starting point that makes reading the large primary literature easier.

We would like to thank the many people who have contributed to our research on attachment and the creation of this book. Mario Mikulincer thanks, in approximate historical order, Victor Florian, Rami Tolmacz, Israel Orbach, Gurit Birnbaum, Ety Berant, Neta Horesh, Orit Nachmias, Gilad Hirschberger, Dana Pereg, Omri Gillath, Nili Lavy, Shiri Lavy, Naama Bar-On, Oren Gur, Eileen Lahat, Galia Diller, Vered Gwirtz, Dar Sarel, Limor Barabi, Rivka Davidovitz, Oz Guterman, Moran Shemesh, Inbal Orbach, and Yonit Doron. Phil Shaver thanks, in approximate historical order, Cindy Hazan, Lee Kirkpatrick, Kim Bartholomew, Kelly Brennan, Linda Kunce, Marie Tidwell, Harry Reis, Julie Rothbard, Daria Papalia, Ken Levy, Catherine Clark, Lynne Cooper, Lilah Koski, Hillary Morgan, Chris Fraley, Mike Cohen, Dory Schachner, Robin Edelstein, Itzi Alonso-Arbiol, Omri Gillath, Rachel Nitzberg, Josh Hart, Erik Noftle, Tom Crawford, and Audrey Brassard. We are very grateful to Kim Bartholomew, Ety Berant, Debbie Davis, Brooke Feeney, Judy Feeney, Gery Karantsas, Brent Mallinckrodt, Ofra Mayseles, Paula Pietromonaco, Jeff Simpson, and two anonymous reviewers for reading all or parts of the first draft of the book and making many useful suggestions. We also thank the Amini Foundation, the Fetzer Institute, the Marchionne Foundation, the National Science Foundation, the Positive Psychology Network, and the Templeton Foundation for supporting our work over the years. We thank Seymour Weingarten, Editor in Chief, and Carolyn Graham, Editorial Administrator, at The Guilford Press, for being such thoughtful and supportive friends to us and other attachment researchers. And we thank Jacquelyn Coggin, Jennifer DePrima, and Deanna Butler at Guilford for careful copyediting, production, and indexing, respectively; we also thank Paul Gordon for designing the book's cover and Dan Weingarten for laying out the inside of the book.

Finally, we dedicate this book to our parents, wives, and children, who have loved us, supported us, and taught us more about attachment and caregiving than we can yet conceptualize or articulate in words.

Contents

III. INTERPERSONAL MANIFESTATIONS OF ATTACHMENT-SYSTEM FUNCTIONING

IV. CLINICAL AND ORGANIZATIONAL APPLICATIONS OF ATTACHMENT THEORY

V. EPILOGUE

APPENDICES

PART I

THE ATTACHMENT BEHAVIORAL SYSTEM

Normative Processes and Individual Differences

CHAPTER 1

The Attachment Behavioral System

Basic Concepts and Principles

My life's work has been directed to a single aim. I have observed the more subtle disturbances of mental function in healthy and sick people and have sought to infer—or, if you prefer it, to guess—from signs of this kind how the apparatus which serves these functions is constructed and what concurrent and mutually opposing forces are at work in it.

—SIGMUND FREUD (1961/1930, p. 208)

As my study of theory progressed it was gradually borne in upon me that the field I had set out to plough so lightheartedly was no less than the one that Freud had started tilling sixty years earlier, and that it contained all those same rocky excrescences and thorny entanglements that he had encountered and grappled with— love and hate, anxiety and defense, attachment and loss.

—JOHN BOWLBY (1969/1982, p. xxvii)

One of the intellectual landmarks of the 20th century was Sigmund Freud's psychoanalytic theory. In a dramatic and highly creative theoretical move, Freud focused attention on the previously hidden and unmapped (except for literature) unconscious dynamics of the human mind. He traced psychological dysfunctions and psychopathologies to abusive, repressive, or dysfunctional childhoods, and bolstered the emerging Western conviction that an individual, through personal insight and deliberate self-reconstruction, can grow beyond the constraints of a particular family or local culture. In a unique way, Freud combined the seemingly incompatible themes of Darwinian evolutionary biology (with its emphasis on selfishness, sex, and aggression), the importance of personal and cultural narratives (life stories, clinical case studies), and the possibility that insight and enlightened rationality can reshape a person's self-control of body, mind, and behavior. Despite the lashing Freud has received from critics, in his own lifetime and down to the present day, no one looking objectively at his achievements can doubt that he was a major force in 20th-century intellectual life.

Following in Freud's footsteps, while also doing battle with some of Freud's intellectual offspring (and in one case a biological daughter, Anna Freud), John Bowlby, a British psychoanalyst working from 1940 to 1990, significantly altered and updated psychoanalytic theory by combining insights from then-current object relations psychoanalytic theories, post-Darwinian ethology, modern cognitive-developmental psychology, cybernetics (control systems theories), and community psychiatry to create attachment theory, an attempt to explain why early childhood relationships with parents have such a pervasive and lasting effect on personality development. Assisted by astute theoretical and methodological insights contributed by his American colleague, Mary Ainsworth, Bowlby laid the foundation for what has become one of the most heavily researched conceptual frameworks in modern psychology.

The purpose of this book is to show how this research has recast our understanding of the adult mind, its goals and strategies for attaining particular life outcomes, and its strong propensity for forming close relationships with other embodied minds and symbolic figures, such as past relationship partners, religious deities, and cultural groups. Unlike Freud's theory, the one proposed by Bowlby and Ainsworth has proven to be eminently testable and subject to adaptation for new purposes, both scientific and therapeutic. By applying some of the best methods of ethology and experimental psychology to the study of children's emotional attachments to parents, Ainsworth set the stage for thousands of subsequent studies, conducted by researchers whose courage and confidence were based partly on Ainsworth's ideas and accomplishments.

Our own perspective on human attachments has arisen in the context of contemporary personality and social psychology, which focuses on adolescent and adult development and social relationships. To extend attachment theory from child development to this new territory, we have had to invent and adapt methods taken from many areas of modern psychology, such as neuroimaging, physiological recording, behavioral observations, questionnaire surveys, and laboratory experiments. The rapid acceptance of our ideas, methods, and research findings has resulted in a large and sprawling literature that, we suspect, is no longer familiar to any one person.

Our goal in this book is to survey this large and unwieldy literature, organize it for readers, and provide a solid foundation for new investigators, as well as for clinicians who wish to apply what has been learned in scientific studies. The literature now ranges from physiological and developmental psychology through academic personality and social psychology to clinical and counseling psychology, and even to applications in organizations and work settings. What began as a theory of child development is now used to conceptualize and study adult couple relationships, work relationships, and relations between larger social groups and societies. Fortunately, although the theory has proven its value in this wide range of settings, its concepts and principles are straightforward and easy to comprehend. It should be possible for any serious reader of this book to understand the theory, evaluate its uses in research and clinical settings, and think of novel ways to extend and apply it.

PERSONAL BACKGROUND

This book can best be understood if we explain briefly how we came, individually, to attachment theory, then began to influence each other and eventually work together. Both of us were attracted to psychoanalytic theory as undergraduates, despite the hard knocks it had taken from critics. Anyone who opens his mind to what goes on in real people's lives, or who reads novels or poems, or watches artful films, realizes that the issues raised by psychoanalysts, beginning with Freud, are extremely important: sexual attraction and desire; romantic love; the development of personality, beginning in infant–caregiver relationships; painful, corrosive emotions such as anger, fear, jealousy, hatred, and shame, which contribute to intrapsychic conflicts, defenses, and psychopathology; and intergroup hostility and war.

When we first began studying academic social and personality psychology, it seemed disappointingly superficial and dry compared with psychoanalysis. But its strong point—and the weak point of psychoanalysis—was a collection of powerful and creative empirical research methods. Psychoanalytic theorists seemed capable of endlessly inventing and debating hypothetical constructs and processes, without being constrained by operational definitions, sound psychometrics, or replicable empirical studies. Both of us began our careers as experimental researchers pursuing existing topics in the field (stress and learned helplessness in Mikulincer's case, self-awareness and fear of success in the case of Shaver), but our interest in psychoanalytic ideas never abated. When Bowlby's books began to appear, we realized that a psychoanalytic thinker could pay attention to the full range of scientific perspectives on human behavior, seek empirical evidence for psychoanalytic propositions, and emend or reformulate psychoanalytic theory based on empirical research. Ainsworth's development of a laboratory "Strange Situation" assessment procedure, which allowed her to classify infants' attachment patterns systematically and relate them to home observations of parent–child interactions, added to our confidence that research on an extension of attachment theory to adults and adult relationships might be possible.

In the mid-1980s, Shaver was studying adolescent and adult loneliness (see, e.g., Rubenstein & Shaver, 1982; Shaver & Hazan, 1984) and noticing both that attachment theory was useful in conceptualizing loneliness (e.g., Weiss, 1973) and that patterns of chronic loneliness were similar in certain respects to the insecure infant attachment patterns identified by Ainsworth et al. (1978). Building on this insight, one of Shaver's doctoral students, Cindy Hazan, wrote a seminar paper suggesting that attachment theory could be used as a framework for studying romantic love—or "romantic attachment," as they called it in their first article on the topic (Hazan & Shaver, 1987).

That article caught the eye of Mikulincer, who had become interested in attachment theory while studying affect-regulation processes related to learned helplessness, depression, combat stress reactions, and posttraumatic stress disorder in Israel. He noticed similarities between (1) certain forms of helplessness in adulthood and the effects of parental unavailability in infancy; (2) intrusive images and emotions in the case of posttraumatic stress disorder (PTSD) and the anxious attachment pattern described by Ainsworth et al. (1978) and Hazan and Shaver (1987); and (3) avoidant strategies for coping with stress and the avoidant attachment pattern described by these same authors. In 1990, Mikulincer, Florian, and Tolmacz published a study of attachment patterns and conscious and unconscious death anxiety, one of the first studies to use the preliminary self-report measure of adult attachment style devised by Hazan and Shaver (1987), and the first to show its connections with unconscious mental processes.

From then on, both of us continued to pursue the application of attachment theory to the study of adults' emotions, emotion regulation strategies, close interpersonal relationships, and the accomplishment of various life tasks, noticing that we were both interested in the experimental study of what might be called attachment-related psychodynamics: the kinds of mental processes, including intense needs, powerful emotions and conflicts, and defensive strategies that had captivated the attention of both Freud and Bowlby. In recent years we have pooled our efforts to craft a more rigorous formulation of our theoretical ideas (e.g., Mikulincer & Shaver, 2003; Shaver &

Mikulincer, 2002a), clarify and extend our model of the attachment system, test it in many different ways, and move it in the direction of positive psychology's emphasis on personal growth and social virtues (e.g., Gable & Haidt, 2005; Seligman, 2002), such as compassion, altruism, gratitude, and forgiveness. In our opinion, attachment theory comfortably incorporates both "positive" and "negative" psychologies by considering all of the psychological forces that arise and collide in the human quest for security and self-control. In this book we summarize what we have learned to date, placing our own work in the context of the large and still growing literature on adult attachment.

ORIGINS OF ATTACHMENT THEORY IN THE LIVES OF BOWLBY AND AINSWORTH

Although our own backgrounds are worth taking into account, it is obviously even more important to know something about Bowlby and Ainsworth, the originators of attachment theory. John Bowlby was born in 1907, in England, to well-off and well-educated parents. His father was a physician, and Bowlby eventually became one, too—a psychiatrist. But long before that, he served as a volunteer at a school for maladjusted children and began to form impressions and opinions that became the seeds of attachment theory. As Bretherton (1992) explained:

> [Bowlby's] experience with two children at the school set his professional life on course. One was a very isolated, remote, affectionless teenager who had been expelled from his previous school for theft and had had no stable mother figure. The second child was an anxious boy of 7 or 8 who trailed Bowlby around and who was known as his shadow (Ainsworth, 1974). Persuaded by this experience of the effects of early family relationships on personality development, Bowlby decided to embark on a career as a child psychiatrist. (p. 759)

These boys' different reactions to inadequate parenting led Bowlby, throughout his later writings, to try to understand the development of what we call "avoidant" and "anxious" attachment styles. This initial focus of his interest is what continues to occupy us and many other researchers who are trying to understand adolescent and adult attachment.

While studying to become a child psychiatrist, Bowlby undertook psychoanalytic training with a then-famous mentor, Melanie Klein, and was psychoanalyzed for several years by Joan Riviere, Klein's close associate. From those mentors Bowlby learned a great deal about the importance of early relationships with caregivers; the tendency of troubled children to deal with painful experiences, especially separations and losses, by defensively excluding them from conscious memory; and the emotions of anxiety, anger, and sadness. Despite absorbing many of Klein's and Riviere's ideas, however, Bowlby seemed from the beginning not to accept their extreme emphasis on fantasies at the expense of reality, and on sexual drives rather than other kinds of relational needs. (See Karen [1994] for a detailed account of this part of Bowlby's professional training.)

Their fundamental disagreement came to a head, at least for Bowlby, when Klein forbade him to speak with or focus attention on a child client's schizophrenic mother, because Klein thought child psychoanalysis should deal with the child's conflicts and fantasies, not with the actual experiences Bowlby thought had probably caused and certainly contributed to them. Recalling these events years later, in 1979, Bowlby said, "It was regarded as almost outside the proper interest of an analyst to give systematic attention to a person's real experiences" (p. 5). In his own work, Bowlby emphasized each child's actual experiences, especially the experience of what he called "maternal deprivation"—separation from or loss of one's mother early in life. One of his first publications (1944), "Forty-Four Juvenile Thieves," used a combination of statistics and clinical case notes to show that juvenile delinquents often came from backgrounds that included loss of the mother, repeated separations from the mother, or being passed from one foster mother to another.

Attachment theory grew gradually out of Bowlby's experiences as a family clinician at the Tavistock Clinic in London and the author of a report for the World Health Organization (WHO) on homeless children following World War II. At the Tavistock Clinic, Bowlby directed a research unit focused on separation from parents. There, he collaborated with a talented social worker, James Robertson, who made powerfully moving films of children who had been forcefully separated from their parents, either because a child had to be hospitalized for medical treatment and the parents were not allowed to visit, or because a parent (usually the mother) had to be hospitalized and the child was not allowed to visit. Besides contributing to Bowlby's early theorizing, these research ventures and films helped to change visitation policies in British hospitals as well as hospitals in other parts of the world.

Bowlby's interest was not only in children who suffered "maternal deprivation" but also in the effects their wounds might have on communities and society more broadly. In 1951 he concluded an essay as follows: "Thus it is seen how children who suffer deprivation grow up to become parents deficient in the capacity to care for their children and how adults deficient in this capacity are commonly those who suffered deprivation in childhood" (pp. 68–69). This insight has been central to attachment research ever since and is now called the "intergenerational transmission" of insecurity (e.g., de Wolff & van IJzendoorn, 1997). Bowlby's suggestions regarding psychotherapy (e.g., summarized in his 1988 book, A Secure Base) can be viewed as an attempt to heal the attachment injuries of children, adolescents, and adults, and at the same time break the intergenerational cycle that otherwise extends the plague of insecurity to subsequent generations.

As Bowlby's clinical observations and insights accumulated, he became increasingly interested in explaining what, in his first major statement of attachment theory, he called "the child's tie to his mother" (Bowlby, 1958). In formulating the theory, he was especially influenced by Konrad Lorenz's (1952) ideas about "imprinting" in precocial birds and the writings of other ethologists and primatologists, including his friend and mentor Robert Hinde (1966). These authors, along with Harry Harlow (1959), had begun to show that immature animals' ties to their mothers were not due simply to classical conditioning based on feeding, as learning theorists (and, using different language, psychoanalysts) had thought. Instead, Bowlby viewed the human infant's reliance on, and emotional bond with, its mother to be the result of a fundamental instinctual behavioral system that, unlike Freud's sexual libido concept, was relational without being sexual. Because Bowlby relied so heavily on animal research and on the notion of behavioral systems, he was strongly criticized by other psychoanalysts for being a "behaviorist." He nevertheless continued to view himself as a psychoanalyst and a legitimate heir to Freud, which is the way he is largely viewed today.

After publishing his 1958 paper on the attachment bond (i.e., the child's tie to his or her mother), Bowlby published two seminal papers: "Separation Anxiety" (1960a) and "Grief and Mourning in Infancy and Early Childhood" (1960b). Over the subsequent decades, each of these foundational articles was developed into a major book, forming a trilogy that is now widely recognized as a major contribution to modern psychology, psychiatry, and social science. The first volume was published in 1969 and revised in 1982: Attachment and Loss: Vol. 1. Attachment. The second volume, Attachment and Loss:

Vol. 2. Separation: Anxiety and Anger, was published in 1973, and the third, *Attachment and Loss: Vol. 3. Loss: Sadness and Depression*, in 1980. These books were accompanied in 1979 by a collection of Bowlby's lectures, *The Making and Breaking of Affectional Bonds*, which is a good place for readers unfamiliar with Bowlby's work to begin, and were capped in 1988 by Bowlby's book about applications of attachment theory and research to psychotherapy, *A Secure Base*. In 1990, he published a biography of Charles Darwin, focusing on the possible effects of the death of Darwin's mother when he was around 10 years of age on Darwin's subsequently poor physical health. (Bowlby attributed his symptoms to hyperventilation, a physiological effect of unresolved grief.) This set of writings is, by any standard, a monumental contribution to our understanding of human relationships and the human mind.

Bowlby's major collaborator, especially in his later years, Mary Salter Ainsworth, was born in Ohio in 1913 and received her PhD in developmental psychology from the University of Toronto in 1939 after completing a research dissertation on security and dependency inspired by her advisor William Blatz's security theory. In her dissertation, *An Evaluation of Adjustment Based on the Concept of Security* (1940), Ainsworth mentioned for the first time the central attachment-theoretical construct of a "secure base":

> Familial security in the early stages is of a dependent type and forms a basis from which the individual can work out gradually, forming new skills and interests in other fields. Where familial security is lacking, the individual is handicapped by the lack of what might be called a secure base from which to work. (p. 45)

Interestingly, in light of Ainsworth's subsequent career, her dissertation included a new self-report measure of security and dependency, as well as coded content analyses of autobiographical narratives. After World War II, Ainsworth participated in Rorschach workshops with Bruno Klopfer, a famous Rorschach expert, because she had been asked to teach a personality assessment course. Out of these workshops came an influential book on the Rorschach Inkblot Test (Klopfer, Ainsworth, Klopfer, & Holt, 1954). Ainsworth was therefore familiar with a variety of research methods and a fruitful theory of security before she ever met John Bowlby.

Ainsworth's husband, Leonard, needed to move to London to complete his doctoral studies, and she moved with him. (In those days, a husband's career was generally considered more important than a wife's career.) Once in London, Mary Ainsworth answered a newspaper advertisement for a research position with Bowlby, having not known about him or his work beforehand. Part of her job was to analyze some of Robertson's films of children's separation behavior. These films convinced her of the value of behavioral observations, which became a hallmark of her contributions to attachment research from then on. When her husband decided to advance his career by undertaking psychocultural research in Uganda in 1953, Mary Ainsworth moved there as well, and began an observational study of mothers and infants, repeatedly visiting them every 2 weeks for 2 hours over a period of several months. Eventually, after returning to North America and working at Johns Hopkins University in Baltimore, Maryland, she published a book in 1967, *Infancy in Uganda: Infant Care and the Growth of Love*. (She was also divorced from her husband Leonard, which caused her to enter a several-year psychoanalysis that she subsequently praised very highly, and that seemed to allow her to move out from under Leonard's harmful shadow and become much more creative and productive. See Isaacson, 2006, for a psychobiography of Ainsworth based on personal correspondence.)

One of the historically significant features of Ainsworth's 1967 book is an appendix that sketches different patterns of infant attachment, which Ainsworth linked empirically with observable maternal sensitivity or insensitivity at home. Although these patterns were not precisely the same as the three types for which Ainsworth later became famous (in this book we call them *secure*, *anxious*, and *avoidant*; see Ainsworth et al., 1978), some definite similarities are evident. The three main patterns of attachment delineated later on, derived from studies of middle-class white infants in Baltimore, involved extensive home observations during the infants' first year of life, supplemented by a laboratory assessment procedure, the "Strange Situation" (now typically capitalized in writings about attachment theory and research, to help readers remember that it is a formal measure, not simply an "odd" situation). Ainsworth et al.'s 1978 book explained how to code an infant's behavior toward the mother in the Strange Situation, and also showed how the three major categories of infant attachment behavior were associated with particular patterns of maternal behavior in the home. The measures and ideas advanced in the 1978 book, in conjunction with Bowlby's theoretical trilogy on attachment and loss, form the backbone of all subsequent discussions of attachment processes and individual differences in attachment style.

Over the years, Ainsworth and Bowlby continued to correspond frequently and meet for extended face-to-face discussions, and both regularly modified their ideas and research efforts in line with the other's discoveries. (One of Bowlby's reasons for creating a revised version of the first [1969] volume of his *Attachment and Loss* trilogy, in 1982, was that he wished to include empirical evidence from Ainsworth's studies. In 1988 he expressly honored Ainsworth and her ideas by titling his book on attachment-oriented psychotherapy *A Secure Base*.) In our opinion, Bowlby's work, no matter how brilliant, would not have had the enormous impact it has had on the discipline of psychology without the theoretical insights and psychometric and empirical contributions of Mary Ainsworth. Many other object relations theories proposed by British psychoanalysts of Bowlby's era did not generate anything like the research literature inspired by attachment theory, partly because they were less clearly stated, less subject to operationalization, and less connected with other scientific literatures.

In 1989, both Bowlby and Ainsworth received the American Psychological Association's Distinguished Scientific Contribution Award. Ainsworth single-handedly completed an article for the *American Psychologist* accepting the award on behalf of both scholars, because Bowlby died before the article was completed (Ainsworth & Bowlby, 1991). Their joint contributions to psychology and psychiatry are remarkable for many reasons, not the least of which is that their work is increasingly cited in psychoanalytic books and articles, despite the cool (and in some cases, hostile) reception Bowlby's ideas initially received from his psychoanalytic colleagues. Not only was he not a behaviorist, but thanks in part to Ainsworth, he also turned out to be the most important psychoanalytic theorist of his or, except for Freud's, any other generation.

NORMATIVE ASPECTS OF THE ATTACHMENT BEHAVIORAL SYSTEM

With the preceding two biographical sections behind us, we can turn to attachment theory itself, placing special emphasis on Bowlby's notion of the "attachment behavioral system." There are two crucial parts of attachment theory, one of which is called "normative" because it deals with normal features of the attachment behavioral system and its development that can be observed in all people, and the other of which concerns "individual differences" in the attachment system's operation. We begin our account of the theory by focusing first on its normative component.

In rejecting the concepts of drive and psychic energy in classical psychoanalytic theory and attempting to replace them with concepts more compatible with the ethological and cognitive psychological theories of his time, Bowlby (1969/1982) borrowed from ethology the concept of *behavioral system*, a species-universal, biologically evolved neural program that organizes behavior in ways that increase the chances of an individual's survival and reproduction, despite inevitable environmental dangers and demands. Theoretically, the attachment behaviors observed when a person encounters threats or stressors—for example, vocalizing distress, seeking proximity or clinging to a caregiver, and relaxing once proximity and support are provided—are due to a hard-wired "attachment behavioral system," just as a caregiver's reactions to a relationship partner's (especially a dependent child's) distress signals and attachment behaviors are due to an innate "caregiving behavioral system." By dividing motivational systems into functional types such as attachment, caregiving, exploration, affiliation, and sex, Bowlby was able to conceptualize links among, and functional and dysfunctional properties of, these systems in a wide variety of life situations and across all phases of life. By conceptualizing each behavioral system as an innate, functional, goal-directed (or as he said, goal-corrected) process, Bowlby was impelled to think about how each system evolved, what function it served in the context of survival and reproduction, and how it was activated, governed, and deactivated in particular situations.

According to the theory, these behavioral systems govern the choice, activation, and termination of behavioral sequences aimed at attaining particular "set-goals"—states of the person–environment relationship that have adaptive advantages for individual survival and genetic reproduction. The adaptive behavioral sequences are "activated" by certain stimuli or kinds of situations that make a particular set-goal salient (e.g., sudden loud noises, darkness, the presence of a stranger or predator) and are "deactivated" or "terminated" by other stimuli or outcomes that signal attainment of the desired goal state (emotional support or protection, in the case of the attachment system). This cybernetic conception of behavioral systems was quite different from theories based on concepts such as "instincts," "drives," or "needs," because there is no assumption that a person experiences, say, increasing needs for attachment over time the way a person becomes hungry over time without food. (Both Freud and Lorenz had imagined that pressure builds up in need systems, causing energy or pressure to leak out or trigger an explosion, but there is no such "balloon-under-pressure" metaphor in attachment theory.) Also, instead of viewing behavior as forced into expression by fluid drives that have to be channeled or repressed, behavior is viewed as "activated" by "signals," and the behavior itself is preorganized into generally functional patterns with identifiable set-goals. Behavior is "terminated" when its set-goal is attained, rather than being exhausted by depletion of psychic energy or libido.

In the following passage, Bretherton (1992) explains the differences between Bowlby's conception of behavioral systems and the views of earlier psychoanalytic and instinct theorists:

> Behaviors regulated by such systems need not be rigidly innate, but—depending on the organism—can adapt in greater or lesser degrees to changes in environmental circumstances, provided these do not deviate too much from the organism's environment of evolutionary adaptedness [EEA, for short]. Such flexible organisms pay a price, however, because adaptable

behavioral systems can be more easily subverted from their optimal path of development. For humans, Bowlby speculates, the environment of evolutionary adaptedness probably resembled that of present-day hunter-gatherer societies. (p. 766)

Conceptually, a behavioral system has six components or aspects: (1) a specific biological function, which in the EEA increased the likelihood of survival or reproductive success; (2) a set of activating triggers; (3) a set of interchangeable, functionally equivalent behaviors that constitute the primary strategy of the system for attaining a particular goal; (4) a specific set-goal—the change in the person–environment relationship that terminates the system's activation; (5) the cognitive processes involved in activating and guiding the system's functions; and (6) specific excitatory or inhibitory neural links with other behavioral systems. Although akin to the evolutionary psychological construct of a mental "module" (e.g., as used in the volume edited by Barkow, Cosmides, & Tooby, 1992), the behavioral system construct is more complex, applies to a broader range of behavior, is "goal-corrected," and is more evident in its behavioral effects. For example, evolutionary psychologists have tended to focus on postulated mental modules that reason in certain ways, detect cheating, cause people to be attracted to sexual partners with "good genes," and arouse jealousy of particular kinds. Bowlby, in contrast, focused on complex and fairly flexible behavior patterns such as seeking proximity to a caregiver (e.g., by crying, smiling, reaching, crawling, or doing whatever else is necessary), exploring the environment curiously and, as a result, building up a complex repertoire of physical and mental skills, and empathizing with people in distress and engaging in a variety of actions to comfort them.

The Biological Function of the Attachment System

The presumed biological function of the attachment system is to protect a person (especially during infancy and early childhood) from danger by ensuring that he or she maintains proximity to caring and supportive others (*attachment figures*), especially in dangerous situations. In Bowlby's view, the innate propensity to seek out and maintain proximity to attachment figures (people he called "stronger and wiser" caregivers) evolved in relation to the prolonged helplessness and dependence on caregivers of human infants who cannot defend themselves from predators and other dangers. According to Bowlby's evolutionary reasoning, infants who maintained proximity to a supportive caregiver were more likely to survive and eventually reproduce, causing genes that fostered proximity seeking and other attachment behaviors in times of danger to be selected for and passed on to subsequent generations.

We now know that the action of these genes is mediated by neuroendocrine hormones and physiological "axes" or systems, such as the neuropeptides oxytocin and vasopressin, the stress hormones adrenaline and cortisol, the amygdala, and the hypothalamic–pituitary–adrenal (HPA) axis, that respond to threats and stressors (for details, see the volume edited by Carter et al., 2005). Interestingly, oxytocin plays a role in both child–parent attachments and later romantic/sexual "pair-bond" attachments (Carter, 2005) and is measurably low in former orphans who were neglected or poorly treated before being adopted into caring families (O'Connor, 2005). (This may be one of the mediators of clinically significant "reactive attachment disorder," which is the technical term for a disorder involving inability to form normal child–caregiver attachments after having been severely neglected or treated abusively early in life.) Another example: Cortisol levels are especially high and labile in both young children and adults who are separated from attachment figures, or are simply asked to think about such separations and losses (e.g., Gillath, Shaver, Mendoza, Maninger, & Ferrer, 2006; Gunnar, 2005). Thus, attachment researchers are well on the way to understanding the physiological processes that account for some of the effects Bowlby and Ainsworth observed in the behavior of clinical cases and participants in laboratory studies.

Although the attachment behavioral system is most evident and perhaps most important early in life, Bowlby (1988) assumed it is active over the entire lifespan and is manifested in thoughts and behaviors related to seeking proximity to attachment figures in times of threat or need. He specifically argued against the idea that dependence on others is immature or pathological at any age, or that grieving a loss is pathological or undesirable. He understood that even fully mature and relatively autonomous adults—especially when they are threatened, in pain, lonely, or demoralized—benefit from seeking and receiving other people's care. He also argued that mature autonomy is attained partly by internalizing positive interactions with attachment figures. In other words, the ability to self-soothe is based largely on having been comforted by caring attachment figures earlier in life for empirical evidence that this is the case even in adulthood (see Mikulincer & Shaver, 2004).

Bowlby, along with Harlow (1959), also rejected psychoanalytic and Pavlovian conceptualizations of social attachment as a secondary effect of being fed by a parent, which Freud and Pavlov attributed to drive reduction and classical conditioning. In line with "object relations" approaches to psychoanalysis (reviewed by Greenberg & Mitchell, 1983), Bowlby viewed human beings as inherently relationship seeking, naturally oriented to seek what Harlow (1959) called "contact comfort" (in his well-known studies of infant monkeys' attachments to and reliance on real and cloth-surrogate mothers), and naturally inclined to seek proximity to familiar, comforting figures in times of threat, pain, or need. That is, Bowlby viewed proximity to and contact with affectionate, trusted, and supportive attachment figures as a natural and functional human phenomenon, and he viewed the loss of such proximity and contact as a natural source of distress and psychological dysfunction. In this book, we show that successful bids for proximity and the attainment of felt security are important aspects of all satisfying close relationships, regardless of a person's age.

Activating Triggers of the Attachment System

Originally, Bowlby (1969/1982) claimed that the attachment behavioral system is activated by environmental threats that endanger a person's survival. Encounters with such threats arouse a need for protection provided by other people and automatically activate the attachment system. When no threat is present, there is no need to seek care from others, so no proximity-seeking tendency is activated, at least not for the purposes of protection. (A person may seek proximity to others for the purpose of some other behavioral system, such as affiliation or sexual mating.) When no threat is present, it is often advantageous not to seek care, but instead to devote time to other activities, such as exploration, food gathering, or mating. In subsequent writings, Bowlby (1973) extended this reasoning by proposing that the attachment system is also activated by "natural clues of danger"—stimuli that are not inherently dangerous but that increase the likelihood of danger (e.g., darkness, loud noises, isolation)—as well as by attachment-related threats such as impending or actual separation from, or loss of, an attachment figure. In his view, a combination of attachment-unrelated sources of threat and lack of access to an attachment figure compounds distress and triggers the highest level of attachment-system activation.

Although the same kinds of processes occur in adulthood, the threshold for activation of the attachment system is generally higher than in childhood, because most adults have developed an array of coping and problem-solving capabilities that can be exercised autonomously, and have developed a strong capacity for symbolic thought. These abilities to self-soothe and regulate emotions allow adults to imagine being calmed by an attachment figure or to postpone comfort seeking until such support is available.

The Primary Attachment Strategy

According to Bowlby (1969/1982), proximity seeking is the natural and primary strategy of the attachment behavioral system when a person needs protection or support. This strategy consists of a wide variety of behaviors that have similar functions (establishing and maintaining proximity to a protective attachment figure) and serve similar adaptive functions (protection from danger, injury, or demoralization). Among these behaviors are signals (interaction bids) that tell a relationship partner one is interested in restoring or maintaining proximity; overt displays of negative emotion (e.g., anger, anxiety, sadness) that call upon a partner to provide support and comfort; active approach behaviors that result in greater physical or psychological contact, including what Harlow (1959) called "contact comfort"; and explicit requests for emotional or instrumental support. According to Bowlby (1969/1982), these behaviors are not all likely to be manifested in every threatening situation. Rather, they are part of a repertoire of behaviors from which an individual can "choose" (consciously or unconsciously) the most appropriate means of attaining protection in a given situation.

In infancy, these strategies of the attachment behavioral system are largely innate (e.g., crying when frightened, reaching out to be picked up and held), but as a person develops and enters more complex social relationships, the goal-corrected behavior motivated by the attachment system has to become increasingly flexible, context-sensitive, and skillful. A child who has been appropriately "coached" (Gottman & Declaire, 1998) and guided by attachment figures in a wide variety of situations is more likely to develop such skills (e.g., expressing emotions appropriately, communicating needs and feelings coherently and clearly, regulating need expression in line with preferences and role demands of an attachment figure) and is therefore more likely to be successful in getting hiss or her needs met in subsequent relationships.

In adulthood, the primary attachment strategy does not necessarily require actual proximity-seeking behavior. It can also include activation of mental representations of relationship partners who regularly provide care and protection. These representations can create a sense of safety and security, which helps a person deal successfully with threats; that is, mental representations of attachment figures can become symbolic sources of protection, and their activation can establish what might be called "symbolic proximity" to supportive others. Mental representations of the self come to include "incorporated" or "introjected" traits of security providing attachment figures, so that self-soothing and soothing by actual others become alternative means of regulating distress (Mikulincer & Shaver, 2004). For example, a student undergoing a difficult examination can call to mind the beneficial support provided on previous occasions by security-providing attachment figures, and can regulate anxiety and focus attention partly by calming herself in some of the same ways her attachment figure previously calmed her.

At the end of the exam, having worked hard and effectively, the student can call her attachment figure on the phone and share the joy of hard work that ends happily. Of course, at times—during painful illnesses or injuries or in the midst of traumatic events—when these strategies are insufficient, even generally secure adults often seek immediate, actual proximity to an attachment figure.

The Set-Goal of the Attachment System

Bowlby (1969/1982) specified the set-goal of the attachment system and described the typical cycle of attachment-system activation and deactivation. The goal of the system is a sense of protection or security (called "felt security" by Sroufe & Waters, 1977b), which normally terminates the system's activation. This sense of felt security is a psychological state with many implications: Feeling secure, a person can devote attention to matters other than self-protection; being well cared for, he can appreciate the feeling of being loved and valued; in some circumstances, he can take risks, being confident that help is readily available. This goal is made particularly salient by encounters with actual or symbolic threats and by appraisals of an attachment figure as not sufficiently near, interested, or responsive. In such cases, the attachment system is activated and the individual is motivated to seek and reestablish actual or symbolic proximity to an attachment figure. These bids for proximity persist until protection and security are attained. When the goal of felt security is attained, the attachment system is deactivated and the individual can calmly and coherently return to nonattachment activities.

This cycle—experiencing threats or distress, seeking protection and comfort from an attachment figure, experiencing stress reduction and felt security, and returning to other interests and activities—provides a prototype of both successful emotion regulation and regulation of interpersonal closeness. Knowing that coping with threats and distress is possible (through affection, gaining assistance, solving pressing problems), and knowing that it can be accomplished in part by assistance from relationship partners, gives a person a model or "script" for regulating negative emotions, maintaining equanimity, and sustaining valuable relationships (Waters, Rodrigues, & Ridgeway, 1998). Part of what is learned and represented in this script is that interpersonal closeness and support for autonomous functioning are mutually sustainable. When one is suffering or worried, it is useful to seek comfort from others; when suffering is alleviated, it is possible to engage in other activities and entertain other priorities. When attachment relationships function well, a person learns that distance and autonomy are completely compatible with closeness and reliance on others. There is no tension between autonomy and relatedness.

Bowlby was primarily interested in infant attachment to the mother. He was a product of his culture and historical era in viewing the mother as the most important and most influential attachment figure. This "monotropy," as he called the tendency to have one particular attachment figure who clearly stands out from all others, has been challenged by feminists, members of modern societies that depend on professional day care workers, and anthropologists. Hrdy (2005), for example, provided extensive evidence for what she calls the "cooperative breeding hypothesis," according to which "allomaternal assistance was essential for child survival during the Pleistocene (p. 9)," when evolution of human attachment behavior is thought to have occurred.

Far from disagreeing with other aspects of attachment theory, Hrdy (2005) views the reliance on allomaternal care as one reason for the evolution of human attachment behavior:

This breeding system—quite novel for an ape—permitted hominid females to produce costly offspring without increasing interbirth intervals, and allowed humans to move into new habitats, eventually expanding out of Africa. Reliance on allomaternal assistance would make maternal commitment more dependent on the mother's perception of probable support from others [such as a male mate or female relatives] than is the case in most other primates. One artifact of such conditional maternal investment would be newborns who needed to monitor and engage mothers, as well as older infants and juveniles who needed to elicit care from a range of caretakers across the prolonged period of dependence characteristic of young among cooperative breeders. (p. 9)

In his writings, Bowlby (1969/1982) also acknowledged that babies become attached to a few significant others during the first year of life and argued that these caregivers are organized into a "hierarchy of attachment figures," but he did not develop these ideas in detail. The issue is important to us because, later in the book, we consider the possibility that attachment-related feelings and behavior can occur in relation to many more people, in more social situations, than attachment researchers who focus exclusively on parent–child relationships would expect.

The Cognitive Substrate of the Attachment System

According to Bowlby (1969/1982), the attachment system operates in a complex goal-corrected manner; that is, a person (infant, child, or adult) evaluates the progress he or she is making toward achieving the set-goal of proximity/protection and then, if necessary, corrects his or her behavior to produce the most effective action sequence. This flexible, goal-directed, and goal-corrected adjustment of attachment behavior requires at least three cognitive operations: (1) processing information about the person–environment relationship, which involves monitoring and appraising threatening events and one's own internal state (e.g., distress, security); (2) monitoring and appraising the attachment figure's responses to one's proximity-seeking attempts; and (3) monitoring and appraising the utility of the chosen behaviors in a given context, so that an effective adjustment of these behaviors can be made in accordance with contextual constraints. These elements of a goal-corrected behavioral system are included in all cybernetic, control system models of self-regulation (e.g., Carver & Scheier, 1981; Miller, Galanter, & Pribram, 1960).

Bowlby (1969/1982, 1973) stressed that the goal-corrected nature of attachment behavior requires the storage of relevant data in the form of mental representations of person–environment transactions. Based on the theoretical writings of Craik (1943) and Young (1964), he called these representations *working models* and seemed to intend the word "working" to carry two senses: (1) The models allow for mental simulation and prediction of likely outcomes of various attachment behaviors (i.e., they provide dynamic, adjustable, context-sensitive representations of complex social situations); and (2) the models are provisional (in the sense of "working" drafts or changeable plans).

Bowlby (1969/1982) distinguished between two kinds of working models: "If an individual is to draw up a plan to achieve a set-goal not only does he have some sort of working model of his environment, but he must have also some working knowledge of his own behavioral skills and potentialities" (p. 112). That is, the attachment system, once it has been used repeatedly in relational contexts, includes representations of attachment figures' responses (*working models of others*) as well as representations of one's own efficacy and value, or the lack thereof (*working models of self*). These working models organize a person's memory about an attachment figure and him- or herself during attempts to gain protection in times of need (Main, Kaplan, & Cassidy, 1985).

Interplay between the Attachment Behavioral System and Other Behavioral Systems

Because Bowlby was interested in human (and other primate) infants' use of attachment figures in situations that evoke fear or distress, he devoted considerable thought to the nature of fear or alarm itself. And because he was interested in what else an infant did when felt security had been established or reestablished, he had to consider all of the other behavioral systems that can become activated when an infant feels safe and unafraid. Like other psychologists who thought about fear and escape behavior, Bowlby realized that there must be an organized behavioral system that links fear arousal with escape behavior. But he also emphasized that a child often escapes *from* threat or danger *to* the safety provided by an attachment figure. As Bretherton (1992) explained,

> Bowlby notes that two distinct sets of stimuli elicit fear in children: the presence of unlearned and later of culturally acquired clues to danger and/or the absence of an attachment figure. Although escape from danger and escape to an attachment figure commonly occur together, the two classes of behavior are governed by separate control systems (observable when a ferocious dog comes between a mother and her young child). Although Bowlby regarded the systems controlling escape and attachment as conceptually distinct, he considers both as members of a larger family of stress-reducing and safety-promoting behavioral systems, whose more general function is that of maintaining an organism within a defined relationship to his or her environment. Rather than striving for stimulus absence, as Freud had suggested, Bowlby posits that humans are motivated to maintain a dynamic balance between familiarity-preserving, stress-reducing behaviors (attachment to protective individuals and to familiar home sites, retreat from the strange and novel) and antithetical exploratory and information-seeking behaviors. (p. 767)

Because fear and proximity seeking must have high priority from the standpoint of biological survival, activation of the attachment system generally deactivates or inhibits other behavioral systems. Under conditions of threat, people turn to others as providers of support and comfort rather than as partners for exploratory, affiliative, or sexual activities. Moreover, at such times they are likely to be so self-focused (so focused on their need for protection) that they lack the mental resources necessary to attend empathically and altruistically to others' needs and provide care. Only when relief is attained and a sense of attachment security is restored can the individual deploy attention and energy to other behavioral systems and engage in nonattachment activities. Because of this reciprocal relation between the attachment system and other behavioral systems, the attainment of attachment security fosters engagement in nonattachment activities such as exploration, sex, and caregiving, and allows an individual to establish distance from an attachment figure, with the belief that he or she will be available if needed.

The dynamic interplay of the attachment system and other behavioral systems can be conceptualized in terms of present-day motivation theories, which focus on the distinction between "prevention" and "promotion" motives (Higgins, 1998), or between inhibitory and excitatory neural circuits (Carver & White, 1994; J. A. Gray, 1987). When viewed in relation to threats or stressors, the attachment system can be viewed as a "prevention" motivational system aimed at protecting a person from injury or "inhibiting" behaviors that lead to or increase the possibility of danger or injury. However, by facilitating closeness to others and the attainment of felt security, which "promotes" the operation of other approach-oriented behavioral systems (e.g., exploration and affiliation), the attachment system can be viewed as a "promotion" system or behavioral "activation" system that facilitates skills acquisition, personal growth, and self-actualization.

IMPORTANT CONCEPTUAL DISTINCTIONS

Although the central concepts and tenets of attachment theory are fairly easy to understand, it is important not to equate them too readily with everyday conceptions of human motivation and social relationships. Attachment figures are not simply any close relationship partner, and the unique features of the former are important to clarify. Moreover, not all interactions with attachment figures are attachment-related interactions; playing tennis with an attachment figure, for example, is not the same as relying on him or her for protection and comfort in times of distress. (Bowlby would have viewed this interaction as governed by the exploration and affiliation systems.) Finally, an attachment relationship is psychologically crystallized in the form of what Bowlby (1969/1982) called an "attachment bond," which is specifically related to using another person as a "stronger and wiser" attachment figure (i.e., as a safe haven and secure base in times of need). There are other forms of emotional bonds between people, for example, based on liking, sexual attraction, common interests, and even parenthood, that are not regarded, theoretically, as attachment bonds. It is important within attachment theory that children are normally "attached" to their parents, but that parents, at least when their children are young, are "caregivers" for the children, not "attached" to them in the sense of being reliant on them for protection or care. (When this reverse form of "attachment" in the technical sense occurs during childhood, attachment theorists consider it to be an inappropriate and psychologically damaging reversal of roles, because it leaves a child uncertain about his or her own safe haven and secure base).

The Uniqueness of Attachment Figures

The concept of attachment figure has a specific meaning in attachment theory. Attachment figures are not just close, important relationship partners. They are special individuals to whom a person turns when protection and support are needed. According to the theory (e.g., Ainsworth, 1991; Hazan & Shaver, 1994; Hazan & Zeifman, 1994), an attachment figure serves three purposes or functions. First, he or she is a target for proximity seeking. People tend to seek and benefit from proximity to their attachment figures in times of need. Second, an attachment figure serves as a "safe haven" in times of need (i.e., he or she reliably provides protection, comfort, support, and relief). Third, an attachment figure serves as a "secure base," allowing a child or an adult relationship partner to pursue nonattachment goals (i.e., activate other behavioral systems) in a safe environment. Based on this narrow definition of an attachment figure, a close relationship partner becomes such a figure only when he or she provides (or is perceived as providing) a safe haven and secure base in times of threat or danger.

A fourth definitional characteristic of an attachment figure is that his or her real or expected disappearance evokes "separation distress" (i.e., people react with intense distress to actual or potential unwanted separations from or losses of an attachment figure). Bowlby's (1969/1982) ideas about separation distress as a defining feature of an attachment figure were inspired by observations by Burlingham and Freud (1944) and Robertson and Bowlby (1952), who noticed that infants and young children who are separated from primary caregivers for extended periods pass through a predictable series of states: protest, despair, and detachment. The initial response to separation from an attachment figure is protest: Infants actively resist separation by crying, clinging, or calling and searching in an attempt to regain contact, or at least physical proximity. If protest does not restore proximity, more pervasive signs of despair, including depressed mood, decreased appetite, and disturbed sleep, replace agitation and anxiety. This despair may subside over time, but when reunited with caregivers after a prolonged separation, infants and young children tend to react with emotional withdrawal or anger mixed with excessive vigilance and anxious clinging. According to Bowlby (1969/1982), this sequence of protest, despair, and detachment is not targeted to every close relationship partner, only to those viewed as attachment figures. Theoretically, separation distress is the normative response to an impending loss of a major source of safety and security.

During infancy, primary caregivers (usually one or both parents, but also grandparents, older siblings, day care workers) are likely to serve attachment functions. Research has shown that when tired or ill, infants seek proximity to a primary caregiver (e.g., Ainsworth, 1973) and are noticeably reassured and soothed in that person's presence (e.g., Heinicke & Westheimer, 1966). In later childhood, adolescence, and adulthood, a wider variety of relationship partners can serve as attachment figures, including siblings, other relatives, familiar coworkers, teachers or coaches, close friends, and romantic partners. They form what Bowlby (1969/1982) called, as mentioned earlier, a person's "hierarchy of attachment figures." There may also be context-specific attachment figures— real or potential sources of comfort and support in specific milieus, such as therapists in therapeutic settings or leaders in organizational settings (e.g., business organizations or the military). Moreover, groups, institutions, and symbolic personages (e.g., God) can become targets of proximity seeking and sources of security. There is evidence that many young children have imaginary friends (e.g., Gleason, 2002); that some married adults who suffer the death of a spouse continue to experience the spouse's presence, and seek his or her assistance and support in times of need (e.g., Klass, Silverman, & Nickman, 1996); and that many adults believe they can and do obtain protection and comfort from gods, angels, saints, and the spirits of deceased ancestors (e.g., Fraley & Shaver, 1999; Kirkpatrick, 2005).

The Uniqueness of Attachment Interactions and Attachment Bonds

Not every interaction between a child and an attachment figure is an attachment interaction. A child and his or her mother can go grocery shopping together, and if the child is never frightened and never feels threatened by separation, both interaction partners can go about their business without attachment issues being salient. A parent and a child can play a game together, laugh at each other's jokes and pranks, and so on, without attachment issues coming to the fore (although these kinds of interactions may help cement or maintain a bond between the two partners, because they provide evidence of affection, psychological and behavioral synchrony, trustworthiness, and special attention). Similarly, adult romantic or marital partners can go to dinner together or take a walk in the park, tease each other good-naturedly, or study history together, and attachment issues, while existing psychologically in the background, may never become salient. Moreover, in relations between an athlete and his or her coach, many of the interactions may be concerned with teaching, criticism, and so on, without the potential attachment aspects of the relationship being salient. Even in a therapeutic relationship, where one person is officially coming to the other for support and guidance, there are moments of information exchange (e.g., about vacations or movies) or mutual joking and kibitzing that do not necessarily serve attachment functions.

Weiss (1998) has made useful distinctions between what Bowlby called "attachment" and affiliation, and has done so even within the context of a particular relationship. An "attachment interaction" is one in which one person is threatened or distressed and seeks comfort and support from the other. An affiliation interaction is one in which both people are in a good mood, do not feel threatened, and have the goals of enjoying their time together or advancing common interests. Importantly, even within a particular relationship—say, between two sisters—there can be both attachment interactions in which one sister (and not always the same one) is needy and the other is temporarily "stronger and wiser," and other, affiliative interactions in which the two consider themselves to be equal. The same goes for romantic or marital partners.

Theoretically, a lasting attachment relationship is based on the formation of what Bowlby (1969/1982) called an "attachment bond." The existence of this bond may not always be evident; when neither partner is threatened, demoralized, or in need, the two may seem quite autonomous, and their interactions may be more affiliative, exploratory, or sexual than attachment-oriented. But when one person is distressed, and especially if separation is threatened or loss occurs (due, at worst, to sudden, unexpected death), the attachment bond becomes evident. There are other kinds of emotional bonds, based on familiarity, shared activities, biological relatedness, and respect, and when these bonds are threatened or broken, a person may be distressed, but usually not to the same extent or for as long as in the case of severed attachment bonds. Most difficult to distinguish for newcomers to attachment theory are emotional bonds associated with two functionally different sides of an attachment relationship—those of the person who is attached, and those of the person who is the care provider. When a parent loses a child, the emotional reaction of the parent is likely to be extreme. But theoretically there are qualitative differences on the attachment and caregiving sides of a severed relationship: The attached person longs for the lost attachment figure's supportive presence and provision of comfort and security; the caregiver who loses a child tends to long for opportunities to care for the child and make restitution for previous failures of adequate care.

Attachment bonds do not develop overnight. Bowlby (1969/1982) and Ainsworth (1973) proposed four phases in the development of infant–caregiver attachments. In the *preattachment* phase (birth to 2 months of age) infants are inherently interested in and responsive to social interaction with virtually anyone. In the next *attachment-in-the-making* phase (from roughly 2 to 6 months of age), infants begin to show preferences, for example, by smiling and vocalizing to and settling more quickly with some caregivers rather than others. In the *clear-cut attachment* phase (beginning at around 6–7 months of age), all of the behaviors that define attachment are selectively directed toward the primary caregiver. This is evident in the infant's efforts to maintain proximity to the caregiver, the use of this person as a haven of safety in time of need and as a secure base for exploration, and reacting to separation from this person with extreme distress. In the fourth phase, *goal-corrected partnership* (beyond about 2 years of age), children can endure longer periods of separation and are increasingly capable of synchronizing their proximity-seeking bids with caregivers' goals and preferences.

In this book we are especially interested in close relationships between adults. According to Bowlby (1979), a long-term romantic (or pair-bond; Hazan & Zeifman, 1999) relationship is the prototype of attachment bonds in adulthood. Following his lead, Shaver et al.

(1988) proposed that romantic bonds in adulthood are conceptually parallel to infants' emotional bonds with their primary caregivers. In their words, "For every documented feature of attachment there is a parallel feature of love, and for most documented features of love there is either a documented or a plausible infant parallel" (p. 73). Love in both infancy and adulthood includes eye contact, holding, touching, caressing, smiling, crying, and clinging; a desire to be comforted by the relationship partner (parent, romantic lover, or spouse) when distressed; the experience of anger, anxiety, and sorrow following separation or loss; and the experience of happiness and joy upon reunion. Moreover, formation of a secure relationship with a primary caregiver or a romantic partner depends on the caregiver/partner's sensitivity and responsiveness to the increasingly attached person's proximity bids, and this responsiveness causes the person to feel more confident and safe, happier, more outgoing, and kinder to others. Furthermore, in both kinds of relationships, when the partner is not available and not responsive to the person's proximity bids, the person can become anxious, preoccupied, and hypersensitive to signs of love or its absence, to approval or rejection. Separations or nonresponsiveness, up to a point, can increase the intensity of both an infant's and an adult's proximity-seeking behavior, but beyond some point they provoke defensive distancing from the partner so as to avoid the pain and distress caused by the frustrating relationship.

All of these parallels led Shaver et al. (1988) to conclude that infants' bonds with parents and romantic or marital partners' bonds with each other are variants of a single core process. Nevertheless, adult pair bonds involve not only the attachment system but also the caregiving and, often, the sexual/reproductive system (Ainsworth & Bowlby, 1991; Hazan & Shaver, 1994). In romantic relationships, people occupy not only the "needy" position and expect to gain security and comfort from their partner but also the "caregiver" position, in which they are expected to provide care and support to their needy partner. In addition, the romantic partner is viewed not only as a source of security and comfort but also, often, as a partner for sexual activities and reproduction.

This kind of role switching is evident even in monogamous or pair-bonded non-human animals, such as prairie voles, titi monkeys, and some species of guinea pigs (C. S. Carter et al., 2005). When describing one such species (the domestic guinea pig, *Cavia aperea f. porcellus*), for example, Sachser (2005) says:

> When placed in an unfamiliar cage, the male's endocrine stress response (e.g., increase in serum cortisol concentrations) is sharply reduced when the bonded female is present. In contrast, the presence of a strange female, or one with whom he is merely acquainted, has little effect. Thus the effect of various types of relationships differs remarkably, and substantial social support is given only by the bonded partner (Sachser et al., 1998). Moreover, in female guinea pigs, presence of the male bonding partner leads to a sharp reduction in the acute stress response. Thus, social support can be provided by social partners in females as well. In contrast to males, however, the female's stress responses can be reduced not only by the bonding partner but also by a familiar conspecific, though in a less effective way (Kaiser et al., 2003). (p. 127)

Hazan and Zeifman (1999) speculated that adolescent and adult romantic relationships that develop into real attachment relationships go through the same stages described by Bowlby and Ainsworth in their discussions of infant–parent attachment. In particular, romantic relationships usually begin with affiliation, flirtation, or uncommitted sexual involvement, which can be viewed as a "preattachment phase," then progress through an "attachment-in-the-making" phase, which involves increasing selectivity and commitment, then to a "clear-cut attachment," which in modern Western societies is often formally celebrated in marriage. This process may take 1–2 years to develop fully, just as in the case of human infants. Research (reviewed by Hazan & Zeifman, 1999) suggests that marriages that end within 2 years result in less grief than ones that end later on, which might be partly a result of the strength of the broken attachment bond.

INDIVIDUAL DIFFERENCES IN ATTACHMENT-SYSTEM FUNCTIONING

In Bowlby's (1969/1982) view, each person's behavioral systems include "ontogenetically learned" components reflecting a particular history of behavioral-system activation in various contexts. Although behavioral systems presumably operate mainly at a sub-cortical level and in a somewhat reflexive, mechanistic manner, their capacity to attain what Bowlby called set-goals depends on experience with the external world. Therefore, to make goal attainment in varied contexts more likely, behavioral systems evolved to include cognitive-behavioral mechanisms, such as monitoring and appraising the effectiveness of behaviors enacted in a particular context, which allow flexible, goal-corrected adjustment of the system's "programming." Over time, after operating repeatedly in a particular relational (usually family) environment, a person's behavioral systems become uniquely tailored to specific relationship partners. A child learns to adjust his or her behavioral systems based on reliable expectations about possible access routes and barriers to goal attainment. These expectations, which operate partly at a conscious and intentional level, become part of a behavioral system's programming and are sources of both individual differences and within-person continuity in a behavioral system's operation. For this reason, attachment theory is in part a theory of individual differences in relationship orientations and personality development.

Attachment Figure Availability, the Sense of Security, and Secondary Strategies

Although nearly all children are born with a normal attachment system, which motivates them to pursue proximity and security in times of need, proximity maintenance and security attainment also depend on the responsiveness of particular relationship partners. As Cassidy (1999) noted, "Whereas nearly all children become attached (even to mothers who abuse them, Bowlby, 1956), not all are securely attached" (p. 7). The quality of interactions with attachment figures in times of need is, according to attachment theory, the major source of individual differences in attachment-system functioning.

When a relationship partner is available, sensitive, and responsive to an individual's proximity-seeking efforts in times of need, the individual is likely to experience felt security—a sense that the world is generally safe, that attachment figures are helpful when called upon, and that it is possible to explore the environment curiously and confidently and to engage rewardingly with other people. This sense implies that the attachment system is functioning well and that proximity seeking is a reliable and effective emotion regulation strategy. Moreover, the individual acquires important procedural knowledge about distress management, which becomes organized around the relational script discussed earlier (Waters et al., 1998). This *secure-base script* includes something like the following if–then proposition: "If I encounter an obstacle and/or become distressed, I can approach a significant other for help; he or she is likely to be available and supportive; I will experience relief and comfort as a result of proximity to this person; I can then return to other activities." The script is a symbolic reflection of the phylogeneti-cally "hard-wired" program at the heart of the attachment system, and as such it requires little in the way of changes in the system's operating parameters.

However, when a primary attachment figure proves not to be physically or emotion-ally available in times of need, not responsive to a person's proximity bids, or poor at alleviating distress or providing a secure base, attachment-system functioning is disrupted and its set-goal is not attained. In such cases, the individual does not experience comfort, relief, or felt security. Rather, the distress that initially activated the system is com-pounded by serious doubts about the feasibility of attaining security: "Is the world a safe place or not? Can I really trust others in times of need? Do I have the resources necessary to manage my own emotions?" These worries about self and others, and the resulting sense of vulnerability, can place the attachment system in a continually activated state, keep a person's mind preoccupied with threats and the need for protection, and interfere with the functioning of other behavioral systems.

Negative interactions with an inadequately available or responsive attachment figure indicate that the primary attachment strategy, proximity seeking, is failing to accomplish its set-goal. As a result, the operating parameters of the attachment system have to be adjusted and certain *secondary attachment strategies* are likely to be adopted. Main (1990) emphasized two such secondary strategies: *hyperactivation* and *deactivation* of the attachment system. Viewed in terms of the famous fight–flight distinction in physio-logical psychology (Cannon, 1932/1939), hyperactivating strategies are "fight" responses to frustrated attachment needs (as mentioned earlier, Bowlby called this kind of response "protest"). Protest is especially likely in relationships where an attachment figure is some-times responsive and sometimes not, placing the dependent, attached individual on a par-tial reinforcement schedule that rewards persistent and energetic proximity-seeking attempts because they sometimes succeed. In such cases, the individual does not easily give up on proximity seeking, and in fact intensifies it so as to demand or force the attachment figure's attention, love, and support. The main goal of these strategies is to get an attachment figure, viewed as unreliable or insufficiently responsive, to pay more attention and provide better protection and support (Cassidy & Kobak, 1988; Main, 1990). Unfortunately, strident demands for support begin to seem both natural and nec-essary, and they can become a cause of further relational conflicts and emotional distress.

Deactivating strategies are a "flight" reaction to an attachment figure's unavailabil-ity, which seem to develop in relationships with figures who disapprove of and punish closeness and expressions of need or vulnerability (Cassidy & Kobak, 1988; Main, 1990). In such cases, a person learns to expect better outcomes if signs of need and vul-nerability are hidden or suppressed, proximity-seeking efforts are weakened or blocked, the attachment system is deactivated despite a sense of security not being achieved, and the person attempts to deal with threats and dangers alone (a strategy that Bowlby, 1969/ 1982, called "compulsive self-reliance"). The primary goal of deactivating strategies is to keep the attachment system turned off or down-regulated so as to avoid frustration and distress caused by attachment figure unavailability.

Attachment Working Models

According to Bowlby (1969/1982), variations in caregiver responses to an attached per-son's bids for proximity and protection not only alter the operation of the attachment system in a particular interaction or short-term series of interactions but also gradually produce more enduring and pervasive changes in attachment-system functioning. Accord-ing to Bowlby (1973), these long-term effects are explicable in terms of the storage in one's long-term associative memory network of mental representations of significant interactions with an attachment figure. This stored knowledge, taking the form of working models or representational models (Bowlby, 1969/1982, 1973), allows a person to predict future interactions with the relationship partner and adjust proximity-seeking attempts without having to rethink each one. Repeated attachment-related interactions result in increasingly stable mental representations of self, partner, and relationships.

The concept of working models is interesting from a social-psychological standpoint, because it is similar to concepts in social psychology such as "cognitive scripts" and "social schemas," which, inspired by digital computer programs and cybernetic machines, originally seemed coolly cognitive, but have since been gradually transformed by theorists into "hot" cognitions (Kunda, 1999). They are hot by virtue of being residues of past emotions and triggers for subsequent, similar experiences. Bowlby also viewed working models as cognitive–affective structures that include affective memories and contribute importantly to expectations and appraisals that evoke emotions (Shaver, Collins, & Clark, 1996). These models include autobiographical, episodic memories (concrete memories of specific interactions with attachment figures), beliefs and attitudes concerning oneself and relationship partners, generic declarative knowledge about attachment relationships and interactions (e.g., the belief that romantic love as portrayed in movies does not exist in real life), and procedural knowledge about how to regulate emotions and behave effectively in close relationships (N. L. Collins & Read, 1994).

According to Main et al. (1985), early working models organize a child's memories about him- or herself and interaction partners during attempts to attain felt security, as well as the typical outcomes of those attempts: success or failure of the primary attachment strategy (proximity seeking) to achieve the security set-goal. In this way, a child can develop working models for successful proximity-seeking efforts, situations in which the attachment system has to be hyperactivated, and situations in which the system has to be defensively deactivated. Each such model consists of episodic memories of an interaction sequence; declarative knowledge about the partner's responses and the efficacy of the individual's actions; and procedural knowledge about the ways in which one responds to such situations and deals with various sources of distress.

Working models guide behavior, cognitions, and feelings, and can bias the ways in which a person cognitively encodes, interprets, and stores memories of subsequent interactions with attachment figures. Because of such biases, working models of self and others reflect only in part the ways the person and a partner actually behaved in a given interaction. They also reflect the underlying regulatory actions of attachment strategies, which can shape cognitions, emotions, and behaviors; that is, working models of self and others are always blends of accurate representations of what actually happened in a relationship (Bowlby [1973] called them "tolerably accurate reflections of the experiences those individuals actually had"; p. 202) and subjective biases resulting from the operation of defensive attachment strategies (e.g., defensive exclusion of painful information from awareness).

Beyond daily interactions with cool, distant, or emotionally unstable parents, which can leave a residue of attachment insecurity (Ainsworth et al., 1978), Bowlby (1980) also talked about various reasons why a child's or an adult's memories might be distorted by defensive exclusion: (1) In some cases (e.g., a relative's suicide) parents do not want children to know, remember, or talk about certain incidents even though the children witnessed them; (2) the children sometimes witness events (e.g., parental violence) that they find too emotionally painful or troubling to think about; and (3) the children may have done or thought about doing something of which they are ashamed. In such cases, defensive exclusion protects a person from psychological pain, but it does so at the expense of the verisimilitude of the person's working models. This kind of distortion can sometimes cause problems later on, when a person activates memories or feelings that cannot be explained, or feels ambivalent about a person who is supposed to be kind and loving but actually arouses feelings of danger.

Like other mental representations, which are presumably underlain by neural circuits or networks, working models form excitatory and inhibitory associations with one another, and the activation of one model primes congruent models while inhibiting incongruent models; that is, experiencing or thinking about an episode of security attainment activates memories of other, successful proximity-seeking attempts and renders memories of hyperactivation and deactivation less accessible. With the passage of time and the recurrent retrieval of related memories, these associative links are strengthened, thereby favoring the formation of more abstract and generalized representations of attachment-system functioning with a specific partner. In this way, models of security attainment, hyperactivation, and deactivation with a specific attachment figure (relationship-specific working models) are created, and they form excitatory and inhibitory links with models representing interactions with other attachment figures. When these links are reinforced and consolidated, even more generic working models are formed—global representations of self and others across different relationships. The end product of this cognitive generalization and consolidation process is a hierarchical associative memory network, in which episodic memories become exemplars of relationship-specific models, and those models become exemplars of generic relational schemas. As a result, with respect to a particular relationship and across different relationships, everyone possesses models of security attainment, hyperactivation, and deactivation, and so can sometimes think about relationships in secure terms and at other times think about them in less secure, more hyperactivating or deactivating terms. Due to differences in relationship histories, dominant working models differ across individuals.

The semantic networks involved in attachment working models have all the properties of any cognitive network (e.g., differentiation, integration, and coherence among the various models; N. L. Collins & Read, 1994). In addition, each working model within the network differs in cognitive accessibility (the ease with which it can be activated and used to guide the attachment system during a particular social interaction). As with other mental representations, the strength or accessibility of each model is determined by the amount of experience on which it is based, the number of times it has been applied in the past, and the density of its connections with other working models (e.g., Baldwin, 1992; N. L. Collins & Read, 1994; Shaver, Collins, & Clark, 1996). At a relationship-specific level, the model representing the typical interaction with an attachment figure has the highest accessibility in subsequent interactions with that person. At a generic level, the model that represents interactions with major attachment figures (e.g., parents and romantic partners) typically becomes the most chronically accessible attachment-related representation and has the strongest effect on attachment-system functioning across relationships and over time.

In addition to a person's history of attachment-related interactions, features of a current situation can also contribute to the activation of a particular working model. For example, clear-cut contextual cues concerning a partner's love, availability, and supportiveness can activate models of security attainment. In addition, working models can be invoked by a person's current motives (e.g., wishing to gain distance from a partner) or current mood (Shaver, Collins, & Clark, 1996). We assume that the chronically accessible overall model coexists with less strong and less personally characteristic working models, and either kind of model can be activated by contextual factors or a person's current mood or internal state. (As we explain in subsequent chapters, these possibilities have been extensively explored in laboratory experiments.)

According to attachment theory, consolidation of a chronically accessible working model is the most important psychological process accounting for the enduring, long-term effects on personality functioning of attachment interactions during infancy, childhood, and adolescence (Bowlby, 1973; E. Waters, Merrick, Treboux, Crowell, & Albersheim, 2000). Given a fairly consistent pattern of interactions with primary caregivers during infancy and childhood, the most representative or prototypical working models of these interactions become part of a person's implicit procedural knowledge, tend to operate automatically and unconsciously, and are resistant to change. Thus, what began as representations of specific interactions with a primary caregiver during childhood become core personality characteristics, are applied in new social situations and relationships, and shape attachment-system functioning in adulthood.

In the following passage, Bowlby (1979) described how these chronically accessible models shape a person's experience:

> [One] tends to assimilate any new person with whom he may form a bond, such as a spouse, or child, or employer, or therapist, to an existing model (either of one or other parent or of self), and often to continue to do so despite repeated evidence that the model is inappropriate. Similarly he expects to be perceived and treated by them in ways that would be appropriate to his self-model, and to continue with such expectations despite contrary evidence. (pp. 141–142)

This tendency to project one's dominant or currently most active working models onto a new relationship partner affects the way a person anticipates, attends to, interprets, and recalls the partner's behavior, thereby confirming well-established expectations and models, and making them more resistant to change.

The Concept of Attachment Style

Most of the research examining individual differences in attachment-system functioning in adults has focused on attachment styles—patterns of expectations, needs, emotions, and social behavior that result from a particular history of attachment experiences, usually beginning in relationships with parents (Fraley & Shaver, 2000). A person's attachment style reflects his or her most chronically accessible working models and the typical functioning of his or her attachment system in a specific relationship (relationship-specific attachment style) or across relationships (global or general attachment style). As such, each attachment style is closely tied to working models and reflects the underlying, organizing action of a particular attachment strategy (primary or secondary, hyperactivating or deactivating).

The concept of attachment style, although not given that name, was first proposed by Ainsworth (1967) to describe infants' patterns of responses to separations from and reunions with their mother in the laboratory Strange Situation assessment procedure, in which infants were originally classified into one of three categories, here called secure, avoidant, or anxious (for short). Main and Solomon (1990) later added a fourth category, "disorganized/disoriented," characterized by odd, awkward behavior and unusual fluctuations between anxiety and avoidance.

Infants classified as secure seem to possess accessible working models of successful proximity-seeking attempts and security attainment. In the Strange Situation, they tend to exhibit distress during separations from mother but then recover quickly and continue to explore the environment with interest. When reunited with mother, they greet her with joy and affection, initiate contact with her, and respond positively to being held, after which they quickly reestablish interest in the toys provided in the experimental setting. During home observations, mothers of these infants are emotionally available in times of need and responsive to their child's proximity-seeking behavior (Ainsworth et al., 1978). It seems reasonable to characterize these mothers as a source of attachment security and as reinforcing reliance on the primary attachment strategy (seeking proximity and comfort when needed).

Avoidant infants seem to possess accessible working models related to attachment-system deactivation. In the Strange Situation they show little distress when separated from their mother and tend to avoid her when she returns. In home observations, their mothers tend to be emotionally rigid, as well as angry at and rejecting of their infants' proximity-seeking efforts (Ainsworth et al., 1978). Anxious infants seem to possess accessible working models related to attachment-system hyperactivation. In the Strange Situation, they are extremely distressed during separation and exhibit conflicted or ambivalent responses toward their mother during reunions (e.g., they may cling one moment and angrily resist comforting the next, which was Ainsworth's reason for sometimes calling them "anxious–ambivalent" or "anxious–resistant"). During home observations, interactions between anxious infants and their mothers are characterized by lack of harmony and lack of caregivers' consistent responsiveness (Ainsworth et al., 1978). Mothers of both avoidant and anxious infants seem to thwart security attainment, thereby fostering their children's adoption of secondary strategies. However, whereas avoidant infants deactivate their attachment system in response to attachment figure unavailability, anxious infants tend to hyperactivate the system to gain a more reliable supportive reaction from their attachment figure (Main, 1990; Main et al., 1985).

Disorganized/disoriented infants seem to suffer from a breakdown of organized attachment strategies (primary, hyperactivating, or deactivating). They either oscillate between strategies or do something bizarre, such as lie face-down on the floor without moving when their mother appears following a separation or sit passively under a table, evincing no clear proximity-seeking strategy at all (Main & Solomon, 1990). These odd behaviors seem to be due to disorganized, unpredictable, and discomfiting behavior on the part of attachment figures who, research shows, are likely to be suffering from unresolved losses or unresolved attachment-related traumas (Hesse, 1999; Lyons-Ruth & Jacobvitz, 1999). When their child approaches them for comfort and reassurance, they sometimes look frightened, look away, or "space out" in a dissociative way, causing the child to stop abruptly, suffer confusion, or adopt whatever momentary strategy seems to reduce discomfort.

In the 1980s, researchers from different psychological fields (developmental, clinical, personality, and social psychology) constructed new measures of attachment style, based on various conceptualizations of the construct, to extend attachment research into adolescence and adulthood. For example, adopting a developmental and clinical approach, Main and her colleagues (George, Kaplan, & Main, 1985; Main et al., 1985; Main & Goldwyn, 1988; see Hesse, 1999, for a review) devised the Adult Attachment Interview (AAI) to study adolescents and adults' mental representations of attachment, or "states of mind with respect to attachment," to their parents during childhood. In the AAI, interviewees answer open-ended questions about their childhood relationships with parents and are classified into three major categories paralleling Ainsworth's infant typology: "secure" (or free and autonomous with respect to attachment), "dismissing" (of attachment), or "preoccupied" (with attachment).

Using the AAI coding system (George et al., 1985; Main & Goldwyn, 1988), a person is classified as secure if he or she describes parents as available and responsive, and verbalizes memories of relationships with parents that are clear, convincing, and coherent. Dismissing (i.e., avoidant) individuals play down the importance of attachment relationships and tend to recall few concrete episodes of emotional interactions with parents. Preoccupied (i.e., anxious) individuals are entangled in worries and angry feelings about parents, are hypersensitive to attachment experiences, and can easily retrieve negative memories but have trouble discussing them coherently without anger or anxiety. Main et al. (1985) called their measurement strategy a "move to the level of representation," because, unlike the Strange Situation, which emphasizes an infant's behavior, the AAI assesses current adult mental representations of childhood attachment relationships as these are articulated in "coherent" or "incoherent" discourse with an interviewer.

Working from a personality and social-psychological perspective, and attempting to apply Bowlby's ideas to the study of romantic relationships, Hazan and Shaver (1987) developed a self-report measure of adult attachment style that asked respondents to characterize their feelings and behavioral tendencies in romantic relationships. In its original form, the measure consisted of three brief descriptions of feelings and behaviors in close relationships that were intended to capture adult romantic analogues of the three infant attachment styles identified by Ainsworth et al. (1978). Participants were asked to read the descriptions, then place themselves into one of three attachment categories according to their predominant feelings and behavior in romantic relationships. The three "types" were described as follows:

1. *Secure*: "I find it relatively easy to get close to others and am comfortable depending on them and having them depend on me. I don't worry about being abandoned or about someone getting too close to me."
2. *Avoidant*: "I am somewhat uncomfortable being close to others; I find it difficult to trust them completely, difficult to allow myself to depend on them. I am nervous when anyone gets too close and others often want me to be more intimate than I feel comfortable being."
3. *Anxious*: "I find that others are reluctant to get as close as I would like. I often worry that my partner doesn't really love me or won't want to stay with me. I want to get very close to my partner and this sometimes scares people away."

In subsequent years, numerous researchers developed similar self-report measures, in some cases to improve the precision of Hazan and Shaver's (1987) measure and in other cases to see whether it is worthwhile trying to capture more of the lower-level concepts in Ainsworth's infant measure (e.g., proximity seeking, separation distress, secure base). Gradually it became evident that there are two dimensions of insecurity underlying all such self-report measures of romantic attachment: avoidance and anxiety (see Chapter 4, this volume, for details). The first dimension, attachment-related *avoidance*, is concerned with discomfort with closeness and depending on relationship partners, preference for emotional distance and self-reliance, and use of deactivating strategies to deal with insecurity and distress. The second dimension, attachment-related *anxiety*, is concerned with a strong desire for closeness and protection, intense worries about partner availability and one's own value to the partner, and use of hyperactivating strategies to deal with insecurity and distress.

People who score low on both dimensions are said to be secure or to have a secure attachment style. This region of low anxiety and low avoidance is defined by a chronic sense of attachment security, trust in partners and expectations of partner availability and responsiveness, comfort with closeness and interdependence, and ability to cope with threats and stressors in constructive ways. Throughout the remainder of this book we refer to people with secure, anxious, or avoidant attachment styles, or people who are relatively secure, anxious, or avoidant. Although our categorical or typological shorthand can incorrectly cause readers to think in terms of discrete types, we will always be referring to fuzzy regions in a two-dimensional space in which people are continuously distributed. Fraley and Waller (1998) used sophisticated psychometric methods to determine whether attachment styles were truly typological or, instead, regions in a continuously distributed two-dimensional space, and their results clearly favored the dimensional conception (again, see Chapter 4, this volume, for measurement details).

CONCLUDING REMARKS

In this chapter we have outlined attachment theory, from its inception in the writings of Bowlby and Ainsworth to the present, with special emphasis on our own extensions of the theory into the adolescent and adult age periods. We have explained that, following Bowlby and Ainsworth, we view the attachment behavioral system as an inborn regulatory system with important implications for personality development and social behavior. The system is activated by perceived threats and dangers, which cause a threatened person to seek proximity to protective others. Attainment of proximity and protection results in feelings of relief and security, as well as positive mental representations of self and relationship partners. Bowlby viewed the healthy functioning of this behavioral system as crucial for emotional stability, mental health, and satisfying, close relationships. Moreover, because healthy functioning of the attachment system facilitates relaxed and confident engagement in nonattachment activities, it contributes to the broadening of a person's perspectives and skills, as well as the actualization of his or her unique potentialities. To borrow a term from another theoretical tradition, humanistic psychology (e.g., Maslow, 1968; C. R. Rogers, 1961), attachment security is not only an important component of healthy love but also a major foundation for self-actualization. We provide extensive evidence for this claim throughout the remaining chapters.

In this chapter, we have also introduced some major individual differences in attachment-system functioning. Although the attachment system is conceptualized as operating mainly at a subcortical, unconscious level and in a relatively automatic, reflexive manner, its activation can yield different response strategies (the primary, proximity-seeking strategy or the secondary, hyperactivating or deactivating strategy) depending on both the quality of the *current* interaction with an attachment figure and internal representations of *past* interactions with the same or other attachment figures. Although these representations (working models of self and others) presumably operate in a more conscious, controlled manner than the innate core of the attachment system, they can become habitual and automatic, and are therefore largely unconscious and can be defensively excluded from awareness. Moreover, they can unconsciously bias information processing about relationships and relationship partners and be a source of within-person continuity in attachment-system functioning.

In the next chapter we present a model of attachment-system functioning in adulthood that we then use to organize our review of the thousands of studies on adult attachment published over the past 20 years. At the end of Chapter 2, we provide a brief overview of the rest of the book.

CHAPTER 2

███ ███ ███

A Model of Attachment-System
Functioning and Dynamics in Adulthood

Once Bowlby and Ainsworth's attachment theory became influential in both developmental and social–personality psychology, thousands of studies were conducted to explore its implications. The resulting literature now needs to be summarized, organized, and coherently conceptualized so that future studies and clinical interventions can build systematically on what is already known. As part of our own work, which focuses on the dynamics of the attachment behavioral system in adulthood and its relation to other behavioral systems, such as exploration, caregiving, and sex, we created a model of attachment-system dynamics and their intrapsychic and interpersonal implications (e.g., Mikulincer & Shaver, 2003; Shaver & Mikulincer, 2002a). In this chapter we describe the model and show how it relates to other theoretical approaches to personality and social behavior. We focus particularly on how attachment-related aspects of personality develop and influence adult emotion regulation and social relationships.

This chapter is the conceptual foundation for those that follow, so we include at the end a brief outline of the rest of the book, showing how subsequent chapters expand on the implications of our model for issues such as self-esteem, emotion regulation, the accomplishment of major life tasks (e.g., identity formation, career choice, work performance, and health maintenance), personal adjustment, couple relationship functioning, mental health, organizational behavior, and psychotherapy.

THE MODEL

To characterize the activation and operation of the attachment system in adulthood, we (Mikulincer & Shaver, 2003; Shaver & Mikulincer, 2002a) proposed a control systems model that integrates the large research literature with the theoretical writings of Bowlby (1969/1982, 1973, 1980), Ainsworth (1991), Cassidy and Kobak (1988), and Main

(1995). Our model is an extension and refinement of previous control systems models of attachment dynamics proposed by Shaver et al. (1988) and Fraley and Shaver (2000). It deals with three issues (indicated by three gray blocks, or modules, in Figure 2.1): (1) proximity seeking following attachment-system activation (the attachment system's primary strategy), (2) beneficial consequences of using this strategy effectively to attain the support of a security-providing attachment figure, and (3) secondary strategies (called anxious hyperactivation and avoidant deactivation) pursued in response to attachment figure unavailability or unresponsiveness. The model also includes the goals of the primary and secondary attachment strategies, associated beliefs and expectations about self and others, and associated rules for managing distress and interpersonal relations. In addition, the model explains what happens when secondary strategies fail to accomplish their aims.

The first component of the model (the upper gray area in Figure 2.1) includes monitoring and appraisal of threatening events—the process responsible for activating the attachment system. The second component (the central gray area) deals with monitoring and appraising attachment figure availability, which is related to individual differences in felt security and the psychological correlates and consequences of secure attachment. The third component (the lower gray area in the figure) involves monitoring and appraising the viability of proximity seeking as a way of dealing with attachment insecurity. This component represents the "choice" to use either a hyperactivating or a deactivating strategy to deal with insecurity; the former strategy is associated with an anxious attachment style and the latter, with an avoidant attachment style. The word "choice" appears in quotation marks, because the process may be largely unconscious and influenced by many previous life experiences, beginning in infancy, that the person did not, and still does not, understand. We call it a choice to emphasize that there are different possible responses to attachment figure unavailability or unresponsiveness, each with its own specific effects.

The model also postulates hypothetical excitatory and inhibitory "neural circuits" (shown as upwardly directed arrows on the left side of Figure 2.1), resulting from recurrent use of hyperactivating or deactivating strategies. These hypothetical circuits affect the monitoring and appraisal of threats and of attachment figure availability. We assume that all components and circuits in the model, not just the "choice" among secondary strategies for dealing with attachment figure unresponsiveness, can operate in the adult mind either consciously or unconsciously, and either deliberately or automatically. Moreover, these components and circuits can operate in parallel, synchronously, or in conflicting ways at conscious and unconscious levels. Finally, although we generally conceptualize hyperactivation and deactivation of the attachment system (associated with anxious and avoidant attachment, respectively) as independent strategies, we acknowledge the existence of "disorganized" or "fearfully avoidant" strategies that involve both anxiety and avoidance (Bartholomew & Horowitz, 1991; Main & Solomon, 1990). Because we view attachment security as a state caused by a person's not needing (except on rare occasions) to use either a hyperactivating or a deactivating strategy, it is obviously possible for a person to use neither strategy very often, just as it is possible for some people to use both strategies often, even if it sometimes results in awkward or inconsistent behavior.

The model is sensitive to both context and personal dispositions (situations and personality traits, as these two classes of variables are typically called in social–personality psychology). Every component of the model can be affected by context (e.g., dangers or threats, current information about attachment figure availability or unavailability, and current information about the viability of seeking proximity to and protection from an

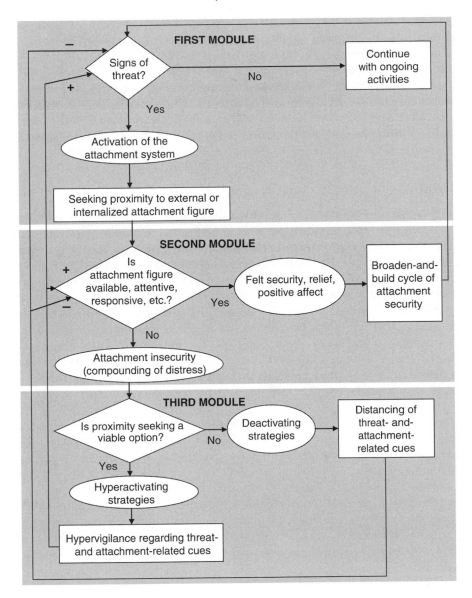

FIGURE 2.1. A model of attachment-system activation and functioning in adulthood.

attachment figure in a particular situation), which initiates "bottom-up" influences on the operation of the attachment system. For example, reminding a person of supportive behavior on the part of a past or present attachment figure can cause even a chronically insecure person to feel momentarily more secure and to behave accordingly. Each component of the model is also affected by a person's prevailing working models of self and other, which bias appraisals of threats, attachment figure availability, and proximity-seeking viability. These biases are part of a "top-down" process by which a person's chronic attachment style (i.e., dominant attachment-related schemas and associated mental and behavioral strategies) shapes the functioning of the attachment system. For example, a chronically anxious person tends to exaggerate threats and remain vigilant for even minor indications of attachment figure unresponsiveness, which in turn keeps the attachment system hyperactivated. Overall, the model emphasizes both reality—the current context in which the attachment system is activated—and fantasies, defenses, and cognitive biases associated with particular attachment schemas, strategies, and styles. In this way, we hope to capture what was correct about both psychoanalytic theory's emphasis on internal biases and Bowlby's (1969/1982) claim, which we quoted in Chapter 1, that attachment working models are "tolerably accurate reflections" of what actually happened (Bowlby, 1973, p. 202).

Activation of the Attachment System

Following Bowlby's (1969/1982) lead, we assume that the continuous monitoring of internal and external events (which range from momentarily recalling past experiences to noticing during a conversation with a relationship partner that he or she no longer seems interested in one's troubles or sexual advances) results in threat-related activation of the attachment system. These triggering events include both physical and psychological threats, such as receiving a frightening medical diagnosis, hearing a radio news flash about a rapidly approaching tornado, or noticing that one's spouse seems strongly attracted to a new office mate. The threats can be either attachment-unrelated (e.g., the medical diagnosis) or attachment-related (e.g., the appearance of a new rival for a spouse's affection), just as in childhood (see Chapter 1) a person can be threatened by a nasty, bleeding cut or by the impending departure of his or her primary attachment figure (e.g., noticing that mother is walking out the door to get in her car and drive to work).

We assume that every event perceived by a person of any age as threatening tends to activate the attachment system. Such activation automatically heightens access to attachment-related mental contents and action tendencies (e.g., images and thoughts of one's attachment figure and strategies for contacting or gaining proximity to him or her), which in turn increases the likelihood of seeking contact with an attachment figure. Although this part of the model deals with the normative (i.e., normal, general) operation of the attachment system, which occurs regardless of individual differences in attachment history or attachment style, it is also affected by the excitatory and inhibitory circuits associated with hyperactivating and deactivating attachment strategies (shown along the left-hand side of Figure 2.1).

The Subjective Nature of Attachment-System Activation

According to the model, attachment-system activation depends on the *subjective appraisal* of threats, not simply on the actual occurrence of threats. Although the presence of genuine threats is obviously important, a person's perception of internal or external events as threatening is the critical trigger for attachment-system activation. This idea fits with most contemporary models of emotion (e.g., Gross, 2007; Lazarus, 1991; Shaver & Mikulincer, 2007) and with Lazarus and Folkman's (1984) model of stress and coping, which emphasizes the role of appraisal in the regulation of distress through coping efforts. We view threat appraisal as a product of both the actual presence of a threat and the individual's expectation that unfolding events may have negative consequences for personal well-being, adjustment, or survival. Although these expectations can be based on a rational, conscious risk analysis of unfolding events, excitatory and inhibitory circuits resulting from secondary attachment strategies may bias them. Moreover, the appraisal process is not always conscious or rational, and the appraising mind may not be aware of its monitoring and appraising activities. When researching these processes, it is sometimes necessary to measure associated physiological reactions (e.g., skin conductance or heart rate) or the accessibility of threat-related thoughts (as revealed in the time taken to decide whether a letter string, such as a-l-o-n-e or n-a-e-o-l, is a word, or to name the color in which a threatening word, such as "alone," is printed).

Another important feature of our model is that *inner* sources of threat (e.g., troubling thoughts, images, fantasies, or dreams) can activate the attachment system. For example, thinking even briefly about one's own mortality can be extremely threatening (J. Greenberg, Pyszczynski, & Solomon, 1997) and can activate the attachment system (Mikulincer, Florian, & Hirschberger, 2003). In such cases, a person does not have to confront a literal threat: Merely being reminded of the general possibility of death is enough to activate the system. And again, these thoughts need not be conscious; they can be activated by a stimulus as minimal as the word "death" presented subliminally (e.g., Mikulincer, Birnbaum, Woddis, & Nachmias, 2000).

Understanding these two processes—subjective appraisal of threats and activation of the attachment system by threat-related thoughts—is crucial for understanding how secondary attachment strategies (hyperactivation and deactivation) bias attachment-system activation. Hyperactivating strategies include vigilance with respect to possible threats, exaggerated appraisals of threats (catastrophizing), and rumination about previous and merely possible threatening experiences that reactivate proximity-seeking efforts and emphasize the urgency of gaining a partner's attention, care, and support. This often causes anxiously attached individuals to activate their attachment system even in the absence of objective threats. Deactivating ("avoidant") strategies, in contrast, include diversion of attention away from threats and inhibition or suppression of threat-related thoughts that might activate the system. Because of these strategic maneuvers, avoidant individuals often distance themselves from threats and keep themselves from thinking about either their need for comfort or protection, or the relief they might experience in the presence or arms of a loving and protective relationship partner. Avoidant people tend to display, as we quoted Bowlby saying in Chapter 1, "compulsive self-reliance."

The Two-Stage Process of Attachment-System Activation

Once a threat is appraised, a two-stage process of attachment-system activation is initiated. In the first stage, the appraisal causes preconscious activation of the system and automatic heightening of access to attachment-related thoughts and action tendencies. In the second stage, this preconscious activation arouses conscious thoughts of seeking proximity to an attachment figure and, in many cases, initiates efforts to seek proximity and protection. In young children, the first stage typically gives way quickly to the second, because the thought of an action, or the need for the consequences of an action, tend to trigger the action without restraint or inhibition. In adults, there may be many steps between the first and second stages, and the second stage may take place only intrapsychically rather than behaviorally.

Preconscious activation of the attachment system consists of heightened availability of attachment-related mental representations, such as representations of security-enhancing attachment figures (including their appearance, comforting words, affectionate behaviors, and personal qualities); episodic (i.e., event-specific) memories of supportive and comforting interactions with these figures; memories of the feelings one experienced when comforted by attachment figures; thoughts related to proximity, love, and support; and mental activation of proximity-seeking goals. These preconsciously aroused mental representations are then available for use in subsequent information processing and action, which means they can shape a person's state of mind and influence his or her behavioral plans even before the thoughts and action tendencies become conscious. This line of theoretical reasoning fits with recent findings from social cognition research showing that accessible ideas, words, and images shape a person's state of mind before he or she notices or acknowledges them in the stream of consciousness (Wegner & Smart, 1997). It is also congruent with Bargh's (1990) "auto-motive" model of motivation, according to which a person's goals can be preconsciously activated and can automatically guide behavior without conscious planning.

In infancy and early childhood, most children probably have a limited repertoire of mental representations of attachment figures and a similarly small repertoire of proximity- and comfort-seeking behaviors. Most young children probably also have a limited number of available attachment figures (although this obviously differs as a function of family size, culture, and other factors), and they are largely limited to the figures provided by the local environment (e.g., the family home, a close adult relative's home, a day care center). In adolescence and adulthood, however, a person may have a wider range of potential comforters and attachment figures, as well as the ability to contact such people or locate a new person who can be converted into an attachment figure. As we explain in more detail in Chapter 3, a great deal of adolescents' and young adults' time and energy is devoted to exploring the trustworthiness of potential attachment figures (e.g., friendly peers; one or more romantic partners; a devoted coach, teacher, or professional mentor). During these years, at least in modern industrialized societies, a person may at times experience loneliness, which attachment researchers view as a form of separation anxiety caused by activation of the attachment system without a specific target (Rubenstein & Shaver, 1982; Weiss, 1973). Loneliness is especially common in adolescence and early adulthood, when many people are not yet confident about their attachment relationships outside the family home.

As mentioned earlier, another difference between infancy and adolescence or adulthood is that in the later age periods, preconscious activation of the attachment system does not necessarily lead to observable proximity-seeking behavior. Age and experience generally bring about an increased ability to gain security from mental representations of security-enhancing attachment figures, without actually having to seek immediate physical proximity to them. In fact, activation of mental representations of people who regularly provide care and protection can create a sense of safety and security, which helps a person deal independently with threats. In other words, activation of the adult attachment system can occur intrapsychically, with or without awareness.

In some cases, a reduction in attachment anxiety can occur simply as a result of reenacting or imagining supportive interactions with attachment figures. We are especially interested in cases in which this process involves memories and mental routines related to actual attachment experiences, but there may also be cases in which satisfaction of attachment needs is accomplished partly in imagination; for example, when a person imagines being loved by a movie star, a character in a book, or an acquaintance who seems kind and lovable but with whom one does not actually have a close relationship. This is the way we interpret many people's ability to gain genuine solace from imagined interactions with God, Jesus, the Buddha, deceased loved ones, and media heroes and heroines.

Like Bowlby (1969/1982), however, we assume that no one at any age is completely or perpetually free of dependence on actual flesh-and-blood attachment figures. There are situations, such as physical and psychological traumas, serious illnesses, important school or job failures, and losses of loved ones, in which symbolic proximity to an internalized or imagined attachment figure may not be sufficient to provide adequate comfort and relief, and under such conditions, attachment-system activation can trigger proximity-seeking behavior regardless of a person's age. There are also developmental periods, such as old age, in which people's physical and psychological resources may be taxed to the point that it becomes necessary to seek proximity to and support from "stronger and wiser" others. In such cases, attachment-system activation is manifested in conscious thoughts, behavioral intentions, and actual proximity- and support-seeking behavior, as we often see in cases in which a middle-aged adult "child," usually a mature daughter, cares for an aging and increasingly infirm parent, who in many ways resembles a dependent child and fully realizes it (e.g., Cicirelli, 1993, 1995; Steele, Phibbs, & Woods, 2004).

Attachment-System Activation and Self-Representations

In 2004, we added another path to the model of attachment-system activation (Mikulincer & Shaver, 2004). In addition to the search for real, external attachment figures or relying on internal, mental representations of past or imagined attachment figures, there is also the possibility of attaining comfort, relief, and increased "felt security" by relying on what we call *security-based self-representations* (i.e., components or subroutines of the self that originated in interactions with available attachment figures but now are experienced as aspects of oneself). According to this new path, activation of the attachment system during times of need can evoke (1) mental representations of oneself (including traits and feelings) derived from interactions with previously available and responsive attachment figures (*self-in-relation-with-a-security-enhancing-attachment figure*) and (2) mental representations of oneself derived from identifying with, or introjecting (to use the psychoanalytic term), features and traits of one or more caring, supportive attachment figures (*self-caregiving representations*). If these representations are available in memory, they can serve a soothing function and increase a person's sense of security. As we explain in more detail in Chapter 6, we devised a way to test these theoretical ideas in the laboratory and found empirical support for them (Mikulincer & Shaver, 2004).

Mental representations of self-in-relation-with-a-security-enhancing-attachment figure are organized around self-aspects (e.g., roles, traits, feelings, behaviors, expectations) that were previously experienced and recorded in memory during interactions with real attachment figures. During such interactions, a person may have construed him- or herself as sturdy, active, and capable based on having coped effectively with whatever threat or danger activated the attachment system. He or she may also feel calm, soothed, and loved because of the attachment figure's availability and kindness (Bowlby, 1973). The associated self-aspects (beliefs and feelings) are stored in semantic memory and are strongly associated with representations of available attachment figures and the positive feelings one has experienced in interactions with them. Moreover, these mental representations and feelings become more available under conditions of threat that activate the attachment system. They then down-regulate or alleviate distress and help a person cope effectively with the challenging situation.

The second category of security-based self-representations—those concerned with self-caregiving—includes self-representations based on identifying with and incorporating into oneself a supportive attachment figure's soothing qualities. To the extent that an attachment figure has demonstrated compassion, empathy, kindness, and encouragement when a person was distressed, these qualities can be modeled internally and assigned to oneself, which aids emotion regulation. This means that a person often treats him- or herself in ways he or she was treated by key attachment figures. A person whose attachment figures have generally been sensitive, caring, and forgiving will adopt a similar approach to him- or herself, and use the skills and personal qualities "borrowed" from attachment figures to comfort the self. When a threat arises, the person automatically activates self-caregiving routines that help him or her cope with distress.

Attachment Style and Attachment-System Activation

The entire process of attachment-system activation described in preceding sections of this chapter can be affected by a person's chronic or dispositional attachment style. We consider these effects in three separate points. First, dispositional attachment patterns can alter the content of the mental representations activated by threat appraisals. For securely attached people, threat appraisals increase the mental accessibility of thoughts about positive interactions with attachment figures—thoughts about proximity, safety, support, love, and relief. For insecurely attached people, however, threat appraisals often increase access to negative thoughts and memories (e.g., thoughts about separations, hurt feelings, rejections, and losses). These insecure people's painful or frustrating experiences with attachment figures have established a strong associative link in their minds between activation of the attachment system and worries about separation or rejection, causing the accessibility of these worries to increase every time proximity-seeking tendencies are activated.

Second, dispositional attachment patterns can affect actual proximity- and support-seeking behavior (Mikulincer & Florian, 1998; Shaver & Clark, 1994). Secure people's histories of interactions with available and responsive attachment figures increase their confidence in proximity seeking as an emotion-regulation strategy and reinforce reliance on this strategy under stressful conditions. In contrast, insecure people have a history of painful interactions with unavailable or rejecting attachment figures, which leads to the worry or conviction that proximity seeking may fail to accomplish its goal, which in turn forces insecure people to deal with unresolved distress through hyperactivating or deactivating attachment strategies.

Third, attachment patterns can determine the use or nonuse of security-based self-representations under distressing conditions. Calling upon this source of personal security and strength should be most common among people with a history of secure attachment, because they, compared with their insecure counterparts, have experienced more security-boosting interactions with attachment figures. This means that secure people can mobilize caring qualities within themselves, qualities modeled on those of their attachment figures, as well as representations of being loved and valued. Moreover, these mental representations can provide genuine comfort, allowing secure people to feel worthy and relatively unperturbed even under stress. In contrast, insecure people, whether they have an avoidant, anxious, or "disorganized" (fearfully avoidant) attachment style, are less likely to be able to call upon mental residues of past positive experiences. In fact, they may find that attachment-system activation reminds them, consciously or unconsciously, of the many times when their attachment figures were unavailable or unresponsive when needed.

Attachment Figure Availability and Security-Based Strategies

Once the attachment system is activated, an affirmative answer to the question posed in the first component of our model (Figure 2.1, upper gray box)—"Is the attachment figure

available?"—results in a sense of felt security. Attachment figure availability also reinforces the use of proximity seeking as a coping strategy in times of need and fosters what
we, following Fredrickson (2001), call a "broaden-and-build" cycle of attachment security, which augments a person's resources for maintaining emotional stability in times of
stress and expands the person's perspectives and capacities. (According to Fredrickson,
this is the general function of positive emotions.) This broaden-and-build cycle also
encourages the formation of intimate and deeply interdependent bonds with others and
maximizes personal adjustment without a need for reality-distorting defenses, such as
narcissistic self-inflation (an avoidant defense) or attempts to merge symbiotically with
others (an anxious defense).

   In the long run, repeated experiences of attachment figure availability have an enduring effect on intrapsychic organization and interpersonal behavior. At the intrapsychic
level, such experiences act as a resilience resource, sustaining emotional well-being, mental health, and personal adjustment, and they cause secure working models of self and
others to be a person's most accessible social schemas. At the interpersonal level, repeated
experiences of attachment figure availability create a secure attachment style, with many
benefits in close relationships (e.g., trust, clear and open communication, ability and willingness to care for others). The broaden-and-build cycle of attachment security can be
viewed as the core advantage of being a secure person.

   As in the system-activation component of our model (the upper gray box), the
answer to the second question (the middle gray box) concerning attachment figure
availability depends on subjective appraisals and can therefore be biased by attachment
strategies. Anxious individuals' hyperactivating strategies intensify the vigilant monitoring of attachment figures' behavior and slant perceptions in the direction of noticing or
imagining insufficient interest, availability, or responsiveness. As a result, the likelihood
of detecting real or imagined signs of disinterest, distance, rejection, or unavailability is
increased, because an attachment figure cannot always be immediately available and
totally at a needy partner's disposal. Avoidant individuals' deactivating strategies interfere with monitoring the availability or unavailability of an attachment figure, increasing
the likelihood that genuine signals of attachment figure availability will be missed
or misperceived. In contrast, security-based strategies facilitate positive appraisals of
attachment figure availability, building on and confirming a positive view of relationship
partners as available and supportive. This stance encourages a securely attached person
to overlook or downplay inevitable instances of temporary unresponsiveness or unavailability.

   These cognitive biases are amplified when attachment-related mental representations
are preconsciously activated. At a preconscious level, expectations concerning attachment
figure availability depend entirely on the kind of internalized figure, available or unavailable, one tends to recall. Insecurely attached people tend to give a negative answer to the
question of attachment figure availability, because they have ready mental access to cognitive representations of unavailable figures. More securely attached people, in contrast,
tend to answer this question positively, because they have many mental representations of
available and supportive attachment figures.

   Despite these cognitive biases, however, reality is still of great consequence in the
appraisal of attachment figure availability. The actual presence of a responsive attachment figure or contextual factors that activate representations of an available figure (e.g.,
being instructed, in one of our experiments, to think about such a person; Mikulincer &
Shaver, 2001) can yield an affirmative answer to the availability question. These contexts,
mainly when they are clear-cut, personally meaningful, and repeated over time and situa-

tions, can counteract even insecure people's tendencies to doubt the availability of attachment figures, and can therefore set in motion a broaden-and-build cycle of attachment security. In other words, an insecure person can be helped to function more securely, both temporarily (as in some of the experiments we describe in later chapters) and chronically (as in successful psychotherapy or other kinds of transformative relationships).

The Broaden-and-Build Cycle of Attachment Security

In our model, the broaden-and-build cycle of attachment security, which results from appraising attachment figures as available and responsive, is viewed as a cascade of mental and behavioral events. This cascade enhances emotional stability; personal and social adjustment; satisfying, close relationships; and autonomous personal growth. The most immediate psychological benefit of attachment figure availability is effective management of distress and restoration of emotional equanimity. According to attachment theory, interactions with available and supportive attachment figures impart a sense of safety, assuage distress, and arouse positive emotions (relief, satisfaction, gratitude). Secure people can therefore remain relatively unperturbed under stress and experience longer periods of positive affectivity, which in turn contribute to sustained emotional well-being and mental health (Bonanno, 2004).

Experiences of attachment figure availability contribute to a reservoir of positive memories of effective distress management and positive mental representations of self and others (the "working models" discussed by Bowlby). Interactions with available and supportive attachment figures sustain a background sense of hope and optimism, making it easy for a person to believe and feel that most of life's problems are solvable and most distress is manageable. These interactions also create positive beliefs about other people and heighten a secure person's confidence in most relationship partners' sensitivity, responsiveness, and goodwill. In addition, secure individuals learn to perceive themselves as strong and competent, valuable, lovable, and special—thanks to being valued, loved, and viewed as special by caring attachment figures.

Appraising attachment figures as available, responsive, and supportive also creates a reservoir of useful procedural knowledge concerning emotion regulation and coping with stress. This knowledge is organized around the "secure-base script" discussed in Chapter 1 (based on H. S. Waters et al., 1998) and includes three regulatory tendencies—acknowledging and appropriately communicating distress; seeking intimacy, closeness, and support; and engaging in instrumental problem solving. During interactions with supportive attachment figures, secure people learn that they can confidently and openly express their vulnerability and neediness, and that this expression yields positive outcomes. They also learn that they can often solve important problems themselves, and that turning to others is an effective way to bolster their own considerable coping capacity. The "emotion-focused coping" components of this script (Lazarus & Folkman, 1984)—acknowledging and expressing feelings and seeking emotional support—work in the service of alleviating distress, so that "problem-focused coping" efforts, such as seeking instrumental support and solving a problem, can proceed successfully.

Besides boosting positive core beliefs and constructive regulatory strategies, experiences of attachment-figure availability can have beneficial effects on social–relational cognitions (beliefs that proximity maintenance is generally rewarding and that attachment relationships are beneficial) and assuage worries about rejection, criticism, or disapproval when one expresses feelings and needs. These beliefs make it easier for a person to get psychologically close to a partner; to express needs, desires, and hopes; and to ask for support when it is needed. They also predispose securely attached people to feel comfortable with intimacy and interdependence; to emphasize the benefits of being together; to feel trust, gratitude, and affection toward relationship partners; and to offer generous interpretations of a partner's ambiguous or disappointing behavior; that is, security-enhancing interactions leave in their wake a network of prosocial behaviors and beliefs, thereby heightening secure people's chances of establishing and maintaining intimate and deeply interdependent relationships.

Possessing these rich resources for dealing with stress makes it less necessary to rely on psychological defenses that distort perception and generate interpersonal conflict. According to our model, people who possess security-enhancing mental representations of attachment experiences generally feel safe and protected without having to deploy defenses. They can devote mental resources that otherwise would be employed in preventive, defensive maneuvers to other behavioral systems and to more promotion-focused, growth-oriented activities. Moreover, being confident that support is available when needed, secure people can take calculated risks and accept important challenges that contribute to the broadening of their perspectives and facilitate the pursuit of individuation and self-actualization.

Proximity-Seeking Viability and Secondary Attachment Strategies

Attachment figure unavailability results in attachment insecurity, compounds the distress aroused by actual dangers and threats, and triggers a cascade of mental and behavioral processes that can jeopardize emotional well-being, personal adjustment, and relationship satisfaction and stability. This painful series of events forces a person to adopt a secondary attachment strategy—hyperactivation, deactivation, or a combination of the two (see the third gray box, bottom section of Figure 2.1). The "decision" between possible strategies (which, as we have already said, can be unconscious and automatic rather than deliberate, and not be a "decision" in the usual sense) depends on subjective appraisal of the expected success or failure of heightened proximity-seeking efforts and on the likely value of proximity if it is pursued.

Attachment figure unavailability can be experienced in different ways and result in different kinds of fears (Mikulincer, Shaver, & Pereg, 2003). A phenomenological analysis of attachment figure unavailability reveals two kinds of psychological pain: (1) the distress caused by failing to achieve or to maintain proximity to an attachment figure, and (2) the sense of helplessness caused by ineffective coregulation of distress and the appraisal of oneself as alone and vulnerable. Although these two kinds of painful feelings are related, their relative strength may vary across situations, relationships, and individuals. Moreover, each kind of feeling predisposes a person to adopt a particular coping strategy.

One state of mind is based on the failure of attachment behaviors to achieve a positive result (closeness, love, or protection) and on being punished (with inattention, rejection, or hostility) for enacting these behaviors. In such a state, seeking greater proximity to the attachment figure is likely to be viewed as futile, if not downright dangerous. A person in this predicament is more or less forced to adopt a deactivating strategy. A very different state of mind emerges when there is a failure to coregulate distress and a person feels inadequate to handle threats autonomously. This state of mind encourages a person to work harder to gain attention, cooperation, and protection from an attachment figure (i.e., to hyperactivate the attachment system). Under such conditions, the person perceives distance from an attachment figure as dangerous, and becomes afraid of what will happen if he or she attempts to cope with the situation and regulate distress alone.

An array of contextual (external) and internal factors contribute to the relative strength of these two different states of mind. The factors that encourage deactivation include, for example, (1) consistent inattention, rejection, or angry responses from an attachment figure; (2) threats of punishment for proximity-seeking signals and behaviors; (3) violent or abusive behavior on the part of an attachment figure; and (4) explicit or implicit demands for greater self-reliance and inhibition of expressions of need and vulnerability. The factors that encourage hyperactivation include (1) unpredictable or unreliable caregiving experienced as out of synch with one's needs and requests for help; (2) intrusive caregiving that interferes with the acquisition of self-regulation skills and punishes a person for trying to cope autonomously; (3) explicit or implicit messages from an attachment figure that one is stupid, helpless, incompetent, or weak; and (4) traumatic or abusive experiences that occur while one is separated from the attachment figure. These factors create an ambivalent state in which approaching the attachment figure is sometimes punishing and sometimes rewarding, but avoidance of this figure seems dangerous. This state of mind may be exacerbated by temperamental deficits in self-regulation and problems in controlling attention and cognition (Rothbart & Ahadi, 1994).

Hyperactivating Strategies

The main goal of hyperactivating strategies is to get an attachment figure, perceived as unreliable or insufficiently responsive, to pay more attention and provide protection or support. These strategies are exaggerations of the primary attachment strategy—intense monitoring of a relationship partner and strong efforts to maintain proximity—and the key distinguishing features of an anxious attachment style. They consist of over-dependence on a relationship partner for comfort; excessive demands for attention and care; strong desire for enmeshment or merger; attempts to minimize cognitive, emotional, and physical distance from a partner; and clinging or controlling behavior designed to guarantee a partner's attention and support. These responses are based on what an anxiously attached person interprets to be past rewards for energetic, even strident, applications of the primary attachment strategy, because such applications, at least at times, seem to succeed (or to have succeeded in the past). Unfortunately, although sometimes successful with at least some interaction partners, these strategies can easily encourage intrusive, coercive, and aggressive behaviors toward a relationship partner that promote relationship dysfunction, partner dissatisfaction, and eventual rejection or abandonment—ironically and tragically, the very outcomes most dreaded by attachment-anxious people.

To gain a partner's attention, care, and support, such people also tend to exaggerate the seriousness of psychological and physical threats and problems, exaggerate their inability to cope autonomously with life demands, intensify the experience and expression of distress, protest any hint of an attachment figure's unavailability or lack of responsiveness, and present themselves in degrading, childish, or excessively needy ways (Cassidy & Berlin, 1994; Mikulincer & Shaver, 2003); that is, attachment-anxious people often deliberately (consciously or unconsciously) emphasize their vulnerabilities, neediness, helplessness, and dependence, while desperately hoping that this exaggeration will capture an attachment figure's attention and concern (Cassidy, 1994). Moreover, because they still hope to gain a partner's care and protection without seeming to blame the partner too severely, attachment-anxious people often take some of the blame for a partner's unreliable care, which, unfortunately, reinforces negative self-images and doubts about their lovability.

These hyperactivating strategies, although originally intended to garner affection and alleviate distress, can increase the frequency and intensity of destructive emotions and the accessibility of threat-related thoughts, making it all too likely that the new, self-manufactured sources of distress will mingle and become confounded with old ones. As a result, attachment-anxious people have difficulty controlling the spread of activation from one affectively negative thought to another, and their minds easily become overwhelmed by a torrent of negative thoughts and feelings. (For this reason, people who produce an uncontrolled stream of negative memories, thoughts, and feelings during the AAI are classified as "enmeshed and preoccupied with attachment"; see Hesse, 1999; Chapter 4, this volume.) The anxious pattern of information processing gives primary attention to the affective tone of information and favors the organization of memory in terms of simple, undifferentiated features, such as the extent to which the information is threatening or implies rejection. As a result, hyperactivating strategies create a volatile, undifferentiated memory network pervaded by negative thoughts and feelings.

Hyperactivating strategies and associated mental processes have negative effects on social perception; they damage an anxious person's self-image by emphasizing helplessness and vulnerability to rejection and encourage negative appraisals of others (who are seen as untrustworthy, unfaithful, or frustrating). Chronic reliance on hyperactivating strategies places anxious individuals at risk for emotional and adjustment problems. It impairs their ability to regulate negative emotions, thereby perpetuating distress, which tends to continue even after objective threats subside. Hyperactivating strategies also have a negative impact on relationship satisfaction and stability, and they interfere with other behavioral systems by impeding their activation and diverting them to serve the goals of the attachment system (e.g., helping someone in order to be thanked, having sex with someone to deter or postpone rejection). These maneuvers make it unlikely that an anxious person will attain the kind of calm security necessary for good health, a clear mind, autonomous creativity, and self-development.

Deactivating Strategies

When proximity seeking is perceived as dangerous or is disallowed, a person tends to adopt deactivating strategies (Cassidy & Kobak, 1988), which include denial of attachment needs and "compulsive self-reliance." They also include the dismissal of threats and of the need for attachment figure availability, because thinking about threats or attachment figures may reactivate a defensively deactivated attachment system. These strategies are the most salient characteristics of avoidant individuals.

At the interpersonal level, deactivating strategies involve inhibition of the primary attachment strategy, proximity seeking. People who rely on deactivating strategies have two main goals in relationships: (1) gaining whatever they need while maintaining distance, control, and self-reliance, and (2) ignoring or denying needs and avoiding negative emotional states that might trigger attachment-system activation. The first goal is manifested in their observable attempts to control and maximize psychological distance from a partner; avoid interactions that require emotional involvement, intimacy, self-disclosure, or interdependence; and deny or suppress attachment-related thoughts and feelings that might imply or encourage closeness, cohesion, or consensus. The second goal is reflected in their reluctance to think about or confront personal weaknesses and relational tensions and conflicts; unwillingness to deal with a partner's distress or desire for intimacy and security; and suppression of thoughts and fears related to rejection, separation, abandonment, or loss.

Deactivating strategies also affect mental organization. Avoidant people try to inhibit or exclude from awareness thoughts or feelings that imply vulnerability, neediness, or dependence, which results in ignoring important information about psychological or physical threats, personal weaknesses, and attachment figure responses. This in turns lowers the accessibility in memory of threatening attachment-related thoughts and inhibits the spread of activation from one such memory to another. It can also create difficulties in the encoding of information that is congruent with defensively excluded cognitions and emotions. Attention is diverted from threatening and attachment-related information, so such information is processed only shallowly, because it does not have strong excitatory neural connections with accessible, central nodes in the memory network. As a result, the information is not fully integrated with other parts of the network and is encapsulated in segregated mental structures, which Bowlby (1980) and George and West (2001) called "segregated systems." The resulting barriers in memory and disrupted action systems contribute to avoidant individuals' failure to deal effectively with many negative experiences.

Deactivating strategies and their associated mental processes have a distorting effect on self-perception and destructive effects on the perception of others. Avoidant individuals defensively inflate their self-conceptions, presumably to feel less vulnerable and less interested in relying on deficient relationship partners. They tend to denigrate partners, dismiss or downplay their needs, and distrust them. Deactivating strategies also impair their ability to regulate negative emotions, causing avoidant individuals to keep anger and resentment alive internally, while attempting not to express them externally. They are also prone to withhold commitment even to close relationship partners, because this might make them dependent or vulnerable to rejection. Avoidant individuals fantasize about sexual partners other than their own primary relationship partner and are more prone than secure individuals to have extrarelationship sex. They also tend to view their relationships as unsatisfying, giving themselves an excuse to flee if a relationship becomes too intimate or demanding. An avoidant person's pervasive down-regulation of feelings and reluctance to express or experience enthusiasm interferes with other behavioral systems by preventing investment in these systems and making sure they (e.g., the caregiving system or the sexual system) do not result in increased intimacy or emotional involvement.

Attachment Disorganization: The Case of Fearful Avoidance

In some cases, intensely insecure people are unable to provide a simple answer to the question, "Is proximity seeking a viable option?" Hence, they have trouble choosing decisively between deactivating and hyperactivating strategies. Simpson and Rholes (2002b) reasoned that such people, whom Bartholomew and Horowitz (1991) called fearful avoidant, "may enact both strategies in a haphazard, confused, and chaotic manner . . . their behavior under stress may be an incoherent blend of contradictory, abortive approach/avoidance behaviors or perhaps paralyzed inaction or withdrawal" (p. 225). Like dismissingly avoidant individuals, fearfully avoidant people often cope by withdrawing and distancing themselves from relationship partners. Unlike their dismissing counterparts, however, who deny being afraid or needing anyone's support, the "fearful avoidants" continue to experience anxiety, ambivalence, and a desire for the relationship partner's love and support. They are avoidant, because they consciously fear the possible negative consequences of closeness to and reliance on others, but they also wish they did not have to feel this way.

This mixed attachment strategy, identified by high scores on *both* the anxiety and the avoidance dimensions (see Chapter 4, this volume), resembles the "disorganized" attachment pattern sometimes observed in Ainsworth's Strange Situation (see Main & Hesse, 1990). Disorganized infants are characterized by simultaneous or rapidly vacillating displays of approach and avoidance behavior toward an attachment figure, and by aimless, disoriented, or confused actions in response to attachment figure unavailability. Fearful avoidance in adolescence or adulthood probably has to be extreme before it parallels disorganization in infancy (which is usually found primarily in abusive or dysfunctional families), but when a person scores quite high on both the anxiety and avoidance scales of a measure of adult attachment, he or she may qualify as disorganized and may well have come from an abusive or neglectful family (e.g., Brennan, Shaver, & Tobey, 1991; Shaver & Clark, 1994).

Theoretically, fearful avoidance derives from a failure to achieve any of the goals of the major attachment strategies: safety and security following proximity seeking (the primary, secure strategy), defensive deactivation of the attachment system (the avoidant strategy), or intense and chronic activation of the attachment system until security-enhancing proximity is attained (the anxious strategy). One important example is the abused child, who can neither achieve security nor simply give up on an abusive parent. Another example is the child of a confused, drug-addicted, or grieving parent whose behavior cannot be predicted and who cannot be relied upon to provide comfort. In such cases, the attachment system is reactivated despite deactivating strategies, attachment-related needs and worries become simultaneously accessible (hence creating ambivalence), and the child becomes trapped in a cycle of conflict-riddled attempts to meet personal needs while avoiding rejection or mishandling. This condition is similar in some ways to posttraumatic stress disorder (M. J. Horowitz, 1982), which also involves attempts to avoid unwanted thoughts and memories, combined with inability to control intrusions of traumatic memories and hyperaroused emotions (see Chapter 13, this volume).

Many adult attachment studies indicate that fearfully avoidant individuals are relatively inhibited and unassertive, and that their lives may have been scarred by physical or sexual abuse or other attachment-related traumas (see Chapters 5 and 9, this volume). Moreover, there is extensive evidence that "fearful avoidants" are the least secure, least trusting, and most troubled of adolescents and adults (Shaver & Clark, 1994). Throughout this book, we review studies that reveal either of two main effects for the anxiety and avoidance dimensions (indicating that the two together have especially destructive effects) or an interaction between the dimensions (indicating that a high score on both dimensions is even more destructive than might be expected from the additive effects of the two forms of insecurity). For example, fearfully avoidant people have especially negative representations of their romantic partners (Chapter 6, this volume), are more likely than others to be involved in highly distressed and violent couple relationships (Chapter 10, this volume), are cognitively closed and rigid (Chapter 8, this volume), exhibit the least empathy for people who are distressed (Chapter 11, this volume), and have the most severe personality disorders and the poorest mental health (Chapter 13, this volume). Taken in conjunction with findings that disorganized infants are the most likely of all four attachment types in infancy to suffer years later from anxiety and dissociative disorders (e.g., Carlson, 1998), these results suggest that life is especially difficult for a person whose scores are high on both anxiety and avoidance.

Model Summary

Our model (Figure 2.1) summarizes the cognitive operations, behavioral strategies, and motivational dynamics of the attachment system in adulthood, as well as the goals of each attachment strategy and their psychological manifestations. Whereas the broaden-and-build cycle of attachment security promotes satisfying, high-functioning intimate relationships, expansion of one's resilience resources, and broadening of one's perspectives and capacities, secondary attachment strategies are mainly designed to manage attachment-system activation and reduce or eliminate the pain caused by frustrated proximity seeking. Hyperactivating strategies keep a person focused on the search for love and security, and constantly vigilant regarding possible threats, separations, and betrayals. Deactivating strategies keep the attachment system in check, with serious negative consequences for psychological and interpersonal functioning. The framework summarized in Figure 2.1 serves as our "working model" for understanding the activation and functioning of the attachment system in adulthood. It also provides a road map for considering the research topics we address in subsequent chapters of this book.

ATTACHMENT THEORY
AND OTHER THEORETICAL FRAMEWORKS

In the remaining sections of this chapter, we consider similarities and differences between attachment theory and four other broad psychological approaches to understanding the human mind and social behavior: psychoanalytic theory, relational interdependence theory, social-cognition theories, and humanistic and "positive psychological" perspectives on personal development. In so doing, we hope to deepen our understanding of the implications of our model and build conceptual bridges to other theoretical approaches.

Psychodynamic Foundations of Attachment Theory

The links between attachment theory and psychoanalysis were evident in Bowlby's early writings (e.g., 1956). As we explained in Chapter 1, he was trained as a child psychiatrist and psychoanalyst, and like other psychoanalytic thinkers he assumed that the explanation of adult behavior lay somewhere in childhood, especially in early social relationships. Although he was dissatisfied with the conventional psychoanalysis of his time, especially the ideas of Anna Freud and Melanie Klein, he still believed that the quality of a child's emotional ties with the mother had powerful effects on normal and abnormal patterns of personal, interpersonal, and social functioning across the lifespan. Moreover, Bowlby organized attachment theory around themes that defined most of the psychoanalytic theories of his time: satisfaction and frustration of basic inner wishes (for security and protection), inner conflicts associated with barriers to wish fulfillment, psychological defenses aimed at avoidance or suppression of negative emotions associated with inner conflicts, and emotional problems related to the overuse of defenses.

These conceptual commonalities become more evident when one considers the basic postulates of contemporary psychodynamic theories (Shaver & Mikuliner, 2005). In a comprehensive and very thoughtful review of contemporary psychoanalysis, Westen (1998) asserted that all contemporary psychodynamic theorists agree on five core postulates: First, a large portion of mental life is unconscious. Second, cognitive and affective processes operate in parallel, so that people can have conflicting motives, thoughts, and feelings toward the same situation or person, and psychological defenses are often used to deal with these conflicts. Third, childhood experiences play a crucial role in the formation of adult personality. Fourth, mental representations of self and others are major components of personality; they often explain a person's behavior in interpersonal and social settings, and account for or contribute to psychological disorders. Fifth, healthy personality development is a journey from social dependence to mature autonomy.

Attachment theorists and researchers agree with all five postulates. According to attachment theory, many components of the attachment behavioral system operate unconsciously. As explained in this chapter, activation of the attachment system can occur unconsciously and shape a person's processing of information before he or she reflects on it consciously. Moreover, deactivating strategies often operate at an unconscious level. Avoidant people seem not to be aware of suppressing or denying attachment needs, and attachment-related thoughts and memories (Cassidy & Kobak, 1988). According to Bowlby (1988) and some of our own research (reviewed later in this book), these suppressed needs, memories, and thoughts continue to remain alive in unconscious, segregated mental systems and at times resurface in experience and action when deactivating strategies prove insufficiently strong given other cognitive or emotional demands on mental resources.

In attachment theory, inner conflict and psychological defense are central to the characterization of secondary attachment strategies. Hyperactivating strategies reflect a compromise between conflicting, ambivalent tendencies toward attachment figures—anger and hostility toward unavailable attachment figures combined with intense needs for protection and love from these frustrating figures (Cassidy & Kobak, 1988). Deactivating strategies are organized around conflicting tendencies at different levels of awareness, with lack of negative emotions and a detached attitude evident at the conscious level, while high levels of unresolved attachment-related distress exist at an unconscious level (Shaver & Mikulincer, 2002a).

Three additional features of attachment theory fit with the remaining postulates of contemporary psychoanalysis. According to Bowlby (1973), childhood experiences with primary caregivers have important effects on attachment-system functioning in adulthood and, as we stated earlier, mental representations of self and others (attachment working models) explain how mental residues of these early experiences become building blocks of a person's later thoughts, feelings, and actions, and have a shaping effect on adult emotion regulation, interpersonal relations, and mental health. Furthermore, according to attachment theory, attachment security provides a foundation for increased exploration, improved self-regulation, and a flexible balance between self-reliance and reliance on others, which in turn facilitates growth toward autonomy and maturity. This developmental progression stands in marked contrast with the overly dependent, infantile position of the highly anxious person and the rigidly self-reliant attitude of the highly avoidant person.

This does not mean, however, that attachment theory can simply be equated with psychoanalysis. In fact, attachment theory offers a unique perspective on the development of working models and their interplay with contemporary interpersonal contexts as determinants of adult feelings and relationship outcomes. Whereas contemporary psychoanalytic theory still views adult mental representations of self and others as mental residues of childhood experiences, Bowlby (1988) believed that the developmental trajectory of working models is not linear or simple, and that these mental representations in adulthood are not based exclusively on early experiences. Rather, they can be updated throughout life and affected by a broad array of contextual factors, such as current interactions with a relationship partner, the partner's attachment style and dynamics, and a person's current life situation, which can moderate or even override the effects of mental residues of past experiences (see Chapter 5, this volume, for research evidence). Thus, attachment theorists do not assert that a person's current attachment orientation must mirror or match his or her attachment orientations with parents during childhood. Rather, the current orientation is a complex amalgam of historical and contemporary factors, and it can be changed by updating and reworking mental representations of self and attachment figures.

The Relational Basis of Attachment Theory

The preceding section highlighted the importance of the relational context in which the attachment system is activated. Although attachment-system functioning involves intrapsychic processes, such as a person's wishes, fears, and defenses, it can be expressed in behavior (e.g., seeking proximity to a relationship partner) and is sensitive to a relationship partner's particular actions and reactions (e.g., availability and responsiveness). In fact, attachment-system functioning involves real and imagined interactions with relationship partners and can be altered by these partners' responses to one's proximity bids. In this respect, attachment theory has much in common with Thibault and Kelley's (1959) interdependence theory, which focuses on a single interpersonal transaction as the unit of analysis and emphasizes the powerful influence of one person's responses on a relationship partner's thoughts, feelings, and behavior.

Attachment theory acknowledges the huge impact of a partner's responses on a person's attachment-related thoughts and behaviors in a particular situation (Shaver & Hazan, 1993). In our model, all three modules of attachment-system functioning can be affected by a partner's behavior. The partner can be a source of danger, therefore triggering attachment-system activation (e.g., by threatening abandonment or violence). Also, a partner can affect the appraisal of both attachment figure availability and the viability of proximity seeking as a means of achieving security. Moreover, a person's relational cognitions and behaviors depend not only on his or her attachment style but also on a partner's attachment behaviors. Indeed, several studies have shown that both partners' attachment styles contribute uniquely to the prediction of both partners' relationship satisfaction (see Chapter 10, this volume, for research evidence). Moreover, a person's attachment anxiety and avoidance can have differential effects on emotions, cognitions, and behaviors depending on the partner's attachment style. For example, an anxious person may hyperactivate his or her attachment system more energetically when trying to compel affection or support from an avoidant relationship partner.

It is important to recall, however, that attachment theory is not exclusively relational in an external behavioral sense. As discussed earlier in this chapter, the attachment system can be activated intrapsychically, without resulting in visible social behavior or requiring responses from an actual relationship partner. In such cases, a person can search for comfort and security in his or her own mental representations, without seeking proximity to or support from anyone outside the self. In our recent analysis of security-based self-representations (Mikulincer & Shaver, 2004), we argued that these mental representations can be effectively called upon even in situations that are not explicitly social. In experimental studies we found that secure people, when under stress, are able to call upon both internalized self-soothing processes and some of their internalized attachment figure's qualities, which then allow them to tolerate failure and frustration induced by a laboratory task, even though the task itself is not social. Another example of strictly internal reactions occurs when an avoidant person processes information related to attachment issues unconsciously, without any observable effect on social behavior.

Because attachment theory has both intrapersonal and interpersonal aspects, it is a prime example of the "person × situation" approach to human behavior that has been popular for years in social/personality psychology. The person in this case is represented by the "hard-wired" programming of the attachment behavioral system, experience-based attachment working models of self and others, and the procedural knowledge implicit in attachment strategies. The situation consists of a relationship partner's responses and other contextual cues that affect a person's appraisal of what is happening in the relationship, thereby influencing his or her subsequent behavior toward the partner. The complexities in this model stem from the fact that major parts of the "person" component were originally based on variations in the availability and responsiveness of primary caregivers in threatening situations (i.e., in the actual social world—a series of "situations"), and major parts of the "situation" component are shaped by the person's attachment behavior, which may affect a partner's expressions of love, intimacy, and care. Ignoring either the person or the situation results in transforming attachment theory into either an interdependence theory or a psychoanalytic theory, transformations that we do not favor.

Social-Cognition Approaches and Attachment Theory

The role assigned by attachment theorists to working models of self and others is similar to the role played by cognitive–affective schemas in social cognition theories (e.g., Baldwin, 1992; Fiske & Taylor, 1991). Both attachment theory and social-cognition theories emphasize the extent to which people subjectively construe social experiences, store representations of these experiences (working models in attachment theory terms; schemas, prototypes, or scripts in social-cognitive language), and use these representations for understanding new social experiences and formulating action plans. In both theoretical approaches, mental representations guide and coordinate emotion regulation, person perception, and goal striving in interpersonal settings. Moreover, attachment theory conceptualizes working models in the same way that social-cognition theorists conceptualize mental representations: They are viewed as being stored in an associative memory network, as having excitatory and inhibitory connections with other representations, and as possessing a certain level of accessibility determined by past experiences and current context.

The commonalities between attachment theory and social-cognition theories have become especially evident in recent adult attachment studies. Attachment researchers have invested a great deal of energy and ingenuity in assessing the effects of attachment style on cognitive structures and processes that had previously been conceptualized and examined in social-cognition research, such as person perception (e.g., Zhang & Hazan, 2002), the accessibility and organization of self-representations (e.g., Mikulincer, 1995), expectations about others' behavior (e.g., Baldwin, Fehr, Keedian, Seidel, & Thompson, 1993), the accessibility of memories of social interactions (e.g., Beinstein Miller & Noirot, 1999), and interpretations of relationship partners' behavior (e.g., Collins,

1996). Moreover, adult attachment research has tended to rely increasingly on research techniques and designs borrowed from social-cognition research, such as implicit memory tasks, semantic priming techniques, and reaction times in lexical decision and Stroop color-naming tasks (e.g., Baldwin et al., 1993; Mikulincer, Gillath, et al., 2001; Mikulincer, Gillath, & Shaver, 2002).

Despite these commonalities, however, it would be a mistake to equate attachment working models with the cognitive structures usually studied in social-cognition research. In their review of the nature, content, and functions of attachment working models, Shaver, Collins, and Clark (1996) identified four differences between these constructs: As compared with other mental representations, (1) working models also contain, express, or activate a person's wishes, fears, conflicts, and psychological defenses, and they can be affected by these psychodynamic processes; (2) working models seem to contain a larger and more powerful affective component than do most social schemas, and tend to be more powerfully shaped by emotion-regulation processes; (3) working models tend to be construed in relational terms and to organize representations of self, others, and social interactions; and (4) working models are broader, richer, and more complex structures, and can include tandem or opposite representations of the same social experience at episodic, semantic, and procedural levels of encoding. Overall, attachment working models, especially in adulthood, cannot be equated with most other social cognitions, because they evolve not only from simple memories of actual experiences but also from dynamic processes of goal pursuit, emotion regulation, and psychological defenses involved with wishes for proximity and security, and fears of separation and helplessness. As a result, attachment working models can distort a person's perceptions of social reality, even though many were formed originally in social situations.

These differences call attention to the dialectical tension between the goal-striving and emotion-regulation functions that attachment working models accomplish. On the one hand, due to the goal-oriented and goal-corrected nature of the attachment system, working models have to be what Bowlby called "tolerably accurate reflections of what actually happened" in attachment relationships; otherwise, people would not be able to plan effective goal-oriented behavior and attain important relational goals. In this respect, working models resemble other cognitive representations that store factual knowledge and semantic and procedural information about reality constraints and demands. On the other hand, due to their emotion regulation function, working models sometimes distort perceptions, thoughts, and actions in order to manage attachment-related fears, worries, and insecurities, and to protect a person from the distress and pain of attachment figure unavailability. This dialectical tension between the goal-striving and emotion regulation functions of working models seems to be unique to attachment theory, which distinguishes it from other social-cognitive theories.

Positive Psychology and Attachment Theory

The broaden-and-build cycle of attachment security calls attention to the optimistic, hopeful, constructive, and actualization-oriented tone of attachment theory, which makes it different from most other psychodynamic, relational, and social-cognition theories. As previously noted, people who possess a stable sense of attachment security generally feel safe and worthy, hold an optimistic and hopeful outlook on life, rely on constructive methods of coping and regulating distress, and interact with others in a confident and open manner. This health- and growth-oriented quality of attachment theory has much in common with the "humanistic psychology" movement of the 1950s and 1960s (e.g.,

Maslow, 1968, C. R. Rogers, 1961) and today's "positive psychology" movement (Aspinwall & Staudinger, 2003; Seligman, 2002). Both humanistic and positive psychology are attempts to balance psychology's traditional focus on conflicts, fears, egoistic defenses, destructive tendencies, and psychopathology with due consideration of human strengths, developmental potentials, and social virtues that contribute to the development of what Carl Rogers (1961) called a "fully functioning person" and Maslow (1968) called "self-actualization."

According to attachment theory, security is a basic human strength. It facilitates the development of other personal qualities that fall under the rubric of "positive" psychological traits, such as resilience, optimism, hope, positive affectivity, curiosity and exploration, healthy autonomy, capacities for love and forgiveness, feelings of interconnectedness and belongingness, tolerance for human differences, and kindness. Moreover, one can easily recognize major similarities between the way the broaden-and-build cycle of attachment security emerges from repeated episodes of attachment figure availability and discussions by humanistic psychologists of the parenting style—unconditional positive regard—that facilitates a child's pursuit of self-actualization. For example, the notion of having an available, caring, and loving attachment figure, then extending the same kindness and benefits to other people resonates with Maslow's (1968) concept of B-perception—nonjudgmental, forgiving, loving acceptance of another human being—and with Carl Rogers's (1961) conception of optimal parenting and psychotherapy based on "unconditional positive regard." The common idea that recurs across the various "positive" theoretical frameworks is that experiences of being loved, accepted, and supported by others constitute the most important form of personal protection and self-confidence. They provide a secure psychological foundation for confronting adversity and maintaining equanimity in times of stress, without interrupting normal processes of growth and self-actualization. They also foster an ethically important tolerance of human differences and what Buddhist writers call "compassion" and "loving-kindness."

Despite the theoretical commonalities between attachment theory and humanistic or positive psychological theories, the two are not identical. Whereas the positive and humanistic approaches focus mainly on growth-oriented, promotion-focused aspects of personality development, attachment theory emphasizes both prevention and promotion aspects of the attachment system. This dual focus is well illustrated in the two basic functions of "safe haven" and "secure base" served by available, responsive, caring, and loving attachment figures. Such figures need to protect a person from threats and dangers, prevent any negative, painful outcomes of unavoidable stressors, and help to downregulate the person's fears and conflicts. At the same time, attachment figures need to provide a "secure base" from which the person can take risks, explore self and environment, and engage in promotion-oriented activities.

Attachment figures' failure to provide either a safe haven or a secure base results in a person's attachment-related doubts and worries, as well as psychological defenses that are attempts to compensate for the lack of security but result in cognitive distortion, rigidity, constriction, alienation, and an increase in interpersonal and intergroup conflict. Unlike positive psychology, attachment theory emphasizes both the "dark" and the "light, bright" sides of human nature and experience, and explains how the attachment system deals with fears, anger, conflicts, and defenses, as well as the equally natural capacities for happiness, love, growth, and self-actualization. We believe it makes sense to explore positive psychology within a framework that also includes "negative psychology," because both are very real aspects of the human mind. We return to this matter at the end of book, in Chapter 16.

CONCLUDING REMARKS AND AN OUTLINE OF SUBSEQUENT CHAPTERS

Having presented the historical background and basic concepts of attachment theory in Chapter 1, we have now organized the major concepts and tenets of the theory in a dynamic model of attachment-system functioning. The model shows how the attachment system is activated in adolescents and adults by threats and stressors, how its primary strategy (proximity seeking or relying on security-based self-representations) works to achieve a sense of felt security and return a person to pursuits motivated and governed by other behavioral systems, and how the sense of security contributes to a broaden-and-build cycle that leads, over time, to personal growth, a fully functioning personality, and self-actualization. The model also shows how failure to attain security forces a person to adopt one of two secondary attachment strategies: hyperactivation or deactivation (or a "disorganized" combination of the two). Choosing either a hyperactivating or a deactivating strategy has important implications for intrapsychic and interpersonal functioning. We have also explained briefly how attachment theory resembles and differs from other major psychological theories.

In the remainder of the book we elaborate on various parts of the model and review empirical studies related to them. In Chapter 3, we review empirical research on the normative processes of attachment system activation, the formation of attachment bonds, and reactions to the availability or unavailability of attachment figures. In Chapter 4 we describe and evaluate various measures developed by attachment researchers over the past several years to assess individual differences in adult attachment styles and strategies. In Chapter 5, we summarize what is known about the developmental origins of these individual differences and the stability or instability of attachment orientations over the lifespan. Chapters 6 through 8 focus on the intrapsychic aspects of attachment-system functioning, including how attachment style is related to measurable mental representations of self and others, emotion regulation and coping with stress, and the regulation of behavior and fulfillment of life tasks, such as forming an identity, finding and developing a career, maintaining personal health, and finding philosophical or religious meaning in life. Chapters 9 through 12 focus on the interpersonal aspects of attachment-system functioning, including how attachment style affects patterns of interpersonal relatedness, couple functioning, caregiving behavior, and sexuality. In Chapter 13, we review research on links between attachment insecurities and various forms of psychopathology. We show in Chapters 14 and 15 how adult attachment theory has been applied to the study of psychotherapy and organizational behavior. Chapter 16 sums up the state of the field and considers some of the deep existential implications of attachment theory and research. Appendices A–G show how many of the researchers who study adolescent and adult attachment measure key constructs. We hope the book as a whole provides a useful launching pad for future research on adult attachment, and its clinical and educational applications.

CHAPTER 3

Normative Attachment Processes

In his trilogy on *Attachment and Loss*, Bowlby (1969/1982, 1973, 1980) explained how the innate, cross-culturally universal attachment behavioral system gets activated in particular situations and functions adaptively. In developmental psychology, these fundamental features of the attachment system are called "normative," because they are the developmental norm. Normative features of the system are ones that require an evolutionary explanation, because they are evident in all people, beginning in infancy, all over the world, and are shared to a large extent with our closest primate relatives (e.g., C. S. Carter et al., 2005; Suomi, 1999).

The attachment system is triggered by threats and dangers, and its main "job" or adaptive function is to motivate a person by activating and directing his or her behavior to seek proximity to and protection from an attachment figure. The actual availability— or in the case of older children, adolescents, and adults, sometimes the internalized, symbolic rather than actual physical availability—of these comforting, caring figures, combined with their responsive provision of protection and support, evokes feelings of safety and security, assures a person of worthiness and lovability, and builds confidence in the effectiveness of seeking help from relationship partners. Over time, repeatedly attaining felt security builds and reinforces a person's coping capacities, creating a flexible repertoire of coping skills that increasingly functions autonomously. This security and self-confidence allow other behavioral systems, such as exploration and affiliation, to operate effectively, adding considerably to a secure person's understanding of self and world, physical and mental health, and life skills. In contrast, unavailability, unresponsiveness, or loss of an attachment figure, resulting in repeated failures to attain proximity and protection, produces intense distress and demoralization, making it necessary to develop secondary attachment strategies and related defenses to regulate feelings of insecurity and worries about rejection or abandonment.

In our model of attachment-system activation and functioning in adulthood (Chapter 2), we characterized these processes in terms of three if–then propositions: First, if threatened, then seek proximity and protection. Second, if an attachment figure is available and supportive, then relax, enjoy, and appreciate the feeling of being loved and secure, and confidently return to other activities. Third, if an attachment figure is unavailable or unresponsive, then either intensify efforts to achieve proximity and protection or deactivate the attachment system and rely on oneself.

In this chapter, we expand on these if–then propositions and review empirical evidence concerning the generic activation and operation of the attachment system in adulthood. Although, as we explained in Chapter 2, the three if–then modules of attachment-system functioning are gradually molded by a person's idiosyncratic social experiences, resulting in fairly stable internal working models and a chronic attachment style, in this chapter we review studies showing how situational threats, actual or symbolic attachment figure availability and responsiveness, and the viability of seeking proximity affect the activation and operation of the attachment system regardless of individual differences in attachment style. Subsequent chapters are devoted, topic by topic, to the many studies of the effects of attachment style (i.e., individual differences in attachment-system parameters) on attachment-system functioning and of related issues such as self-esteem, emotion regulation, personal adjustment, interpersonal behavior, relationship functioning, and mental health. These studies are easier to understand once the normative aspects of the attachment behavioral system have been explained.

ATTACHMENT-SYSTEM ACTIVATION

In our control system model of attachment-system dynamics (Figure 2.1 in Chapter 2, this volume), activation of the attachment system occurs when appraisal of physical or psychological threats causes preconscious activation of attachment-related mental representations (e.g., of security-enhancing attachment figures and memories of the feelings experienced during supportive interactions with these figures), conscious thoughts about proximity and support seeking, and, in many cases, behavioral efforts to attain comfort and protection from an actual attachment figure. In adolescence and adulthood, attachment-system activation also includes choosing a specific security provider from a hierarchy of attachment figures (e.g., parents, friends, romantic partners). In the following sections we review evidence concerning preconscious activation of attachment-related mental representations, the tendency to seek comfort and protection from an actual attachment figure, and the choice of a specific relationship partner as a security provider.

Preconscious Activation

Two series of studies (Mikulincer et al., 2000; Mikulincer, Gillath, & Shaver, 2002) examined preconscious activation of the attachment system in adulthood. Participants were subliminally primed with threat-related words (e.g., *failure*) or neutral words (e.g., *hat*), and the accessibility of thoughts about attachment themes or mental representations of attachment figures were assessed using two kinds of cognitive tasks: a lexical decision task (deciding quickly whether particular letter strings are words) and a Stroop color-naming task (quickly naming the color in which each word is printed, which requires temporarily ignoring or suppressing the meaning of the word). These tasks indicate, indirectly, how accessible particular mental contents are at a given moment, so they allow us to measure the effects of symbolic threats on the availability of attachment-related mental content, and to do this without study participants being aware of either the thoughts themselves or our assessment of them.

This research strategy is based on the previous discovery that a cognitive process can occur unconsciously and influence a person's performance without noticing it in his or her subjective stream of consciousness (Wegner & Smart, 1997). Thus, we can measure the extent to which an unconscious threat activates certain mental contents and processes, such as mental processes related to seeking support from attachment figures, without research participants guiding or controlling the flow of mental events consciously (e.g., Bargh, Chen, & Burrows, 1996).

In Mikulincer et al.'s (2000) studies, the accessibility of thoughts about attachment themes was assessed in a lexical decision task. On each of many trials, participants read a string of letters on a computer screen and were asked to indicate as quickly as possible, by pushing particular response keys, whether the letter string was or was not a word. Reaction times (RTs) served as a measure of the accessibility of thoughts related to the target words: The quicker the RT, the higher the cognitive accessibility (D. E. Meyer & Schvaneveldt, 1971). The strings of letters in these studies included proximity-related words (e.g., *love, hug*), separation-related words (e.g., *separation, rejection*), neutral words (e.g., *office, table*), positive non-attachment-related words (e.g., *honesty, efficacy*), negative non-attachment-related words (e.g., *cheat, lazy*), and nonwords created by scrambling the letters of actual words (e.g., *btale* [*table*], *vleo* [*love*]). Before each string of letters was presented, a threat word (e.g., *failure, death*) or a neutral word (*hat*) was flashed on the screen for 20 milliseconds, which is not long enough to be perceived consciously. In cognitive psychology, this is called subliminal "priming," because the subliminal stimulus "primes" particular mental contents, just as priming an old-fashioned pump causes water to flow.

The findings supported the hypothesized effects of threats on attachment-system activation; that is, a subliminally presented threat word, in comparison with a subliminally presented neutral word, led to faster identification (implying greater cognitive accessibility) of proximity-related words (*hug, love*, etc.) This effect was specific to proximity-related words and did not generalize to separation-related words, neutral words, or negative or positive emotion words that had no attachment connotation. Moreover, this heightened accessibility of proximity-related thoughts occurred regardless of individual differences in attachment style (although these individual differences also had effects, as we discuss in later chapters), suggesting that everyone was subject to preconscious activation of the attachment system.

Following these studies, Mikulincer, Gillath, and Shaver (2002) conducted three experiments focusing on the accessibility of the names of people described by participants as attachment figures (i.e., people to whom they turned for closeness, protection, and security). Participants filled out the WHOTO scale (Hazan & Zeifman, 1994), which identifies a person's primary attachment figures by asking for the names of people who are preferred as providers of proximity (e.g., "Whom do you like to spend time with?"), a safe haven (e.g., "To whom do you turn for comfort when you're feeling down?"), and a secure base (e.g., "Whom do you feel you can always count on?"). Participants also named close others who were not necessarily attachment figures (e.g., father, sister, friends), as well as people they knew who were not particularly close (e.g., coworkers, casual friends) and people they did not know at all (from a long list of names we provided). They then performed either a lexical decision task or a Stroop color-naming task to measure the cognitive accessibility (reflected by RTs) of mental representations of attachment figures following subliminal presentation of either a threatening or a neutral word.

In the lexical decision task, participants were exposed to the names of their own attachment figures, names of close people who were not mentioned in the WHOTO scale (and therefore were not, in our estimation, attachment figures), names of known persons, names of unknown persons, and nonwords. They were asked in each case to indicate as quickly as possible whether each string of letters was or was not a person's name. Faster lexical decision RTs for a particular name were interpreted as indicating greater momentary accessibility of name-related (or named person–related) mental representations. In the Stroop color-naming task (Stroop, 1938), participants were exposed to the same four categories of names, each printed in one of several colors, and asked to indicate the color in which each name was printed. (Different colors were randomly assigned to different names.) Extensive previous research had demonstrated that cognitive activation of a specific mental representation increases attention to representation-congruent stimulus features, which slows a person's ability to suppress the reading of the word while detecting and indicating its color (e.g., Mathews & MacLeod, 1985); that is, interference with color identification (slower RTs) indicates implicit activation of stimulus-related cognitive networks. Before each trial in both the lexical decision task and the Stroop task, a threat prime (the word *failure* or *separation*) or a neutral word (*hat*, *umbrella*) was presented for 20 milliseconds (i.e., subliminally).

Across three different conditions, study participants reacted to a threat-prime word (either failure or separation) with heightened access to the names of the people they had listed on the WHOTO scale as attachment figures. As compared with neutral subliminal words, subliminal priming with threat words produced (1) faster identification of names of attachment figures in the lexical decision task and (2) slower color-naming RTs in the Stroop task. In both cases, fast lexical decisions and slow color-naming responses were interpreted as indicating heightened activation of mental representations of attachment figures in threatening contexts. Importantly, priming with threat words had no effect on mental representations of close others or known persons who were not mentioned in the WHOTO scale. Thus, heightened accessibility under threatening conditions depended on the extent to which a person was viewed as a safe haven and secure base.

These findings imply that the adult mind turns rapidly and unconsciously to mental representations of attachment figures when threats loom, and also that people identified as attachment figures in the WHOTO scale are psychologically special. They are distinguished from other people when threats are detected, which means that most adults can name the members of a special group of close others who accomplish attachment functions and whose mental representations are called up mentally in threatening situations. This is powerful evidence that the attachment system and mental representations of attachment figures exist in adulthood and are psychologically significant.

The Actual Seeking of Proximity and Support

There is ample evidence, emanating from many different theoretical traditions, that encountering a serious danger or threat motivates efforts to gain proximity to and support from other people (e.g., Lazarus & Folkman, 1984; Schachter, 1959). This is one of many senses in which people are "social animals." For example, studies examining Schachter's fear-leads-to-affiliation hypothesis have consistently found that anticipation of a noxious event heightens the tendency to affiliate with other people, especially ones who understand the nature of the threat (for a review, see Shaver & Klinnert, 1982). Although this finding was originally interpreted in terms of social comparison (i.e., trying to understand a threat by comparing one's own feelings with those of other people), Kirkpatrick and Shaver (1988) suggested that stress increases proximity seeking as a means of alleviating distress. In addition, the major theories of stress and coping agree that a frequently used means of dealing with threats is to seek social support (see Zeidner & Endler, 1996, for a review of theories). In fact, most coping inventories include items that deal with efforts to obtain support from relationship partners or members of one's social network (for a review of coping inventories, see Schwarzer & Schwarzer, 1996).

In a naturalistic study of behavioral reactions to a major attachment-related threat, separation from a close relationship partner, Fraley and Shaver (1998) saw many examples of proximity-seeking behavior. They unobtrusively observed couples waiting in the departure lounges of a public airport and noted, over time, whether the partners were separating from each other (because one person was flying to another city) or were not separating (because they were both about to fly somewhere together). Fraley and Shaver found that couples who were separating were more likely than couples who were not separating to seek and maintain physical contact (e.g., by mutually gazing at each other's faces, talking intently, and touching). Theoretically speaking, the threat of separation activated these people's attachment systems and caused them to engage in proximity-seeking behavior.

The connection between experiencing stress and seeking support from attachment figures has also been documented in a diary study of couples (Collins & Feeney, 2005). Both members of each couple completed a nightly diary for 3 weeks, recording stressful life events, support-seeking behaviors, predominant mood, and thoughts and feelings about the relationship. In line with attachment theory, participants reported seeking more instrumental and emotional support from their partner on days when they experienced more stress. Moreover, the study yielded important information about activation of the caregiving system (see Chapter 11, this volume) and beneficial effects of attachment-figure availability (discussed later in this chapter). Collins and Feeney observed that people knew they had provided more support on days when their partner reported experiencing more stress. And on days when participants perceived their partner as more supportive, they felt more valued and more secure in the relationship.

Recently, a series of experimental studies showed that the anxiety aroused by thinking about one's mortality causes people to seek proximity to attachment figures as a way to reduce distress (for a review, see Mikulincer, Florian, & Hirschberger, 2003). For example, Florian, Mikulincer, and Hirschberger (2002, Study 1) asked people to write about either their own death (the "mortality salience" condition) or a neutral topic (watching TV). Following a distracter task, all participants then rated the extent to which they were committed to their romantic partner (e.g., "I am completely devoted to my partner"), as well as their moral commitment to marriage (e.g., "Marriages are supposed to last forever"). People in the mortality salience condition reported greater psychological commitment to their romantic partner than did participants in the neutral condition. However, there was no significant effect of mortality salience on moral commitment. Florian et al. concluded that death reminders increase the sense of love and closeness to a romantic partner, but not the sense of cultural obligations concerning marriage. (This makes sense theoretically, because the attachment behavioral system evolved biologically long before marriage became a cultural institution.)

Of course, Florian et al.'s (2002) findings do not necessarily mean that the attachment system, as we have conceptualized it, becomes activated following "mortality salience." In fact, establishing closeness and commitment can serve purposes other than protection and security, such as promoting common interests or encouraging sexual intercourse (hence, reproduction). To demonstrate attachment-system activation, it is necessary to show that proximity seeking serves a protective function. This kind of demonstration can be accomplished in two ways. First, if proximity seeking buffers a person from distress, seeking proximity to an attachment figure following death reminders should reduce the need for other defensive maneuvers that protect against death anxiety, such as validating one's cultural worldview. (Many studies have shown that mortality salience heightens people's defense of their political and religious beliefs, and causes them to reject or oppose others who threaten those beliefs; see Mikulincer, Florian, & Hirschberger, 2003.) Second, if proximity seeking shields people from death awareness, interference with proximity seeking should increase the mental accessibility of concerns about death.

In two studies, Florian et al. (2002) provided evidence for the protective function of proximity seeking following death awareness. In Study 2, Florian et al. assigned people randomly to a mortality salience or a neutral condition, then divided them randomly into two subgroups based on a manipulation of the salience of romantic commitment. Participants in the romantic commitment condition were asked to describe emotions associated with committing themselves to a romantic partner. Participants in the no-commitment condition were asked similar questions about a neutral topic (listening to the radio). All of them then rated the severity of punishment that was appropriate for various social transgressions, which was meant to assess a common worldview defense—punishing people who transgress social norms (Rosenblatt, Greenberg, Solomon, Pyszczynski, & Lyon, 1989). The results showed that mortality salience (compared with the neutral condition) increased participants' harsh judgments of purported social transgressions in the no-commitment condition, but it had no effect on punishment severity when romantic commitment had been made salient; that is, asking people to think about their romantic commitment reduced the need to use other defenses against the threat of death.

In Study 3, Florian et al. (2002) divided participants randomly into three conditions according to the kinds of thoughts that were made salient (problems in a romantic relationship, academic problems, and neutral topics). All participants then completed J. Greenberg, Pyszczynski, Solomon, Simon, and Breus's (1994) word-completion task, which measures the implicit accessibility of death-related thoughts. When given partial words and asked to complete them (e.g., _ R A V _), participants in the "problems in romantic relationship" condition produced more death-related words (e.g., *grave* rather than *brave*) than did participants in the "academic problems" and neutral conditions. Thus, thinking about difficulties in close relationships heightens death-thought accessibility, probably because of the threat posed by relationship problems to the protective function of proximity seeking.

There is also evidence that proximity seeking can override the need for other defenses against death awareness. Hirschberger, Florian, and Mikulincer (2003) asked whether proximity seeking following death awareness can overcome threats to self-esteem—for example, complaints or criticisms from one's relationship partner. Study participants were assigned to a mortality salience or to a control condition and asked to imagine having dinner at their partner's parents' home, then receiving one of three kinds of evaluations from their partner—admiration ("I'm very proud of you. You were so friendly and nice tonight"), a complaint ("Tonight you seemed to be really withdrawn, and you didn't even offer to help my mother"), or a criticism ("As usual, you were totally self-absorbed all evening and didn't help my mother. You are an egotist! What kind of a person are you?"). They were then asked, following a distracter task, to rate their willingness to engage in emotionally intimate interactions with their partner in a situation like the one imagined.

Participants who had been exposed to a mortality salience induction were more interested in emotional intimacy than were participants in the neutral condition. Moreover, whereas in the neutral condition a partner's admiration led to a stronger desire for intimacy than a partner's complaint or criticism, this difference was not significant in the mortality salience condition. In fact, death reminders increased the desire for emotional intimacy even after a partner complained or criticized, implying that death awareness makes people willing to pay the price of diminished self-esteem to maintain emotional closeness with a romantic partner. This conclusion is reinforced by Wisman and Koole's (2003) observation that death reminders heightened preference for sitting close to other people in a group discussion, rather than sitting alone, even if this seating preference required exposing their worldviews to potential attack (they knew that other participants would disagree with their beliefs).

Overall, findings from these studies clearly indicate that proximity seeking is a shield against existential threats, and that most people prefer to maintain proximity to others following death reminders rather than try to validate their beliefs or enhance their self-esteem. We suspect that reliance on worldview defenses or self-esteem inflation occurs mainly when proximity seeking fails to accomplish its protective function. And, as we discuss in Chapters 6 and 7, these ethnocentric and egoistic defenses are typical of insecurely attached people.

Choosing among Potential Attachment Figures

When a person's attachment system is activated by threats or stressors, a particular relationship partner is usually targeted as an attachment figure and viewed as a potential comforter and security provider. Even during infancy, although proximity seeking is automatically aimed at the primary caregiver, usually the mother, most children have other relationship partners who can be turned to as attachment figures, often including their father, grandparents, older siblings, day care workers, neighbors, and so on. Of course, the size and diversity of the network of attachment figures differs as a function of family size, culture, and attitudes and values (e.g., Bretherton, 1985; Main & Weston, 1981; van IJzendoorn & Sagi, 1999). This network tends to increase dramatically in size and diversity during adolescence and adulthood. Beyond parents and other family members, adolescents and adults can seek proximity and comfort from friends, romantic partners, spouses, teachers, mentors, clergy, managers at work, and others (Ainsworth, 1991; Weiss, 1982). In old age, proximity seeking can be targeted at one's children and grandchildren, as well as residential social workers, nurses, and therapists (e.g., Antonucci, Akiyama, & Takahashi, 2004).

Bowlby (1969/1982) discussed the issue of multiple attachment figures, noting that "almost from the first, many children have more than one figure to whom they direct attachment behavior" (p. 34). However, this does not mean that all attachment figures are interchangeable or that a person has no special affinity toward particular attachment figures, preferring them above all others. "It is a mistake to suppose that a young child diffuses his attachment over many figures in such a way that he gets along with no strong attachment to anyone, and consequently without missing any particular person when the person is away" (Bowlby, 1969/1982, p. 308). Rather, attachment figures appear to be organized in a "hierarchy" (Bretherton, 1985), with a particular figure being targeted as the principal safe haven and secure base, and the others being regarded as subsidiary attachment figures who can provide safety and security in the absence of the principal figure. According to Cassidy (1999), this strong tendency to prefer a particular attachment figure, or what Bowlby (1969/1982) called "monotropy," has two adaptive advantages: (1) It increases the likelihood that the targeted caregiver will assume primary responsibility for the child's welfare, and (2) it allows the child to make quick, automatic proximity-seeking responses in times of need, without losing precious time deciding which attachment figure should be selected in a given situation.

In support of this view, several studies have found that although infants can seek and derive comfort and protection from multiple attachment figures, when their principal attachment figure (usually the mother) is present, they prefer to seek comfort from her and are calmed only when they attain proximity to her (e.g., Ainsworth, 1967; Lamb, 1976; Rutter, 1981). Similarly, Ainsworth (1982) observed that "the child would tolerate major separations from subsidiary figures with less distress than comparable separations from the principal attachment figure. Nor could the presence of several attachment figures altogether compensate for the loss of the principal attachment figure" (p. 19).

The notion of a hierarchy of attachment figures raises important questions. Does the hierarchy change with age and development, depending on life tasks, challenges, and opportunities characteristic of each age period? Does it depend on relational factors, such as the duration of a relationship with a specific figure, the kind of relationship (e.g., friendship, student–teacher relationship, sexual relationship), or the quality of care a particular figure provides? Does the hierarchy depend on personal factors, such as current needs and strivings (e.g., needs for autonomy, competence, or belongingness)? Only recently have attachment researchers begun to address these questions, collecting preliminary evidence regarding the complexity of adults' hierarchies of attachment figures.

Adopting a lifespan perspective, attachment researchers have identified a developmental trajectory according to which peers gradually replace parents as principal attachment figures (e.g., Ainsworth, 1991; Hazan & Zeifman, 1994; Weiss, 1982). Although parents are usually the primary attachment figures in infancy and childhood, close friends and romantic partners often become principal attachment figures during adolescence and adulthood. This does not mean that parents are completely relinquished as attachment figures or removed from the attachment hierarchy, but they typically change their position and function (Allen & Land, 1999; Weiss, 1993). This process of accepting peers as principal attachment figures usually involves a gradual transition from parents to same-sex close friends, then to romantic partners and, eventually, to a spouse (Hazan & Zeifman, 1994, 1999; Nitzberg, Shaver, & Conger, 2007). According to Hazan and Zeifman (1994), proximity seeking in adulthood is often directed toward a romantic partner or spouse to whom one is emotionally attached but with whom, in addition, one is sexually involved. As a result, sex becomes bound up with adult romantic attachment. However, as we explain in Chapter 12, proximity seeking for the sake of safety and social support—even to express romantic love—does not necessarily require sexual desire or sexual involvement (L. M. Diamond, 2006; Weiss, 1982).

In the first systematic research on developmental changes in the hierarchy of attachment figures, Hazan and Zeifman (1994) conducted two studies using the WHOTO scale (briefly described earlier in this chapter) to assess participants' preferred principal target for the attachment-related functions of proximity, safe haven, and secure base. In the first study, participants ages 6–17 preferred to spend time with peers rather than parents, regardless of age. In other words, proximity seeking was already targeted at peers during elementary school. However, the targeting of peers as principal providers of a safe haven and secure base typically occurred later, during adolescence and young adulthood. Peers replaced parents as sources of comfort and support between the ages of 8 and 14, and replaced them as a secure base only late in adolescence. Using the WHOTO scale, Fraley and Davis (1997) and Mayseless (2004) also discovered that young adults were in the midst of transferring the secure base function from parents to friends and romantic partners.

In a second study, Hazan and Zeifman (1994) found that adults to whom they administered the WHOTO scale preferred friends or romantic partners rather than parents when they sought closeness or a safe haven. With regard to the secure base function, they preferred their romantic partner, if they were involved in a long-term romantic relationship or marriage. However, if no such relationship existed, adults still preferred parents rather than friends as secure-base providers. These findings were conceptually replicated in a large sample of 812 adults ranging in age from 16 to 90 (N. A. Doherty & Feeney, 2004). Beyond documenting again the preeminent caregiving roles played by romantic partners and parents throughout most of adulthood, N. A. Doherty and Feeney obtained novel information about the attachment functions played by siblings and children. Like friends, siblings were typically nominated as important sources of companionship, comfort, and support (see J. A. Feeney & Humphreys [1996] for similar findings on sibling relationships). Young children were more preferred for proximity than for a safe haven or secure base, but adult children typically became safe havens for their aging parents.

Schachner (2006) compared a sample of long-term single adults with a matched sample of married peers (around 40 years of age, on average). The married adults, not surprisingly, were more likely to view their spouse as their principal attachment figure, but beyond a certain age, they also mentioned their children. The long-term single adults were more likely to rely for a safe haven and secure base on a sibling and/or a close friend. Overall, the number of attachment figures was about the same, on average, for married and long-term single adults, but the constellations of different kinds of attachment figures in each group's hierarchy were somewhat different. (Also not surprisingly, the long-term single adults were somewhat lonelier on average; less likely to be satisfied with their sex lives; more likely to masturbate; less likely to have children, although some did have them; and more likely to have had troubled relationships with parents while growing up.)

Adopting a slightly different approach to measurement, Trinke and Bartholomew (1997) constructed a scale to assess attachment networks rather than just principal attachment figures. Young adults were asked to list multiple attachment figures for the proximity seeking, safe haven, and secure base functions, and to rank the figures in order of importance. With respect to the safe haven and secure base functions, Trinke and Bartholomew also asked about both desired and actual use of specific attachment figures. The most common principal attachment figure for members of this young adult sample, defined by the highest composite rank, was mother (36% of participants), followed by romantic partner (31%), best friend (14%), father (11%), and sibling (8%). However, 62% of the participants who were involved in a serious romantic relationship named their romantic partner as a principal attachment figure. In a conceptual replication of Hazan and Zeifman's (1994) findings, Trinke and Bartholomew (1997) found that romantic partners were more preferred as a safe haven (both desired and actual) than as a secure base, whereas parents were more preferred as a secure base than as a safe haven.

Taken together, findings published to date indicate that romantic partners occupy the top rung in most people's attachment hierarchies during young adulthood, but parents are still preferred as a secure base for exploration and growth. (Whether this is the case in other cultures has yet to be determined.) As adults age, they are even more likely to rely on a romantic or marital partner, if they have one, as a principal attachment figure, but siblings and friends are important as well. As adults get older, if they have grown children, they increasingly rely on them as attachment figures.

Choosing a particular person as an attachment figure during adulthood is affected by a variety of relational factors. For example, length of a romantic relationship is associated with choosing the romantic partner as a principal attachment figure (J. A. Feeney, 2004a; Fraley & Davis, 1997; Hazan & Zeifman, 1994; Trinke & Bartholomew, 1997). In fact, Hazan and Zeifman (1994) found that consolidation of a full-blown attachment to a romantic partner (i.e., using the partner for proximity maintenance and as a safe haven and secure base) takes approximately 2 years. In addition, feelings of trust, intimacy, and commitment in a romantic relationship have been found to affect the seeking of proximity, support, and security within the confines of the relationship (N. A. Doherty & Feeney, 2004; J. A. Feeney, 2004a; Fraley & Davis, 1997). Interestingly, Colin (1996) listed a similar set of relational factors that determine the structure of infants' and young children's attachment hierarchies.

There is preliminary evidence concerning the malleability of people's attachment hierarchies during adulthood. For example, J. A. Feeney, Hohaus, Noller, and Alexander (2001) studied the transition to parenthood, asking pregnant women and their husbands to complete a version of the WHOTO scale before and after the birth of their first child. These couples were compared to married couples who did not have children. The results replicated previous findings showing that the spouse was nominated as a principal attachment figure in the vast majority of both transition and control couples. However, transition couples (mainly wives) reduced their use of spouses and friends as attachment figures from prenatal to postnatal periods, and increased their reliance on parents following the birth of the baby. This fits with Weiss's (1993) idea that parents serve as attachment figures "in reserve" and are called into active service whenever their adult child passes a developmental milestone or encounters serious difficulties. During these demanding periods, adults renew their relationships with former primary caregivers and begin to acknowledge and appreciate their assistance and support.

Overall, studies conducted to date indicate that adults have multiple attachment figures and that viewing a particular relationship partner as the principal attachment figure depends on the individual's developmental stage and current needs, and on the nature of the relationship with the potential attachment figure. These complexities are amplified by individual differences in attachment style, which bias the choice of attachment figures (see Chapter 9, this volume). In any case, attachment-system activation in adulthood includes both automatic preconscious processes (heightened accessibility of attachment-related mental content) and more controlled, reflective processes, such as deciding whether to engage in the actual seeking of proximity and support, as well as selecting the person to whom bids for proximity and support will be directed.

The Broaden-and-Build Effects of Attachment Figure Availability

Once the attachment system is activated and a person seeks actual or symbolic proximity to an external or internalized attachment figure, he or she usually senses or decides whether this attachment figure is sufficiently available and responsive. This decision is part of the second if–then module in our control systems model of attachment dynamics (Figure 2.1). This module includes a cascade of mental and behavioral processes triggered by appraising the degree of attachment figure availability and responsiveness. When the appraisal is positive, it contributes to what we call a broaden-and-build cycle of attachment security. As we described in Chapter 2, this cycle includes positive emotions (comfort, relief, love, pride), promotes positive perceptions of both self and others, and encourages comfortable, confident engagement in intimate relationships and growth-oriented activities (e.g., exploration, education, helping others). In other words, this cycle helps to explain the documented benefits of interacting with available and responsive attachment figures: healthy personality development, satisfying close relationships, and good personal and social adjustment.

Experiencing Positive Affect

According to attachment theory, the physical availability and supportiveness of an attachment figure in times of need impart a sense of safety and felt security that significantly reduces distress. In adulthood, this infusion of positive affect can result simply from thinking about responsive and supportive attachment figures or retrieving memories of warm and comforting interactions with these people. Temporarily activating mental representations of attachment figures makes these figures symbolically available and augments a person's sense of felt security. In the following paragraphs we review research documenting the soothing effects of (1) the physical availability of an attachment figure, (2) the actual or perceived supportiveness of this figure, and (3) conscious or unconscious thoughts about supportive, security-enhancing figures who are not physically present.

With regard to the physical availability of an attachment figure, attachment research consistently shows that tired, ill, or distressed infants are likely to be soothed in the presence of a primary caregiver (e.g., Ainsworth, 1973; Heinicke & Westheimer, 1966). In adulthood, experimental studies show that the mere presence of a close relationship partner during a stressful experience has a similar soothing, distress-alleviating effect (e.g., K. M. Allen, Blascovich, Tomaka, & Kelsey, 1991; Edens, Larkin, & Abel, 1992; Kamarck, Manuck, & Jennings, 1990). In these experiments, participants were asked to perform stressful mental arithmetic tasks while their physiological signs of distress (cardiovascular responses, galvanic skin responses) were assessed. Findings indicated that physiological arousal was reduced more when participants performed the stressful tasks in the presence of a best friend (and, in one study, a pet dog!) than when they performed the same tasks in the presence of the experimenter alone. However, it is important to mention that this effect was present only when friends were unable to observe and evaluate the participants' task performance. (Interestingly, pet dogs were more comforting in certain respects than human companions, because dogs are unable to evaluate their owners' mathematical ability; K. M. Allen et al., 1991.)

Conceptually similar findings were obtained in a naturalistic study of cohabitating and married couples (Gump, Polk, Kamarck, & Shiffman, 2001). Both members of each couple wore ambulatory blood-pressure monitors during their waking hours for a week, and blood pressure was recorded at least once an hour. At each of the assessments, participants were asked to report what they were doing and feeling, and whether anyone was with them at the time. Across the week, blood pressure was lower when participants were interacting with their romantic partner than when interacting with other people or alone. Interestingly, this effect was observed even during nonintimate exchanges with the partner, implying that the partner's mere presence had beneficial effects.

In a related study, Coan, Schaefer, and Davidson (2006) studied married women who underwent a laboratory stressor (threat of electric shock) while their brains were scanned by an fMRI (functional magnetic resonance imaging) machine. During each scan, a woman was either holding her husband's hand, holding the hand of an otherwise unfamiliar male experimenter, or holding no hand at all. Spousal handholding reduced stress responses, as seen in brain regions associated with stress and distress (right anterior insula, superior frontal gyrus, and hypothalamus). The researchers also found that the reduction in stress responses was greater in better functioning marriages, probably because of the greater sense of security induced by physical contact with an especially loving, comforting, and supportive husband.

The positive emotional effects of a close relationship partner's physical availability have also been documented in naturalistic studies of reunion with a spouse following wartime or job-related separations (e.g., Gerstel & Gross, 1984; Piotrkowski & Gornick, 1987). These reunions were generally experienced as exciting and exhilarating, and tended to evoke joy and happiness. In some cases, however, the fantasies and expectations concerning the reunion were so high that the actual reunion was disappointing or disorienting (Vormbrock, 1993). This finding suggests, although with disheartening implications in this particular case, that symbolic availability of an internalized attachment figure (thinking about a happy reunion with an attachment figure) can be a strong source of positive feelings—perhaps stronger than reality itself.

Regarding the importance of the perceived supportiveness of an attachment figure, many investigators have found that people who appraise their partners as supportive during stressful experiences feel less distressed and are less likely to develop emotional and somatic problems as a result (for reviews and meta-analyses, see S. Cohen, Gottlieb, & Underwood, 2000; S. Cohen & Wills, 1985; Finch, Okun, Pool, & Ruehlman, 1999; Schwarzer & Leppin, 1989). Research also indicates that perceived partner support acts as a stress buffer, bolstering perceived coping abilities and reducing catastrophic appraisals of stressful events, intrusive worries and futile rumination, and maladaptive coping responses (e.g., S. Cohen & McKay, 1984; Lepore, Silver, Wortman, & Wayment, 1996; Thoits, 1986). Moreover, appraising partners as more supportive buffers physical pain, such as labor pain, cardiac pain, and postoperative pain (see MacDonald & Leary [2005] for a review). There is also evidence that supportive interactions with close relationship partners attenuate stress-related arousal of the autonomic nervous system and the hypothalamic–pituitary–adrenal (HPA) axis during stressful experiences (see S. Cohen et al. [2000] for a review).

In an observational study of dating couples who were videotaped while one partner disclosed a personal concern to the other, Collins and Feeney (2000) found that actual partner supportiveness reduced the distress experienced by the support recipient; that is, people whose romantic partner provided more responsive support (as judged by independent coders) felt better after disclosing a personal problem than they did beforehand. Moreover, couples who experienced more supportive interactions (as judged by both the couple members themselves and by independent coders) reported having better relationships overall. Similar findings were obtained when perceptions of secure base support were assessed within close friendships ("I feel that my friend provides me with choices and options," "My friend listens to my ideas and thoughts"). The higher the friend's perceived supportiveness, the stronger the support recipients' feelings of safety, security, relationship satisfaction, and global positive affect (Deci, La Guardia, Moller, Scheiner, & Ryan, 2006).

Recently we used social cognition research paradigms, including well-validated priming techniques, to experimentally activate mental representations of supportive attachment figures and see what emotional effects they have (Mikulincer, Hirschberger, Nachmias, & Gillath, 2001; Mikulincer, Gillath, et al., 2001; Mikulincer, Gillath, et al., 2003; Mikulincer & Shaver, 2001). These techniques included subliminal presentation of pictures suggesting attachment figure availability (e.g., a Picasso drawing of a mother cradling an infant in her arms; a couple holding hands and gazing into each other's eyes); subliminal presentation of the names of people nominated by participants as security-enhancing attachment figures; guided imagery concerning the availability and supportiveness of an attachment figure; and visualization of the faces of security-enhancing attachment figures. We compared the effects of these primes with the effects of emotionally positive but attachment-unrelated pictures or emotionally neutral pictures, and consistently found that portrayals of attachment figure availability improved participants' moods.

Mikulincer, Hirschberger, et al. (2001) also found that priming with representations of supportive attachment figures infused formerly neutral stimuli with positive affect, even when the priming was done subliminally. For example, subliminal presentation of the names of people nominated by participants as security-enhancing attachment figures (using the WHOTO scale), compared with the names of close others or mere acquaintances who were not nominated as attachment figures, led to greater liking of previously unfamiliar Chinese ideographs. Moreover, Mikulincer, Hirschberger, et al. reported that subliminal priming with representations of available attachment figures led to more positive evaluations of neutral stimuli even in threatening contexts, and it eliminated the detrimental effects that threats otherwise had on liking for neutral stimuli. It therefore seems that symbolic availability of internalized attachment figures has a calming and soothing effect, similar to effects observed during actual interactions with available and responsive relationship partners.

Sustaining a Sense of Self-Worth

A core proposition of attachment theory is that actual or anticipated interactions with available and responsive attachment figures contribute to the formation of positive self-representations. This idea resonates with previous psychodynamic and object relations theories (e.g., Blatt & Behrends, 1987; Kohut, 1971, 1977; Schafer, 1968), which highlight the importance of "internalization"—the process by which people adopt, as their own, personal qualities that were originally experienced in their close relationships or noted in their relationship partners. According to Schafer (1968), "Internalization refers to all those processes by which the subject transforms real or imagined regulatory interactions with his environment, and real or imagined characteristics of his environment, into inner regulation and characteristics" (p. 9). Supporting this notion of internalization, developmental studies have revealed that the quality of the mother–child relationship is the best predictor of the positivity of the child's self-concept (e.g., Verschueren & Marcoen, 1999).

Similar ideas appear in classic theories of the self (e.g., C. H. Cooley, 1902; James, 1890; C. R. Rogers, 1961; Sullivan, 1953) and in more recent social-cognitive perspectives on the self (e.g., Aron, Aron, & Norman, 2001; Baldwin, 1992; Higgins, 1987). For example, C. H. Cooley (1902) viewed self-evaluation as an interpersonal process involving three parts: "the imagination of our appearance to the other person, the imagination of his judgment of that appearance, and some sort of self-feeling, such as pride or mortification" (p. 184). More recently, Andersen and Chen (2002) contended that "given the profound importance of significant others in people's lives, the self and personality are shaped largely by experiences with significant others" (p. 621). Pursuing this idea, Hinkley and Andersen (1996) found that implicit memories of feelings experienced in connection with a close relationship partner affect a person's self-evaluations when interacting with someone new who resembles the previous partner. Specifically, study participants freely listed more positive self-traits (controlling for baseline self-evaluation at a pretest session) after learning about a new person who resembled an accepting and supportive relationship partner than after learning about a positively valued person who did not resemble a previous partner.

The importance of interactions with accepting and loving relationship partners for the construction of a positive self-image is also emphasized in the currently popular "sociometer" theory of self-esteem (M. R. Leary, Tambor, Terdal, & Downs, 1995). According to this theory, self-esteem serves as a sociometer (a social barometer) measuring the extent to which one is accepted or rejected by others. When a person interacts with an accepting, loving other, he or she experiences a positive boost in self-esteem; when ignored or rejected, he or she experiences a painful drop in self-esteem. A good deal of research (not to mention everyday experience) supports this association between acceptance–rejection and self-esteem (for reviews, see M. R. Leary, 1999; M. R. Leary & Baumeister, 2000). For example, laboratory manipulations that convey others' acceptance, approval, or interest consistently increase participants' self-esteem (e.g., M. R. Leary et al., 1995; M. R. Leary, Cottrell, & Phillips, 2001; Snapp & Leary, 2001). Moreover, a relationship partner's acceptance in real-life settings is associated with positive self-evaluations (e.g., Baumeister, Wotman, & Stillwell, 1993; M. R. Leary et al., 1995). Also, feeling accepted and valued by relationship partners predicts subsequent positive changes in self-esteem (Srivastava & Beer, 2005).

Recent studies indicate that the relational basis of self-esteem is so strong and pervasive that feeling accepted and loved by others automatically increases one's sense of self-worth, even when one is not aware of it. For example, Baccus, Baldwin, and Packer (2004) paired self-relevant information with cues of others' acceptance and assessed subsequent changes in self-esteem. Participants provided information about themselves (e.g., name, birthday, home town), then performed a reaction time (RT) task in which they clicked on a word appearing on a computer screen as quickly as possible. After clicking on each word, a picture of a person was presented on the screen for a few seconds. In the experimental condition, every time a self-relevant word (e.g., the participant's name) appeared, it was followed by a picture of a smiling, accepting face. In the control condition, self-relevant words were randomly paired with pictures of smiling, frowning, and neutral faces. As indicated by two different measures of state self-esteem, participants in the experimental condition provided more positive self-evaluations than those in the control condition. These findings support the notion that when people think about themselves, automatic and unconscious representations of others' acceptance and love are likely to strengthen their positive self-evaluations.

Two other experimental studies show that mental representations of security-enhancing attachment figures can instill a sense of self-worth that is sufficient to render defensive self-inflation maneuvers unnecessary (Arndt, Schimel, Greenberg, & Pyszczynski, 2002; Schimel, Arndt, Pyszczynski, & Greenberg, 2001). In these studies, thoughts about attachment figure availability (e.g., thinking about an accepting and loving other) or neutral thoughts were encouraged, and participants' use of particular self-enhancement strategies was assessed. Schimel et al. studied defensive biases in social comparison—searching for more social comparison information when it was likely to suggest that one has performed better than other people (Pyszczynski, Greenberg, & LaPrelle, 1985). Arndt et al. (2002) studied defensive self-handicapping—emphasizing factors that impair one's performance in an effort to protect against the damage to self-esteem that might result from attributing negative outcomes to one's lack of ability (Berglas & Jones, 1978). In both studies, momentary strengthening of mental representations of attachment figure availability weakened the tendency to make self-enhancing social comparisons or self-handicapping attributions.

Along similar lines, Kumashiro and Sedikides (2005) suggested that "close positive relationships may bolster and shield the self to the point where, even following unfavorable feedback, accurate information about personal liabilities is sought out despite its self-threat potential" (p. 733). In two separate studies, participants performed a difficult cognitive task and then were asked to visualize either a responsive close friend or a distant or negative partner. Following the priming procedure, all participants received negative feedback about their performance and were asked about their interest in obtaining further information about the task and the underlying cognitive ability it tapped. In both studies, participants who were primed with a responsive close relationship partner expressed more interest in receiving information about their newly discovered liability than participants in other conditions; that is, having visualized a security-enhancing relationship partner, participants seemed to be so confident of their self-worth that they were willing to explore and learn about potential personal weaknesses. These findings are consistent with Bowlby's (1988) notion that therapists who serve as a secure base for their clients can help the clients explore painful issues, including the ways in which clients' own behavior contributes to their problems (see Chapter 14, this volume).

Overall, research indicates, in line with attachment theory, that interactions with available, caring, and loving attachment figures in times of need constitute a primary source of an authentically positive sense of self-worth. People can find enough reassurance, indications of personal worth, and signs of acceptance in these positive interactions to reduce or eliminate the need to inflate their self-esteem defensively or reject negative information about themselves. As we show in Chapter 6, the well-established internal representations of attachment figure availability held by securely attached people supersede the need for defensive self-enhancement and render it unnecessary. Besides being a hopeful sign for individual human beings, these findings provide hope in the long run for a safer, less defensively hostile, and more peaceful world.

Mitigating Relational Worries and Facilitating Pro-Relational Behavior

Besides boosting self-esteem, regularly experiencing attachment figure availability can assuage worries about being rejected, criticized, or abused. It can thereby bolster a person's willingness to get close to a partner; express needs, desires, hopes, and vulnerabilities; and ask for support when needed; that is, interactions with available, caring, and loving attachment figures facilitate pro-relational behaviors that are conducive to establishing and maintaining satisfyingly intimate and deeply interdependent relationships. This positive relational process begins with appraising an attachment figure's sensitivity and responsiveness, and the consequent formation of positive beliefs and expectations about this person's good qualities and intentions. One gradually becomes convinced that such a good and caring figure is unlikely to betray one's trust, will not react negatively or abusively to expressions of need, and will not reject bids for closeness. With such confidence, it is relatively easy for a person to behave prosocially and become more deeply involved in a relationship.

This characteristic flow of relational feelings and behaviors is conceptualized in H. T. Reis and Shaver's (1988) intimacy model, which portrays intimacy as a dynamic process that begins when one person reveals personally significant aspects of him- or herself to a partner. Subsequent steps in the process are then shaped by the partner's responses. A sensitive, accepting, supportive, and encouraging response facilitates the expression of deeper personal needs and concerns, which gradually leads to development of an intimate relationship. In contrast, a distant, disinterested, disapproving, or rejecting response discourages and interferes with intimacy and destroys the chances for an intimate relationship. According to the model, a responsive and accepting partner engenders three kinds of feelings in an intimacy seeker that strengthen his or her confidence in the partner's good intentions, thus encouraging more intimate interactions: a feeling of being understood (i.e., feeling that the partner accurately perceives and understands what is important to the speaker), a feeling of being validated (i.e., feeling that the partner appreciates and respects the speaker), and a feeling of care (i.e., sensing that the partner is concerned about one's welfare and responsive to one's needs). These three kinds of feelings are important components of the broaden-and-build cycle of attachment security discussed in this and previous chapters.

In creating their control system model of risk regulation in close relationships, Murray, Holmes, and Collins (2006) reached similar conclusions about the role of attachment figure availability in the formation and maintenance of intimate relationships. They assumed that dependence on a partner's responsiveness—at times when the attachment system is activated and one expresses needs for proximity and support—can automatically activate worries about rejection and disapproval ("How I can be sure my partner will accept my bid for support?"). Because most people do not want to be rejected or to endanger their sense of self-worth, they carefully assess a partner's regard and responsiveness before engaging in intimate or interdependent behavior. They rely on another if–then rule: "If I am feeling a partner's regard and acceptance, then I can increase interdependence; but if I am experiencing or expecting the partner's rejection, then I should retreat from interdependence." Thus, when a person expects a partner to be available and responsive, based on previous interactions or momentary memories of supportive interactions, he or she can openly express needs and confidently engage in intimacy-promoting behavior. Although this model is more focused on the risk of rejection than on the benefits of partner responsiveness, Murray et al. recognize, in line with attachment theory, that interactions with available and responsive partners are critical in forming intimate relationships.

There is both correlational and experimental evidence for the surge of positive relational feelings and behaviors produced by actual or imagined interactions with an available, accepting, and responsive dating or marital partner (for reviews, see Murray et al., 2006; H. T. Reis, Clark, & Holmes, 2004; H. T. Reis, in press). For example, daily diary studies reveal that people experience stronger feelings of closeness and intimacy on days when they perceive their partner to be accepting and responsive to their bids for intimacy (e.g., Laurenceau, Barrett, & Pietromonaco, 1998; Laurenceau, Barrett, & Rovine, 2005; Lin, 1992). In one diary study, H. T. Reis (in press) found that daily ratings of relatedness with a romantic partner depended more on the extent to which people felt understood and appreciated by their partner than on the extent to which they engaged in joint activities and had fun. Reis also reviewed a series of correlational studies of dating and married couples in which appraisals of a validating partner (e.g., "Because of the way my partner acts with me, I am able to be my true self") or an affirming partner (e.g., "My partner treats me in a way that is close to the person I ideally would like to be") contributed to dyadic satisfaction. In addition, Duemmler and Kobak (2001) found that appraisals of a dating partner's supportiveness predicted increases in relationship commitment over an 18-month period, and Gore, Cross, and Morris (2006) found that undergraduates' perceptions of their roommate's responsiveness (e.g., "I can count on this person for help with a problem") predicted increases in relationship satisfaction over a 1-month period.

There is also evidence that perceptions of a partner's responsiveness encourage support seeking and intimacy-promoting behavior, such as open and confident disclosure of private thoughts and feelings to a partner (e.g., M. S. Clark, Reis, Tsai, & Brissette, 2005; Collins & Feeney, 2000; Gore et al., 2006; Larose, Boivin, & Doyle,

2001). For example, M. S. Clark et al. (2005) asked participants to rate a series of relationship partners as either somewhat distant (e.g., a neighbor) or close (e.g., a romantic partner) in terms of the extent to which each was sensitive and responsive to their needs. Participants were then asked how willing they would be to express to that partner various emotional states (either positive or negative states that had been caused by that person, or by someone or something else). The more favorable the appraisals of a partner's sensitivity and responsiveness, the more willing participants were to express openly their positive and negative feelings to that person. Similar findings have been obtained in studies of marital interactions in which one partner's sensitive and responsive listening encourages the other partner's emotional openness and self-disclosure (see Gottman [1994] for a review).

Using priming techniques, attachment researchers have found that momentary activation of mental representations of available and supportive attachment figures has beneficial effects on expectations of a partner's behavior (Pierce & Lydon, 1998; Rowe & Carnelley, 2003). In Rowe and Carnelley's study, participants were primed with representations of attachment figure availability or unavailability (writing for 10 minutes about a relationship in which they had felt secure or insecure), then completed a questionnaire assessing general expectations about relationship partners' behavior. Priming with examples of partner availability led to more positive expectations for the current relationship than priming with insecure representations. In Pierce and Lydon's study (1998), young women were subliminally exposed (for 15 milliseconds) to security-related words (e.g., *caring*, *supportive*), insecurity-related words (e.g., *rejecting*, *hurtful*), or no words. They then read a hypothetical scenario in which they had unexpectedly become pregnant, and were asked to describe how they would cope with this event. Compared with the no-word condition, priming with security-related words caused an increase in seeking emotional support as a way of coping with the unwanted pregnancy. Security priming also reduced self-blame, and neither this nor the other obtained effects could be explained by variations in mood.

These simple priming effects are likely to be relatively short-lived and unstable (Bargh, 1989), with subliminal priming of single words lasting only a few seconds (Versace & Nevers, 2003). However, Rowe and Carnelley (2006) recently found that repeated priming of security-related representations can lead to long-lasting positive effects on relational beliefs. In an initial (baseline) session, participants answered a self-report scale assessing general expectations about relationship partners' behavior. Then, on three occasions (across 3 days), participants were exposed to a secure or a neutral prime (e.g., recalling or imagining interactions with an attachment figure in which they felt secure, or recalling or imagining a neutral event, such as shopping at a supermarket). Two days later, all participants once again provided their general expectations about relationship partners' behavior, not preceded by any prime. Rowe and Carnelley noted more positive changes in expectations about relationship partners' behavior following repeated priming with security-related stimuli than following repeated priming with neutral stimuli. These findings offer still preliminary but very encouraging evidence that repeated priming with security-related stimuli may be an effective way to create long-lasting changes in relational beliefs and behaviors.

Broadening Capacities and Perspectives

As we explained in Chapter 1, Bowlby (1969/1982) proposed that a dynamic interplay between the attachment system and other behavioral systems (such as exploration, caregiving, affiliation, and sex) contributes to the development of personal knowledge and skills, opens a person's mind to new possibilities and perspectives, and helps a person adapt flexibly to a wide variety of situations and actualize his or her natural talents. One reason for these beneficial effects is that security-enhancing interactions reduce anxiety, vigilance, and preoccupation with attachment, allowing a person to devote more attention and effort to growth-oriented activities. Moreover, these interactions impart a sense of safety and protection that allows a person to take calculated risks and accept important challenges. With these interactions in mind, people can feel confident that support is available when needed, that their relationship partners will accept and love them even if they make some ill-fated decisions, and that the world is a safe place for exercising skills and actualizing one's potential.

Bowlby (1973) and Ainsworth (1991) were especially interested in the relation between attachment and exploration, conceptualized as the fields of operation of two separate behavioral systems. They portrayed attachment insecurity as a major hindrance to optimal exploration and learning. A child or an adult who feels threatened and inadequately protected or supported finds it difficult to explore objects and environments, and acquire new information that challenges or expands existing beliefs and understandings. Considered more generally and extended over a longer period of development, this same interference disrupts information search and prevents adaptive accommodation of existing knowledge structures to new data. Just as being harassed or distracted at school interferes with normal cognitive development, being forced by one's social environment to focus only on threats and feelings of attachment insecurity distorts and interferes with cognitive openness.

This line of reasoning implies that an available and supportive attachment figure enhances a person's curiosity and encourages relaxed exploration of new, unusual information despite the uncertainty and confusion temporarily caused by such information. Supporting this idea, infants and young children tend to explore their environment mainly when they know their primary attachment figure is nearby, emotionally available, and responsive (e.g., Ainsworth et al., 1978; Ricciuti, 1974).

The availability and supportiveness of relationship partners are also important for cognitive functioning and personal development in adulthood. As Collins, Guichard, Ford, and Feeney (2006) insightfully noted, "Individuals routinely assign credit for their accomplishments and successes to the support of the significant people in their lives—people who have encouraged them to grow as individuals and strive to reach their full potentials" (p. 177). Indeed, adolescents and adults who perceive their parents or friends to be available and supportive in times of need perform better on difficult cognitive tasks, concentrate better during task performance, and get better grades on school and college examinations (e.g., Cutrona, Cole, Colangelo, Assouline, & Russell, 1994; DeBerard, Spielmans, & Julka, 2004). In addition, high school and college students who receive more parental care and affection also report more positive attitudes toward learning and perform better in school (e.g., Heaven, Mak, Barry, & Ciarrochi, 2002; Lopez, 1997). Similar beneficial effects have been noted in the domain of work and careers: Adolescents with more supportive parents or friends have more positive attitudes toward career-related exploration and a stronger sense of self-efficacy in choosing a career (e.g., Blustein et al., 2001; Schultheiss, Kress, Manzi, & Glasscock, 2001).

In an examination of the connection between attachment figure availability and exploration within the context of romantic relationships, B. C. Feeney (2004) videotaped dating couples during discussions of one partner's personal goals. Analysis of the videotapes revealed that participants were more likely to discuss personal goals openly and explore alternative ways to achieve these goals with partners who were coded by independent observers as more supportive and responsive. In fact, participants tended to modify or distort their goals during the discussion with partners coded as displaying more intrusive and controlling remarks and behaviors. In addition, participants who perceived their partners to be supportive and encouraging during the discussion reported a more positive mood and higher self-esteem following the discussion (controlling for prior global self-esteem and mood).

Following the discussion, B. C. Feeney (2004) asked one couple member to work on a computerized puzzle game while the partner's apparent supportiveness was systematically manipulated by delivering messages ostensibly written by the partner. Participants were assigned to one of four message conditions. In the supportive/nonintrusive condition, they received two emotionally supportive messages during the game (e.g., "good luck" and "good job"). In the supportive/intrusive condition, the same supportive messages were more frequently and intrusively delivered during the game. In the intrusive/controlling condition, participants received frequent messages that provided answers to the puzzle or suggested what to do next. In the control condition, no message was delivered during the game. Findings indicated that participants in the supportive/nonintrusive condition experienced higher self-esteem and a more positive mood after the game than participants in the other conditions. In addition, compared to the control condition, intrusive (controlling or supportive) messages damaged puzzle performance, although participants in the controlling condition were actually given some of the correct answers. Participants generally rejected and resented insensitive messages that threatened their own problem-solving efforts.

Research also indicates that experimental priming of mental representations of available and supportive attachment figures has beneficial effects on exploration and cognitive openness. For example, J. D. Green and Campbell (2000) primed representations of attachment figure availability or unavailability (by asking people to read sentences describing secure or insecure close relationships) and found that the secure prime led to greater endorsement of exploration-related behavior and greater liking for novel pictures (Escher art prints) than did insecure primes. Moreover, Mikulincer and Arad (1999, Study 3) reported that people who were asked to visualize a responsive and supportive relationship partner (compared to those who visualized a rejecting partner) showed increased cognitive openness and were more likely to revise knowledge about a relationship partner following behavior on the part of the partner that seemed inconsistent with prior actions.

Experimental priming of mental representations of available and responsive attachment figures also affects negative, prejudicial attitudes toward outgroups (Mikulincer & Shaver, 2001). In five separate studies, we found that momentarily activating mental representations of attachment figure availability (by subliminally presenting security-related words, such as *love* and *closeness*, or by asking participants to read a story or visualize the face of a supportive relationship partner) eliminated negative responses to a variety of outgroups (as perceived by heterosexual, secular Israeli Jewish students): Israeli Arabs, ultra-Orthodox Jews, Russian immigrants, and homosexuals. That is, mental representations of available attachment figures promoted more tolerant and accepting attitudes toward people who did not belong to the study participants' own social group.

Theoretically, the security-enhancing, "broadening" effects of attachment figure availability should promote better functioning of the caregiving system, which expresses itself not only in greater intergroup tolerance but also in willingness to provide care to others who are suffering or otherwise in need. In line with this prediction, some of our recent studies have shown that priming mental representations of attachment figure availability (e.g., by asking people to recall personal experiences, read a story, or view a pictorial display of supportive behavior; or by exposing them to security-related words) increases empathy, compassion, and generous, altruistic responses to needy others (Mikulincer, Gillath, et al., 2001, 2003; Mikulincer, Shaver, Gillath, & Nitzberg, 2005). We discuss these studies in greater detail in Chapter 12, this volume.

Summary and Commentary

In recent years, under the banner of "positive psychology," there has been a resurgence of interest in issues such as personal authenticity, self-actualization, virtuous and compassionate behavior, and optimal self-development (e.g., Aspinwall & Staudinger, 2003; Seligman, 2002). To date, although interesting, this turn toward positive psychology has lacked a coherent theoretical foundation. A variety of investigators are exploring important phenomena, such as authentic self-esteem, optimism, compassion, and personal growth, but without much grounding in a general understanding of the human mind and its roots in close relationships. Perhaps we are biased by tunnel vision or overcommitment to a theory that has proven useful in generating novel research findings (Bowlby's attachment theory, 1969/1982), but so far the theory has seemed to us to provide an excellent foundation for positive psychology (Mikulincer & Shaver, 2005a) and to be a rich wellspring of hypotheses and insights. As reviewed here, actual or imagined (i.e., symbolic) interactions with supportive attachment figures move a person toward the ideal advocated by positive psychologists—a calm, confident person with an authentic, solid sense of personal value; a person who is willing and able to establish intimate, caring relationships and take risks to help others and to broaden his or her skills and perspectives. Following Bowlby's (1988) lead, we conclude that attachment figure availability acts as a growth-enhancing psychological catalyst, fostering prosocial motives and attitudes and promoting personal development and improved relationships.

ATTACHMENT FIGURE UNAVAILABILITY AND SECONDARY ATTACHMENT STRATEGIES

Beyond emphasizing the constructive and growth-enhancing consequences of interactions with supportive attachment figures, attachment theory also illuminates how people attempt to cope with unavailable or unresponsive attachment figures. This is the focus of the third if–then module in our control systems model of attachment dynamics (Figure 2.1). In this section, we focus on three issues related to this module: (1) emotional effects of attachment figure unavailability, (2) ways in which people cope with the loss of an attachment figure, and (3) adoption of secondary strategies involving hyperactivation or deactivation of the attachment system.

Emotional Impact of Attachment Figure Unavailability

The idea that attachment figure unavailability is highly distressing is one of the central tenets of attachment theory. As we reviewed in Chapter 1, ethological observations of infants who were separated from mother (e.g., Heinicke & Westheimer, 1966; Robertson & Bowlby, 1952) convinced Bowlby (1969/1982) that the absence of an attachment figure arouses anxiety, anger, protest, and yearning. An infant, finding itself without an attentive caregiver, cries, thrashes, attempts to reestablish contact with the absent figure by calling and searching, and resists other people's well-intentioned soothing efforts. If the separation is prolonged (e.g., by the mother's extended stay in a hospital or, at worst, by her death), the infant grieves disconsolately, and anxiety and anger gradually give way to despair (Bowlby, 1980).

Similar reactions, although not as intense, are often observed among adolescents and adults who feel rejected, disapproved of, or criticized by their close relationship partners. For example, in a meta-analysis of 48 published studies, as well as their own, Finch et al. (1999) found that distressing interactions (marked by a partner's criticism, hostility, or rejection) had adverse effects on psychological well-being and resulted in anxiety, anger, and sadness. Research also shows that young adults who are rejected by a romantic partner or experience unrequited love feel miserably sad and entertain doubts about their personal worth and desirability as a relationship partner (e.g., Ayduk, Downey, & Kim, 2001; Baumeister et al., 1993; J. A. Feeney, 2005). According to MacDonald and Leary (2005), these rejection experiences are so upsetting that they amount to social pain that is quite close to physical pain. Indeed, in an fMRI study of the effects of social rejection and exclusion by strangers, Eisenberger, Lieberman, and Williams (2003) observed heightened activation of brain regions associated with physical pain (e.g., the anterior cingulate cortex); that is, the painful effects of rejection can be measured even when the rejecters are (initially cooperative) strangers.

The negative emotions provoked by attachment figure unavailability in adulthood can be seen following the breakup of a romantic relationship or temporary separations from loved ones. For those who are abandoned without warning, the breakup of a love relationship can be devastating, and the reaction can be so intense that it amounts to grief (e.g., B. Carter & McGoldrick, 1988; Frazier &Cook, 1993; G. A. Miller & Rice, 1993). For example, in a diary study of emotions recorded over a 28-day period, Sbarra and Emery (2005) found more emotional volatility and higher levels of sadness and anger in the days following the breakup of a dating relationship than in days before the breakup. Such reactions are especially likely following a marital separation or divorce, which—in line with attachment theory—can provoke intense anxiety, sorrow, loneliness, emptiness, and despair (e.g., Birnbaum, Orr, Mikulincer, & Florian, 1997; Mearns, 1991; Weiss, 1975, 1976), as well as doubts about one's inherent love-worthiness (e.g., Gotlib & Hammen, 1992; J. D. Gray & Silver, 1990). Even temporary and justifiable separations from a spouse can be distressing for both the departing and the stay-at-home partner (e.g., see Vormbrock, 1993, for a review of studies of wartime and job-related separations).

Of course, the most dramatic emotional effects of attachment figure unavailability occur following the death of an attachment figure (see the M. Stroebe, Hansson, Stroebe, & Schut [2001] *Handbook* for reviews). This kind of loss is one of the most devastating experiences in most people's lives and is likely to bring forth a torrent of anxiety, sadness, loneliness, guilt, anger, and longing for the deceased (e.g., Parkes, 1985; Zisook, Schuchter, Sledge, Paulus, & Judd, 1994). It can cause a person to feel like dying in order to rejoin the lost partner. It can disrupt psychological functioning for months and lead to depression, posttraumatic stress disorder (PTSD), and impaired physical health (e.g., Futterman, Gallagher, Thompson, & Lovett, 1990; S. A. Murphy et al., 1999; Zisook et al., 1994). Cross-cultural research indicates that despite variations in mourning rituals and expressions of grief across cultures, death of an attachment figure evokes profound pain and disorientation everywhere in the world, and has done so during all periods of recorded history (e.g., W. Stroebe & Stroebe, 1987).

The integration of academic research findings with a person's own experiences is vividly and movingly portrayed in Joan Didion's (2005) recent book about her husband's sudden and unexpected death from a heart attack, *The Year of Magical Thinking*. Being a well-read intellectual, Didion tried to understand her reactions by reading a book published by the National Academy of Science's Institute of Medicine, *Bereavement: Reactions, Consequences, and Care* (Osterweis, Solomon, & Green, 1984):

> Dolphins, I learned from J. William Worden . . ., had been observed refusing to eat after the death of a mate. Geese had been observed reacting to such a death by flying and calling, searching until they themselves became disoriented and lost. Human beings, I read but did not need to learn [because she was going through these experiences herself], showed similar patterns of response. They searched. They stopped eating. They forgot to breathe. They grew faint from lowered oxygen, they clogged their sinuses with unshed tears and ended up in otolaryngologists' offices with obscure ear infections. They lost concentration. . . . They lost cognitive ability on all scales. . . . They forgot their own telephone numbers and showed up at airports without picture ID. They fell sick, they failed, they even . . . died. . . . I began carrying identification when I walked in Central Park in the morning, in case it happened to me. (pp. 46–47)

According to attachment theory, these reactions are due to an upsurge of attachment needs that are no longer being satisfied by the deceased spouse (Bowlby, 1980; Weiss, 1993). Therefore, the intensity of grief is a function of the place and importance of the deceased spouse in the bereaved person's hierarchy of attachment figures. Parkes and Weiss (1983) suggested that individuals who lose the person on whom they most depend to provide a "safe haven and secure base" are the most vulnerable to despair. In support of this idea, more intense grief is observed among people who describe themselves as more strongly attached to the person they have lost (e.g., Van Doorn, Kasl, Beery, Jacobs, & Prigerson, 1998; Wayment & Vierthaler, 2002). In Didion's case, she and her husband, writer John Gregory Dunne, had spent decades writing and sharing ideas and insights almost every day. Both worked at home, read extensively and discussed what they read, and edited each other's manuscripts. She found, as she encountered one odd experience after another during her "year of magical thinking," that she immediately wanted to share and compare feelings with Dunne, who, of course, was no longer available to participate in the discussion.

Coping with Loss: The Adaptive and Maladaptive Nature of Secondary Strategies

The unavailability of an attachment figure is not only a source of distress but also a sign that the primary attachment strategy—proximity seeking—is not working and that a secondary strategy—hyperactivation or deactivation, or both—needs to be adopted if equanimity is going to be restored (see Chapter 2, this volume). Although secondary strategies can be invoked even in brief periods of rejection or separation, Bowlby (1980) paid special attention to the use of these strategies during bereavement. When an attachment figure dies, the primary attachment strategy, seeking proximity, definitely does not work. Hence, mourning provides an excellent, if saddening, research laboratory in which to study secondary attachment strategies.

Disordered Mourning

In his discussion of loss and bereavement, Bowlby (1980) suggested that secondary attachment strategies are involved in the two major forms of disordered mourning—"chronic mourning" and "prolonged absence of conscious grieving" (p. 138). Chronic mourning is characterized by overwhelming anxiety and sorrow, prolonged difficulty in reestablishing normal life, ruminative thoughts and worries about the missing partner, and maintenance of an intense and active attachment to the deceased even years after the loss. An apparent absence of grief is characterized by lack of overt expressions of sadness, anger, or distress; detachment from the missing partner; and continuation of normal life without major disruptions. Most clinicians agree with Bowlby's conceptualization of disordered mourning, although they tend to call the absence of grief "delayed grief," "inhibited mourning," or "absent mourning" (see the Stroebe et al. [2001] *Handbook*). According to Bowlby (1980), chronic mourning results from pervasive and prolonged hyperactivation of the attachment system, whereas absence of grief stems from a defensive shutdown of attachment-related thoughts and actions.

As we explained in Chapter 2, hyperactivation of the attachment system motivates people to do whatever is necessary to gain an unavailable attachment figure's attention and care. Hyperactivated individuals are vigilant with respect to signs of attachment figure availability or unavailability. They yearn and ask for closeness and love, intensify expressions of distress and signals of vulnerability so as to elicit support, and sometimes blame themselves for failing to possess the resources and skills necessary to command a partner's engagement. They are often overly invested in and dependent on a relationship with an insufficiently available or responsive attachment figure; hence, they are too preoccupied with attachment-related fears and worries to concentrate on other activities. Following the loss of an attachment figure, this hyperactivating stance becomes even more intense, rendering a person vulnerable to chronic mourning and depression. Research indicates that these reactions can even increase the likelihood of mortality following loss of a spouse, as Joan Didion mentioned in the passage we quoted (see also Stroebe et al., 2001).

In contrast, deactivation of the attachment system involves denying attachment needs, suppressing attachment-related thoughts and emotions, inhibiting of desires to attain proximity to an insufficiently available attachment figure, and striving to remain self-reliant and independent (see Chapter 2, this volume). Deactivation also involves distancing oneself from causes of distress and shunning emotional investment in close relationships, if such investment threatens to reactivate the attachment system. Following the loss of an attachment figure, this deactivating method of coping can cause a person to steer clear of all feelings related to the loss and to avoid doing the usual mental labor required for resolution and reorganization. It also requires dismissing the importance of the lost relationship and trying never to think about the deceased—all key features of the absence of grieving. According to Bowlby's (1980) analysis of this defensive strategy, attention is directed away from painful thoughts and feelings about the loss ("defensive exclusion") to such an extent that memories, thoughts, and feelings become mentally segregated or dissociated, although they continue to influence a person's feelings and behavior, without the person realizing it.

Bowlby (1980) thought prolonged absence of grieving could produce difficulties in adjustment and symptoms of physical deterioration if the lost figure had been someone to whom the bereaved individual was deeply attached, whether acknowledged or not. In such cases, suppression proves difficult, because even subtle reminders of the deceased (such as seeing someone with a similar appearance or hearing someone mention a cause to which the deceased was devoted) can reactivate suppressed memories and feelings. Moreover, if the mourner shared many everyday activities with the deceased, these activities will become painful reminders of the loss. According to Fraley and Shaver (1999), "Repeated activation of inexplicable and partially suppressed negative emotions may eventually have a negative impact on psychological well-being or physical health" (p. 743). Bowlby (1990) illustrated these negative consequences in his final book, *Charles Darwin: A New Life*, in which he drew a connection between Darwin's forced suppression of grief following his mother's death when he was 8 years old and the repeated occurrence later on of "hyperventilation syndrome" (including light-headedness, gastric pains, vomiting, and heart palpitations). (Darwin's straightlaced father disallowed grieving in his house following his wife's premature death.)

It is important to realize, however, that the negative emotional and physical sequelae of absence of grieving are likely to emerge only if the mourner was deeply attached to the lost partner and relied on the partner to provide a safe haven and secure base. Bereaved individuals who rarely sought proximity and comfort while the partner was alive, and remained emotionally detached from the partner even while living with him or her, are less likely to experience intense anxiety or grief, to develop segregated or dissociated memories and emotions, or to be bowled over by the eruption of unwanted memories and feelings when reminded of the deceased. In such cases, absence of grieving may reflect a true absence of distress rather a defensive reaction against the pain of a meaningful loss. Compatible with this possibility, many people who exhibit few signs of grief shortly after the loss of a partner do not display signs of distress, maladjustment, or poor health months or years later (for a review, see Bonanno, 2001). As we discuss in Chapter 7, dismissingly avoidant people, who tend to remain detached and self-reliant even when involved in long-term relationships, including marriage, often do not show strong signs of distress or maladjustment following the death of a partner.

Attachment Reorganization and Grief Resolution

Beyond noting the role of secondary attachment strategies in disordered mourning, we propose that some degree of hyperactivation and deactivation is necessary for grief resolution. Adjusting to the loss of an attachment figure requires undertaking two major psychological tasks: (1) accepting the death of the loved one, returning to everyday activities, and rearranging or "editing" the attachment figure hierarchy, by forming new attachments or upgrading old ones; and (2) maintaining a symbolic attachment to the deceased and integrating the lost relationship into a revised model of reality. These two tasks are part of what Bowlby (1980) called "attachment reorganization"—the rearrangement of representations of self and deceased, combined with "editing" the hierarchy of attachment figures. Attachment reorganization, like the adolescent transition described earlier in this chapter, requires a gradual transfer of attachment functions from the deceased to other security-providing figures, so that proximity seeking can be addressed to these real figures. Moreover, just as many adolescents use their parents as attachment figures "in reserve," mourners can transform the functions of the deceased, so that he or she becomes an internal, symbolic source of security rather than a flesh-and-blood, real-world source. The person's continuing sense of security then depends on both the symbolic bond with the deceased and new or renewed attachment bonds with living figures.

Probably every adult eventually becomes familiar with and reliant on both kinds of security providers.

How can hyperactivation and deactivation contribute to normal attachment reorganization? We suspect that by motivating a mourner to experience the deep pain of loss, reactivate memories of the deceased, and yearn for this person's proximity and love, attachment-system hyperactivation provides a context for exploring the meaning and importance of the lost relationship and finding new ways to maintain a symbolic bond with the deceased. When hyperactivation is properly regulated, a mourner can work to incorporate the past into the present, without splitting off important elements of personal and social identity related to the lost attachment figure. In our view, deactivating strategies can also contribute to the reorganization process by enabling momentary detachment from the deceased and down-regulating the intrusion of painful thoughts and feelings. With this assistance, the bereaved individual can explore the new reality, return to mundane activities, and realize that life presents new and attractive opportunities following a loss. If this deactivation is directed mainly at attachment to the deceased rather than proximity seeking and social connections of all kinds, it can even facilitate the formation of new attachment bonds and the adaptive transfer of attachment functions.

Without a degree and at least some periods of attachment-system hyperactivation, a mourner is not fully capable of understanding the depth and meaning of the loss. But without a degree of deactivation, the mourner may remain stuck in grief, unable to transfer attachment functions to new figures. Attachment reorganization requires both kinds of secondary strategies, operating either in a dynamic balance or a graceful "oscillation," to use M. Stroebe and Schut's (1999) term. According to M. Stroebe, Schut, and Stroebe (2005),

> Oscillation occurs in the short term (transient fluctuations in the course of any particular day) as well as across the passage of time, because adaptation to bereavement is a matter of slowly and painfully exploring and discovering what has been lost and what remains: what must be avoided or relinquished versus what can be retained, created, and built upon. (p. 52)

With the passage of time and the successful transfer of attachment functions, this oscillation is gradually reduced, and the broaden-and-build cycle of attachment security is restored by the actual availability of new attachment figures and the continual symbolic availability of the deceased.

Thus, an attachment perspective on the bereavement process implies that secondary strategies can have both adaptive and maladaptive consequences. As in infancy, these strategies are basically adaptive responses to an attachment figure's inattention, unavailability, or unresponsiveness. But if their activation fails to bring about a happy resolution—following either a painful separation or the complete loss of an attachment figure—they are likely to become an obstacle to the establishment of new security-providing relationships. In the case of a child who relies on one of the secondary strategies because a parent's behavior requires it, the difficulties will show up in later close relationships. In the case of an adult who adopts one or the other secondary strategy as a long-term method of coping with loss, it may damage the person's mental and physical health, as well as interfere with the development of new and healthy relationships. (Relevant research is reviewed throughout this book.)

The success of the dynamic oscillation between hyperactivation and deactivation probably depends on the extent to which (1) the deceased was a major source of security, and (2) new relationship partners are willing and able to provide security and comfort. When the lost figure was unavailable and rejecting while alive, hyperactivation seems likely to entrap the bereaved person in a welter of distress, confusion, and ambivalence (like a child returning to an abusive parent when there is no alternative figure available). Encountering new relationship partners who are emotionally distant and unresponsive can also prevent the transfer of attachment functions and the formation of new attachment bonds. In both cases, reorganization may fail. Moreover, deactivation can be overgeneralized, leading to undifferentiated inhibition of attachment needs and proximity-seeking behaviors. Thus, if a person needs help with grieving, the helper should allow the person to oscillate within normal bounds, and help the person to reorganize his or her attachment hierarchy and gradually enter new relationships with reasonable hope and good judgment. For most mourners, all of this—the oscillation, the reorganization, and the renewed life structure—come about fairly naturally, if nevertheless painfully.

Bowlby (1980) also thought that chronic attachment insecurities jeopardize attachment reorganization. Whereas anxiously attached individuals are likely to have difficulty deactivating thoughts and feelings related to the deceased, avoidant individuals are likely to have difficulty grieving openly and maintaining useful symbolic bonds with the deceased. In both cases, attachment-related worries, fears, and defenses can interfere with adaptive oscillation between hyperactivation and deactivation, cause a person to rely much more on one secondary strategy than the other, and thereby complicate the grief process. In Chapter 7 we review the relevant research.

Bowlby's (1980) analysis fits well with various subsequent dual-process models of bereavement (e.g., Rando, 1992; S. S. Rubin, 1991; M. Stroebe & Schut, 1999). For instance, M. Stroebe and Schut viewed adjustment to loss as a dynamic oscillation between what they called "loss orientation" and "restoration orientation." Loss orientation is conceptually similar to attachment-system hyperactivation and includes yearning, rumination, separation distress, and reappraisal of the meaning and implications of the loss. Restoration accomplishes the same functions as attachment-system deactivation— attending to life changes, doing new things, distracting oneself from the loss, denying or avoiding grief, and forming new relationships. Following Bowlby's lead, M. Stroebe and Schut also proposed that disordered patterns of mourning—chronic grief and delayed or inhibited grief—result from disturbances in the oscillation process and the one-sided adoption of rigid forms of either loss or restoration orientations.

Despite the logical soundness of Bowlby's ideas, no systematic longitudinal research has been conducted on oscillation between hyperactivation and deactivation. Most of the relevant research has focused on attachment-style differences in coping with and adjusting to loss (see Chapter 7, this volume) without examining the dynamic process of attachment reorganization. However, there is some evidence that both hyperactivation and deactivation contribute to grief resolution. For example Schut, Stroebe, de Keijser, and van den Bout (1997) found that men who habitually tended to avoid confronting their grief benefited from counseling that encouraged them to deal with neglected aspects of the loss. They also found that women who habitually dwelled on the meaning and implications of the loss benefited from counseling that emphasized learning how to deal again with mundane activities. In other words, the appropriate treatment seems to require deemphasizing one secondary strategy while strengthening the other.

In a longitudinal study of reactions to the death of a spouse, Shuchter and Zisook (1993) found that widows and widowers adapted to the new reality without relinquishing their symbolic attachment to the deceased 2, 7, and 13 months after the loss. According to these authors, mourners maintained this bond by transforming "what had been a relationship operating on several levels of actual, symbolic, internalized, and imagined relatedness to one in which the actual (living and breathing) relationship has been lost, but the other forms remain or may even develop in more elaborate forms" (p. 34). These symbolic forms include being comforted by the "fact" that the spouse was in heaven, experiencing the spouse's presence in daily life and dreams, talking with the spouse regularly in one's mind (or aloud when alone), or keeping the deceased's belongings. Conceptually similar findings were reported by Roberto and Stanis (1994) in a study of reactions of older women to the death of their friends.

There is also evidence, however, that continuing bonds with the deceased without acknowledging the reality of the death, and without reorganizing the attachment hierarchy, can deter adjustment and endanger mental health (for a review, see Bonanno, 2001). For example, Field, Nichols, Holen, and Horowitz (1999) found that a tendency to maintain the deceased's possessions similar to the way they were when he or she was alive (assessed 6 months after the loss) predicted increases in grief symptoms 18 months later. Moreover, whereas greater involvement with the deceased's possessions was predictive of more expressions of helplessness and despair during a monologue role play in which participants were asked to speak to the deceased, reports of getting greater comfort through memories of the deceased were associated with less helplessness during the "empty chair" monologue role play; that is, the beneficial consequences of continuing bonds seem to depend on the extent to which the deceased is transformed into a symbolic rather than actual, physical source of protection and comfort.

These examples underline the need for more studies of the attachment reorganization process, the adaptive oscillation between secondary strategies, and the internal and external factors that sustain recovery and reorganization or lead to disordered forms of mourning. Such studies should be guided by the understanding of normative attachment processes, as well as the accumulating evidence regarding attachment-style differences in emotion regulation (see Chapter 7, this volume). Ultimately what is needed is a more complete picture of normative grieving, appropriately conceptualized, as well as an understanding of how the grieving process is affected by individual differences.

The Choice of Secondary Strategies

According to our control system model of attachment-system functioning (Chapter 2, this volume), appraisals of the viability of proximity seeking as a protective strategy can consciously or unconsciously determine the choice of a specific secondary attachment strategy. Appraising proximity seeking as likely to capture a partner's attention and regain the partner's support results in an up-regulation (hyperactivation) of the attachment system. This kind of response tends to occur in relationships with unpredictable or unreliable partners who place a person on a partial reinforcement schedule for persistence or insistence: At some times, on an unpredictable schedule, the partner responds to hyperactivated proximity seeking and emotional prodding. In contrast, appraising proximity seeking as unlikely to alleviate distress results in deactivation of the attachment system. This response tends to occur in relationships with partners who disapprove of or even punish expressions of needs for attention and affection.

Unfortunately, adult attachment researchers have not yet studied the hypothesized causal pathway running from appraisal of proximity-seeking viability to the adoption of a particular secondary attachment strategy. The vast majority of adult studies have been based on an individual-differences perspective and have examined whether and how historical factors, such as parental abuse, parental death, or parental divorce (see Chapter 5, this volume), or recollections of parental attitudes and behaviors during childhood (see Chapter 6, this volume), contribute to adults' attachment insecurities. Although these findings have enriched our knowledge of the correlates and possible antecedents of anxious and avoidant attachment in adulthood, they do not provide direct evidence concerning the dynamic process that culminates in the adoption of a particular secondary strategy in a given situation. That is, we still do not know why a person (regardless of chronic attachment style) sometimes anxiously seeks proximity and love from a frustrating partner and at other times avoids intimacy and interdependence with such a partner. Experimental studies manipulating the appraisal of proximity-seeking viability or diary studies assessing daily fluctuations in such appraisals would provide valuable information about the selection of a particular secondary attachment strategy.

Given the dearth of relevant evidence, we recently conducted an experiment in which we manipulated the predictability and reliability of an unavailable relationship partner and examined the effect on a behavioral indicator of proximity seeking: disclosure of private thoughts and feelings to others (self-disclosure). Participants (72 Israeli undergraduates) arrived at the laboratory simultaneously with an opposite-sex confederate, and the two were then placed in different rooms, where they performed a series of tasks. In the first task, participants read 24 sentences describing relational behaviors of three opposite-sex target individuals (eight sentences per target), all identified by their first name, and were asked to learn this information. One of the targets was consistently described, across all eight sentences, as intimacy-averse, emotionally distant, cool, rejecting, and unsupportive. Another target was portrayed as unreliable and unpredictable—sensitive and supportive in three of the eight sentences but rejecting, inattentive, and unsupportive in the remaining five sentences. Regarding the third target (a neutral figure), participants received attachment-unrelated information concerning household chores, joint activities, and attitudes toward the person's extended family.

Next, participants performed a computerized lexical decision task in which they were subliminally primed (for 20 milliseconds) with the name of one of the three target partners described earlier. Following this priming procedure, participants received a sheet of paper containing a story ostensibly written by the confederate, describing personal information that he or she wanted to disclose to them. For half of the participants, the story included intimate, emotionally engaging information concerning the recent death of the confederate's brother in a car accident (the high self-disclosure condition). For the remaining participants, the story included less intimate information about the university courses the confederate was currently taking (the low self-disclosure condition). After reading the story, all participants were given the Self-Disclosure Index (SDI; L. C. Miller, Berg, & Archer, 1983) and asked to rate the extent to which they were comfortable disclosing intimate information to the confederate.

If one's mental representation of a consistently intimacy-averse, emotionally distant relationship partner encourages one to adopt avoidant deactivating strategies, it should inhibit proneness to disclose intimate information even to a highly disclosing confederate. Moreover, if the mental representation of an unpredictable, unreliable partner encourages one to choose anxious, hyperactivating strategies, it should encourage the sharing of intimate information even with a nondisclosing confederate. As can be seen in Figure 3.1, the findings were in line with these predictions. Whereas neutral priming led to greater willingness to disclose personal information (higher SDI scores) to the high- than to the low-disclosing confederate, priming with the name of an intimacy-avoidant partner resulted

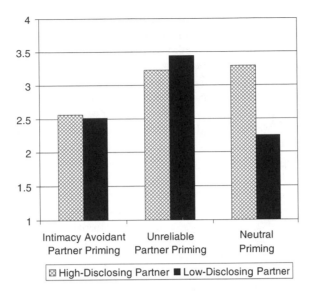

FIGURE 3.1. Mean self-disclosure scores as a function of priming conditions and partner's disclosure level.

in relatively low levels of self-disclosure to both high- and low-disclosing confederates (a previously documented tendency of avoidant individuals; see Chapter 9, this volume). In contrast, priming with the name of an unpredictable, unreliable partner resulted in relatively high levels of self-disclosure to both high- and low-disclosing confederates (a well-documented tendency of attachment-anxious people; see Chapter 9).

This study, an initial step in exploring factors that influence the adoption of particular secondary strategies, provides a small example of the theoretical questions and methodological strategies that can be explored in future studies. As shown throughout this book, the field has accumulated a great deal of knowledge about the cognitive, emotional, and behavioral correlates of attachment styles. We now need more information about whether and how momentary activation of attachment insecurities can cause similar cognitive, emotional, and behavioral reactions, and how heightened insecurity interacts with dispositional attachment styles.

CONCLUDING REMARKS

In this chapter, we have considered three fundamental, interrelated normative principles of attachment theory that are crucial for understanding attachment processes. The first principle concerns the adaptive, regulatory functions of proximity and support seeking: When a person encounters threats and dangers, whether stemming from environmental demands or internal experiences (e.g., worries, pain), the attachment system is activated and certain goals become salient—to gain proximity to, and protection and comfort from, attachment figures. The second principle concerns the beneficial effects of available and responsive relationship partners on a person's emotional state, self-image, behavior in close relationships, and engagement in growth-oriented activities. As shown throughout the chapter, many mental and social processes studied by personality and social psychologists working outside the attachment framework are affected and moderated by attachment figure availability. The third principle concerns the intense distress and urgent coping demands imposed by the unavailability or loss of an attachment figure.

These demands often cause hyperactivation or deactivation of the attachment system, which are natural reactions to the loss or unavailability of an attachment figure, but once established as habitual coping strategies, they contribute to psychological and social difficulties. Because of the centrality of these principles to any broad characterization of the human mind, especially its social or relational aspects, attachment theory helps tie together many of the basic concepts and findings of personality, social, developmental, and clinical psychology.

Some social psychologists, mainly those focusing on interdependence theories of close relationships, have criticized attachment theory for being overly focused on individual differences and personality processes, while ignoring or dismissing social processes in given situations or attributable to a particular relationship partner (e.g., Holmes & Cameron, 2005; Murray et al., 2006). We hope the theoretical ideas and research presented in this chapter belie that criticism: Attachment theory makes specific predictions about (1) how situational threats, indications of attachment figure availability, and proximity-seeking viability momentarily affect the activation and functioning of the attachment behavioral system regardless of a person's attachment style; and (2) how these momentary effects extend to a person's self-esteem, emotion regulation, personal adjustment, interpersonal behaviors, relationship functioning, and mental health. We also hope the material presented in this chapter further clarifies the shared features of attachment theory and interdependence theories.

Nevertheless, it is important to note that attachment theory also acknowledges the contributions of a person's attachment working models and chronic attachment style to the activation and functioning of the attachment system. As we mentioned in Chapter 2, attachment theory is a prime example of the person × situation approach to understanding human behavior. It considers both general processes likely to occur in certain kinds of situations and individual differences in responses arising from a person's history of attachment interactions. We devote the remaining chapters to these individual differences and the thousands of adult attachment studies that demonstrate the importance of the attachment style construct for understanding the complexities of a human mind shaped by and immersed in a social world.

CHAPTER 4

███ ███ ███

Measurement of Attachment-Related Constructs in Adulthood

Measurement of individual differences in attachment began with Ainsworth's (1967) book on infant–mother attachment in Uganda. She observed the naturally occurring behavior of 28 mother–infant dyads in their homes in country villages and developed preliminary ideas about the different kinds of attachment and attachment behavior that might exist during infancy. After leaving Uganda and beginning an intensive year-long study of 26 mother–infant dyads in Baltimore, Ainsworth published a chapter (Ainsworth & Wittig, 1969) describing the now-famous laboratory Strange Situation assessment procedure, which can be used to complement, or even substitute for, observations made in research participants' homes.

The Strange Situation involves a set of eight scripted, 3-minute laboratory episodes in which a caregiver (mother, in the early studies) and a 12- to 18-month-old infant enter a laboratory room equipped with two chairs (one for the mother and one for a later-arriving stranger) and some attractive toys arrayed on a rug. At first, the infant and care-giver get settled in the room, then a series of interactions occur—between the infant and the mother (or, in later studies, the infant and another familiar caregiver, such as the father or the grandmother) and between the infant and the stranger (a laboratory assis-tant). The series of eight episodes includes two reunions with the mother (or caregiver) following separations and is filmed or digitally videotaped for later coding. Ainsworth et al. (1978) created a detailed coding system for the films, and many researchers have since learned the coding system to a high degree of reliability.

Following Ainsworth's early studies, many other measures of infant and child attach-ment were developed (see reviews by Kerns, Schlegelmilch, Morgan, & Abraham, 2005; J. Solomon & George, 1999). Some involve Q-sort descriptions of a child's attachment behavior provided by parents or researchers; others involve doll play story completion tests; and still others, for older children, involve interviews and self-report questionnaires. In this book we are interested primarily in adult attachment, so we do not describe the infant and child attachment measures, except for the coding system used by Ainsworth and her colleagues (1978) in connection with the Strange Situation. Instead, we provide a sufficiently detailed overview of adult attachment measures, so that we can (1) refer to them in subsequent chapters, often using simple acronyms; and (2) reproduce some of them in appendices, so that readers can examine them, keep them in mind when thinking about study results, and use or adapt them in their own research and clinical work.

As we explain in this chapter, there are both interview, or narrative, and self-report measures of adult "states of mind with respect to attachment" and "attachment styles," and multiple exemplars of each approach. Because our research is based primarily on self-report measures, we describe those first and more completely, but we also provide enough information about the interview measures so that readers can understand results based on them, which we review in later chapters. There are good published descriptions and discussions of all the measures, and we provide references for readers who wish to explore them further.

We begin with a description of Ainsworth et al.'s (1978) infant attachment coding system and its underlying structure. We then turn to self-report measures of adult attachment and attachment styles, followed by a brief discussion of interview and narrative measures. Finally, we discuss similarities and differences between various kinds of measures and explain what kinds of research are still needed to clarify and refine our understanding of attachment-related measures. More information about some of the measures can be found in Appendices A–G.

AINSWORTH'S CODING SYSTEM

As we mentioned in Chapter 1, Ainsworth et al. (1978) focused on three patterns of infant–mother attachment, which they initially called A, B, and C to avoid premature fixation on potentially misleading verbal labels. This stratagem did not really work, just as Cattell's (1957) earlier efforts to avoid everyday names for common personality traits did not succeed (he used idiosyncratic terms such as "affectothymia," "threctia," and "alaxia" for warmth, shyness, and trust, respectively). Psychologists who study human beings simply cannot avoid putting their conceptual constructs into words borrowed from ordinary language. Ainsworth's A, B, and C categories are sometimes called (1) avoidant, insecure–avoidant, or anxious–avoidant; (2) secure; and (3) anxious, anxious–ambivalent, insecure–ambivalent, anxious–resistant, or insecure–resistant. In this book we generally use the simplest possible names: avoidant, secure, and anxious. Sometimes we subdivide the avoidant category into dismissing and fearful subtypes, based on influential research by Bartholomew and Horowitz (1991). It is wise to remember, however, that the studies we review are based on particular operationalizations of theoretical constructs. It is worthwhile to keep both the measures and the constructs in mind, because there are more measures than constructs, and the measures do not necessarily correspond with each other, or with particular understandings of the constructs.

The A, or avoidant, infant is marked in the Strange Situation by relative disinterest in mother and her whereabouts, lack of wariness about the stranger, and little or no fussing when mother leaves the room for 3 minutes and then returns. Avoidant infants may actively turn away from the mother when she returns following the final and most stressful separation. They seem to maintain both emotional and physical distance from their mother, even though their elevated heart rate reveals underlying anxiety or distress (Sroufe & Waters, 1977a).

The C, or anxious, infant is marked by high vigilance concerning the mother's presence and her availability or unavailability, frequent verbal or physical contact with her, noticeable wariness with respect to the stranger, intense distress when the mother leaves the room and, in many cases, anger and resistance when she returns. This seeming inconsistency between wanting mother close, then showing anger and resistance following separation from her, is the reason for the terms "ambivalent" and "resistant" in some of the labels for this attachment pattern. We think it is preferable to consider this reaction a sign of protest and retributive anger rather than ambivalence. (A person of any age can truly love and need another without ambivalence, yet still be angry about betrayals and unexplained separations.)

The B, or secure, infant is marked by easy and warm interactions with the mother, genuine interest in exploring the Strange Situation and examining novel toys, mild but not persistent or excessive wariness toward the stranger, noticeable upset when mother leaves the room, and obvious relief, warm greetings, and proximity seeking when she returns. Secure infants seem to accept mother's apologies and hugs following a separation and quickly return to exploration. These three patterns are the foundation on which the entire literature on individual differences in attachment is based.

Various coding scales were designed by Ainsworth to rate the notable aspects of infants' behavior in the Strange Situation (the scales and instructions for their use are included in appendices of Ainsworth et al.'s [1978] book). Most of them tap one of the following theoretical constructs: proximity seeking, contact maintenance, avoidant behavior, resistance (protest and angry lack of cooperation); distance interaction (i.e., communicating across a space without approaching); exploratory locomotion (or movement); exploratory manipulation (e.g., of toys); and crying. A certain profile of scores on these dimensions across the eight episodes of the Strange Situation (e.g., including separation from the mother, being alone in the room, interacting with the stranger, and reuniting with the mother) is used to place each infant into a particular category (A, B, or C). The main emphasis is placed on only a few of the scales, especially the ones concerning an infant's behavior during reunion episodes.

Of special interest here are the analyses presented by Ainsworth et al. (1978, Chapter 6, "An Examination of the Classificatory System: A Multiple Discriminant Function Analysis"). There, the authors showed quantitatively, not just verbally, how the three infant attachment patterns relate to the various coding scales. A slightly modified version of the main graph in that chapter appears here as Figure 4.1. The discriminant analysis used by Ainsworth et al. was intended to determine how well one or more weighted linear combinations of coding scales could accurately assign infants to one of the three (A, B, or C) categories proposed.

The answer is that *two* linear functions did an excellent job. As can be seen in Figure 4.1, almost all of the 105 infants studied by Ainsworth et al. (1978) before their book was published were placed in their appropriate qualitative (i.e., typological) category based on two linear combinations, or discriminant functions. As can also be seen, one of the functions (labeled Function I, or Avoidance, in Figure 4.1) separates avoidant infants from secure and anxious ones, and the other function (labeled Function II, or Anxiety, in Figure 4.1) separates anxious infants from secure and avoidant ones.

The coding scales that correlated most highly with the Avoidance dimension (Function I) were (1) avoiding mother during Episodes 5 and 8 of the Strange Situation (the two reunion episodes), (2) not maintaining contact with mother during Episode 8 (even if mother tried to pick the child up), (3) not seeking proximity during Episode 8, and (4) engaging in more exploratory behavior and more distance interaction (verbal and non-

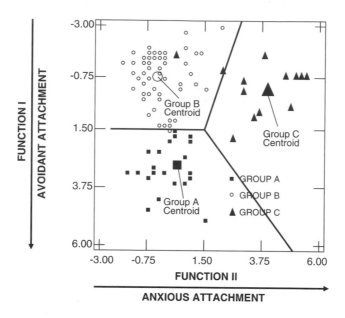

FIGURE 4.1. An adaptation of Figure 10 from Ainsworth, Blehar, Waters, and Wall (1978), with the names of the two attachment dimensions (avoidant attachment and anxious attachment) added. Copyright 1978 by Erlbaum. Adapted by permission.

verbal communication with the stranger while mother was absent) in Episode 7. All of these scales indicate avoidance of the mother, lack of closeness to her, and relatively little distress during her absence (with or without the presence of a stranger). The coding scales that correlated most highly with the Anxiety dimension (Function II) were (1) crying (all through Episodes 2–8, but especially in Episode 6, when the infant was left alone for 3 minutes), (2) greater angry resistance to the mother during Episodes 5 and 8 (the reunions), (3) greater angry resistance to the stranger during Episodes 3, 4, and 7 (when the stranger tried to comfort or play with the infant), and (4) reduced exploration in Episode 7, when the solitary infant was joined by a stranger.

   Thus, from the very beginning, Ainsworth's three infant–mother attachment patterns could be conceptualized as regions in a two-dimensional space, the two dimensions being Avoidance (self-reliance, emotional suppression, and discomfort with closeness and dependency) and Anxiety (crying, failing to explore confidently in the absence of the mother, and angry protest directed at the mother during reunions after what the infant probably experienced as abandonment). In general, however, most researchers who read about Ainsworth's research paid more attention to the A, B, and C categories than to the two dimensions. Attachment theory came to be viewed as a typological theory from then on, even though Bowlby had not formulated it as such.

   When Hazan and Shaver (1987) decided to assess similar patterns of adult "romantic attachment," they began with a three-category typological measure. And when Main and her students (e.g., Main et al., 1985) devised the Adult Attachment Interview (AAI) they used it to classify mothers of A, B, and C category infants into parallel D, F, and E adult categories. They called the categories "Dismissing of attachment," "Free and autonomous with respect to attachment," and "Enmeshed and preoccupied with attachment," presumably because this allowed them to extend the ABC system to a DEF (actually, DFE) system. But other authors quickly cut the names down to size: dismissing, secure, and preoccupied, respectively. It then took years for researchers to reconsider the dimensions underlying the categorical assessment systems (e.g., see Fraley & Spieker [2003a, 2003b] with respect to the infant categories, and Kobak, Cole, Ferenz-Gillies, Fleming, & Gamble [1993] and Fyffe & Waters [1997] regarding the adult AAI categories).

SELF-REPORT MEASURES OF ATTACHMENT STYLE AND ATTACHMENT-RELATED CONSTRUCTS

Hazan and Shaver's Adult Attachment Prototypes

When Hazan and Shaver (1987) began their work on what came to be called romantic attachment "styles" (M. B. Levy & Davis, 1988), they adopted Ainsworth's three-category typology as a framework for conceptualizing individual differences in the ways adults think, feel, and behave in romantic relationships. In their initial studies, Hazan and Shaver (1987, 1990) developed brief, multisentence descriptions of each of the three proposed attachment types—avoidant, secure, and anxious (see Chapter 1, this volume). They were based on an intuitive extrapolation of the three infant patterns summarized in the final chapter of Ainsworth et al.'s (1978) book. Respondents were asked to think back across their history of romantic relationships and say which of the three descriptions best captured the way they *generally* experienced and acted in romantic relationships. Subsequently, various writers called this a "conscious" measure, a measure of "internal working models," and a measure of models of "self and other," but it is important to notice that (1) the measure asks only about the respondent's self, and except for slight mentions of self-knowledge derived from what relationship partners have said, does not explicitly assess "model of others"; (2) the measure asks about feelings, tendencies, and behavior in relationships, not about whatever might be inside a person's conscious or unconscious mind that accounts for these feelings, tendencies, and behaviors. Whatever does account for them must be determined by, and inferred from, empirical research; it is not evident in the measure itself. Thus, the measure does not explicitly assess "models" of anything except perhaps a model of the way a person views his or her experiences and reactions in close relationships, which is not very close to what Bowlby (1969/1982) meant by "working models."

In their initial studies, Hazan and Shaver (1987, 1990) found that people's self-reported romantic attachment patterns related to a number of theoretically relevant variables, including beliefs about love and relationships (working models of romantic relationships, perhaps), recollections of early experiences with parents (these findings are reviewed in Chapters 6 and 10, this volume), and experiences in work (or "exploration") contexts (see Chapter 15, this volume). Many personality and social psychologists adopted Hazan and Shaver's categorical, forced-choice measure because of its brevity, face validity, and ease of administration. Nonetheless, a few early investigators quickly, and correctly, recognized the measure's limitations (e.g., Collins & Read, 1990; M. B. Levy & Davis, 1988; Mikulincer et al., 1990; Simpson, 1990).

For example, categorical measures are implicitly based on the assumption that variation among people within a category is unimportant or does not exist, and that individuals within a category do not differ in the extent to which they can be characterized by a particular pattern. (It was obvious from the beginning, however, as shown in Figure 4.1, that infants labeled A, B, or C *did* differ on the underlying anxiety and avoidance dimensions, but this was generally ignored.) In addition, as Baldwin and Fehr (1995) pointed out, the test–retest stability of the categorical measure was only 70% (equivalent to a Pearson's *r* of approximately .40) and did not decrease as a function of the magnitude of the test–retest interval. This suggested that the instability was due to measurement error resulting from classification artifacts, not to "true" change in attachment security over time (Fraley & Waller, 1998; Scharfe & Bartholomew, 1994).

To address these issues, attachment researchers began to use continuous rating scales. For example, M. B. Levy and Davis (1988) asked participants to rate how well each attachment pattern described their general experience of romantic relationships. Test–retest reliability estimates for ratings of the three alternatives tended to be about .60 over intervals ranging from 1 to 8 weeks (Baldwin & Fehr, 1995; J. A. Feeney & Noller, 1996). Subsequently, other researchers decomposed Hazan and Shaver's (1987) three prototype descriptions to form separate items that could be individually rated on Likert-type response scales (e.g., Collins & Read, 1990; J. A. Feeney & Noller, 1990; Mikulincer et al., 1990; Simpson, 1990). Moreover, some of these researchers extended the focus of the scales to a person's attachment orientation in close relationships *in general* rather than in romantic relationships exclusively (e.g., Mikulincer et al., 1990), while others used them to assess a person's attachment orientation in a specific relationship (e.g., Baldwin, Keelan, Fehr, Enns, & Koh Rangarajoo, 1996). In our opinion, all of these efforts were legitimate, and all produced interesting research findings. We describe a few of the most frequently used measures in the following sections, so that readers can refer back to them when we name them by their acronyms in subsequent chapters.

Adult Attachment Questionnaire

Simpson (1990) was one of the first to convert the statements in Hazan and Shaver's three prototypes into separate Likert-type items. By breaking the prototype descriptions into separate propositions, he was able to create 13 such items. Simpson, Rholes, and Phillips (1996) later expanded the Adult Attachment Questionnaire (AAQ) from 13 to 17 items to increase the internal consistency of the attachment anxiety subscale. (The most recent version of the measure is reproduced in Appendix A.) Participants are asked to rate (on a 7-point scale) the extent to which each item is descriptive of the way they feel in romantic relationships (in general, not with a specific partner). Some of the items are worded in a negative direction to control for acquiescence response bias.

In contrast to Hazan and Shaver's (1987, 1990) early prototype measure, the AAQ represents adult attachment style in terms of two dimensions. Factor analyses have confirmed that the AAQ items load on two independent factors, attachment anxiety and avoidance (e.g., Brennan, Clark, & Shaver, 1998; Simpson, 1990). The two factors yield two unit-weighted scales with adequate internal consistency. For example, Simpson et al. (1996) computed Cronbach's alpha coefficients separately for men and women, and obtained values of .70 and .74 for avoidance, and .72 and .76 for attachment anxiety. Scale scores are computed by averaging item scores, and higher scores indicate higher attachment anxiety or avoidance. As shown throughout this book, the two AAQ scales have good construct and criterion validity and are associated with self-report measures of relationship functioning, as well as behavior in laboratory interactions with close relationship partners (e.g., Rholes, Simpson, & Blakely, 1995; Simpson, Rholes, & Nelligan, 1992; Simpson et al., 1996). Brennan et al. (1998) found that the AAQ Avoidance scale correlated .81 with one of two major orthogonal factors (also labeled avoidance) in their analysis of numerous self-report attachment style measures, and the AAQ anxiety score correlated .77 with the other major factor (also labeled anxiety). Thus, the AAQ assesses the constructs we refer to throughout this book as attachment anxiety and avoidance.

Adult Attachment Scale

While Simpson was working on his measure, Collins and Read (1990), in an independent venture, also decomposed Hazan and Shaver's (1987, 1990) prototype descriptions to create separate items and added other items concerning (1) beliefs about whether one's partner (viewed as an attachment figure) is available and responsive when needed and (2) how one reacts to separations from one's partner. This resulted in an 18-item Adult Attachment Scale (AAS). Collins (1996) later revised the original 18 AAS items to increase the internal consistencies of its subscales. (The most recent version of the measure is reproduced in Appendix B.)

Using factor analysis, Collins and Read (1990) found that their items formed three factors, which they called discomfort with closeness, discomfort with depending on others, and anxious concern about being abandoned or unloved. Unit-weighted scales based on these factors yielded adequate, though not high, alpha coefficients (ranging from .69 to .75) and moderate temporal stability over a 2-month period (ranging from .52 to .71). The internal consistency of the three factors was improved in the revised version of the AAS, with alpha coefficients ranging from .78 to .85 (Collins, 1996). In both the original and revised versions of the AAS, the two discomfort scales are fairly highly correlated. This is important theoretically, because Brennan et al. (1998) found that discomfort with closeness correlated .86 and discomfort with depending on others correlated .79 with the major avoidance factor common to most self-report attachment scales (the third AAS subscale, Anxiety, correlated .74 with Brennan et al.'s anxiety factor). Thus, both kinds of discomfort are highly related to an underlying avoidance dimension and are largely independent of the anxiety factor.

Collins and Read (1990) found theoretically sensible associations between the three AAS subscales and a large battery of self-report scales tapping working models of self and others, and relationship functioning. The construct and criterion validity of the AAS have since been demonstrated in many studies reviewed throughout this book. Although we generally subsume discomfort with closeness and dependency into a general avoidance construct, it is worth mentioning that Shaver, Belsky, and Brennan (2000) obtained interesting and slightly different results for the two AAS subscales when examining associations with rating scales used to code the AAI, so the distinction between the two kinds of avoidant discomfort might sometimes be worth making.

Attachment Style Questionnaire

The ASQ is another multi-item questionnaire designed to assess adult attachment style. J. A. Feeney, Noller, and Hanrahan (1994), noting the deficiencies of Hazan and Shaver's (1987, 1990) initial measure, went back to the attachment literature and tried to build a measure "from the ground up," so to speak, in order not to miss any important nuances in Bowlby's and Ainsworth's writings. They also worded their items in a less "romantic" way than Hazan and Shaver had done (and than Simpson [1990] and Collins and Read [1990] did by virtue of basing their scales on Hazan and Shaver's measure). This made the ASQ more suitable for adolescents who had not had much experience in romantic relationships.

J. Feeney et al. (1994) created an initial pool of 65 items, and through structural analyses reduced the number to 40 (see Appendix C). Participants were asked to rate (on a 6-point scale) the extent to which each item described their feelings and behavior in "close" (not necessarily romantic) relationships. The 40 items formed five factor-based scales: lack of confidence (in self and others), discomfort with closeness, need for approval and confirmation by others, preoccupation with relationships, and viewing relationships as secondary (to achievement in various domains, such as school or career). Discomfort with closeness and viewing relationships as secondary are clearly related conceptually to avoidant attachment, and in Brennan et al.'s (1998) factor-analytic study, the correlations of these two scales with the avoidance factor were .90 and .61, respectively. Preoccupation with relationships and need for approval and confirmation by others are conceptually related to anxious attachment, and they loaded .86 and .62, respectively, on Brennan et al.'s (1998) anxiety factor. The lack of confidence scale was composed in such a way (combining both self and other judgments, but emphasizing lack of trust in others) that it also loaded mostly on avoidance (.70).

J. Feeney et al. (1994) reported alpha coefficients for the five scales, ranging from .76 to .84 in a large sample of undergraduates, and stability coefficients ranging from .67 to .78 across a 10-week period. As can be seen throughout this volume, researchers have used the ASQ to measure attachment style in many samples of adolescents and adults, providing further evidence of its reliability and validity. A study by Fossati et al. (2003a) supported the five-factor structure of an Italian version of the ASQ in both clinical and nonclinical samples, while also finding that the five scales loaded on two larger factors, attachment anxiety and avoidance. Like Collins and Read's (1990) three-subscale AAS, the ASQ may prove especially useful in studies where specific facets of anxiety and avoidance matter.

Bartholomew's Measures

The various attempts to create multi-item scales (AAS, AAQ, ASQ) reveal that there are two major dimensions underlying self-report measures of attachment style: anxiety (about separation, abandonment, or insufficient love) and avoidance (of intimacy, dependency, and emotional expressiveness). These two dimensions are conceptually similar to the ones emphasized by Ainsworth et al. (1978) and schematized in Figure 4.1.

Bartholomew (1990) provided an interpretation of these dimensions in terms of Bowlby's (1969/1982) ideas about internal working models of self and others. She proposed that the anxiety dimension be conceptualized as "model of self" (positive vs. negative) and the avoidance dimension be conceptualized as "model of others" (positive vs. negative). She pointed out that combinations of the two dimensions can be viewed as defining four, rather than three, attachment patterns in a two-dimensional space (see Figure 4.2): People with positive models of self and others are "secure" (or secure with respect to attachment); those with positive models of others and negative models of self are "preoccupied" (a term borrowed from the AAI Enmeshed and preoccupied category); those with a negative model of others but a positive model of self are "dismissing" (a name for one kind of avoidance, also borrowed from the AAI); and those with negative models of both self and others are "fearful" (or fearfully avoidant). In most nonclinical samples there are more secure and fearful people than preoccupied and dismissing ones, suggesting (according to Bartholomew's theorizing) that most people possess affectively congruent (i.e., both positive or both negative) models of self and others.

Following Main et al.'s (1985) lead, Bartholomew (see Bartholomew & Horowitz,

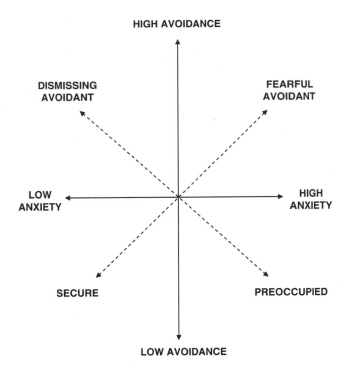

FIGURE 4.2. Diagram of the two-dimensional space defined by attachment anxiety and avoidance, showing the quadrant names suggested by Bartholomew (1990).

1991) created a peer attachment interview to assess people's location in the four-category typology, and following Hazan and Shaver's (1987) lead, she also developed the Relationship Questionnaire (RQ), a short measure containing multisentence prototype descriptions of the four theoretical types. The four "types" were described as follows:

1. *Secure*: "It is easy for me to become emotionally close to others. I am comfortable depending on them and having them depend on me. I don't worry about being alone or having others not accept me."
2. *Fearful*: "I am uncomfortable getting close to others. I want emotionally close relationships, but I find it difficult to trust others completely, or to depend on them. I worry that I will be hurt if I allow myself to become too close to others."
3. *Preoccupied*: "I want to be completely emotionally intimate with others, but I often find that others are reluctant to get as close as I would like. I am uncomfortable being without close relationships, but I sometimes worry that others don't value me as much as I value them."
4. *Dismissing*: "I am comfortable without close emotional relationships. It is very important to me to feel independent and self-sufficient, and I prefer not to depend on others or have others depend on me."

The wording of three of the four prototypes (secure, preoccupied, and fearful) is very similar to the wording of Hazan and Shaver's (1987) three prototypes (secure, anxious, and avoidant). However, the compulsive self-reliance and independence emphasized in

Bartholomew and Horowitz's (1991) dismissing prototype were not well represented in Hazan and Shaver's measure. This may explain why early studies based on prototype ratings (e.g., M. B. Levy & Davis, 1988) found secure and avoidant to be at opposite ends of a single dimension, whereas anxiety was a separate, orthogonal dimension; that is, Hazan and Shaver accidentally defined avoidance in a way that made it more similar to a fearful rather than to a dismissing form of avoidance. This possibility was tested by Brennan et al. (1991), who compared ratings of Hazan and Shaver's (1987) three prototypes with ratings of Bartholomew and Horowitz's (1991) four prototypes. Both measures reduced to the same two dimensions: one running from secure to fearful (or to what Hazan and Shaver called "avoidant") and the other running from preoccupied (or anxious, or anxious–ambivalent) to dismissing. These subtle structural issues may have had important effects on early research, but it is difficult to tell in retrospect, because most investigators used only a single measure of attachment style rather than comparing measures.

As in the case of Hazan and Shaver's (1987) prototype measure, respondents completing the RQ choose the description that best characterizes them, but they also rate how well each of the four descriptions fits them, and this allows researchers to use both continuous and categorical indicators. (This is what M. B. Levy and Davis [1988] did with Hazan and Shaver's [1987] prototypes.) In general, the reliability estimates for the RQ self-classifications (kappas of around .35) and ratings (test–retest r's around .50) are comparable to those for Hazan and Shaver's three-category classifications (Scharfe & Bartholomew, 1994).

Later, Griffin and Bartholomew (1994a) developed the Relationship Styles Questionnaire (RSQ), a 30-item inventory that contains items based on both Hazan and Shaver's (1987) prototypes and the RQ prototypes. (Some of the items were probably also based on Bartholomew's extensive interviewing experience.) The RSQ (shown in Appendix D) can be used to create a score for a person on each of the four attachment patterns (secure, preoccupied, fearful, and dismissing). It can also be used to place a person in the two-dimensional space (Figure 4.2) within which the patterns reside (model of self and model of other, in Bartholomew's terms; anxiety and avoidance in our terms). Due to its length, the RSQ is somewhat more reliable than the RQ, but the internal consistency coefficients are still low for the four prototype scales. They are somewhat higher for the two composite dimensions.

Experiences in Close Relationships Scale

As already mentioned, Brennan et al. (1998) factor-analyzed the nonredundant items from all self-report attachment measures that had been created by the late 1990s, using a large sample of over 900 university students. The goal was to boil all of the existing measures down to measures of Ainsworth's two major dimensions, maximizing internal consistency without unduly narrowing the constructs being assessed. Brennan et al. found that two major higher-order factors (anxiety and avoidance) were common to most of the measures (as we have already indicated by showing how highly other measures correlated with the two factors).

The items on the attachment anxiety factor are reminiscent of Ainsworth et al.'s (1978) coding scales describing anxiously attached infants; that is, they emphasize both fear of abandonment and anger about separations. For example: "I worry about being rejected or abandoned"; "I need a lot of reassurance that close relationship partners really care about me"; "When I don't have close others around, I feel somewhat anxious and insecure"; "I resent it when my relationship partners spend time away from me." The items on the avoidant attachment factor are, similarly, reminiscent of Ainsworth et al.'s (1978) coding scales describing avoidantly attached infants. They emphasize lack of closeness and emotional suppression; for example: "I find it difficult to allow myself to depend on close relationship partners"; "I prefer not to show others how I feel deep down"; "I try to avoid getting too close to others"; "I don't mind asking close others for comfort, advice, or help" (reverse-scored).

Based on their factor analysis, Brennan et al. (1998) proposed two 18-item scales, one to assess Attachment Anxiety and the other to Assess Avoidant attachment. These scales make up the Experiences in Close Relationships scale (ECR) measure of attachment style, which is reproduced here in Appendix E. This measure has been used in hundreds of studies since 1998, always with high reliability (the alpha coefficients are always near or above .90, and test–retest coefficients range between .50 and .75, depending on the time span and the nature of the sample). The correlation between the two scales is often close to zero, as intended (to fit with Bartholomew's [1990] conceptual analysis and Ainsworth et al.'s [1978] discriminant analysis), but the two scales seem to be more highly correlated when they are administered to members of long-term couples. (As far as we know, this informal observation of ours has not been evaluated quantitatively in a study that examines the size of the correlation as a function of being in a relationship or not, and as a function of relationship length for people involved in a relationship.) The wording of the ECR items and the instructions can be altered slightly to apply to a particular relationship, to one's general orientation in romantic relationships, or to one's general or global "attachment style" in various kinds of relationships.

The validity of the ECR has been demonstrated in numerous studies, including ones that included both experimental manipulations and behavioral observations. (These studies are summarized in later chapters of this book.) We have used the ECR in most of our studies, and it has performed similarly in Israel and the United States (i.e., in both Hebrew and English). It has been translated into many other languages, always producing more than adequate reliability coefficients and good evidence of construct validity. Because we have used this measure in our own work, it is a benchmark for us when we evaluate other measures and other people's studies. We do not believe, however, that it is the be-all and end-all of self-report attachment measures. The ECR Anxiety scale contains only one reverse-scored item, making it, we assume, vulnerable to acquiescence response bias. Both scales contain some items that refer to "partners" (plural) and others that refer to "partner" (singular)—an accidental result of taking the items from different scales and accepting whichever ones loaded highly on the two major factors. As mentioned earlier in this chapter, the ECR measures the anxiety and avoidance dimensions rather than their 45° rotations: the secure–fearful and preoccupied–dismissing dimensions. As we discuss later, it would be desirable to have equally precise and efficient measures of all four dimensions.

In one attempt at improvement, Fraley, Waller, and Brennan (2000) used item response theory to evaluate the extent to which the two ECR scales discriminate with equal sensitivity across their full ranges. The answer appeared to be "no," so Fraley et al. suggested using different items taken from Brennan et al.'s (1998) large item pool to replace some of the original ones, mostly to yield better discrimination at the secure ends of the two scales. The resulting measure is called the ECR-R (R for revised). Its new items are shown in Appendix F. The reliability estimates and stability of the two-factor structure of the ECR-R items are comparable to those of the original ECR items (e.g., Sibley, Fischer, & Liu, 2005; Sibley & Liu, 2004). Personally, we have not been persuaded to trade the ECR for the ECR-R, because we do not like the wording of some of the new items, and the two new scales seem to correlate slightly more with each other than the originals did (at least this has happened when we have included both scales in our studies), with no gain in validity. Also, the new and old parallel scales always correlate around .95 with each other, because they share most of their items, so findings for the new and old scales are usually quite similar in meaning.

Nevertheless, the research that generated the ECR-R showed correctly that the ECR, by focusing so intently on anxiety and avoidance, may be deficient in assessing security, except as the vague absence of avoidance and anxiety. Klohnen and John (1998) conducted interesting preliminary research on an adjective-based measure of all eight octants of the two-dimensional space shown in Figure 4.2. This approach suggested how the entire space might be mapped with more than two scales, but to date this measure has not been perfected or used very often. There are several other self-report adult attachment style measures as well (e.g., Carver, 1997; Onishi, Gjerde, & Block, 2001; Sperling, Berman, & Fagen, 1992), each with its own emphases and assets, but to date they have not risen to prominence. In addition, many investigators have extended the self-report measurement of attachment style in various directions: to friendships (see Chapter 9, this volume), to the client–therapist relationship (see Chapter 14, this volume), and to the study of group and organizational processes (see Chapter 15, this volume). We therefore expect and welcome further developments in the measurement of attachment-related constructs.

In the following sections we consider a few other self-report measures, all related to family and other nonromantic attachment relationships. These measures were not designed to classify people into attachment style categories or assess their location in the space defined by Ainsworth et al.'s (1978) two dimensions of attachment insecurity (anxiety and avoidance). Rather, they were intended to assess the extent to which a person feels secure or insecure in his or her relationship with parents and friends, his or her appraisals of these figures, or his or her recollections of childhood experiences with parents.

Inventory of Parent and Peer Attachment

Around the same time that Hazan and Shaver (1987) were working on their measure of adult romantic attachment, Armsden and Greenberg (1987) developed the Inventory of Parent and Peer Attachment (IPPA) to assess adolescents' perceptions of their relationships with parents and friends (not specifically targeting romantic partners). They reasoned that in adolescence "the 'internal working model' of attachment figures may be tapped by assessing (1) the positive affective/cognitive experience of trust in the accessibility and responsiveness of attachment figures, and (2) the negative affective/cognitive experiences of anger and/or hopelessness resulting from unresponsive or inconsistently responsive attachment figures" (p. 431). Accordingly, the IPPA consists of 25 items tapping three broad constructs with respect to the mother, the father, and peers: degree of mutual trust (e.g., "My mother respects my feelings"), quality of communication (e.g., "I like to get my mother's point of view on things I'm concerned about"), and degree of anger and alienation (e.g., "My mother expects too much from me"). The three dimensions are highly correlated within each relationship type (parents, peers) and are commonly aggregated to yield composite indexes of security versus insecurity with respect to parents and peers. Reliability estimates for the composite IPPA subscales are high (e.g., Armsden & Greenberg, 1987; Armsden, McCauley, Greenberg, Burke, & Mitchell, 1990). The measure has been used extensively to assess security in adolescents, as we note repeatedly in subsequent chapters.

The measure was not designed to differentiate among the attachment patterns delineated by Ainsworth and her colleagues: "It is not clear what the developmental manifestations of 'avoidant' or 'ambivalent' would be in adolescence, or if other conceptualizations of insecure attachment would be more appropriate" (Armsden & Greenberg, 1987, p. 447). Brennan et al. (1998) found that the IPPA Communication subscale (measured only with reference to peers) loaded negatively on their avoidance factor (–.72), as did the IPPA Trust subscale (–.72). The IPPA Alienation and Anger subscale loaded equally (.53) on the avoidance and anxiety factors. Thus, except for its anger facet, the IPPA does not measure attachment anxiety very well, but it measures general insecurity fairly well, with special emphasis on avoidance.

Parental Attachment Questionnaire

Also used in many studies of the quality of adolescents' attachment to their parents is the Parental Attachment Questionnaire (PAQ; Kenny, 1987a), a 55-item self-report scale suitable for adolescents and young adults. It contains three scales—Affective Quality of Relationships, Parental Fostering of Autonomy (the secure base function), and Parental Provision of Emotional Support (the safe haven function)—derived from factor analyses of an item pool developed by Kenny (1987a). The items, rated on a Likert-type scale, assess a person's description of his or her parents ("My parents live in a different world"), his or her relationship with parents ("My parents have trust and confidence in me"), and associated feelings and experiences ("I enjoy telling [my parents] about the things I have done and learned"). Usually, both parents are rated as a set (if there are two parents), but it is easy to adapt the scale to obtain separate ratings of each parent. Kenny (1987a) reported full-scale internal consistencies of .93 and .95 for samples of college students. Internal consistency and stability coefficients for the PAQ subscales are also high (e.g., Kenny, 1987a, 1990).

Reciprocal and Avoidant Attachment Questionnaires for Adults

Some measures can be used to assess an adult's attachment to a parent or to any other attachment figure. An example is the Reciprocal Attachment Questionnaire for Adults (RAQA; West & Sheldon, 1988; West & Sheldon-Keller, 1992, 1994), which operationalizes various aspects of adult attachment—proximity seeking (e.g., "I feel lost if I'm upset and my attachment figure is not around"), separation protest (e.g., "I feel abandoned when my attachment figure is away for a few days"), feared loss (e.g., "I'm afraid that I will lose my attachment figure's love"), availability (e.g., "I am confident that my attachment figure will try to understand my feelings"), and reliance on the attachment figure (e.g., "I talk things over with my attachment figure"). It also operationalizes general patterns of attachment—angry withdrawal (e.g., "I get frustrated when my attachment figure is not around as much as I would like"), compulsive caregiving (e.g., "I put my attachment figure's needs before my own"), compulsive self-reliance (e.g., "I feel it is best not to rely on my attachment figure"), and compulsive care seeking (e.g., "I would be helpless without my attachment figure").

An unusual feature of the RAQA is that it asks a person to respond with respect to whoever happens to be his or her most important attachment figure, regardless of that person's age or form of relatedness to the respondent. In this respect, the RAQA is somewhat similar to the WHOTO scale (Hazan & Zeifman, 1994; discussed in Chapter 3, this volume), which asks respondents to provide the names of relationship partners who serve the various functions of an attachment figure. However, it is important to note that the

WHOTO scale does not assess anxiety or avoidance; rather, it provides information about a person's hierarchy or network of attachment figures.

West and Sheldon-Keller (1992) also created a separate questionnaire, the Avoidant Attachment Questionnaire for Adults (AAQA), for adults who claim not to have a primary attachment figure. This instrument contains four subscales: Maintains Distance in Relationships (e.g., "I'm afraid of getting close to others"), High Priority on Self-Sufficiency (e.g., "My strength comes only from myself"), Attachment Relationship Is a Threat to Security (e.g., "Needing someone would make me feel weak"), and Desire for Close Affectional Bonds (e.g., "I long for someone to share my feelings with").

The subscales of the RAQA have adequate internal consistency and test–retest reliability. Factor analyses of the items indicate that a two-factor solution provides a fairly good fit to the interitem correlations (West & Sheldon-Keller, 1994). In the Brennan et al. (1998) factor-analytic study of self-report attachment measures, availability and feared loss loaded on both the anxiety and avoidance factors (–.39 and –.66 for availability, .64 and .41 for feared loss), suggesting that they measure overall security. Use of the attachment figure as a secure base loaded only on the avoidance factor (–.79), and separation protest loaded only on the anxiety factor (.48). Proximity seeking loaded negatively on the avoidance factor (–.36) and positively on the anxiety factor (.59), suggesting that it distinguishes between preoccupied and dismissing attachment categories in Bartholomew's (1990) scheme. Overall, the scales in the RAQA seem easy to place in the two-dimensional space mapped by Brennan et al. (1998), which we interpret as parallel to the Ainsworth et al. (1978) conceptual space, and as a reflection of hyperactivating and deactivating attachment strategies (discussed in Chapter 2, this volume).

Other Family- and Attachment-Related Self-Report Measures

We mention three other self-report measures of attachment to parents, because many researchers seem to want, retrospectively, to measure attachment to parents during childhood. We do not believe this can be done with great accuracy, but it is nevertheless sometimes worthwhile to assess either major attachment-related experiences in childhood, such as being abused or abandoned, or current (adult) mental representations of attachment experiences in childhood.

Beginning with a 1985 article by Ricks, several attachment researchers have used an unpublished scale, the Mother–Father–Peer scale (MFP; Epstein, 1983) to assess adolescents' and adults' recollections of their childhood relationships with parents. The MFP includes three scales: Acceptance–Rejection (by mother, father, and peers), Independence–Overprotection (by mother, father, and peers), and Defensive Idealization (of mother and father). Sample items include "When I was a child, my mother could always be depended on when I really needed her help and trust" (mother acceptance), "When I was a child, my mother often said she wished I had never been born" (mother rejection), and "My mother was close to a perfect parent" (defensive idealization). According to Ricks (1985, p. 221), "Epstein has found that mother acceptance in childhood [as reported by adults] is more highly correlated with sense of worthiness in adulthood . . . than with any other of a wide range of personality variables assessed, including ego strength, neuroticism, [and] introversion." Ricks used the MFP scale and found that mothers of secure infants (in the Strange Situation) had more positive recollections of childhood relationships with their mothers, fathers, and peers than did mothers of insecure infants.

Another measure that assesses key aspects of (remembered) attachment-related experiences during childhood, the Attachment History Questionnaire (AHQ), first copyrighted by Pottharst and Kessler in 1982, was described in print by Pottharst (1990b). The questionnaire assesses family history (including losses, parental divorce, and separations from parents), patterns of family interactions, parental discipline techniques, and friendship and social support history. Most of the items are based on Bowlby's writings. Fifty-one of the items are answered on 7-point response scales, in addition to which there are several open-ended questions and checklists. A factor analysis was conducted on the 51 scaled items, and four factors emerged: secure base (e.g., trusted parents, amount of love from mother), parental discipline (e.g., not allowed to see friends, parents took things away), threats of separation (e.g., parents threatened to leave, parents threatened to call police), and peer affectional support (e.g., dependability of friends, having been supported by friends). In many studies the subscales were combined to yield a single security score, with an alpha coefficient around .90. A book edited by Pottharst (1990a), *Explorations in Adult Attachment,* describes several studies based on this measure. They consistently showed that AHQ insecurity is related to negative outcomes (e.g., being the mother in a family in which father and daughter have an incestuous relationship, abusing one's children, becoming a prostitute, and having severe emotional problems following loss of a spouse). Few researchers have taken advantage of the promising preliminary steps taken by Pottharst to measure a person's memories of attachment relationships, and this topic still needs both psychometric and substantive research.

Even less fully developed was the simple measure used by Hazan and Shaver (1987) to assess adults' recollections of their childhood experiences with parents. They asked, "During your childhood, were you and your mother ever separated for what seemed like a long time? (If yes, for how long? What was the reason for the separation? How old were you at the time?) Did she ever threaten to leave you or send you away? (If yes, how often?)" The same questions were asked about the father. Also, for each parent, respondents were asked to check which of the following adjectives, if any, described his or her "attitudes, feelings, and behavior toward you": loving, demanding, caring, sympathetic, overprotective, affectionate, strict, unresponsive, disinterested, critical, respectful, understanding, rejecting, abusive, attentive, intrusive, accepting. Participants were also asked which of the following adjectives, if any, described each parent: happy, weak, confident, unpredictable, insecure, selfish, responsible, respected, troubled, sad/depressed, strong, nervous, fair, warm, flexible, unfair, likeable, immature, cold, hostile, funny, inconsistent. Finally, they were asked to say which of the following adjectives, if any, described their parents' relationship: affectionate, happy, argumentative, distant, troubled, comfortable, violent, unhappy, strained, caring, supportive, good-humored.

Hazan and Shaver (1987) conducted a discriminant analysis to see whether two linear combinations of adjectives could distinguish among the three prototypical romantic attachment patterns (secure, anxious, and avoidant). The analysis was successful, and the best discriminators between secure and insecure attachment patterns (with correlations between adjective selection and the function in parentheses) were a relationship between the parents that was affectionate (.44), caring (.32), and not unhappy (−.34); a mother who was respectful toward her child (.43), confident (.35), accepting (.33), responsible (.31), not intrusive (−.42), and not demanding (−.40); and a father who was caring (.41), loving (.40), humorous (.40), and affectionate (.30). Clearly, these results fit well with attachment theory and were subsequently replicated by J. A. Feeney and Noller (1990) in another country (Australia). Given that a person had one of the two insecure romantic attachment styles, the more anxious (rather than avoidant) ones described their mother as more humorous (.43), likable (.38), respected (.37), and not rejecting (−.30), implying that the avoidant people had parents who were more rejecting and less humorous. The more anxious (rather than avoidant) people described their father as more unfair (.47). The findings from these studies were quite preliminary, and many have not been adequately followed up, but considering the results based on the MFP scale, the AHQ, and Hazan and Shaver's adjective checklist, it is clear that self-report measures of childhood experiences with parents are systematically related to adult attachment insecurities (see Chapter 6, this volume, for a more detailed review).

GENERAL ISSUES RELATED TO SELF-REPORT ATTACHMENT MEASURES

Several questions and challenges have arisen with respect to self-report measures of attachment style, and here we address them briefly to give readers and future researchers some perspective. They should be kept in mind while reading later chapters, which focus more on study outcomes than on measurement per se.

Categories versus Continuous Scores

The first issue concerns whether adult attachment patterns are best conceptualized and measured in terms of types or dimensions (e.g., Fraley & Waller, 1998; Griffin & Bartholomew, 1994b). As we mentioned earlier in this chapter, Hazan and Shaver (1987) began by trying to assess Ainsworth et al.'s (1978) types in the context of adult romantic relationships. Subsequent taxometric research demonstrated, however, that adult attachment patterns assessed with self-report measures are best characterized in dimensional terms (Fraley & Waller, 1998). Fraley and Waller described the many problems that arise when categorical models are used to assess what are actually dimensional phenomena, and they recommended that researchers use dimensional measures. Their analyses suggested that many published and theory-confirming findings based on self-report attachment measures would have been even stronger if dimensional rather than categorical measures had been used. Categorical measures throw away important information about individual differences within categories (for examples, see Brennan et al., 1998).

In research that we ourselves have conducted since Fraley and Waller's (1998) chapter was published, we have used dimensional measures, such as the ECR, and have employed dimensional scores in regression analyses as continuous predictors, rather than conducting analyses of variance with categorical predictor variables (i.e., three or four attachment "types"). With hierarchical regression analysis it is possible to determine whether interactions between the two dimensions add anything to their main effects, as would happen, for example, if a particular region of the two-dimensional space described by Ainsworth et al. (1978) was strongly responsible for a particular effect. For example, if an effect were due to fearful people rather than to people who were simply avoidant, then it would produce a significant interaction between anxiety and avoidance in a regression analysis. Although this does sometimes happen in our studies, we generally find one or two main effects but no significant interactions.

We should also mention that the complex formula provided by Brennan et al. (1998) for obtaining categorical classifications from scores on the ECR dimensions discards important information, and we do not recommend using it. Brennan et al. developed it to show that categories based on dimensions are more accurate and informative than research participants' own self-assigned classifications based on qualitative measures such as Hazan and Shaver's (1987) three-category measure or Bartholomew and Horowitz's (1991) four-category RQ. The categorization formula was meant for a particular analysis in Brennan et al.'s (1998) study, not for general use by other investigators, and we no longer use it ourselves.

Prototype Ratings versus Dimensions

A second issue is the use of continuous ratings of individual attachment patterns (e.g., secure, anxious, avoidant, fearful) or dimensional scores (model of self, model of others; anxiety, avoidance). Although the former method is better than nothing when one is forced to use only four items in a brief questionnaire, Fraley and Waller (1998) discussed the issue in detail and concluded that it is better to use the two RSQ or ECR scales rather than the four RQ ratings whenever one has sufficient time and space for a longer measure. (In most cases it is easy to use both, which sometimes helps connect one's findings to those in the literature based on only one or the other measure.)

Conceptualization of the Two Major Dimensions of Attachment Style

A third issue is how best to conceptualize the two dimensions underlying self-report measures of adult attachment. Bartholomew (1990; Bartholomew & Horowitz, 1991) conceptualized them in terms of the beliefs (working models) that people hold about themselves and close others, whereas Hazan and Shaver (1987) conceptualized them in terms of self-reports about attachment-system functioning in close relationships. The latter conceptualization is closer to the one presented in Chapter 2, where we relied on the concepts of hyperactivation and deactivation of the attachment system. Pursuing Bartholomew's conceptualization, many researchers have attempted to specify the actual beliefs held by people with different attachment orientations (e.g., Baldwin et al., 1993; Collins, 1996; Klohnen & John, 1998). Pursuing Hazan and Shaver's (1987) conceptualization, we (e.g., Mikulincer & Shaver, 2003; Shaver & Mikulincer, 2007) have put more emphasis on the functional organization of the attachment system and its role in affect and behavior regulation in interactions with relationship partners (see Chapters 7–9, this volume).

According to the model we presented in Chapter 2, self-report measures of attachment dimensions assess the tendency to hyperactivate and/or deactivate the attachment system when the availability (either physical or symbolic) of a supportive attachment figure is in question. People who score high on the anxiety dimension tend to increase their sense of vulnerability, their expressions of need, or their anger at unresponsive relationship partners. People who score high on the avoidance dimension tend to decrease their sense of vulnerability, suppress any tendency to express need, and make an effort to go it alone. People who score high on both dimensions—the ones Bartholomew (1990) called fearful (or fearfully avoidant)—may vacillate between the two strategies, continue to feel vulnerable while withdrawing behaviorally, or become "disorganized and disoriented" (Main & Solomon, 1990), which amounts to forgoing any coherent attachment strategy.

When one takes the behavioral system, or behavioral strategy, perspective rather than the model of self and model of others perspective, one realizes that further specification of the concerns, appraisals, and emotional processes that underlie adult attachment experiences and behavior need not be limited to positive and negative beliefs about self and others. Moreover, it becomes easier to see that "preoccupied" people, who are clearly high on attachment anxiety, do not necessarily have a positive model of others. As may be seen throughout this book, they tend to be jealous, distrustful, easily angered, and sometimes violent—reactions that are not well characterized as "positive" toward others. Nor do dismissingly avoidant people have simple positive models of self. In fact, when their defenses are interfered with (e.g., Mikulincer, Dolev, & Shaver, 2004), they are revealed to have actively suppressed negative self-conceptions.

Our general point is that although researchers from both the "internal working models" and "behavioral systems" perspectives currently assess individual differences using scales that measure the same empirical dimensions (the two dimensions shown throughout this chapter to underlie most self-report measures of attachment style), there are differences in the way the dimensions are conceptualized and different perspectives on which associated constructs should be measured, and how the attachment measures themselves should be used and revised. It is not yet clear how best to conceptualize the dimensions, although for the time being we have chosen the "behavioral systems" approach rather than the "internal working models" approach. We accept that there are working models, but we do not believe they are directly measured by the major self-report attachment scales. Keeping working models conceptually distinct from measures of attachment-related emotions and behavior allows us to retain the complexity in Bowlby's (1969/1982) discussions of working models, which he thought could exist at different levels of consciousness and be in conflict across these different levels.

Optimal Configuration of the Dimensions

Another issue is that once one accepts that dimensional measures of attachment are superior to categorical measures, one still has a choice regarding how best to conceptualize the two-dimensional space shown in Figure 4.2. Brennan et al. (1998) oriented their two dimensions to match Bartholomew's (1990) two dimensions, even though this would not have been necessary given that the "model of self" and "model of other" conceptualization of the dimensions (and of the space) might be misleading. Other authors have suggested that it would be better to rotate the axes of the measurement space and assess individual differences in security versus insecurity (along the secure-to-fearful axis in Figure 4.2) and anxiety versus avoidance (the dismissing-to-preoccupied axis in Figure 4.2) rather than differences along the anxiety and avoidance dimensions (e.g., Asendorpf, Banse, Wilpers, & Neyer, 1997; Banse, 2004; Elizur & Mintzer, 2003). For example, Asendorpf et al. (1997) consistently found that their data from dating and married couples fit a model in which a primary secure–fearful dimension was crossed by a secondary preoccupied–dismissing dimension.

A 45° rotation of the ECR dimensions fits well with the process model proposed by Shaver and Mikulincer (2002a; Mikulincer & Shaver, 2003; see Figure 2.1, this volume), a model in which appraisals of a threat, attachment figure availability, and the feasibility of hyperactivating and deactivating strategies occur in sequence. The rotated axes are also congruent with the two dimensions obtained by Brennan et al. (1991) when they factor-analyzed ratings of Hazan and Shaver's (1987) three prototype ratings and Bartholomew and Horowitz's (1991) four prototype ratings, and they correspond well with the two dimensions of the Kobak et al. (1993) Q-sort method of scoring the AAI and the Fyffe and Waters's (1997) discriminant function–based two-dimensional scoring system for the AAI, described later in this chapter.

As mentioned earlier in passing, the problem of mapping the two-dimensional space suggests the potential value of creating a measure that validly assesses all four axes shown in Figure 4.2. This was attempted by Klohnen and John (1998), but their measure has not found wide acceptance, and we have not been able to achieve a clean circumplex structure in our preliminary attempts to use it. There is also a question about how well simple adjectives can measure attachment styles as distinct from more general personality traits. The creation of a better four-axis measure remains, therefore, a worthy project for future research.

In some ways, the process model we proposed in Chapter 2 calls for multiple kinds of scales. In the second module in the model, the key issue is perceived attachment figure availability and the associated sense of felt security (or lack thereof). It might be useful to devise a unidimensional scale to measure felt security (similar to existing scales designed to measure other inner resources or strengths; e.g., optimism, hope, mastery, and self-efficacy). This scale would be designed to differentiate between relatively secure and relatively insecure people, and would be valuable in studies in which the main issue is the dispositional sense of security and the broaden-and-build cycle of security that emanates from it, rather than the forms and effects of attachment anxiety and avoidance. In the next module of the process model, researchers could use the ECR, ECR-R, or one of the similar measures reviewed earlier in this chapter to assess the two main dimensions of attachment insecurity, anxiety, and avoidance. This kind of scale could be used in studies of broadly "normal" samples, in which the main issue is the effect of a particular kind of "organized" or "strategic" attachment insecurity on some other variable or outcome.

Although we might interpret high scores on both the anxiety and avoidance dimensions as an adequate index of fearful avoidance or disorganized attachment given that the severe forms of this pattern are likely to be prevalent in clinical samples and in studies motivated by clinical issues, it might be worthwhile to create more specialized scales to probe specific forms or manifestations of disorganized attachment or failed attachment strategies. These scales might distinguish between people with organized attachment strategies (including "normal" hyperactivating or deactivating tendencies) and those with a disorganized pattern of attachment.

These different kinds of measures would undoubtedly be correlated with each other, but they might be sufficiently different and distinct in their other correlates to be useful in mapping the full array of normal and abnormal attachment orientations. They might also help create bridges between attachment research, other theoretical approaches to close relationships, and clinical psychology and psychiatry. Hence, they are worthy topics for future research.

General and Relationship-Specific Attachment Orientations

Yet another issue is the need to choose the kind of social relationship, or relationship category, to be targeted by self-report measures of attachment style. It is possible, for example, to ask about relationships with parents and romantic partners, about a particular relationship with one romantic partner, or about all close relationship partners (in the present or in one's entire history). Adult attachment research, as reviewed throughout this book, clearly indicates that attachment style can be meaningfully measured at a fairly abstract level, and that secure and insecure attachment orientations are relevant to much more than primary attachment relationships. This fact seems to bother some authors (e.g., E. Waters, Crowell, Elliott, Corcoran, & Treboux, 2002), because they think of attachment as a process that occurs only in a very few kinds of relationships. To us, however, expanding the applicability of the attachment style construct opens the door to important conceptual links between attachment theory and other topics of interest to psychologists.

As we explained in previous chapters, attachment working models have been conceptualized as hierarchically arranged, running from, at bottom, episodic memories of interactions with particular relationship partners through representations of kinds of attachment relationships (e.g., child–parent, romantic, close friendship), to generic representations of attachment relationships (e.g., Collins & Read, 1994; Shaver, Collins, & Clark, 1996). Researchers (e.g., Cozzarelli, Hoekstra, & Bylsma, 2000; Klohnen, Weller, Luo, & Choe, 2005; La Guardia, Ryan, Couchman, & Deci, 2000; Pierce & Lydon, 2001) are increasingly aware of the need to include both generic and relationship-specific measures of attachment orientations in their studies, a need further highlighted by the recurrent finding that these measures tap distinguishable but correlated constructs. (It had already been shown, years before, that an infant's attachment pattern with its mother could differ from the same infant's pattern with its father or a day care worker; see Chapter 5, this volume.)

Bowlby (1969/1982) had little research to guide him when he wrote about mental representations of attachment-related experiences: Bruner's (1973) operationalization of well-defined categories (e.g., cards containing red triangles and green squares), Piaget's (1953) ideas about cognitive schemas, and early examples of control systems theory or cybernetic control theory applied to military devices (early "smart bombs"). Today we have many information-processing theories (e.g., J. Anderson, 1994) that enable us to conceptualize working models in terms of associative neural networks that change subtly or dramatically depending on context and recent experiences. In such neural network theories, the "hierarchy" notion mentioned in the previous paragraph is cast in terms of different and context-sensitive subsets of neural networks. There are not necessarily any clear "types" or "levels." Thus, our notion of hierarchical levels is an abstraction, a theoretical convenience, not a concrete description of a psychological or neurological reality.

In reality a series of networks, each containing thousands or millions of neurons, together can represent either specific experiences or averages of many experiences, or mixtures of abstractions and specific experiences, depending on what is being thought about at a particular moment, or what has been mentioned or experienced recently. Presumably, just as repeated experiences in other domains lead to excitatory and inhibitory connections between many nodes in a neural network, which at the experiential and behavioral levels represent fairly stable, familiar concepts and patterns of thinking and feeling, repeated experiences with attachment figures, especially the most important experiences, create central tendencies in neural networks that can be conveniently referred to as generic working models. These central tendencies, however, can be modified by many contextual factors and can color interactions with people (and groups of people) who are not attachment figures themselves.

This conception of working models has implications for measurement. The outcome of a particular measurement effort depends on which networks are accessed by, or constructed during, the measurement procedure. Particular questions and instructions in either an interview or a self-report questionnaire can affect responses. If we ask research participants to describe a particular ongoing relationship, we may get different results than if we ask about close relationships in general. If we ask about an adult's relationship with his or her mother now, we may get different results than if we ask about the earliest memories he or she has of relating to mother during childhood. The fact that in our studies we obtain systematic, theory-consistent findings using generic self-report attachment measures—results based on diverse reactions, including behaviors, physiological responses, and reaction times in cognitive tasks (i.e., not just self-reports)—indicates that the generic level of measurement is psychologically meaningful. But this does not mean that generic measures are equivalent to measures of childhood relationships with particular parents, or current relationships with specific relationship partners.

A study by Overall, Fletcher, and Friesen (2003) provided evidence concerning the cognitive organization of attachment representations. These authors asked people to complete self-reports of attachment style for three specific relationships within each of three domains—family, friendship, and romantic relationship. They then examined whether all of these measures were organized within (1) a single, global working model summarizing attachment orientations across relationships and domains; (2) three independent working models for the domains of family, friendship, and romantic relationship; or (3) a hierarchical arrangement of specific and global working models. Confirmatory factor analyses showed that the hierarchical model fit the data best, indicating that ratings of attachment orientations for specific relationships are nested within, or organized under, relationship domain representations, which in turn are nested within, or organized under, a single, global attachment working model. Further studies should be conducted to extend this pioneering work. Although, as we have said, the results do not reveal how the brain actually represents these hierarchical relations among attachment representations, they do suggest that thinking about attachment measures in terms of hierarchical levels is still useful.

NARRATIVE AND INTERVIEW MEASURES OF ATTACHMENT

We turn now to a brief discussion of the use of narrative and interview measures of adult attachment. The use of narratives is based on the idea that "mental processes vary as distinctively as do behavioral processes" (Main et al., 1985, p. 78) and that representational processes are reflected in language. According to Crowell, Fraley, and Shaver (1999) the scoring of narrative measures such as the Adult Attachment Interview (AAI) is based

> on the concept of attachment security—that is, the ability of an individual to use an attachment figure as a secure base from which to explore and a safe haven in times of distress or danger (secure), versus the inability to do so (insecure). The assessments ultimately derive their validity from observations of attachment behavior in natural settings. Each measure was designed to have the same basic structure—that is, to include an assessment of the continuum from secure to insecure, and secondarily to assess differences among insecure strategies. (p. 438)

Adult Attachment Interview

In what Main et al. (1985) called "a move to the level of representation" (in contrast to the Strange Situation's emphasis on infant *behavior*), they interviewed adults about their childhood experiences with attachment figures (using questions updated by George, Kaplan, and Main in 1996). They were interested not only—in fact, not even primarily—in people's actual answers to questions about these experiences but also to indications that working models, viewed as complex affective–cognitive structures and processes, were either allowing or not allowing access to attachment-related information in memory

(Main et al., 1985, p. 77). In the AAI, an adult is interviewed about "his or her general view of the relationship with parents; ordinary experiences with parents in which the attachment system is presumed to be activated (upset, injury, illness, separation); experiences of loss; and finally the meaning that the adult attributes to these experiences" (Crowell, Fraley, & Shaver, 1999, p. 438). In their initial studies, Main and her coworkers (1985) already knew the Strange Situation classifications of their adult interviewees' infants, and they were looking, in part, for features of the adults' interviews that might "predict" (or actually, postdict) the infants' classifications.

The AAI is tape-recorded and transcribed, and the transcripts are coded, like Strange Situation videotapes, according to a complex scoring system meant to capture both the content of what the interviewee says—for example, that the mother was loving, neglectful, or abusive—and unintended qualities of the person's discourse, such as incoherence, inconsistency, and emotional disorganization. Scoring is based primarily on a person's ability to give an integrated, believable account of his or her experiences and the implications of these experiences for the person's development and performance as a parent, which the measure's developers took to be reflections of a person's "current state of mind with respect to attachment" (Hesse, 1999; Main et al., 1985). The interview and its scoring system have been repeatedly refined over a period of 20 years but never published. The procedure is taught at special workshops, and the number of trained scorers is still relatively small. The most complete and useful published description of the interview and coding system is the one provided by Hesse (1999).

Main and Goldwyn's Scoring System

AAI classifications are based on two sets of scales—parental behavior scales and state of mind scales—that characterize an interviewee's childhood experiences with each parent, in the coder's opinion. The parental behavior scales, used separately for mother and father, are [parent was] loving, rejecting, neglecting, involving, or pressuring. They are scored in terms of the coder's best judgment, not necessarily based literally on what an interviewee says (because he or she might be defensively withholding information or misunderstanding the implications of his or her own statements, hesitations, and inconsistencies). The state of mind scales assess discourse coherence and are labeled: idealization, insistence on lack of recall, active anger, derogation of parents or of attachment, fear of loss, metacognitive monitoring, and passivity of speech. Based on these features, a coder judges the overall coherence of the transcript and the interviewee's "coherence of mind." Scale score patterns, or profiles, are used to assign an interviewee to one of three major categories: secure ("Free and autonomous with respect to attachment") or one of the two major insecure categories ("Dismissing of attachment" or "Enmeshed and preoccupied with attachment"). Individuals classified as secure (i.e., autonomous)

> maintain a balanced view of early relationships, value attachment relationships, and view attachment-related experiences as influential in their development. In parallel to the direct approach of the secure infant, the autonomous adult's approach to the interview is open, direct, and cooperative, regardless of how difficult the material is to discuss. The interview itself contains coherent, believable reports of behavior by parents. . . . Because security is inferred from coherence, any kind of childhood experience may be associated with being classified as autonomous, although in many cases parental behavior is summarized as loving, and there are clear and specific memories given of loving behavior by the parents. (Crowell, Fraley, & Shaver, 1999, p. 439)

Dismissing adults, in contrast, are uncomfortable being interviewed about their childhood relationships, typically deny the influence of early attachment relationships on their current personality, have difficulty recalling specific events (often hesitating before answering), and often idealize or attempt to put a positive spin on what to a coder seem to be negative experiences. A coder moves toward a dismissing classification if the person seems to have been rejected by one or both parents or pushed away, despite his or her claim that the parents were loving. Adults classified as preoccupied seem anxious and/or angry when discussing childhood relationships with parents and still enmeshed in these experiences, and they tend to give long-winded answers marked by confusion or inconsistency. Some seem to have had intrusive parents, including ones who demanded to be taken care of instead of providing good care themselves.

People can also be classified as "unresolved" (with respect to losses, traumas, or abuse), in addition to being assigned to one of the other three categories. Unresolved adults report attachment-related traumas of loss and/or abuse, manifest confusion and disorganization in the discussion of trauma-related experiences, and tend to suffer from severe attachment insecurities. There is also a "cannot classify" designation for people whose coding scale profiles do not resemble any of the standard profiles (e.g., they might be incoherent to different degrees, or in different ways, when discussing mother and father [Hesse, 1999] or show signs of otherwise distinct patterns during different parts of the interview).

Q-Sort Scoring System

The Adult Attachment Q-Sort is an alternative method of scoring the AAI (Kobak, 1993; Kobak et al., 1993). It emphasizes the relation between affect regulation and attachment representations by examining the use of secure versus insecure emotion regulation strategies and minimizing (deactivating) versus maximizing (hyperactivating) strategies. A forced normal distribution of 100 descriptors sorted into nine categories along a single continuum is used by coders to create scores on two conceptual dimensions: security–insecurity and deactivation–hyperactivation (roughly speaking, the diagonal axes of Figure 4.2). Security is inferred from coherence and cooperation during the interview and convincing memories of supportive attachment figures (as judged by coders). Deactivation corresponds to dismissing strategies, whereas hyperactivation corresponds to the excessive detail and active anger often seen in the transcripts of preoccupied adults. The deactivating and hyperactivating strategies lie at opposite ends of a single dimension, which is assumed to be orthogonal to the secure–insecure dimension. An individual's transcript is rated by multiple coders, which allows average intercoder reliability to be increased to any desired level by increasing the number of coders. The scoring system is probably easier to learn than the one originally developed for the AAI. The individual's average item scores can be correlated with expert-based prototypic scores for the two major dimensions. The resulting correlations can be used to classify an adult into the usual AAI categories (not counting "unresolved" and "cannot classify"). When this is done, approximately 80% of individuals receive the same classification with the Q-sort system as with the original system (kappa = .65).

Another method of scoring the AAI on continuous dimensions, based on a discriminant analysis similar to the ones conducted by Ainsworth et al. (1978) for the Strange Situation and by Hazan and Shaver (1987) for their romantic attachment measure, was explored by Fyffe and Waters (1997). They created two linear combinations of coding scales (e.g., mother loving and coherence of transcript) based on samples from five AAI studies involving over 350 adults. One function distinguished between the autonomous (secure) category and all insecure categories (with 89% accuracy), and the other distinguished the dismissing category from the preoccupied category (with 96% accuracy). The coder rating of "coherence of transcript" correlated .96 with the security function, indicating that the secure–insecure judgment made by coders was virtually identical with their coherence judgment.

Reflective Functioning

Fonagy, Steele, Steele, Moran, and Higgitt (1991) developed a method of scoring the AAI in terms of something they called "reflective self," or "reflective functioning," an adult's quality of understanding his or her own and other people's mental states (e.g., intentions, motives). In a study of 200 parents, self-reflective functioning as assessed from AAI transcripts correlated highly with the usual "coherence of mind" score, but it was an even better predictor of an interviewee's infant's Strange Situation security than was coherence. This is interesting theoretically, because it suggests that a parent's reflective functioning contributes to his or her accurate understanding and effective parenting of a young child (i.e., it is an aspect of good caregiving).

Psychometric Properties of the AAI

In an early meta-analysis, Bakermans-Kranenburg and van IJzendoorn (1993) found that the distribution of AAI classifications in nonclinical samples was 58% autonomous (secure), 24% dismissing, and 18% preoccupied. About 19% of individuals also received an unresolved classification in association with a major classification. Within these normative samples, about 11% of people classified as autonomous, 26% of the dismissing group, and 40% of the preoccupied group were also classified as unresolved. Of people classified as unresolved, 38% had a major classification of autonomous, 24% of dismissing, and 38% of preoccupied. These results suggest, in line with many subsequent studies, that being unresolved with respect to loss, trauma, or abuse is more common among people with a primary classification of preoccupied. The base rate of insecurity in clinical and at-risk samples is much higher than in nonclinical samples: 8% autonomous, 26% dismissing, 25% preoccupied, and 40% unresolved (Bakermans-Kranenburg & van IJzendoorn, 1993).

High stability of attachment classifications (78–90% for three classification groups across periods ranging from 2 weeks to 18 months) has been observed in a number of studies using the original AAI scoring system (e.g., Bakermans-Kranenburg & van IJzendoorn, 1993; Benoit & Parker, 1994). There are no consistent gender differences in AAI classifications, although in some studies there are more preoccupied women and more dismissing men (see Shaver, Papalia, et al. [1996] for similar results using self-report measures). AAI security is generally not associated with IQ or discourse coherence when people discuss topics other than attachment history (Hesse, 1999). There is an association between AAI scores and self-reports of how one was parented (de Haas, Bakermans-Kranenburg, & van IJzendoorn, 1994), but the correlation is not so high as to suggest that self-reports could substitute for interview codes.

Current Relationship Interview

In the last decade, several interviews have been developed to assess adult attachment within close relationships: the Current Relationship Interview (CRI; Crowell & Owens,

1996), the Couple Attachment Interview (CAI; Alexandrov, Cowan, & Cowan, 2005), the Family and Peer Attachment Interview (Bartholomew & Horowitz, 1991), the Attachment Style Interview (Bifulco, Lillie, Ball, & Moran, 1998); the Marital Attachment Interview (Dickstein, Seifer, St. Andre, & Schiller, 2001), and the Romantic Relationship Interview (Furman, Simon, Shaffer, & Bouchey, 2002). These interviews and their coding systems have been adapted from the AAI and provide three or four categorical classifications of a person's state of mind with respect to current attachment to a close relationship partner (e.g., dating partner, spouse, or friend). There is evidence that these interviews are associated with relational cognitions and behaviors, and indices of relationship quality and stability. Moreover, they relate strongly to AAI classifications. This suggests, if common method variance is ignored, that "state of mind with respect to attachment" to parents during childhood is the foundation on which state of mind with respect to one's current close relationships and relationship partners during adulthood is constructed.

In this section, we focus on the CRI, because it is the most frequently used interview procedure for assessing adult attachment in couple relationships (e.g., Crowell, Treboux, Gao, et al., 2002; Crowell, Treboux, & Waters, 2002; Roisman, Collins, Sroufe, & Egeland, 2005; Treboux, Crowell, & Waters, 2004). The CRI asks an adult interviewee to describe his or her couple relationship and provide examples of using the partner as a secure base and of providing a secure base for the partner. Like the AAI, it is scored by coders from a transcript, and coder ratings are used to characterize (1) the interviewee's behavior and thinking about attachment-related issues (e.g., valuing of intimacy and independence); (2) the partner's behavior; and (3) the interviewee's discourse style (e.g., anger, derogation, idealization, passivity of speech, fear of loss, and overall coherence).

The secure–insecure distinction in the CRI is based on coherent reports of being able to use the partner as a secure base and to provide a secure base, or the coherently expressed desire to do so. Individuals who cannot coherently discuss these issues are divided into two categories: persons who avoid discussion of these behaviors or dismiss their significance (similar to the AAI and RQ dismissing category) and those who appear to be preoccupied with the relationship and intent on controlling it. As explained by Crowell, Fraley, & Shaver (1999, p. 445):

> These factors are given primacy in the determination of attachment security, rather than the individual's reported feelings about the relationship or the behaviors of the partner. Thus, whereas most individuals who are classified as secure with the CRI have good relationships with their partners, this is not a requirement for such a classification. Rather, they must value attachment and coherently describe their relationships with respect to the secure base elements. Similarly, a number of individuals classified as insecure with the CRI are satisfied with their current relationships. They are classified as insecure because they are incoherent in describing the secure-base phenomenon within the relationship.

An "unresolved" designation is given to a transcript, in addition to one of the three major classifications, if a previous romantic relationship is exerting a disruptive or disorganizing influence on the individual's language or reasoning. This is similar to the designation of "unresolved with respect to loss" in the AAI.

The distribution of CRI classifications is similar to that of AAI classifications, and the distribution of couple classifications is such that the most common patterns are ones in which both partners are secure or both are insecure, similar to what has been found using self-report attachment style measures (e.g., Crowell, Treboux, et al., 2002; Treboux et al., 2004). The CRI shows good temporal stability over a period of 18 months (Crowell, Treboux, et al., 2002) and is generally unrelated to intelligence, education, gender, duration of a person's current couple relationship, or self-reported depression (e.g., Crowell, Treboux, & Waters, 2002; Treboux et al., 2004). Across different samples, the correspondence between the AAI and the CRI is high and ranges from 55 to 71%. CRI classifications have predicted self-reports of relationship quality, violence, and satisfaction, and they mediate the association between AAI scores and these relational variables (e.g., Treboux et al., 2004).

Adult Attachment Projective

In an extension of the projective methodology used in some child attachment research (e.g., story completion tests) to the study of adult attachment, George and West (2001) developed the Adult Attachment Projective (AAP). Instead of relying on autobiographical narratives of childhood experiences or current relationships, George and West believe that "the shifting balance of adaptive and defensive processes, guided by mental representations of attachment, can be evidenced in adults' story responses to pictures of hypothetical attachment situations" (pp. 31–32).

The AAP consists of eight drawings, one neutral scene and seven pictures of attachment situations dealing with illness, solitude, separation, loss, and abuse. For example, the "departure" picture depicts an adult man and woman facing each other, with suitcases positioned nearby, and the "cemetery" picture depicts a man standing by a gravesite headstone. The interviewee is asked to look at each picture and tell a story (what is happening, what led up to the depicted situation, what might happen next, and what the story subject might be feeling or thinking). The entire set of eight stories is taped, transcribed, and coded by a trained, reliable coder. As with the AAI and CRI, coding the narrative transcripts requires lengthy training.

The AAP assesses the same four adult attachment classifications as the AAI. In the first step, coders rate two aspects of narrative discourse: coherence of the stories, based on the same coding rules as the AAI, and the extent to which the interviewee allows unsought intrusions of autobiographical memories into his or her stories (this kind of intrusion is interpreted as a sign that the interviewee is overwhelmed by attachment-related distress). In the second step, coders rate attachment-related aspects of the story, such as the extent to which the character (1) is portrayed as capable of taking effective steps to manage distress or cope with stress, (2) expresses a desire to interact with others, and (3) engages in mutual, reciprocal interpersonal interactions. Coders also examine stories for markers of attachment-system deactivation (e.g., negative evaluation of others, distancing, rejection, dismissal of relationships), attachment-system hyperactivation (e.g., anger, unfinished thoughts, indecision, worry, emotionality), and unresolved attachment (isolation, helplessness, emptiness, lack of control, odd or disturbing themes). Based on these ratings, coders place an interviewee in one of the four attachment categories.

George and West (2001) and van Ecke, Chope, and Emmelkamp (2005) reported high interrater reliabilities for both secure–insecure classifications and the four attachment types. George and West (2001) also reported high convergence between the AAP and the AAI for the four attachment classifications ($r = .94$, kappa = .86). The measure is fairly new and has not yet been widely used, so it remains to be independently validated.

COMPARING NARRATIVE AND SELF-REPORT ASSESSMENT TECHNIQUES

An important question in adult attachment research is whether attachment patterns are best assessed with self-reports or interviews. A related issue is whether different methods converge on the same phenomenon (e.g., Bartholomew & Shaver, 1998; Crowell & Treboux, 1995). Although some investigators use both kinds of methods (e.g., Simpson, Rholes, Orina, & Grich, 2002; Treboux et al., 2004), the two approaches have generated two fairly distinct lines of research (as discussed by Rholes & Simpson, 2004; Shaver & Mikulincer, 2002a, 2002b). The two lines both derive from Bowlby's and Ainsworth's writings, and both deal with secure and insecure strategies of emotion regulation and behavior in close relationships. But researchers working in the two different traditions tend to identify with different subfields of psychology (developmental and clinical in one case, personality and social in the other), and largely ignore each other's work. Most social psychologists do not use the AAI or the CRI and have not attempted to link their self-report measures developmentally with earlier assessments of attachment quality in Ainsworth's Strange Situation. Most developmental and clinical psychologists who use the AAI do not also use social psychologists' self-report measures or laboratory experimental methods developed by social cognition researchers.

The two lines of attachment research have remained separate partly because of the research questions motivating investigators—intergenerational transmission of attachment patterns versus social-cognitive dynamics affecting feelings and behavior in adult close relationships. Also, investigators in the two traditions have largely accepted the idea that the AAI and self-report attachment measures are unrelated. This belief is based on the substantial differences between the AAI and self-report attachment measures in targeted relationships (parent–child vs. adult couple relationships), method (coded interview transcripts vs. brief self-reports), and analytic focus (structural properties of discourse coherence and believability when discussing attachment experiences vs. the content of a person's perceptions, feelings, and self-observed behavior). The belief that the two kinds of measures assess different constructs is mainly based on comparisons at the categorical level, and to the extent that categories are inappropriate (Fraley & Waller, 1998) or are defined somewhat differently across different measures, relations between more detailed aspects of different measures can be overlooked when categories prove not to correspond well (e.g., Crowell & Treboux, 1995).

Another barrier to integrating the two lines of research is AAI researchers' supposition that self-report measures cannot plumb the psychodynamic depths revealed by the AAI. As Jacobvitz, Curran, and Moller (2002) asserted: "The AAI classification coding system assesses *adults' unconscious processes for regulating emotion.* . . . Unlike the AAI, the self-report measures of attachment tap adults' *conscious appraisals* of themselves in romantic relationships" (p. 208, emphasis in original). Such researchers believe that because self-report measures involve conscious, deliberate answers to explicit questions, they are probably limited to indexing conscious mental processes.

Moreover, AAI researchers (e.g., Belsky, 2002; Bernier & Dozier, 2002; Jacobvitz et al., 2002; E. Waters et al., 2002) believe that their approach is superior in delineating the information-processing strategies of dismissing and preoccupied adults, evoking rich narrative accounts of attachment relationships that reflect interviewees' internal working models, relating attachment working models to social behavior, and discovering how adult attachment patterns emerge from a person's attachment history. Such researchers also suspect that self-report measures of attachment style suffer from a lack of discriminant validity insofar as they correlate with other self-report measures, including scales measuring trait anxiety and depression.

Reasoning along similar (or mirror image) lines, personality/social psychologists tend to doubt that the complex scoring procedures for the AAI and CRI are necessary for probing key attachment-related dynamics, and they suspect that measures such as the AAI and CRI are related to each other and to certain kinds of behavior because they share method variance with each other and with those behavioral measures. (The AAI and CRI are, in a sense, coded samples of dyadic social behavior involving accurate listening, cooperating with an interviewer, and talking coherently about attachment-related memories and feelings. The same processes are presumably involved in constructive parent–child interactions and interactions of marital partners.)

In the following section, we review findings concerning the convergence of narrative and self-report measures of attachment. We also examine the research literature in the self-report (plus experimental manipulations) tradition, to which we belong, to see if the AAI researchers' criticisms stand up to the evidence.

Evidence for Convergence (or Lack of Convergence) between Assessment Methods

Over the past decade, 10 published studies have examined associations between the AAI and self-report measures of adult attachment (Bouthillier, Julien, Dubé, Bélanger, & Hamelin, 2002; Creasey & Ladd, 2005; Crowell, Treboux, & Waters, 1999; de Haas et al., 1994; Holtzworth-Munroe, Stuart, & Hutchinson, 1997; Shaver et al., 2000; Simpson et al., 2002; Stanojević, 2004; Treboux et al., 2004; E. Waters et al., 2002). Overall, the findings are not consistent. Whereas some studies have found that self-reports of attachment anxiety and avoidance are not significantly associated with AAI classifications (e.g., Simpson et al., 2002; Waters et al., 2002), others have found significant, but only moderate, associations between self-report and interview measures of attachment patterns (e.g., Creasey & Ladd, 2005; Shaver et al., 2000). Moreover, whereas some researchers found that these associations were significant only for self-reported avoidance (Bouthillier et al., 2002; Holtzworth-Munroe et al., 1997; Treboux et al., 2004), others found significant associations only for self-reported anxiety (Creasey & Ladd, 2005; Crowell, Treboux, & Waters, 1999).

In a study of over 100 married women, Shaver et al. (2000) found that the two AAS avoidance scales (assessing discomfort with closeness and dependence on partners) could be predicted from AAI coding scales with multiple R's around .50. Interestingly, the most heavily weighted predictor was "coherence of mind" (beta = .40), the essence of AAI security. The anxiety dimension was predictable, with an R of .30, due mainly to the AAI coding scale assessing whether or not the father was portrayed by a female interviewee as loving. Analyses running in the other direction revealed that every AAI coding scale except one was predictable from self-report items. For example, the R for predicting "coherence of mind" was .40, and one of the major predictors was the theoretically central item, "I am not sure that I can always depend on others to be there when I need them."

These results differed from those in other comparison studies by looking at the coding scales in the AAI and particular items in the AAS, rather than simply comparing attachment patterns at a categorical level. Shaver et al. (2000) concluded that at a detailed level, the two assessment procedures were more related than several other researchers had said they were (based on categories). They also speculated that the AAI, which was initially validated in terms of its ability to predict the Strange Situation classification of a parent's infant might be a measure of caregiving rather than attachment orientation (see Chapter 11, this volume, for a discussion of caregiving). We mention these associations not to imply that scores on the two kinds of measures are similar in meaning, which they most certainly are not, but to show that both are related in sensible ways to the central concepts of attachment theory.

Implicit, Unconscious Correlates of Self-Reports of Attachment Style

A number of authors have questioned the ability of self-report measures of attachment style to relate to implicit, unconscious aspects of attachment-system functioning (e.g., Crowell & Treboux, 1995; Hesse, 1999; Jacobvitz et al., 2002). We agree that it is possible for some people to defensively report that they are not worried about rejection and separation, when actually they are worried, and for some not to have conscious access to such worries even though the worries exist. However, although attachment style scales can be biased by social desirability concerns and other motivational tendencies and cognitive limitations, there are good reasons for continuing to use them to index implicit aspects of attachment-system functioning, as Crowell, Fraley, and Shaver (1999) have explained. First, most adults have sufficient experience in close relationships to provide valuable information about their relational cognitions, feelings, and behavior. Their characteristic responses may reflect unconscious processes, even though these processes cannot be perceived and reported on directly. Second, conscious and unconscious processes typically operate in the same direction to achieve a goal, and unconscious motives are often manifested in conscious appraisals (Chartrand & Bargh, 2002). Third, even with people who defensively deny attachment needs or claim they do not suffer from attachment insecurities, "it is possible to use attachment theory to derive the kinds of conscious beliefs that defensive people may hold about themselves" (Crowell, Fraley, et al., 1999, p. 453). For these reasons, we are often able to predict from self-reports how a person is likely to behave under certain conditions, even if the people providing the reports are not able to make the same predictions. This kind of prediction is commonly made in studies based on other kinds of self-report scales, such as measures of narcissism (Morf & Rhodewalt, 2001); it is not unique to the attachment domain.

Beyond these conceptual considerations, research using self-report measures of attachment style has already revealed many theoretically predictable associations between self-reported attachment style and indices of implicit, unconscious processes. As we show throughout this book, self-reports of attachment anxiety and avoidance are associated with implicit mental processes assessed in a wide variety of cognitive tasks, such as lexical decision tasks, the Stroop color-naming task, the Implicit Association Task, and semantic priming tasks (e.g., Baldwin et al., 1993; Baldwin & Meunier, 1999; Mikulincer et al., 2004; Mikulincer, Gillath, & Shaver, 2002; Zayas & Shoda, 2005). In these studies, self-reports of attachment anxiety correctly predict implicit, unconscious preoccupation with attachment-related worries, whereas self-reports of avoidant attachment predict unconscious activation of negative representations of others and unconscious suppression of worries related to separation and rejection. In short, although self-report measures depend on conscious self-observations, they validly point to individual differences in unconscious mental processes as well.

In another line of research, investigators have assessed physiological correlates of self-reported attachment style. Self-reports are associated in theoretically predictable ways with activation of the autonomic nervous system, as indexed by heart rate, blood pressure, and skin conductance (e.g., E. M. Carpenter & Kirkpatrick, 1996; L. M. Diamond & Hicks, 2005; Fraley & Shaver, 1997; Kim, 2006). We review such findings throughout this volume.

Recently, Berant, Mikulincer, Shaver, and Segal (2005) adopted another strategy for examining the unconscious correlates of self-reported attachment style. They administered a self-report attachment measure, together with the well-known Rorschach Inkblot Test (1942)—one of the most frequently used projective methods for assessing a person's implicit cognitive representations, unconscious motives, and underlying mental organization (Exner, 1993). We found, as predicted, that self-reported attachment anxiety, which is assumed to reflect hyperactivation of negative emotions, rumination on distress, and negative models of self, were associated with Rorschach test codes indicating distress and emotional outbursts, lack of ability to regulate and control emotional experience, and distorted perception of oneself as helpless, weak, disgusting, and unlikable. Moreover, self-reported avoidant attachment, which is theoretically associated with deactivation of negative emotions and defensive maintenance of self-esteem, was associated with Rorschach test codes reflecting inhibition of emotional expression, a tendency to hide behind a false facade, and a grandiose, inflated self-image.

Once again, therefore, a measure designed to tap unconscious processes, one used frequently in clinical settings, produced results compatible with both attachment theory and the validity of self-report measures of attachment style. In later sections and chapters we review studies that include measures of Thematic Apperception Test (TAT) narratives and systematically coded dreams. Although not yet definitive, such studies strongly suggest that self-reports of attachment style are predictably associated with measures of implicit and automatic mental processes. Thus, we reject the criticism that self-report measures of attachment style reflect mainly response biases or conscious attitudes and fail to correlate with implicit, unconscious aspects of attachment-system functioning.

Dismissing and Preoccupied Information-Processing Strategies

Another criticism of self-report measures of attachment style is that they do not tap the same information-processing strategies assessed by the AAI (e.g., Bernier & Dozier, 2002; Crowell & Treboux, 1995; Hesse, 1999). Specifically, self-report scales are viewed as inadequate ways to assess what Main and colleagues (1985) called "dismissing" and "preoccupied" states of mind. Bernier and Dozier (2002, p. 173) concluded, for example, that "the AAI and self-reports of adult attachment tap related but distinct manifestations of the attachment system." We readily agree that self-reports of attachment style are not identical with coded dimensions of the AAI. This does not mean, however, that attachment style scales fail to relate to the information-processing strategies assessed by the AAI. In fact, recent studies that have examined the strategies characteristic of dismissing and preoccupied attachment using techniques other than the AAI have turned up theoretically predicted associations with self-report scales.

For example, one important AAI coding scale that identifies a dismissing state of mind is "idealization of the primary attachment figure" (Main et al., 1985). According to Hesse (1999), "This scale assesses the discrepancy between the overall view of the parent taken from the subject's speech at the abstract or semantic level, and [the coder's] inferences regarding the probable behavior of the parent" (p. 403). Shaver and Mikulincer (2004) found that self-reports of avoidance predicted idealization of the mother in a sample of Israeli undergraduates. Idealization was measured in terms of the discrepancy between adjectives chosen by each study participant to describe his or her mother and written memory narratives about the relationship with the mother.

A second AAI coding scale used to identify a dismissing state of mind is "lack of memory for childhood" (Main et al., 1985). According to Hesse (1999), "This scale assesses the speaker's insistence upon her inability to recall her childhood, especially as this insistence is used to block further queries or discourse" (p. 403). Using methods borrowed from cognitive psychology (e.g., memory retrieval times, forgetting curves), researchers who use self-report measures of avoidant attachment have found them to be related to poor memory of childhood experiences and other attachment-related information (e.g., Edelstein et al., 2005; Mikulincer & Orbach, 1995; Fraley, Garner, & Shaver, 2000; see Chapter 7, this volume).

A third AAI coding scale that defines the dismissing state of mind is "active derogating dismissal of attachment-related experiences and/or relationships." In Hesse's (1999) words, "This scale deals with the cool, contemptuous dismissal of attachment relationships or experiences and their import" (p. 403). Relevant to this scale, there is extensive evidence that self-reports of avoidance are related to derogating, negative evaluations of close relationships and relationship partners (e.g., Bartholomew & Horowitz, 1991; Collins & Read, 1990; see Chapter 6, this volume).

Adult attachment research also provides consistent evidence that self-reports of attachment anxiety are associated with one of Main and colleagues' (1985) defining characteristics of the preoccupied state of mind: experience and expression of dysfunctional anger toward attachment figures (e.g., Mikulincer, 1998b; Rholes, Simpson, & Orina, 1999; Woike, Osier, & Candela; 1996; see Chapter 7, this volume, for a review). Overall, these studies indicate that self-reports of attachment avoidance and anxiety are fairly accurate predictors of the information-processing strategies thought to be assessed by the AAI.

Narratives about Attachment Figures, Interactions, and Relationships

Some critics argue against the use of self-report measures because of their failure to evoke the rich, multifaceted material that appears in people's narratives about attachment experiences and relationships (e.g., Crowell & Treboux, 1995; Hesse, 1999). In their view, self-report attachment scales cannot probe a person's defenses or idiosyncratic attachment history, and researchers who use simple self-report scales fail to acknowledge that attachment-related processes are woven into contexts, experiences, and memories that differ importantly from person to person. We agree, of course, that the scores people receive on self-report attachment scales are not generated from detailed descriptions of their attachment figures and relationships. We acknowledge that coded interviews, such as the AAI and the CRI, are more useful than simple questionnaires in characterizing a person's unique narratives and specific mental representations. This does not mean, however, that attachment style scales are unrelated to such narratives and cannot serve as useful indicators of the way adults recount attachment-relevant descriptions and stories.

In support of this view, there are associations between attachment style scales and the thematic content and structure of narratives about significant others and interpersonal experiences (e.g., Avihou, 2006; Gilad, 2002; K. N. Levy, Blatt, & Shaver, 1998; Raz, 2002). These findings are based on a variety of qualitative methods, such as coding descriptions of significant others (parents, romantic partners), coding narratives of inter-personal interactions, coding dream narratives, and coding stories generated in response to projective tests (see Chapters 6 and 9, this volume, for details). Moreover, the findings are consistent across a variety of scoring systems, such as Blatt, Wein, Chevron, and Quinlan's (1992) object-representation scales, the core conflictual relationship themes scoring system (CCRT; Luborsky & Crits-Christoph, 1998), and the Social Cognition and Object Relations Scales (SCORS; Westen, 1991), which measure substantive and structural aspects of a person's representations of self, significant others, and close rela-tionships. These studies provide impressive evidence for the validity of self-report attach-ment scales as predictors of personal narratives and mental representations.

Behavioral Observations and Self-Reported Attachment Style

Another purported strike against self-report attachment scales is that they are a long way from actual social behavior (e.g., Crowell, Treboux, et al., 1999); that is, self-reports of attachment style, being subjective and nonbehavioral, are unlikely to be associated with behavior in close relationships. In contrast, AAI coders believe not only that they are clas-sifying people's mental and behavioral responses in an interview but also that they are doing so in ways that the people themselves could not match and, in some cases, with which they would not agree. This argument is raised especially vigorously in relation to dismissingly avoidant people, who are believed "to distort, disorganize, or limit access to memories, feelings, intentions, and recognition of options" (Main, 1991, p. 146). According to this view, an avoidant stance can bias self-reports of attachment style and reduce the correspondence of these reports with actual behavior. For example, people who act avoidantly in close relationships may be unaware of their avoidance or may defensively deny their cool detachment; therefore, they may rate themselves lower than they should on self-report items intended to detect avoidance. A similar critique might apply to anxiously attached individuals: They might be reluctant to answer honestly about their anxiety, because it could be viewed as weakness or as socially undesirable.

This criticism is amplified by the fact that research on attachment style has been dominated by correlational studies examining associations between self-report measures of attachment and other self-reports obtained from the same individuals. As a result, some of the high correlations between attachment scales and other self-report measures may be attributable to shared method variance, including shared social desirability bias and other response sets. Despite the plausibility of this critique, evidence is accumulating that self-reports of attachment style are predictably related to interpersonal behavior. Moreover, some adult attachment studies have included observer evaluations in addition to self-reports, and have documented considerable correspondence between the two sources of information (e.g., Collins & Feeney, 2000; Simpson et al., 1992; and many others discussed throughout this book).

Another set of studies revealed high levels of convergence between self-reported attachment styles and external observers' ratings of participants' traits (e.g., Banai, Weller, & Mikulincer, 1998; Bartholomew & Horowitz, 1991; Griffin & Bartholomew, 1994a; Onishi et al., 2001). For example, Banai et al. (1998) compared a participant's own ratings of attachment style with those made about him or her by two same-sex friends, two opposite-sex friends, and a stranger who took part in a 5-minute getting-acquainted conversation with the participant. In this study, both discrete and continuous self-descriptions of a person's attachment anxiety and avoidance were significantly related to the parallel descriptions of the person provided by same-sex friends, opposite-sex friends, and a new acquaintance. Even more important, high correlations were found among the five external observers' ratings. In addition, the strength of the correlations between self-descriptions and descriptions provided by other people was similar to that found in studies of other well-known traits (e.g., Funder & Colvin, 1988). These findings indicate that self-reports of attachment anxiety and avoidance reflect real and socially observable personal attributes, and that their status is similar to that of other observable personality traits. Moreover, they suggest that a person's attachment orientation, as measured by self-report scales, is evident to interaction partners even in the very early stages of a relationship.

Beyond this empirical evidence, the logic of critics' argument against self-reports is at odds with the generally accepted conceptualization of attachment-related strategies of affect regulation (Cassidy, 1994). First, the contention that avoidant individuals are reluctant to endorse avoidant items, because such items are socially undesirable, is inconsistent with the documented goals of interpersonal distance and emotional detachment that guide deactivating strategies (Mikulincer & Shaver, 2003). For avoidant people, being distant and cool toward a relationship partner is not a problem but a desirable way to manage close relationships. Second, the contention that anxious individuals might be reluctant to endorse items indicating anxious attachment is also at odds with theoretical accounts of hyperactivating strategies, which entail presenting oneself as weak, distressed, and vulnerable so as to elicit relationship partners' sympathy and support (Mikulincer & Shaver, 2003).

The Discriminant Validity of Self-Report Measures of Attachment Style

Beyond delineating the "nomothetic net" (Cronbach & Meehl, 1955) of theory-consistent empirical associations that establish the construct validity of self-report attachment style scales, attachment researchers also need to be concerned about these scales' discriminant validity. Do they overlap too much with measures of constructs viewed as theoretically unrelated to attachment organization? If so, it could be argued (e.g., E. Waters et al., 2002) that self-report measures actually measure something other than variations in attachment-system functioning. According to Bernier and Dozier (2002), "Perhaps the most widespread concern regarding attachment research is that we are tapping into a general personality construct that does not need attachment theory's rich and nuanced developmental conceptualizations to be explained" (p. 176).

Fortunately, the issue of discriminant validity has received empirical attention in adult attachment research (e.g., Griffin & Bartholomew, 1994b; Noftle & Shaver, 2006; Shaver & Brennan, 1992). Many studies clearly demonstrate that self-reports of attachment anxiety and avoidance, although correlating with a broad network of cognitive, emotional, and behavioral manifestations of hyperactivating and deactivating strategies (as shown throughout this volume), are not simply redundant with these constructs. Correlations between self-reports of attachment style and constructs derived from other theoretical or descriptive frameworks rarely exceed .50 (indicating less than 25% shared variance) and are usually considerably lower. This conclusion holds for associations between self-reported attachment anxiety and measures of neuroticism, trait anxiety, global distress, emotional intensity, emotion-focused ways of coping, self-esteem, self-efficacy, threat appraisal, relationship quality and satisfaction, cognitive representations of others, and intergroup attitudes (for reviews, see Chapters 6, 7, 10, and 13, this volume). It also holds for associations between self-reported avoidant attachment and measures of defensiveness, social desirability, coping by distancing, support seeking, mental representations of self and others, relationship quality, reactions to others' needs, and exploration and cognitive openness (for reviews, see Chapters 6, 7, 9, 10, and 11, this volume).

Several studies have demonstrated that self-reports of anxiety and avoidance explain theory-relevant cognitions, emotions, and behaviors even after controlling statistically for other personality constructs. For example, studies we review in Chapter 10 have found that self-reports of attachment style were associated prospectively with relationship length, satisfaction, and commitment, even after controlling for the "Big Five" personality traits—Extraversion, Neuroticism, Openness to Experience, Agreeableness, and Conscientiousness—depression, dysfunctional beliefs, self-esteem, or sex-role orientation. Moreover, behavioral observation studies by Simpson and Rholes's research team showed that the association between self-reports of attachment style and interpersonal behaviors, such as support seeking, support giving, and conflict resolution, were not explained by the Big Five traits, self-esteem, or relationship quality (e.g., Simpson et al., 1992, 1996; Simpson et al., 2002).

In many of our own studies, associations between self-reports of attachment style and creative problem solving, intergroup hostility, reactions to others' needs, accessibility of mental representations of attachment figures, rejection sensitivity, and appraisal of interpersonal competencies are all significant after controlling for positive mood, self-esteem, or trait anxiety (e.g., Mikulincer, Gillath, & Shaver, 2002; Mikulincer & Shaver, 2001). These findings indicate that the nomothetic net of theory-consistent correlates of attachment style cannot be explained by other constructs that are theoretically distant from attachment processes and organization.

The Developmental Origins of Self-Reported Attachment Style

Another frequently mentioned criticism of self-report studies of attachment is that they fail to examine the developmental roots of individual differences in anxiety and avoidance (e.g., Belsky, 2002; Bernier & Dozier, 2002); that is, although these studies provide important information about the cognitive, emotional, and behavioral manifestations of self-reported attachment patterns in adulthood, they fail to examine whether variations in these self-reports are systematically associated with childhood experiences. We agree that Bowlby (1969/1982) was deeply interested in personality development, and that a core proposition of attachment theory is that attachment patterns are a function of lived experiences, especially actual experiences within the family of origin in the first few years of life. Therefore, a rigorous test of the construct validity of attachment style scales should trace adult differences in anxiety and avoidance to childhood experiences.

In Chapter 5, we review evidence linking self-reports of adult attachment style to attachment-related experiences in childhood. These studies have consistently found, for example, that the childhood experiences theoretically expected to have a long-term disturbing effect on the development of attachment security, such as sexual or physical abuse, parental drinking problems, parental death, or parental divorce, are associated with heightened reports of attachment anxiety and avoidance in clinical and community samples (e.g., Brennan & Shaver, 1998; Brennan et al., 1991; Mallinckrodt, McCreary, & Robertson, 1995). Moreover, Sampson (2003) reported a 20-year correlation coefficient of .44 between observed parental support at age 2 and self-reported comfort with depending on romantic partners in early adulthood, the latter being measured by one scale in the AAS. In a recent analysis of longitudinal data from a 6-year study of adolescents and their parents, Nitzberg et al. (2007) found that both self-reported attachment style and observed behavior in interaction with dating, romantic, and eventually marital partners were related to each other at each time point study and predictable from observable interactions with parents earlier in the study.

CONCLUDING REMARKS

There are now many measures inspired by Bowlby and Ainsworth's attachment theory. They reflect different foci (parenting, romantic relationships, other relationships) and different methods (self-reports, interviews, projective narratives). Although the different measures do not all converge on the same constructs or the same level of analysis, there is good evidence that all have value, are related coherently to attachment theory, and often are related to each other. Because our own work has been based primarily on self-report measures of attachment style, combined with many other methods of measuring correlated behavior, conscious and unconscious mental processes, defenses, physiological processes, and so on, we have given disproportionate attention to self-report measures and their critics and defenders. As will be seen throughout this book, there are several studies of the same hypotheses that use different methods, and in most cases the different methods yield similar conclusions. Much more work is needed to understand and improve attachment measures. But given that our main goal in this book is to examine and organize existing empirical findings, we will be referring to methods described in this chapter, because they are the main ones that have been used to date. Probably many of the landmark studies will need to be repeated, in improved forms, when new and better attachment measures are developed. Meanwhile, we make do with the ones we have.

CHAPTER 5

■ ■ ■

Individual Differences
in Attachment-System Functioning

Development, Stability, and Change

> No variables, it can be held, have more far-reaching effects on personality development
> than have a child's experiences within his family; for, starting during the first months in
> his relation with his mother figure, and extending through the years of childhood and
> adolescence in his relations with both parents, he builds up working models of how
> attachment figures are likely to behave towards him in any of a variety of situations; and
> on those models are based all his expectations, and therefore all his plans, for the rest of
> his life.
>
> —JOHN BOWLBY (1973, p. 418)

Attachment theory is a multifaceted theory of personality structure, functioning, and development, as well as a theory of interpersonal behavior, emotional bonds, and close relationships. In our model (Chapter 2) and in most of the studies related to it, we have focused on attachment-system functioning in adulthood and variations in system parameters that affect intrapsychic processes and behavior in close relationships. Numerous studies of adult attachment are summarized in the other chapters of this book. However, because Bowlby (1973) and Ainsworth (1991) were deeply interested in the development of attachment patterns from infancy to adulthood, and because they sought to understand the cognitive and interpersonal factors responsible for continuity and discontinuity in these patterns throughout life, we devote this chapter to the developmental roots of adult attachment patterns. We do so by pursuing two of Bowlby's (1973) key propositions: (1) Attachment patterns are a function of lived experiences, especially actual experiences within one's family of origin during childhood, and (2) attachment patterns are fairly stable from infancy to adulthood, but are nevertheless open to change.

To characterize the development of attachment patterns, Bowlby (1973) drew an analogy between developmental trajectories and a complex railway system like the one in Great Britain at the time he was writing:

[The system] starts as a single main route which leaves a central metropolis in a certain direction but soon forks into a range of distinct routes. Although each of these routes diverges in some degree, initially most of them continue in a direction not very different from the original one. The further each route goes from the metropolis, however, the more branches it throws off and the greater the degree of divergence of direction that can occur. Nevertheless, although many of these sub-branches do diverge further, and yet further, from the original direction, others may take a course convergent with the original; so that ultimately they may even come to run in a direction close to, or even parallel with, routes that have maintained the original direction from the start. In terms of this model, the critical points are the junctions at which the lines fork, for once a train is on a particular line, pressures are present that keep in on that line; although, provided divergence does not become too great, there remains a chance of a train taking a convergent track when the next junction is reached. (pp. 413–414)

According to this analogy, at birth a person has a multitude of pathways along which he or she might develop, as well as a variety of attachment patterns he or she might construct and revise throughout life. Early experiences with caregivers determine the set of behavioral strategies a child uses to regulate proximity to attachment figures (e.g., sensitive and responsive parental caregiving reinforces confident and comfortable reliance on proximity seeking) and the quality of his or her working models of self and others (Bowlby, 1973). These early experiences may be particularly influential in shaping the parameters of the attachment system, and the organization and enactment of attachment behavior in subsequent relationships; that is, early experiences with parents may help to determine which of many possible developmental pathways a person actually takes and which attachment pattern tends to characterize his or her interactions with close relationship partners later in life.

In expounding the railway analogy, Bowlby (1973) contended that once the attachment system becomes organized by early experiences with primary caregivers, a number of psychological mechanisms make it likely that early working models of self and others will be sustained. He was influenced by Piaget's (1953) theory of cognitive development, according to which the mind, whenever possible, assimilates new information to existing knowledge structures. (The same idea is a mainstay of contemporary theories of social cognition. See Fiske & Taylor, 1991, for an overview.) People of all ages appraise, interpret, and remember attachment interactions in ways that conform to their beliefs and expectations. For example, people with a secure attachment history are likely to dismiss, ignore, or forgive temporary signs of a partner's inattentiveness or unavailability, but people with an anxious history are likely to be on the lookout for signs of inattentiveness and to be both hurt and angry when they detect such signs (see Chapters 9 and 10, this volume). Moreover, people frequently behave in ways that elicit expectation-consistent reactions from attachment figures, which in turn reinforce existing working models. For example, anxious, clinging behavior often annoys a partner and causes the partner to become more avoidant, thus confirming an anxiously attached person's chronic fear of rejection and abandonment (see Chapter 10, this volume).

Moreover, as Bowlby (1973) noted, people often attract relationship partners who fit their working models of others, and form attachments that maximize the congruence between current attachment experiences and preexisting models (see Chapter 10, this volume). These tendencies reinforce the models, which then continue to have a powerful shaping effect on experiences in close relationships. This process constrains some people to the developmental trajectory they established during infancy and childhood, allowing for a degree of predictability of adult attachment patterns from what can be observed in infancy and childhood.

However, Bowlby (1969/1982) also argued, as we explained in Chapter 1, that attachment working models are tolerably accurate reflections of what actually happened to a person in close relationships, and they are always subject to revision and updating in response to subsequent social experiences. This idea was also part of the theory of cognitive development by Piaget (1953), who conceptualized cognitive development as a process of accommodation of mental schemas to important new information that cannot be assimilated by existing schemas. Hence, even though people are likely to assimilate new information to existing working models, if possible, they are also able to update these models to accommodate new information when attachment-relevant experiences (e.g., losing an attachment figure, learning of a trusted partner's secret infidelity, or forming a new attachment bond with an unusually caring partner) challenge the validity of their self- and social schemas. This openness to reality, which makes it possible to change attachment patterns during any phase of life, has been noted by other attachment theorists. Sroufe (1978), for example, while writing about the tendency for there to be continuity in attachment patterns, said: "We would not expect a child to be permanently scarred by early experiences or permanently protected from environmental assaults. Early experiences cannot be more important than later experience, and life in a changing environment should alter the qualities of a child's adaptation" (p. 50).

Borrowing from Waddington's (1957) epigenetic landscape model, Bowlby (1973) emphasized that attachment representations are both "environmentally stable" and "environmentally labile." On the one hand, attachment representations need to be somewhat "environmentally stable" to ensure a degree of continuity over time in a person's understanding of his or her social experiences, despite fluctuations in the social environment. On the other hand, attachment representations need to be somewhat "environmentally labile" if they are going to allow a person to stay in tune with changes in the social environment, age-related changes in kinds of relationships, and encounters with previously unfamiliar relationship partners.

According to Bowlby (1973), the development of adult attachment patterns is constrained by two forces: (1) "homeothetic forces" (Waddington, 1957) that buffer changes in attachment patterns from infancy to adulthood, making it less likely that they will deviate from early working models; and (2) "destabilizing forces" that encourage deviation from early working models given powerful experiences that demand revision and updating of attachment representations. Hence, adult attachment patterns are rooted in both early interactions with primary caregivers and later attachment experiences that challenge the validity of the early working models. This is what makes personal development and successful psychotherapy possible.

The main question here is how these two antagonistic forces act together to shape attachment patterns. Some theorists have formulated a "prototype" approach that leaves room for both stability and change in attachment patterns (e.g., Fraley, 2002; Owens et al., 1995; Sroufe, Egeland, & Kreutzer, 1990; van IJzendoorn, 1996). They distinguish between two kinds of working models that jointly determine a person's attachment pattern at a given developmental stage: current working models and early "prototype" models. Current working models can be revised and updated throughout childhood, adolescence, and adulthood by attachment-relevant experiences that deviate from previous experiences and existing knowledge. However, the prototype working models formed during the first few years of life continue to exist and exert a shaping influence on attachment patterns across the lifespan. The process is analogous to learning one or more foreign languages, while retaining an "accent" based on a native language, or learning to play golf after years of playing baseball or softball. In golf, it is debilitating to use an elbow-cocked baseball swing, yet many people find a well-practiced cocked-elbow style difficult to resist.

The main alternative to the prototype view is the "revisionist" (Fraley, 2002) or "continuous change" view; that is, a person's working models might be similar to his or her adaptation to constantly changing technology. Most adults who live in modern industrialized societies have experienced and adapted to many such changes. Older persons among us have used early telephones, which initially required turning a crank on a wooden box and talking to an intervening human operator to make a connection. This was followed by early handheld dial-up phones, which had to be connected to a telephone network via wires. It did not take most people long to give up reaching for a crank when they wished to make a call on a handheld phone, and everyone learned to dial numbers rather than recite them to a human operator. Later, as all readers of this book know, mobile digital telephones came into existence, and it was no longer necessary to use a wire-connected phone. Few people had trouble shifting from rotary dials and wires to push-button calls and an absence of wires. Changing attachment styles, and the associated working models of self and others, might conceivably have been like adapting to new forms of technology: The new behaviors and expectations might have been easy to acquire without much interference from old habits. In a review of longitudinal attachment studies, however, Fraley (2002) found that the evidence favors a prototype model. Although the effect of early attachment patterns on later patterns was not large, it was quite persistent and seemed never to erode completely, as simple old habits often do. Thus, we began our own consideration of the developmental stability issue with a slight bias toward the prototype view.

According to this view, working models formed during infancy are sensorimotor, procedural, and nonlinguistic in nature. They reflect parent–infant interactions that took place before sophisticated linguistic and introspective capacities were developed. (Similar ideas appear in Sullivan's [1953] writings on "prototaxic" and "parataxic" modes of early experience, modes that cannot easily be overridden or replaced by later, more sophisticated "syntaxic" forms of experience.) These preverbal working models (which include unconscious expectations and reflex-like reactions to certain kinds of threats) tend to be reactivated during later close relationships, where they unconsciously influence a person's expectations, fears, defenses, and behavior. This unconscious influence can be inferred from a person's proneness to seek out or to recreate interpersonal experiences that fit with early prototype models, and to appraise, interpret, and recall interactions in prototype-consistent ways. A person is often not aware of what he or she is doing in such cases, or why.

Since the notion of powerful sensorimotor, nonverbal memories might seem intuitively implausible to some readers at a time when psychodynamic notions are doubted or downplayed in psychology, it might be worthwhile to consider how an articulate writer, novelist Aharon Appelfeld (2004), describes the, to him, odd way in which his 3 years as a child on the run from Nazis seem to be ingrained in his physiology decades later:

[I] remember the moment when I first stood before a tree laden with red apples. I was so astonished that I took a few steps back. More than my conscious mind does, my body seems to remember those steps backwards. If I ever make a wrong movement, or unexpectedly stumble backward, I see the tree with red apples. [He ate one and then fell asleep.] When I awoke, [it was dusk and I didn't know what to do], so I got up on my knees. This position, too, on my knees, I feel to this very day. Any time I'm kneeling, I remember the sunset glowing through the trees and I feel happy. (p. 51)

Later in the book he continues: "I say 'I don't remember,' and that's the whole truth. The strongest imprints those years have left on me are intense physical ones. The hunger for bread. . . . Dreams of hunger and thirst haunt me almost on a weekly basis" (p. 89).

> Everything that happened is imprinted within my body and not within my memory. . . . For years after the war, I would walk neither in the middle of the sidewalk nor in the middle of the road. I always clung to the walls, always staying in the shade, and always walking rapidly, as if I were slipping away. . . . Sometimes I find myself in a dark alley—as one can in Jerusalem— and I'm sure that the gate will soon be closed and I won't be able to get out. I quicken my pace and try to get away. (p. 90)

Figure 5.1 is a schematic representation of the prototype view of attachment working models. Being unchanged by later attachment experiences, prototype working models contribute a stable core to later models, increasing the likelihood that attachment patterns later in life will reflect infant patterns. However, attachment patterns at a given developmental stage are also a function of past and current attachment-relevant experiences. These experiences can be compatible with model stability if they converge with the prototype models (e.g., insecurely attached people's experiences of rejection, abuse, separation, or loss), but experiences that deviate significantly from these models can induce change (e.g., insecure people's encounters with sensitive and responsive relationship partners).

In this chapter we consider the development, stability, and change of attachment patterns across the lifespan as conceptualized in the prototype approach. First we examine evidence concerning the stability of infant attachment patterns across childhood, adolescence, and adulthood, and evaluate the impact of early, formative experiences with parental caregivers on later attachment patterns. Second, we consider discontinuities in attachment patterns between infancy and adulthood, and evaluate the impact that attachment-relevant experiences during childhood and adolescence have on the development of adult attachment. Third, we examine evidence for the stability of attachment patterns during adulthood and the extent to which they can be reshaped by new kinds of social experiences.

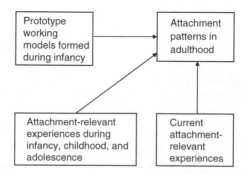

FIGURE 5.1. A schematic representation of the prototype view of the development of adult attachment patterns.

CHILDHOOD ROOTS OF ADULT ATTACHMENT

The first module of the prototype approach concerns the formative influences that early attachment experiences exert on later attachment styles. According to this approach, infant attachment patterns are cores or templates for attachment patterns throughout life. By the same logic, the antecedents of infant attachment patterns can contribute significantly to attachment representations and behaviors across the lifespan and can be viewed as the childhood roots of adult attachment. However, although these ideas imply continuity of attachment styles across the lifespan, the prototype approach includes the notion that prototype-discrepant experiences during childhood, adolescence, and adulthood can reduce the degree of continuity observed; that is, we cannot expect more than a moderate degree of stability in attachment patterns between infancy and adulthood, although the stability should be higher for people who grow up in stable social environments (e.g., with the same parents, in the same neighborhood).

What are the antecedents of prototype working models, the roots of infants' attachment patterns? In Bowlby's (1973) theory and Ainsworth et al.'s (1978) early studies of infant attachment in the home and in the Strange Situation, parental availability, sensitivity, and responsiveness during times of need were considered to be the antecedents of infant attachment security or insecurity. However, with the progress of attachment theory and research, parents' own attachment patterns (and related caregiving patterns); the personal, familial, and broader social contexts of parental caregiving (e.g., parental stress, parental mental health, family economic problems); and children's innate characteristics (e.g., temperamental irritability or proneness to distress) were recognized as possible contributors to the quality of infant attachment. These factors are likely to influence or moderate parental availability, sensitivity, and responsiveness, in which case the roots of an infant's attachment pattern may be quite dense and broadly distributed.

Van IJzendoorn and Bakermans-Kranenburg (1997) included many such factors in their model (reproduced here in Figure 5.2). In their view, parental caregiving is the direct antecedent of an infant's attachment pattern, with more sensitive and responsive parents inducing a more secure pattern of infant attachment. Parents' own attachment patterns can affect infant attachment by influencing parental sensitivity and responsiveness. For example, more secure parents tend to be more sensitive and responsive to their child's attachment needs and signals (see Chapter 11, this volume, for an extensive review), thereby increasing the child's attachment security. The personal, familial, and social contexts of parental caregiving and the infant's innate temperament can affect the links between parents' attachment patterns, parental caregiving, and infant attachment. For example, a supportive husband may make it easier for his wife to react sensitively to their infant's attachment signals, allowing even an insecure mother to provide adequate support to her baby. In contrast, some irritable infants may frustrate mothers' attempts to calm and soothe them, thereby weakening or breaking the link between parental sensitivity and infant attachment security.

In the following section we review evidence concerning the continuity of attachment patterns from infancy to adulthood. We also consider the theoretically hypothesized effects of parental attachment and caregiving styles, the social and economic context of parents' caregiving efforts, and infants' innate characteristics on infant–parent attachment. We also consider whether these variables affect attachment style differences throughout childhood, adolescence, and adulthood.

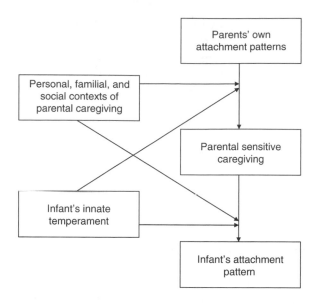

FIGURE 5.2. An adaptation of van IJzendoorn and Bakerman-Kranenburg's (1997) schematic representation of the antecedents of infant attachment patterns.

Continuity of Attachment from Infancy through Adulthood

Early studies of the continuity of infant attachment focused on the second year of life and examined the stability of attachment classifications in the Strange Situation (secure, avoidant, anxious, and—only later, after the category was added—disorganized) over periods ranging from 1 to 12 months. Research exploring the continuity issue beyond the second year was slow in coming, because the Strange Situation can be reliably used only with children ranging in age from 9 to 24 months, and no other procedure for assessing attachment patterns in older children was developed until the mid-1980s. In the first systematic study of early continuity of infant classifications, E. Waters (1978) observed children's attachment responses to separation and reunion from their mother in the Strange Situation at 12 and 18 months of age and found that 96% of 50 children were independently placed in the same category at both assessments. However, this impressive stability might have been achieved by preselecting children who were known to live in stable homes during the 6-month study period (E. Waters, 1978).

Following this lead, several studies examined the stability of Strange Situation classifications during the second year of life (see Scharfe [2003, Table 4.1, pp. 66–67] for a detailed description of these studies). Overall, between 45 and 90% of the children were judged to exhibit the same pattern of attachment to mother across periods ranging from 1 to 12 months. (Whereas this is fairly high, one has to remember that a certain degree of match would occur by chance alone. Because most infants in most studies are judged to be securely attached, one could achieve a 50 or 60% hit rate simply by guessing that every child in a particular study was secure.) In a meta-analysis of these studies, Fraley (2002) found a mean correlation of .32 ($N = 896$), indicating a moderate level of stability in attachment patterns across the second year of life. Three of these studies (Belsky, Campbell, Cohn, & Moore, 1996; Main & Weston, 1981;

Owen, Easterbrooks, Chase-Lansdale, & Goldberg, 1984) also assessed the stability of infant attachment to the father over 7–8 months and found degrees of concordance ranging from 46 to 87%.

With the development of other procedures for assessing attachment patterns in older children (e.g., parental Q-sort methods, story completion tests), attachment researchers who collected data on infant attachment patterns in the Strange Situation at 12 months began to ask whether these patterns remained stable after 3, 4, or 6 years (see Scharfe [2003, Table 4.1, pp. 66–67] for a detailed description). These studies revealed moderate levels of stability in attachment classification over periods ranging from 3 to 6 years. Fraley (2002) meta-analyzed five of these studies and found a mean correlation of .35 ($N = 161$) for studies that examined attachment patterns at 1 and 4 years, and a mean correlation of .67 ($N = 131$) for studies that examined stability over 6 years. (This correlation was high because of one radically high outlier.) Overall, the findings resemble the correlations observed in studies examining attachment stability from 12 to 24 months, implying that the same moderate level of continuity is observed in older children as well.

In the last decade, attachment researchers who administered the Strange Situation to infants in the late 1970s and early 1980s, and reassessed the participants as much as 18–20 years later, have been able to examine the continuity of attachment patterns all the way to adulthood. All of these studies used the AAI to assess attachment patterns at age 19 or 20 and compared participants' AAI classifications with classifications based on the Strange Situation two decades earlier. The findings are quite divergent.

On the one hand, four of these studies (Hamilton, 2000; Iwaniec & Sneddon, 2001; Main, 2001; E. Waters, Merrick, Treboux, Crowell, & Albersheim, 2000) found significant associations between Strange Situation and AAI classifications, with concordance rates ranging from 61 to 64% (again, this has to be evaluated against the concordance rate expected by chance). On the other hand, three studies (Lewis, Feiring, & Rosenthal, 2000; Weinfeld, Sroufe, & Egeland, 2000; Zimmermann, Fremmer-Bombik, Spangler, & Grossmann, 1997) failed to find a significant association between infant and adult attachment, with less than 40% concordance between the two measures (not much different from chance). However, two more recent studies of the same sample assessed by Weinfeld et al. (2000)—the large Minnesota sample—found a significant Strange Situation–AAI match when participants were 26 years old (Sroufe, Egeland, Carlson, & Collins, 2005) and a significant match between Strange Situation classifications and CRI (close relationship) classifications at 20–21 years of age (Roisman et al., 2005). Moreover, Fraley's (2002) meta-analysis of studies using the AAI at ages 19–20 revealed a mean correlation of .27 ($N = 218$) with Strange Situation scores, indicating moderate continuity from infancy to young adulthood and replicating already reviewed findings on continuity of infant attachment during childhood.

Beyond meta-analyzing 27 studies that had examined attachment stability across various time spans in infancy, childhood, adolescence, and young adulthood, Fraley (2002) constructed a dynamic mathematical model based on the prototype view (i.e., assuming that a stable prototype of infant attachment is carried through time, but with prototype-discrepant events and relationships tempering the prototype's influence over time) and tested its goodness of fit with longitudinal data. He compared this model with the alternative "revisionist" (continuous change) model, which did not assume the existence of an initial prototype that had a lasting influence. Fraley's conclusion is a good summary of the findings we have just reviewed:

The prototype model provided the best fit to the data, indicating that a prototype-like process may contribute to attachment stability across the life course. The estimated model indicates that early prototypes exert a moderate influence on subsequent interactions and that these interactions are easily incorporated into concurrent beliefs about the world. Furthermore, the prototype model predicts that the continuity between early attachment security and attachment security at any point later in the life course will be equivalent to a correlation of approximately .39. In summary, there is a moderate degree of stability in attachment from childhood to adulthood, and the pattern of stability observed is better accounted for by a prototype-like process than a revisionist one. (p. 135)

Parental Caregiving

Attachment studies have examined the contribution of early parenting (parental sensitive responsiveness) to attachment patterns throughout life. Most such studies have focused on the association between maternal sensitivity during mother–infant interactions and infant attachment assessed in the Strange Situation. However, a few recent longitudinal studies provide initial evidence concerning the very long-term effects of parental caregiving during infancy and childhood on later adult attachment (K. E. Grossmann, Grossmann, & Waters, 2005, summarized the major longitudinal studies). Taken together, these studies emphasize the important role of parental sensitive responsiveness to the development of infant attachment security and support the hypothesis that adult attachment is rooted in early experiences of parental caregiving.

In the earliest studies of infant attachment, Ainsworth et al. (1978) identified several maternal behaviors during home observations of mother–child interactions associated with the attachment security exhibited by an infant in the Strange Situation. These behaviors included, for example, being responsive to the infant's crying, timing of feeding, sensitivity to the infant's signals and needs, psychological accessibility when the infant was distressed or asked for support and comfort, cooperation, and acceptance of the infant's needs and behavior. Ainsworth et al. developed rating scales to assess maternal sensitivity versus insensitivity, acceptance versus rejection, cooperation versus interference, and psychological accessibility versus ignoring—all used in the mothers' and infants' homes— and found that these scales significantly differentiated between secure and insecure infants in the Strange Situation. In subsequent decades, dozens of studies followed up Ainsworth et al.'s findings, while linking infant attachment security to other aspects of maternal caregiving (e.g., expressions of positive affect, emotional availability, encouragement of exploration) and also the quality of paternal caregiving (for reviews, see L. Atkinson, Niccols, et al., 2000; Belsky, 1999; de Wolff & van IJzendoorn, 1997; and Goldsmith & Alansky, 1987).

Since Ainsworth et al.'s (1978) study, three major meta-analytic reviews have been published on the link between maternal sensitivity and infant attachment security assessed in the Strange Situation. Goldsmith and Alansky's (1987) meta-analysis included 13 studies (based on 691 mother–child dyads), de Wolff and van IJzendoorn (1997) meta-analyzed 66 studies (including 4,176 dyads), and Atkinson, Niccols, et al. (2000) meta-analyzed 41 studies (2,243 dyads). The three studies yielded quite similar, significant, but only moderate size mean correlations (.32, .24, and .27) between maternal sensitivity and infant attachment security. Although these effect sizes are fairly small, and suggest that there are other factors involved, de Wolff and van IJzendoorn (1997) showed that the 0.24 effect size they obtained implies that mothers who are sensitive and responsive increase the likelihood of their infant being securely attached from 38% to 62%. However, the three meta-analyses also found substantial effect size variability across studies. This variability resulted from different methods of assessing maternal sensitivity (with studies using broad, holistic ratings of sensitivity yielding stronger correlations than studies counting specific maternal behaviors). Some variability was attributable to the time span separating the assessments of maternal caregiving and infant attachment: The larger the time interval, the smaller the correlation. This is an important finding, because it casts some doubt on the long-term effects of early parental care.

Experimental intervention studies aimed at improving parental sensitivity to infants have provided further evidence for a link between parenting and infant attachment. These experiments are extremely important, because random assignment of parents to control and intervention groups allows researchers to determine whether experimentally induced changes in parenting have a causal impact on infant attachment. In a meta-analytic review of 23 experimental intervention studies (including 1,255 mother–child dyads), Bakermans-Kranenburg, van IJzendoorn, and Juffer (2003) reported a small to moderate, but statistically significant, mean effect size (0.20) linking interventions aimed at improving maternal sensitivity (compared to control groups), with a higher probability of secure infant attachment. Importantly, the same authors found that this effect was mediated by improved maternal sensitivity. There was a strong effect size (equivalent to a correlation of .45) between experimentally induced changes in maternal sensitivity and subsequent infant attachment security (that is, interventions that were more successful in improving maternal sensitivity were also more effective in enhancing infant security). In a subsequent article, Bakermans-Kranenburg, van IJzendoorn, and Juffer (2005) meta-analyzed a subsample of 15 studies (based on 842 dyads) that included infant attachment disorganization (the attachment category that seems to be most predictive of later mental health problems) among the outcome categories. They found a significant effect size (0.23) linking interventions aimed at improving maternal sensitivity with a lower rate of infant disorganized attachment.

Based on the accumulated evidence linking sensitive maternal care with infant attachment security, van IJzendoorn and Bakermans-Kranenburg (2004) concluded that "the causal role of maternal sensitivity in the formation of the infant–mother attachment relationship is a strongly corroborated finding. Correlational, experimental, and cross-cultural studies have replicated the association between sensitivity and attachment numerous times, and through different measures and designs" (p. 248).

Longitudinal studies examining the association between parental care during infancy and childhood and attachment patterns in offspring during adolescence or adulthood are scarce, but their findings provide some evidence for the formative influence of early experiences on later adult attachment. For example, Beckwith, Cohen, and Hamilton (1999) assessed maternal sensitivity (attentiveness, responsiveness, and supportiveness) during mother–child interactions when the children were 1, 8, and 24 months old, then assessed their attachment to their mothers (using the AAI) when they were 18 years old. Supporting the prototype hypothesis, higher levels of maternal sensitivity and responsiveness during early childhood were associated with less avoidant and more secure AAI classifications late in adolescence. Relying on data from the Minnesota Longitudinal Study (Sroufe et al., 2005), Roisman, Madsen, Hennighausen, Sroufe, and Collins (2001) found that more sensitive and responsive parenting during parent–child interactions when study participants were 13 years old was associated with more secure attachment at age 19. Similarly, J. P. Allen and Hauser (1996) found that secure attachment to mother at age 25 was associated with the mother's encouragement of relatedness and autonomy during social interactions when the study participants were 14 years old.

K. Grossmann, Grossmann, and Kindler (2005) have supplied the most comprehensive and systematic findings concerning the longitudinal implications of parental caregiving during infancy and childhood. In what is known as the Bielefeld Project, K. Grossmann et al. followed 49 participants from birth to age 22 and assessed both the mother's and the father's sensitive responsiveness several times during infancy and childhood. They also administered the AAI to the offspring at age 22. Childhood experiences with the mother and the father during infancy and childhood predicted attachment patterns 20 years later. Specifically, secure attachment at age 22 was positively associated with (1) the father's sensitivity during the first 3 years of life, mainly when the mother also showed relatively high levels of sensitivity and responsiveness, and (2) supportive experiences with either the mother or the father during later childhood (between ages 6 and 10). The authors concluded that both mothers' and fathers' sensitivity and supportiveness (each in its own right and taken together) during infancy and childhood are important predictors of adult attachment classification.

Parental Attachment

Once attachment measures had moved "to the level of mental representations," to use Main et al.'s (1985) phrase, the field began to discover that a parent's "state of mind with respect to attachment," measured with the AAI, is another good predictor of his or her offspring's attachment security or insecurity. Main et al. proposed that parental sensitivity and responsiveness are a reflection, or consequence, of parents' state of mind with respect to attachment; that is, parents' attachment working models shape their caregiving behavior and affect their ability and willingness to provide a safe haven and secure base for their child, which in turn contribute to the child's attachment security. There is now extensive evidence that parents with a "secure state of mind" are more willing and able to respond sensitively to their child's need for proximity, comfort, safety, and assistance with emotion regulation (see Chapter 11, this volume, for a review). This finding indicates that there is "intergenerational transmission of attachment" (e.g., van IJzendoorn, 1995), by which secure or insecure parental "states of mind" are transmitted to children via caregiving patterns. Insightful comments about the transmission process appeared in Bowlby's (1951) early writings, before there were systematic empirical data on the subject: "Thus it is seen how children who suffer deprivation grow up to become parents deficient in the capacity to care for their children and how adults deficient in this capacity are commonly those who suffered deprivation in childhood" (pp. 68–69).

In the first systematic study of the "intergenerational transmission of attachment," Main et al. (1985) found a strong association between the mother's secure state of mind as measured by the AAI and the security of her 1-year-old child in the Strange Situation. Numerous researchers subsequently replicated this finding, in each case showing a concordance rate of 60 to 85% between mother's state of mind and infant's attachment classification in the Strange Situation. (It is worth noting, however, that in most studies the three attachment categories are collapsed to two, secure and insecure, making the chance rate of concordance fairly high.) Similar findings have been obtained with prospective, retrospective, and concurrent designs (e.g., Benoit & Parker, 1994; Fonagy, Steele, & Steele, 1991; van IJzendoorn, Kranenburg, Zwart-Woudstra, van Busschbach, & Lambermon, 1991). A few studies have also found significant degrees of concordance between paternal state of mind and infant attachment to the father in the Strange Situation (e.g., Steele, Steele, & Fonagy, 1996; van IJzendoorn et al., 1991). In a meta-analytic review of 18 studies (based on 854 mother–child dyads), van IJzendoorn (1995) reported a strong mean effect size (1.06 standard deviation units, corresponding to about 75% concordance) linking the mother's secure state of mind with the infant's attachment security. The father's state of mind was also significantly associated with the infant's attachment classification in the Strange Situation, but this association was notably weaker than the one observed for mothers and infants.

Van IJzendoorn's (1995) meta-analysis also revealed what he called a "transmission gap." Although a meta-analysis of the 10 studies available at the time revealed a strong mean effect size of 0.72 linking parental state of mind with respect to attachment and sensitive responsiveness to children's needs and signals during parent–child interactions, van IJzendoorn concluded (after considering data linking parental sensitivity to infant attachment) that some parts of the influence of parental state of mind on offspring attachment classification occurred through processes other than parental sensitive responsiveness.

This "gap" opened the door for other possible transmission mechanisms. For example, parents' ability to reflect on their child's emotions and inner states (what Fonagy, Steele, et al. [1991] called "reflective function," as explained in Chapter 4, this volume) has been found to mediate the connection between parental state of mind and infant attachment security (e.g., Fonagy, 1996; Slade, Grienenberger, Bernbach, Levy, & Locker, 2005). In addition, other investigators have found that parents' frightening/frightened behaviors or a mixture of hostility and helplessness (which Lyons-Ruth, Bronfman, & Parsons [1999] called "atypical maternal behaviors") explained the link between the mother's insecure/unresolved status in the AAI and infant attachment disorganization (e.g., Goldberg, Benoit, Blockland, & Madigan, 2003; Lyons-Ruth, Yellin, Melnick, & Atwood, 2005; Schuengel, Bakermans-Kranenburg, & van IJzendoorn, 1999). Among older children, attachment patterns can also be transmitted via parents' direct teaching about relationships and relational behavior.

The "transmission gap" also opened the door for possible genetic explanations of intergenerational transmission of attachment patterns, which challenged Bowlby's almost exclusive emphasis on the importance of early experiences with parents. Of course, genetic explanations could still play a role even if there were no transmission gap. Specifically, there could be some genetic basis for both parental sensitivity and individual differences in attachment patterns. (We deal with these explanations later in this chapter, when we consider the effects of a child's innate characteristics on the formation of attachment patterns.) Moreover, parental sensitivity could be, in part, conditioned by child temperament (van IJzendoorn & Bakermans-Kranenburg, 1997). For example, Knafo and Plomin (2006) showed that genetic factors largely mediate some associations between parenting behaviors (e.g., parental negative affect and coercive disciplinary practices) and child outcomes (e.g., prosocial child behavior).

Parental state of mind with respect to attachment is also an important precursor of attachment patterns in offspring during middle childhood, adolescence, and adulthood. In childhood (between 3 and 7 years of age), for example, three studies have found significant concurrent links between children's attachment patterns in story completion tasks and their mother's state of mind assessed with the AAI (Gloger-Tippelt, Gomille, Koenig, & Vetter, 2002; Goldwyn, Stanley, Smith, & Green, 2000; Miljkovitch, Pierrehumbert, Bretherton, & Halfon, 2004). Miljkovitch et al. also assessed paternal state of mind but found no significant concordance between the father's AAI and the child's attachment classifications.

Seven studies have examined concurrent associations between self-reported parental attachment style or AAI-assessed state of mind and offspring attachment style during young adulthood (Benoit & Parker, 1994; Besser & Priel, 2005; Cook, 2000; J. A. Feeney, 2002b, 2006; Mikulincer & Florian, 1999a; Obegi, Morrison, & Shaver, 2004). Whereas Benoit and Parker (1994) relied on the AAI for assessing parental and offspring states of mind, the remaining six studies used self-report attachment scales (e.g., the RQ or the Attachment Style Questionnaire [ASQ]). Despite this methodological difference, the findings are consistent across the seven studies. For example, Benoit and Parker found 75% correspondence between 81 pregnant women's AAI classifications and their own mothers' AAI classifications. All six studies based on self-report attachment style scales found significant associations between mothers' and adult offsprings' scores on avoidance, and four of them (Besser & Priel, 2005; Cook, 2000; J. A. Feeney, 2002b, 2006) found significant associations on the attachment anxiety dimension. With the exception of Besser and Priel's (2005) study, the other five studies also included assessments of the fathers' attachment styles, but only Cook (2000) and J. A. Feeney (2002b, 2006) found significant associations (for both the avoidance and the anxiety dimensions).

Although these seven studies provide suggestive evidence for parental sources of adults' attachment styles, they cannot be viewed as strong support for the prototype hypothesis, according to which parents' attachment patterns influence their infant's attachment pattern, which in turn becomes a prototype for adult attachment. A direct test of this hypothesis would require assessing parental attachment styles, or states of mind with respect to attachment, when study participants were infants or, ideally, before they were born, then assessing offspring attachment styles when the offspring reached adolescence or adulthood. Unfortunately, the studies we just reviewed assessed parental attachment styles or states of mind when the offspring were young adults, and although there is some degree of stability in attachment patterns over periods of years (as documented earlier in this chapter), we cannot be sure a parent's attachment style, or state of mind, when the offspring reaches young adulthood is the same as it would have been when the young adult was an infant.

Only one longitudinal study provides preliminary evidence regarding the intergenerational transmission of adult attachment patterns through the lens of the prototype hypothesis (Steele & Steele, 2005). In 1987–1989, Steele and Steele asked 63 expectant parents to complete the AAI during the third trimester of the mother's first pregnancy, and 12–18 months later they assessed the offsprings' attachment patterns in the Strange Situation. They assessed these attachment patterns again in middle childhood (5–6 years of age), using story completion tasks; later in childhood (11–12 years), using an interview focused on family relations and friendships; and in adolescence (16 years) with the AAI.

Although the last wave of measurement is still in progress, Steele and Steele (2005) have already published valuable findings concerning the long-term effects of prebirth parental state of mind with respect to attachment and offspring's attachment orientations at ages 5–6 and 11–12. Mother's prebirth attachment security predicted her 5- to 6-year-old child's ability to resolve social and emotional dilemmas and to describe resourcefully and explain emotional states. In addition, 11-year-old children who expressed more coherent representations of self and others while telling stories about family relations and friendships were more likely to have had mothers with secure states of mind 11 years earlier. For boys only, these intergenerational associations were also found for their fathers. Of course, there is a need for more longitudinal studies examining the validity and generalizability of these findings. But even being cautious, we cannot help being impressed by the long-term influence that parental attachment status exerts on the development of offsprings' attachment patterns over periods of years. We have to be even more cautious in interpreting the causal pathway, however, because the children continued to have the same parents over the period studied, so some of the causal force may stem from long, consistent relationships, not simply from what happened during infancy.

Contextual Sources of the Transmission Gap: The Ecology of Attachment Security

The transmission gap that van IJzendoorn (1995) noted between parental state of mind, parental caregiving, and infant attachment ushered in what van IJzendoorn and Bakermans-Kranenburg (1997), harking back to Main et al.'s (1985) move to the representational level, labeled "a move to the contextual level." This new "move" involved attachment researchers paying more attention to what Belsky (1999, 2005) called the "broad ecology of attachment security." The transmission gap implies that some securely attached parents do not show sensitive responsiveness in interactions with their children, and some infants who interact with sensitive parents do not get classified as secure in the Strange Situation. These cases cannot be explained by an intergenerational transmission of attachment patterns, and they call for a careful examination of other potential antecedents of parental care and infant attachment, such as parental characteristics other than attachment patterns (e.g., personality traits, mental health), and the familial and social contexts in which the parent–child dyad is embedded (e.g., the marital relationship and nonparental providers of infant care). According to Belsky and Isabella (1988), "Factors beyond the specific interactions that transpire between mother and infant also serve to influence the development of attachment security, if only because they are likely to affect the very behavioral exchanges that take place between mother and infant" (p. 45).

This theoretical "move" to include context implies that every personal, familial, or social factor that interferes with parental sensitive responsiveness (e.g., maternal depression, financial problems, marital discord) may moderate the link between parental attachment and parental caregiving, thus contributing to insecure infant attachment despite signs of parents' secure states of mind. The link can also be moderated by factors that facilitate a parent's mental and behavioral organization, self-regulation, and enactment of sensitive and responsive caregiving (e.g., social support, good parent training), thereby promoting more secure patterns of infant attachment even among fairly insecure parents. In addition, the association between parenting and infant attachment can be moderated by the quality of the infant's interactions with nonparental caregivers (e.g., grandparents, older siblings, day care workers), which can either intensify or weaken the effects of parental caregiving on infant attachment. For example, low-quality nonparental care can intensify the detrimental effects of parental attachment insecurities and a lack of parental sensitivity, and dilute the security-enhancing influences of a "good enough" (Winnicott, 1953) parent–child relationship. If we take the prototype hypothesis seriously, all of these contextual factors that influence infant attachment security may also have long-term effects on later attachment security or insecurity, including adult attachment style.

In one of the first attempts to examine the ecology of infant attachment, Belsky and Isabella (1988) followed up 56 mother–infant dyads from the last trimester of pregnancy until the infants were 1 year old. During pregnancy, mothers were asked about their own child-rearing history, personality (e.g., ego strength), marital quality, work–family relations, and social support (friendliness and helpfulness of neighbors). Assessments of marital quality, work–family relations, and social support were repeated 1, 3, and 9 months postpartum, and infants' attachment security was assessed in the Strange Situation at 1 year of age. The investigators found that the mother's ego strength and interpersonal affection; a stable, high-quality marital relationship; and supportive and friendly neighbors contributed significantly and uniquely (i.e., independent of other factors) to infant attachment security. When all of these factors were considered together, a clear picture emerged, in which a more positive family ecology (positive maternal characteristics, less marital deterioration, supportive neighbors) increased the likelihood of the infant being securely attachment to his or her mother.

In a subsequent study, Belsky (1996) examined the importance of family ecology in explaining infants' attachment to their fathers in the Strange Situation. He computed a measure of overall family resources by adding positive personality traits of each parent (high extraversion, high agreeableness, low neuroticism), a measure of positive infant temperament, and facilitating social context variables (social support satisfaction, number of supportive people, and lack of work–family interference). He found that the greater the family resources, the more likely infants were to become securely attached to their fathers. This overall composite measure of family resources also contributed significantly to an infant's attachment security with the mother (Belsky, Rosenberger, & Crnic, 1995).

Dozens of subsequent studies have replicated and extended these findings (for reviews see L. Atkinson, Paglia, et al., 2000; Belsky, 1999). In 2000, Atkinson, Paglia, et al. conducted an integrative meta-analytic review on the contribution of three distal factors—social support/marital satisfaction, maternal stress, and maternal depression—to infant attachment classification. The meta-analysis and several subanalyses were conducted on 35 studies (of 2,064 mother–infant dyads) and revealed moderate but significant mean effect sizes for mother's appraisals of social support and marital satisfaction (0.15, based on 15 studies of 851 dyads), mother's reports of stressful life events during pregnancy and the first year of her infant's life (0.19; 13 studies of 768 dyads), and maternal depression (0.18; 15 studies of 953 dyads). Across most of the studies, a mother's sense of available support and marital satisfaction, as well as lower levels of maternal stress and depression, increased the probability of the infant being securely attached. Although the strength of the association between the three distal factors and infant attachment security varied across studies depending on how, when, and in what context these factors were measured, Atkinson, Paglia, et al.'s findings highlight the importance of the personal, familial, and social contexts in which the parent–child relationship is embedded for filling in the "transmission gap."

Attachment research also provides important information about the role of non-parental care in the development of infant attachment security or insecurity. For example, Belsky (1988; Belsky & Rovine, 1988) found that more than 20 hours a week of nonmaternal care in day care centers during the first year of life lowered the probability of an infant being securely attached to his or her mother in the Strange Situation. In addition, infant attachment security with father was hindered in families relying on more than 35 hours a week of nonmaternal care. However, one should be aware that self-selection can account for these findings; that is, parents of children with extensive day care experience may have differed from those without extensive day care from the outset. Belsky's findings provoked and were refined by the National Institute of Child Health and Human Development (NICHD) Study of Early Child Care (NICHD Early Child Care Research Network, 1994), in which more that 1,300 children living in different regions of the United States were followed from 1 month to 54 months of age. In this very large and ambitious study, nonmaternal care had no direct effect on infant attachment, but it acted as a "secondary" risk factor, which compounded the detrimental effects of deficiencies in maternal sensitive responsiveness. Low levels of maternal sensitivity resulted in insecure infant attachment mainly when children were also exposed to poor caregiving in day care centers or more than 10 hours a week in day care centers, or more than one nonmaternal care arrangement during the first 15 months of life.

Similar detrimental effects of nonmaternal care have been found in Israeli kibbutzim with communal sleeping arrangements (i.e., a situation in which children spent only a few hours in the afternoon with parents and during the rest of the day and night were under the care of other professional caregivers called *metapelot*). Infants from kibbutzim with communal sleeping arrangements were less likely than infants from kibbutzim with family sleeping arrangements to exhibit a secure attachment to mother in the Strange Situation (Sagi, van IJzendoorn, Aviezer, Donnell, & Mayseless, 1994). Moreover, communal sleeping arrangements weakened the intergenerational transmission of attachment (Sagi et al., 1997). Whereas the typical 76% correspondence between maternal and infant attachment patterns was found in kibbutzim with family sleeping arrangements, the correspondence was only 40% in kibbutzim with communal sleeping arrangements. This reduced level of concordance derived mainly from several securely attached mothers whose infants, subject to communal sleeping arrangements, exhibited insecure attachment. This finding led van IJzendoorn and Bakermans-Kranenburg (1997) to conclude that "intergenerational transmission of attachment is not context-free, and . . . cultural childrearing practices may block the transmission of security" (p. 156).

Having shown that a wide array of distal factors tends to constrain the associations between parental state of mind, parental caregiving, and infant attachment, we next ask whether and how these factors also constrain attachment orientations in adolescence and adulthood. Unfortunately, no published longitudinal study has examined the long-term effects on adult attachment of the personal, familial, and social contexts in which the parent–infant relationship was embedded during the first year of life. In the next section, we review a large number of studies showing that changes in family and social contexts throughout childhood and adolescence have an impact on adult attachment and weaken the continuity of attachment style between infancy and adulthood. But these studies cannot be viewed as valid tests of the prototype hypothesis, because they assess changes in familial and social contexts across the lifespan rather than the contexts present during the first year of life that might have affected the development of infant attachment.

A number of attachment researchers concurrently assessed some of the relevant contextual factors together with self-reports of adult attachment style and found similar associations to those found in infant attachment studies. For example, maternal depression and parental marital discord were concurrently associated with young adult offspring attachment insecurities (Besser & Priel, 2005; J. A. Feeney, 2006; K. Henry & Holmes, 1998; Kesner & McKenry, 1998; Mikulincer & Florian, 1999a). In addition, in line with Sagi et al.'s (1994) findings on infant attachment, Shaver and Mikulincer (2004) and Scharf (2001) reported that young adults raised with communal sleeping arrangements in Israeli kibbutzim scored higher on self-report measures of attachment anxiety and avoidance, or showed a higher incidence of insecure attachment in the AAI, than young adults who grew up in kibbutzim where family sleeping arrangements were the norm. Again, these studies are not sufficient to make a strong case for the prototype hypothesis, because they did not assess maternal depression, marital discord, or attachment patterns when participants were infants. They do suggest, however, that longitudinal studies might turn up theoretically expected childhood antecedents of adult attachment orientations.

Potential Genetic Explanations of the Intergenerational Transmission of Attachment

As mentioned earlier, genetic factors might be involved in the intergenerational transmission of attachment patterns. First, parents and children share 50% of their genes, so intergenerational transmission of attachment style might be based on transmission of genes from one generation to the next. Second, innate differences in infant temperament and reactivity to stress (Rothbart & Derryberry, 1981; Thomas & Chess, 1977) might elicit different parental responses and reduce the concordance of attachment patterns. A highly irritable infant, for example, might make it more difficult for parents to respond sensitively to the infant's attachment-related signals, disrupting the expected link between independently assessed parental attachment style (or state of mind with respect to attachment) and parental caregiving. Third, some children might be so prone to distress that even sensitive and responsive parents might fail to soothe, calm, or comfort them, breaking the link between parental sensitive responsiveness and infant attachment security. As Rothbart and Derryberry (1981) suggested, "The role of the mother as a source of security or comfort depends not only on her sensitivity to the infant's signals, but also on the infant's requirements for such security" (p. 67). Fourth, some of the personal, familial, or social contexts that affect parental sensitive responsiveness might also be affected by genetic factors (e.g., maternal depression, marital discord).

Attachment theorists (Belsky, 1997; Main, 1999; van IJzendoorn & Bakermans-Kranenburg, 1997; Vaughn & Bost, 1999) have gradually recognized the possible importance of children's innate characteristics in explaining parental sensitivity and infant attachment security. For example, Belsky (1997) proffered a hypothesis of differential susceptibility, according to which some children might be especially susceptible to insecure attachment when confronted with a parent's unavailability and insensitivity, whereas other children might be somewhat genetically protected from the negative consequences of such parenting. However, even if attachment theorists assign some importance to genetic, temperamental factors, they still view parental state of mind and parental caregiving as the major antecedents of individual differences in infant attachment. In effect, they view infant temperamental differences as contextual–ecological factors, such as parent personality or other social and familial factors, that may impinge on the infant–parent relationship (van IJzendoorn & Bakermans-Kranenburg, 1997). As far as we know, however, there have been no systematic studies of the role of genetics in the complex interplay of parental attachment style, parenting behavior, child characteristics, child attachment orientations, and the broader social environment.

Following Rothbart and Derryberry's (1981) lead, numerous researchers have explored whether infants' temperamental characteristics (e.g., irritability, proneness to distress, negative reactivity) can explain individual differences in attachment patterns observed in the Strange Situation (e.g., Belsky, Fish, & Isabella, 1991; Belsky & Rovine, 1987; Egeland & Farber, 1984; Nachmias, Gunnar, Mangelsdorf, Parritz, & Buss, 1996). In an extensive review of these studies, Vaughn and Bost (1999) concluded that the evidence for a contribution of infant temperament to infant attachment patterns is less consistent than the evidence for the contribution of parental caregiving behavior. Moreover, they concluded that "attachment security cannot be considered as redundant with temperament in the explanation of personality and/or in explanations of qualities of interpersonal action" (p. 218). However, Vaughn and Bost also concluded that although temperamental factors do not directly explain infant attachment, they might still influence parental caregiving when parents' social or psychological resources are strained. In three different studies, for example, infant irritability was associated with more insecure patterns of infant attachment in low-resource but not high-resource families (Crockenberg, 1981; Susman-Stillman, Kalkose, Egeland, & Waldman, 1996; van den Boom, 1994). In these cases, infant irritability was an additional stressor for low-resource parents, which might have interfered with parental sensitivity and increased the likelihood of insecure infant attachment.

There is also accumulating evidence that although genetic factors might contribute to individual differences in attachment during infancy and childhood, attachment patterns are still also affected by nongenetic factors. For example, Dozier, Stovall, Albus, and Bates (2001) assessed infants placed in foster care between birth and 20 months of age and found a correspondence of 72% between the foster mother's AAI attachment classification and the infant's attachment classification in the Strange Situation. As reviewed earlier, this concordance rate is similar to the level van IJzendoorn (1995) found among biological mother–infant dyads. This finding emphasizes both the important role of caregiver state of mind with respect to attachment in shaping infant attachment, even following a disruption in care during the first year of life, and the nongenetic mechanisms underlying intergenerational transmission of attachment. A similar nongenetic mechanism is needed to explain Sagi et al.'s (1995) finding that biologically unrelated kibbutzim infants raised by the same *metapelet* showed 70% concordance with the *metapelet*'s AAI classification.

Another relevant piece of evidence comes from studies assessing the consistency or inconsistency of a child's attachment behavior in the Strange Situation across multiple caregivers, including mothers, fathers, child care providers, and kibbutzim *metapelet* (e.g., Belsky & Rovine, 1987; Easterbrooks, 1989; Fox, Kimmerly, & Schafer, 1991; Howes & Hamilton, 1992; Sagi et al., 1985). The results consistently show that although there is some nonrandom consistency in a child's attachment pattern with different caregivers, especially between attachments to the mother and father, a child can exhibit different patterns of attachment with different caregivers. Based on a meta-analytic review, Fox et al. (1991) concluded that concordance rates increase as the various caregivers share child-rearing values and practices, and the child experiences a similar caregiving environment across the various figures. These studies provide further evidence for social instead of or in addition to genetic determinants of children's attachment patterns. If the patterns were entirely genetically determined, they presumably would not differ markedly with different caregivers.

In an attempt to provide more direct evidence concerning the heritability of attachment patterns, some researchers have assessed concordance of attachment patterns in monozygotic (MZ) and dizygotic (DZ) twins. Their studies provide statistical estimates of genetic and environmental (parental caregiving, familial context) contributions to individual differences in attachment patterns. Given that MZ twins share roughly twice as many genes as DZ twins, greater concordance of attachment patterns in MZ twins than in DZ twins indicates that genetic influences are present. The higher the difference between MZ and DZ twins, the stronger the genetic determination of attachment patterns. Moreover, given that both MZ and DZ twins are typically reared together by the same parents in the same socioeconomic status (SES) and familial context, similar levels of concordance of attachment patterns in MZ and DZ twins would indicate the influence of a "shared environment" that has the same influence on both twins in either kind of twin pair.

Four published studies examined concordance of attachment patterns in samples of MZ and DZ twins during infancy and childhood (Bakermans-Kranenburg, van IJzendoorn, Bokhorst, & Schuengel, 2004; Bokhorst et al., 2003; Finkel & Matheny,

2000; O'Connor & Croft, 2001). In the Louisville Twin Study, Finkel and Matheny (2000) assessed attachment patterns at ages 18 months and 24 months with an adapted separation–reunion procedure originally designed for assessing temperament and found greater concordance of attachment patterns in MZ twins (66%) than in DZ twins (48%). They concluded that 25% of individual differences in attachment patterns can be attributed to genetic factors. Moreover, due to the low level of concordance found in DZ twins, the remaining variance may be more attributable to unexplained environmental factors than to shared environment. However, two subsequent studies based on the standard Strange Situation assessment procedure (Bokhorst et al., 2003) or the attachment Q-sort assessment procedure (Bakermans-Kranenburg, van IJzendoorn, et al., 2004) found almost no role at all for genetic factors in explaining attachment patterns. In these two studies, individual differences in attachment were largely explained by shared environment.

Similar findings were reported (O'Connor & Croft, 2001) in a study of preschool children's attachment patterns. The degree of concordance in attachment patterns (measured in a preschool version of the Strange Situation) was equally high in MZ (70%) and DZ (64%) twins. Moreover, twin correlations on continuous measures of attachment security were similar for MZ twins (.48) and DZ twins (.38). O'Connor and Croft concluded that the findings were consistent with a substantial influence of shared environment (32% of explained variance) and a modest role for genes (14%).

Brussoni, Jang, Livesley, and MacBeth (2000) examined concordance of self-reports of attachment orientations (on the RSQ) in young adult pairs of MZ and DZ twins. Their findings revealed that genetic effects accounted for 37, 43%, and 25% of the variance in the secure, fearful, and preoccupied adult attachment styles, respectively. For these styles, shared environmental effects were negligible. Only for the dismissing avoidant style did shared environment explain 29% of the variance, with genetic factors explaining less than 1%. Similar findings were reported by T. Crawford, Livesley, et al. (in press). In their study, twin correlations on the ECR Attachment Anxiety scale were greater in MZ twins (.44) than in DZ twins (.24), but twin correlations on the ECR Avoidance scale were similar for MZ twins (.29) and DZ twins (.33). In addition, structural equation models revealed that genetic factors accounted for 40% of the variance in attachment anxiety but had essentially no influence on avoidant attachment (accounting for less than 1% of the explained variance).

These two studies indicate that genetic factors may contribute to adult attachment styles measured by self-report scales. Moreover, compared with the relatively low genetic component found in twin studies of infant attachment, these two studies raise the interesting possibility of changes in heritability with age. It is possible that for some personal characteristics, including attachment orientations, genetic influences become more pronounced as children become older and leave home, because the constraints of the family environment might inhibit the expression of temperamental tendencies. In addition, as one gets older, one can have more control over one's relationships (e.g., by autonomously choosing one's relationship partners), allowing one's genetic dispositions to show more clearly. In infancy and early childhood, the quality of relationships with attachment figures may be largely controlled by adult caregivers. During adolescence and adulthood, however, a person's experience and behavior in close relationships may be more influenced by genetic dispositions. It is also possible, however, that self-report measures are more affected by genetic factors than are interview or behavioral measures, a possibility that has yet to be studied. Overall, the findings from twin studies of adult attachment are interesting and thought provoking, but more systematic longitudinal studies are needed, in which temperamental factors, early experiences with parents, and the ecology of attachment in infancy are all assessed and the people are followed up for years, preferably using multiple measures.

There have also been very few studies exploring possible molecular genetic markers associated with attachment patterns, and the early findings to date are not consistent. On the one hand, Lakatos et al. (2000, 2002) found a significant association between the dopamine D_4 receptor (DRD4) gene polymorphism and the probability of an infant being judged disorganized in the Strange Situation. Moreover, the odds ratio (OR) for disorganized attachment increased 10-fold in the presence of a specific allele (the −521 T allele) in the promoter region of the DRD4 gene. The DRD4 gene has already been associated with pathologically impulsive behavior, substance abuse, and attention-deficit/hyperactivity disorder (ADHD), so it seemed possible that a similar genetic mechanism underlies attachment disorganization and self-regulatory problems. On the other hand, Bakermans-Kranenburg and van IJzendoorn (2004) failed to replicate these findings in a sample of 132 infants. Moreover, when their sample was combined with Lakatos et al.'s (2000, 2002) sample, no significant association was found between the DRD4 gene or the presence of specific alleles and attachment disorganization in the Strange Situation. Bakermans-Kranenburg and van IJzendoorn (2004) concluded that these findings cast doubt on a "pure" or simple genetic explanation of disorganized attachment, and they explicitly called for more studies exploring how the interaction of genetic vulnerabilities and environmental risks (e.g., poor parental caregiving) might contribute to insecure forms of attachment, especially disorganization.

CHANGE IN ATTACHMENT PATTERNS FROM INFANCY TO ADULTHOOD

According to Bowlby (1973), the development of an adult attachment orientation, though rooted in early parent–infant interactions, should not be conceptualized as fixed or frozen during the first year of life. As described earlier (Figure 5.1), the assumption of malleability is included in the prototype approach to attachment style continuity (e.g., Owens et al., 1995; van IJzendoorn, 1996), which acknowledges the existence of both a core attachment prototype formed in infancy, and a degree of flexibility and openness to subsequent experiences. According to this approach, attachment patterns at a given point in life are a complex product of a working model prototype formed during infancy, revisions in attachment representations due to changing social circumstances and other factors throughout development, and current attachment-relevant experiences that result in further updating of attachment representations.

What are the life events or environmental changes that produce revisions in attachment representations? According to Bowlby (1973), at any point in life—infancy, childhood, adolescence, or adulthood—important and long-lived changes in the quality of interactions with primary attachment figures, due either to changes in their sensitive responsiveness or to discrepancies between the responses of earlier caregivers (e.g., parents) and new attachment figures (i.e., close friends, romantic partners, therapists), can produce discontinuities in attachment patterns. Moreover, every change in the personal, familial, and social contexts that impinge on the availability, sensitivity, and responsiveness of key attachment figures (e.g., death of a parent, parental stress, parental divorce, difficulties in parents' work life) can affect the quality of attachment interactions, thereby inducing revision and updating of working models. These changing circumstances include not only negative life events that damage a person's sense of attachment security (e.g., experiences of attachment figure unavailability, abuse, separation, or loss), but also positive life events, such as the return of a loving parent after a prolonged separation, finding a supportive partner, or entering psychotherapy (Bowlby, 1988), which can cause positive revisions in working models or boost a previously diminished sense of attachment security.

In the following pages, we review evidence concerning changes in attachment patterns between infancy and adulthood. Specifically, we focus on two kinds of studies: (1) those examining changes in attachment patterns during childhood, and (2) those examining the impact of attachment-related experiences during childhood and adolescence on eventual adult attachment style.

Change in Attachment Patterns during Childhood

One of the major causes of discontinuity in attachment orientation during childhood is a mother's experience of stress and distress that draws psychological resources away from caregiving and interferes with the organization and delivery of sensitive and responsive care. Even in studies assessing the stability of Strange Situation classifications between 12 and 18 months of age (e.g., Egeland & Farber, 1984; Egeland & Sroufe, 1981; Vaughn, Egeland, Sroufe, & Waters, 1979), children who moved from security to insecurity during the 6-month study period were more likely to have mothers who reported stressful life events during that period. These studies also revealed that children became more secure if their mothers reported a reduction in stressful life events, and an increase in marital and parental satisfaction during the study period (e.g., Egeland & Farber, 1984). In a more recent study of attachment stability at 14, 24, and 58 months of age, Bar-Haim, Sutton, Fox, and Marvin (2000) found that mothers of children who became less secure over time reported more negative life events and fewer positive life events during the study period than did mothers of children who remained secure over time.

Changes in maternal employment and resulting discontinuities in patterns of children's care (e.g., entry into day care or an increase in day care hours) during early childhood have also been found to destabilize children's attachment patterns. For example, children tend to become less secure during the second year of life if their mothers return to work for the first time during the study period (e.g., Owen et al., 1984). In addition, children who experienced an abrupt introduction to day care when they were about 12 months of age were likely to become less secure by 21 months of age (Rauh, Ziegenhain, Muller, & Wijnroks, 2000). However, a larger study of the effects of day care on children's attachment (NICHD Early Child Care Research Network, 2001) found that this detrimental effect of day care was significant only when mothers showed relatively low levels of maternal sensitivity and did not appropriately prepare their children for the transition. These results support the idea that changes in maternal employment per se do not alter children's attachment patterns, but do so only when they are accompanied by poor maternal care. In fact, the stable presence of a sensitive attachment figure can buffer negative effects of changes in children's environments. Moreover, the inclusion of another supportive figure (e.g., a grandmother) in the caregiving network tends to keep children securely attached even after their mothers return to work (e.g., Egeland & Sroufe, 1981).

Attachment studies also indicate that common family transitions (e.g., the arrival of a sibling), which can introduce changes in maternal availability, sensitivity, and responsiveness, tend to affect children's attachment to mother. In two different studies, for example, Teti, Sakin, Kucera, Corns, and Eiden (1996) and Touris, Kromelow, and Harding (1995) measured firstborn children's attachment to mother before and after the birth of a sibling. Although this was associated with considerable change in mother–firstborn interactions, both studies found that children were just as likely to move toward security as insecurity; that is, the arrival of a sibling is an influential occurrence but it does not necessarily have a negative effect on firstborn children's attachment security. Teti et al. (1996) explored factors that moderated the negative effects and found that the arrival of a sibling is likely to move firstborn children toward insecurity when mothers reported increasing levels of distress and marital discord, and a deterioration of their involvement with the firstborn child. These findings imply that family transitions move a child toward insecurity mainly when the changes are compounded by other personality and familial factors that derail maternal sensitive caregiving. In other words, it is negative change in the caregiving environment and not the arrival of a sibling per se that seems to disturb the firstborn's sense of security.

Maternal vulnerabilities can also disrupt children's attachment security. For example, children who moved toward insecurity between 12 and 18 months of age were more likely to have mothers who suffered from substance abuse and high levels of stress, depression, and antisocial behavior (aggression, anger) than were children who remained secure across the study period (Edwards, Eiden, & Leonard, 2004; Egeland & Farber, 1984; Vondra, Hommerding, & Shaw, 1999). Vondra et al. also found that mothers of children who moved toward attachment disorganization during the second year of life had an extremely chaotic lifestyle and the highest levels of suspiciousness and poor anger control. As we show later, these personal vulnerabilities are also a source of instability in adult attachment (e.g., Davila, Burge, & Hammen, 1997). Therefore, it seems likely that vulnerable mothers can erratically move from secure to insecure states of mind, as well as from sensitive caregiving to cold and rejecting responses to their children, thereby creating an unstable caregiving environment that pushes their children toward insecurity and, in extreme cases, disorganized attachment.

"Lawful Discontinuities" in Attachment Orientation from Childhood to Adulthood

Some of the 20-year longitudinal studies we reviewed earlier provide evidence of lawful discontinuities in attachment patterns between infancy and adulthood (K. Grossmann et al., 2005; Hamilton, 2000; Lewis et al., 2000; Sagi-Schwartz & Aviezer, 2005; E. Waters et al., 2000; Weinfeld et al., 2000). These studies assessed infant attachment in the Strange Situation at 12 months of age and adult state of mind with respect to attachment two decades later. They also gathered data concerning attachment-relevant life events during the 20-year study period. For example, K. Grossmann et al. (2005), Hamilton (2000), and E. Waters et al. (2000) assessed whether participants experienced attachment-relevant negative events (e.g., death of a parent, parental divorce, a parent developing a life-threatening illness, a parent with a psychiatric disorder, physical or sexual abuse by a family member) during childhood or adolescence. Lewis et al. (2000) focused on parental divorce as one of the major events that can interfere with parental availability; Weinfeld et al. (2000) assessed maternal reports of stressful life events during 11 time periods between child ages of 18 months and 19 years, maternal depression during early childhood and adolescence, maltreatment during childhood, and family functioning at age 13; Sagi-Schwartz and Aviezer (2005) assessed changes in sleeping arrangements among kibbutzim dwellers.

Overall, these studies show that attachment-relevant stressful life events occurring during childhood or adolescence produce discontinuities in attachment patterns and increase the likelihood that what were once securely attached infants will be classified as insecure in the AAI (K. Grossmann et al., 2005; Lewis et al., 2000; E. Waters et al., 2000). Interestingly, although Hamilton (2000) did not find any association between these events and discontinuities in attachment, probably because of a high Strange Situation–AAI concordance (77%), her findings illustrate how life circumstances affect secure and insecure attachment in both infancy and adulthood. She found that study participants who were classified as secure in both the Strange Situation and the AAI grew up in intact families that suffered few stressful life events. In contrast, participants who were classified as insecure at both assessments experienced parental divorce early in childhood and were exposed to marital violence, financial stress, and substance-abusing parents.

Taken together, the studies indicate that parental divorce and other stressful events during childhood and adolescence predict attachment insecurities in young adulthood. This conclusion is reinforced by a study by Beckwith et al. (1999), who found that 73% of 18-year-old adolescents classified as preoccupied (anxious) in the AAI had experienced parental divorce before 8 years of age, whereas only 28% of the secure adolescents had experienced a family breakup. We cannot tell from this study, however, whether parental attachment insecurity affected both the breakup and the children's attachment orientations, or whether the breakup occurred independent of parental attachment style, meaning that the children were affected solely by the experience of divorce (which to us seems unlikely based on studies discussed in subsequent chapters of this volume).

Weinfeld et al.'s (2000) longitudinal analyses revealed that maternal depression, child maltreatment, and poor family functioning during childhood and adolescence are significant predictors of attachment insecurities revealed in the AAI at age 19. However, these insecurity-inducing factors differed in the way they affected discontinuities in attachment patterns. Maternal depression increased the likelihood that securely attached infants would be classified as insecure adults in the AAI. Maltreatment and poor family functioning increased the likelihood that insecurely attached infants would be classified as insecure adults in the AAI; that is, lack of maltreatment and good-enough family functioning tend to move insecure infants toward more secure attachment representations by age 19. Weinfeld et al. believed that maltreatment during childhood and adolescence was concordant with prototypical parent–infant negative interactions and therefore supported the continuity of insecure attachment over time. With regard to the positive change produced by family functioning, Weinfeld et al. concluded that "the families of insecure participants who changed to security seemed to balance the needs of the family, the individuals, and the task better; they allowed for comfortable expressions of opinion and unfettered cooperation toward task goals" (p. 701).

Sagi-Schwartz and Aviezer (2005) assessed the continuity of attachment from 12 months to 17 years of age among kibbutzim dwellers who moved from communal sleeping arrangements to a family sleeping arrangement, and examined the impact of attachment-relevant stressful life events and the point in development when sleeping arrangements changed (before age 6 or afterwards). They discovered that either the experience of attachment-relevant negative events or early change in sleeping arrangements (before age 6) increased the likelihood that securely attached infants would later be classified as insecure adults in the AAI. In fact, a combination of stressful events and early change in sleeping arrangements produced the highest frequency of secure-to-insecure changes in attachment classification. Since parental divorce was the most frequently reported stressful event, Sagi-Schwartz and Aviezer reasoned that a family sleeping arrangement (meaning that children were under the care of their parents) might have compounded the strain of distressed parents and interfered with sensitive caregiving. "Thus for some families change [in sleeping arrangements] may be a stressor and a major challenge that could have interfered with their ability to preserve the family unit and attend to their children's needs" (p. 179).

Beyond these longitudinal studies, numerous cross-sectional studies have examined the extent to which individual differences in self-reports of attachment style in young adulthood are associated with retrospective reports of attachment-relevant life events during childhood and adolescence. Some of these studies have documented the security-disrupting effects of maltreatment and experiences of physical or sexual abuse. With only one exception (Merrill et al., 2005), the findings indicate that retrospective reports of maltreatment and experiences of sexual or physical abuse within or outside the family during childhood and adolescence are associated with attachment insecurity in young adulthood (P. C. Alexander, 1993; Mallinckrodt, McCreary, & Robertson, 1995; Roche, Runtz, & Hunter, 1999; Shapiro & Levendosky, 1999; Shaver & Clark, 1994; Sternberg, Lamb, Guterman, Abbott, & Dawud-Noursi, 2005; Styron & Janoff-Bulman, 1997; Swanson & Mallinckrodt, 2001; Twaite & Rodriguez-Srednicki, 2004; Wekerle & Wolfe, 1998). For example, P. C. Alexander (1993) found a much higher proportion of insecure attachment in women who were sexually abused within their families than in a control group of nonabused women. This association was replicated in clinical and community samples.

There is also evidence that attachment insecurity in adulthood is related to loss of a parent to death (Brennan & Shaver, 1998; Shaver & Mikulincer, 2004) and to parental divorce (K. Henry & Holmes, 1998; Lopez, Melendez, & Rice, 2000; Shaver & Mikulincer, 2004). For example, we (Shaver & Mikulincer, 2004) reported that Israeli young adults who experienced paternal death or parental divorce before age 4 were less secure than young adults who grew up in intact families or whose parents divorced after age 4. However, other studies have failed to find an association between parental divorce and self-reported attachment style in adulthood (Brennan & Shaver, 1993; Hayashi & Strickland, 1998; E. M. Hill, Young, & Nord, 1994; Tayler, Parker, & Roy, 1995). Brennan and Shaver (1993) argued that the reason for this lack of association is that some intact families are also troubled and can produce offspring with insecure attachment styles, whereas some postdivorce arrangements (remarriage and construction of a more harmonious family) can promote security. In support of this view, parental marital conflict is associated with adolescent attachment insecurity among adolescents who grew up in "intact" families (J. A. Feeney, 2006; K. Henry & Holmes, 1998; Mikulincer & Florian, 1999a). Moreover, Brennan and Shaver (1993) found that participants whose mothers remarried after divorce were more securely attached than those whose mothers remained single after divorce (which might have created contextual forces pressing for insecurity or might have been a reflection of the mother's insecure attachment style).

Attachment studies have also examined the security-disrupting effects of parental alcoholism. S. Brown (1988) viewed parental alcoholism as a risk factor for the development of attachment insecurity in children, because a parent's compulsive need for alcohol and his or her insensitivity while under the influence of alcohol interferes with meeting children's needs. It can also augment marital distress and increase the risks of physical and sexual abuse. According to Brown (1988), even when there is a nonalcoholic parent, he or she is often more preoccupied with the needs and threats of the alcoholic spouse than with the needs of the child. There is extensive evidence that young adults of alcoholic parents are more likely than young adult offspring of nonalcoholic parents to classify themselves as insecurely attached or report high levels of attachment insecurity in their relationships with parents or romantic partners (Brennan et al., 1991; Cavell, Jones, Runyan, Constantine-Page, & Velasquez, 1993; El-Guebaly, West, Maticka-Tyndale, & Pool, 1993; Kelley, Cash, Grant, Miles, & Santos, 2004; Kelley et al., 2005; Vungkhanching, Sher, Jackson, & Parra, 2004; but see Mothersead, Kivlighan, & Wynkoop, 1998, for nonsignificant findings). Using the AAI, Jaeger, Hahn, and Weinraub (2000) also found that young-adult daughters of alcoholic parents were more likely to have an insecure state of mind with respect to attachment than young-adult daughters of nonalcoholic parents.

Although the cross-sectional nature of these studies and the failure to assess infant attachment preclude any firm conclusions about attachment style discontinuity, they do show that adult attachment is rooted in childhood and adolescent experiences of parental caregiving, separation, and loss. Together with the longitudinal studies reviewed earlier, the findings fit with Bowlby's emphasis on the attachment system's openness to influence and accommodation throughout childhood and adolescence.

Carlson, Sroufe, and Egeland (2004) reanalyzed the data they collected from study participants' infancy to young adulthood and provided evidence for the joint contribution of infant attachment and childhood and adolescent experiences to adult attachment. Specifically, they computed structural equation models of the associations between Strange Situation classifications at 12 months, attachment representations and socioemotional functioning during early childhood (4.5 years of age), middle childhood (8 years), and early adolescence (12 years), and AAI classifications at 19 years. Interestingly, although Strange Situation classifications were not directly associated with AAI classifications 19 years later, infant attachment was found to be indirectly related to adult attachment via its effects on attachment representations and socioemotional functioning throughout childhood and adolescence; that is, infant attachment in the Strange Situation had significant influences on attachment representations and socioemotional functioning during early childhood, which in turn contributed to later representations and functioning during middle childhood and adolescence. And adolescents' representations and functioning contributed to AAI classifications at age 19.

According to Carlson et al. (2004), the findings suggest that continuity of attachment patterns from infancy to adulthood is a dynamic process resulting from successive transactions between the person and the environment across the lifespan. Infant attachment security or insecurity is carried from one time point to another by attachment representations that are also responsive to socioemotional functioning in a wide variety of settings (family, school, peer relationships) and current attachment-relevant experiences, so that later attachment representations are always a reflection of the early prototype and the accumulated subsequent experiences. This interpretation fits with Bowlby's (1973) railway system metaphor in which people travel a specific developmental route early in life, then encounter multiple branch points across childhood and adolescence that can lead to either a similar or a different outcome in adulthood.

CONTINUITY AND DISCONTINUITY IN ADULT ATTACHMENT

Do attachment patterns remain stable in adulthood? Can attachment-relevant experiences (e.g., divorce, death of a romantic partner) and developmental transitions (e.g., marriage, parenthood) lead to substantial changes in attachment patterns? Theoretically, the answers to these important questions are likely to be "yes." Adult attachment patterns tend to be well-formed personality structures that remain relatively stable over time and across different relationships. At the same time, the adaptive accommodation and updating of working models in response to new attachment-relevant experiences continue to occur during adulthood, or else adults would not be able to continue to make accurate appraisals of their changing selves and changing life circumstances.

Bowlby (1973) discussed the increasing stability of attachment patterns across childhood, adolescence, and into adulthood as follows:

> [The] model proposed postulates that the psychological processes that result in personality structure are endowed with a fair degree of sensitivity to the environment, especially to family environment, during the early years of life, but a sensitivity that diminishes throughout childhood and is already very limited by the end of adolescence. Thus the developmental process is conceived as able to vary its course, more or less adaptively, during the early years, according to the environment in which development is occurring; and subsequently, with the reduction of environmental sensitivity, as becoming increasingly constrained to the particular pathway already chosen. (pp. 415–416)

More than 30 published studies have examined the stability of attachment patterns during adulthood (see Table 5.1 for a summary of methods and findings). These studies used either interview methods (e.g., AAI, Current Relationship Interview [CRI]) or self-report scales and computed either stability coefficients of continuous attachment scores or concordance rates of categorical attachment classifications. Most of these studies examined the stability of attachment patterns over short periods of time, ranging from 1 week to 1 year. However, some studies collected stability data over 2, 4, or 6 years (see Table 5.1). Moreover, Klohnen and Bera (1998) examined the stability of adult attachment in a sample of women (the Mills College sample) over 25 years. Women completed a self-report attachment scale at age 52, and the researchers derived earlier attachment scores using adjective checklists that the women had completed at ages 27 and 43.

The findings summarized in Table 5.1 reveal moderate to high stability of adult attachment patterns over periods ranging from 1 week to 25 years. For continuous ratings of attachment styles or dimensions, the test–retest correlations range between .47 and .70, with an average coefficient around .56. For categorical attachment classifications, test–retest concordances ranged between 44% and 90%. On average, around 70% of the participants received the same attachment classification or chose the same attachment category at different time points. These relatively high levels of stability remain roughly the same after 1, 2, 4, 6, and even 25 years (see Table 5.1). For example, Klohnen and Bera (1998) found similar stability coefficients over 16 years (.58 from age 27 to 43) and 25 years (.55 from age 27 to 55). Fraley and Brumbaugh (2004) meta-analyzed 24 of these studies, compared them to the meta-analysis Fraley (2002) conducted on studies of childhood attachment, and concluded that the stability of attachment patterns in adulthood was higher (.54) than that observed in childhood attachment (.39). Moreover, they noted that the data fit well with a prediction made by the prototype model, according to which a core attachment pattern is maintained over time.

The findings are consistent with Bowlby's (1973) idea that adult attachment patterns can remain stable over long periods of time. However, at the same time, the fact that the average test–retest correlation is around .56 leaves considerable room for change and suggests that adult attachment patterns are still somewhat sensitive to changing life cir-

TABLE 5.1. A Summary of Findings Concerning the Stability of Adult Attachment Orientations

Study	N	Measure	Time lapse	Estimated stability coefficient
Studies assessing stability of attachment types				
Pistole (1989)	67	HS types	1 week	.52
Bakermans-Kranenburg & van IJzendoorn (1993)	83	AAI	2 months	.63
Senchak & Leonard (1992)	335	HS types	12 months	.48
Baldwin et al. (1993)	16	HS types	4 months	−.13
Benoit & Parker (1994)	84	AAI	12 months	.67
Keelan et al. (1994)	105	HS types	4 months	.60
Kirkpatrick & Hazan (1994)	172	HS types	4 years	.40
Sagi et al. (1994)	59	AAI	3 months	.79
Baldwin & Fehr (1995)	517	HS types	1–40 weeks	.42
Crowell, Treboux, & Waters (2002)	161	AAI	21 months	.62
Lopez & Gormley (2002)	207	RQ	7 months	.37
Studies assessing stability of attachment ratings				
M. B. Levy & Davis (1988)	63	HS ratings	2 weeks	.57
Collins & Read (1990)	101	AAS	2 months	.64
Hammond & Fletcher (1991)	102	HS ratings	4 months	.47
J. A. Feeney & Noller (1992)	172	HS ratings	2 months	.67
Shaver & Brennan (1992)	242	HS ratings	8 months	.68
West & Sheldon-Keller (1992)	35	RAQ	4 months	.75
J. A. Feeney, Noller, & Callan (1994)	70	15-item scale	8 months	.62
J. A. Feeney, Noller, & Hanrahan (1994)	295	ASQ	10 weeks	.76
Scharfe & Bartholomew (1994)	72	RQ	8 months	.51
Brennan & Shaver (1995)	128	HS ratings	8 months	.57
Fuller & Fincham (1995)	44	HS ratings	24 months	.62
Davila et al. (1997)	155	HS ratings	6 months	.52
			24 months	.48
Klohnen & Bera (1998)	142	Adjective ratings	5 years	.71
			9 years	.58
			27 years	.55
Davila et al. (1999)	344	AAS	6 months	.68
			12 months	.71
			18 months	.58
			24 months	.61
E. R. Smith et al. (1999)	60	ECR	3 months	.77
Pierce & Lydon (2001)	304	RQ (global)	11 months	.52
Pierce & Lydon (2001)	304	RQ (within relationships)	11 months	.57
Ruvolo et al. (2001)	322	RQ	5 months	.49
Cozzarelli et al. (2003)	442	RQ	24 months	.38
Davila & Cobb (2003)	86	RQ	12 months	.63
Davila & Sargent (2003)	154	AAS	2 months	.81
Simpson, Rholes, Campbell, & Wilson (2003)	212	AAQ	6 months	.64
J. P. Allen et al. (2004)	101	AAI—security	2 years	.61
Sibley & Liu (2004)	142	ECR-R	6 weeks	.90
Zhang & Labouvie-Vief (2004)	370	ECR	2 years	.44
			6 years	.35

Note. HS, Hazan and Shaver.

cumstances. Baldwin and Fehr (1995) estimated that around 30% of adults experience statistically significant changes in their attachment patterns across relatively short time spans (less than 1 year). However, it is important to note that some portion of this variation can be explained by the unreliability of the attachment measures on which their conclusions were based. Not only are the reliabilities of most adult attachment measures far from perfect, but also the cross-time stability of attachment patterns in adulthood, whether measured by interviews or self-report questionnaires, seems to be about the same *regardless of the time span between assessments*, which suggests that the changeability of attachment patterns is partly a reflection of measurement error (Scharfe & Bartholomew, 1994).

A handful of studies have explored whether changes in adult attachment style can be explained by attachment-relevant experiences that challenge existing working models. For people who enter the adult world with a secure attachment style, these destabilizing experiences include experiences of rejection, disapproval, or criticism, the breaking of an attachment bond, and separation or loss of an attachment figure. For insecure people, the formation of a stable, secure attachment bond with a romantic partner; positive interpersonal interactions; a good marriage; successful psychotherapy; becoming a loving and caring parent; and encounters with available, sensitive, and supportive relationship partners can contradict their negative models of self and others. As in childhood and adolescence, these changing life circumstances can encourage people to reflect upon and reevaluate their attachment behavior and working models.

Unfortunately, the evidence to date is not strongly consistent. On one hand, Kirkpatrick and Hazan (1994) found that over a period of 4 years, secure people tended to become less secure after the breakup of a romantic relationship, whereas insecure people tended to become more secure after initiating a new romantic relationship. Hammond and Fletcher (1991), J. A. Feeney and Noller (1992), and Ruvolo, Fabin, and Ruvolo (2001), who followed up dating couples for periods ranging from 2 to 5 months, found that relationship difficulties or breakups led to a decrease in attachment security. In 2-year longitudinal studies of newlyweds, Davila, Karney, and Bradbury (1999) and Crowell, Treboux, and Waters (2002) found that people became more secure (as indicated by either self-report scales or the AAI) during the transition to marriage. Simpson, Rholes, Campbell, and Wilson (2003) found a similar change toward increased security across the transition to parenthood among women (but not men). In an 8-week diary study, Davila and Sargent (2003) also found that positive interpersonal experiences (signs of a partner's attention, love, and acceptance) on a given day tended to increase feelings of attachment security on that day (compared with the prior day's security level). On the other hand, several studies have failed to find associations between attachment-relevant life events and changes in adult attachment patterns (Baldwin & Fehr, 1995; Cozzarelli, Karafa, Collins, & Tagler, 2003; Davila & Cobb, 2003; Davila et al., 1997; Scharfe & Bartholomew, 1994).

What accounts for these inconsistencies? One possibility is that some authors did not consider individual differences in the subjective appraisal of interpersonal events. As we discuss in subsequent chapters, people differ in the way they appraise and interpret life events, and this cognitive construal of experience can have a more potent effect on working models than the mere occurrence of an attachment-relevant event. For example, some people construe divorce as a painful loss, whereas others view it as a relief, if not a cause for celebration. According to Davila and Cobb (2004), "Whereas there might be objective features of events that contribute to whether they will disconfirm attachment models, a person would need to construe an event as providing evidence of disconfirmation.

Hence, the effect of events on change in attachment models might be cognitively mediated through subjective perceptions" (pp. 143–144). The same reasoning led Lazarus and Folkman (1984) to argue two decades ago that a stressful event is a "stressor" only if it is appraised as such; its implications for mental health depend on people's appraisal and coping processes.

In support of this view, Davila et al. (1999) found that the transition to marriage moved newlywed husbands and wives toward attachment security mainly if they appraised their marital relations positively (i.e., had high marital satisfaction). Simpson, Rholes, Campbell, and Wilson (2003) reported that the transition to parenthood was more likely to move anxiously attached women toward security if they perceived their spouses as available, supportive, and accepting during pregnancy. In addition, whereas women who sought less spousal support during pregnancy became more avoidant across the transition to parenthood, husbands who perceived themselves as providing more spousal support during pregnancy became less avoidant. In their 8-week diary study, Davila and Sargent (2003) found that negative events on a given day reduced felt security on that day mainly when people viewed these events as involving some kind of interpersonal loss. Thus, we conclude that changes in self-reported attachment orientation are systematically related to the meaning people assign to attachment-relevant life events, and to the way they perceive themselves and their relationship partners during these events.

Another possible explanation of the inconsistencies observed in studies of changes in adult attachment styles is that the changes reflect not only adaptive accommodation of working models to changing life circumstances but also random fluctuations in attachment strategies (which infant attachment researchers call "disorganization") resulting from inner problems and vulnerabilities (for similar analyses of personal vulnerability and variability in personality traits, see Block, 1961; C. R. Rogers, 1961). According to Davila et al. (1997), some people exhibit changes in attachment style over time, or report fluctuating feelings of security, because they never developed clear prototype working models and now possess inconsistent, conflicting, or confusing attachment representations. This lack of clarity and coherence of attachment representations can result from diverse vulnerability factors (e.g., frightening/frightened parents, abusive parents, parental psychopathology, or personal psychopathology) and can render adult attachment patterns unstable mainly when the interpersonal context is also unstable. Davila et al.'s analysis implies that change in attachment patterns is a joint function of changing life circumstances and the clarity and coherence of one's attachment prototype and working models.

Few studies have examined this possibility, but those few consistently show that individual vulnerability factors are associated with more dramatic changes in adult attachment patterns over time (J. P. Allen, McElhaney, Kuperminc, & Jodl, 2004; Cozzarelli et al., 2003; Davila & Cobb, 2003; Davila et al., 1997, 1999; J. A. Feeney, Passmore, & Peterson, in press). For example, Davila et al. (1997) found that late adolescent women who changed attachment patterns over 6 or 24 months (either from secure to insecure or from insecure to secure) had more psychological vulnerabilities (parental divorce, history of psychopathology, and personality disorders) than those who remained secure during the 2-year study period. Moreover, the level of vulnerabilities of women who changed attachment patterns was similar to the levels of those who were stably insecure. According to Davila et al., this implies that fluctuations in adult attachment patterns are a reflection of a core sense of insecurity. Cozzarelli et al. (2003) also found that women who moved toward insecure attachment over a 2-year period after undergoing abortion were more likely to have a history of depression or abuse, and Davila and Cobb (2003) found that a history of psychopathology and a diagnosis of personality disorder were associated with lack of clarity in models of self and others, which in turn was associated with changes in self-reported attachment style over a 1-year period. In a recent study, J. A. Feeney et al. (in press) found that for adults who were adopted as infants (but not for a comparison sample), recent relationship difficulties (e.g., conflict with romantic partners) were associated with increases in attachment insecurity.

Overall, existing studies provide important information about continuity and discontinuity in adult attachment style. Although adult attachment patterns, as Bowlby (1973) proposed, are less "environmentally labile" than childhood attachment patterns, they are still somewhat malleable in response to attachment-relevant experiences and life transitions. Moreover, some vulnerable adults tend to show very unstable, randomly fluctuating attachment patterns that may point to disorganization of the attachment system. Future research should examine these erratic fluctuations in adult attachment patterns and their possible roots in attachment disorganization in infancy and childhood. Studies should also be designed to determine whether and how therapeutic interventions or other positive interpersonal experiences can increase attachment style stability in vulnerable adults.

CONCLUDING REMARKS

The developmental trajectory of childhood, adolescent, and adult attachment is not linear or in any other way simple. There are numerous, complex determinants of adult attachment style, especially as it is manifested under varying life circumstances. Adult attachment patterns are likely to be rooted in early experiences with parents and associated prototype working models formed during infancy and early childhood. But they are also affected by attachment-relevant experiences during later childhood and adolescence, recent experiences in adult relationships, and a broad array of contextual factors that moderate the effects of internalized representations of past experiences. Studies fairly consistently yield a moderate degree of stability in attachment patterns from infancy to adulthood and a moderate to high degree of stability throughout the adult years, but they also reveal lawful discontinuities in attachment patterns in response to changing life circumstances. The data suggest that changing attachment relationships in adulthood can change the organization and functioning of the attachment system. If this were not the case, psychotherapy—including the kind conducted by Bowlby himself—would be fruitless.

Discussions about continuity and discontinuity in attachment style are further complicated by the fact that a person's current state of mind with respect to attachment and contextual factors that make specific working models or memories accessible can affect his or her attachment style at a given moment (Baldwin et al., 1996; Mikulincer & Shaver, 2003). The attachment style a person displays at a given moment is not the only one that he or she might display on other occasions, in other social circumstances. Bowlby (1969/1982) talked about multiple, even conflicting, attachment working models, some of which are more conscious than others. Experimental social psychologists have shown that people typically have multiple models of attachment applying to particular relationships or kinds of relationships (e.g., Baldwin et al., 1996). Therefore, although people may have chronically accessible, fairly general attachment representations, perhaps reflecting their childhood prototype working models, and although these models can be fairly stable over time, they also possess less immediately accessible working models that can be activated by inner or outer forces (thoughts, images, dreams, or environmental stimuli that prime specific working models). These less accessible working models, which can be contextually activated in experimental settings (e.g., as shown by Baldwin et al., 1996; Mikulincer & Shaver, 2001), have measurable effects on momentary self-conceptions, defenses, and behaviors, and are a source of temporary changes in attachment patterns.

In line with this reasoning, every theoretical model of attachment dynamics should include ideas concerning both contextual and more long-lasting changes in the functioning of the attachment system. These ideas are particularly relevant to creating adequate attachment-oriented psychotherapies and for understanding factors in the client–psychotherapist relationship that foster symptom alleviation and personality change (Shaver & Norman, 1995). In this context, our studies on the positive effects of the contextual activation of security-enhancing mental representations (e.g., Mikulincer, Gillath, et al., 2001; Mikulincer & Shaver, 2001) can be viewed as an initial step in developing a research program on attachment and psychotherapy. Such a program should examine the functioning of the psychotherapist as a security-enhancing attachment figure, changes in the client's attachment dynamics caused by attachment to and internalization of this figure, and the ways in which these processes advance psychotherapeutic aims (see Chapter 14, this volume, for an extensive review of evidence on these issues).

There will undoubtedly be future discoveries about independent and interactive determinants of attachment patterns. It seems likely that the role of genes is still clouded by insufficient measurement procedures. The transmission of security or insecurity from parents to children may be affected by children's imitation of parents—a transmission process that is too rarely considered. That is, secure children may be similar to secure parents in their social behavior, methods of affect regulation, and styles of caregiving not only because they have been well treated, but also because the parents have been models of security, equanimity under pressure, positive affect, considerate kindness, compassion, and empathy. We already know enough, however, to be sure that genes will never be the whole story and that attachment patterns can be different with different relationship partners and at different times in life. In other words, the gist of Bowlby's original insights and of Ainsworth's early observations, in people's homes and in the Strange Situation, is still valid and in fact is increasingly supported by scientific research.

PART II

INTRAPERSONAL ASPECTS OF ATTACHMENT-SYSTEM FUNCTIONING

CHAPTER 6

Attachment-Related Mental
Representations of Self and Others

One of Bowlby's (1969/1982) key ideas was that actual experiences with attachment figures during times of need are cognitively encoded, processed, and stored in the form of mental representations of self and others (attachment working models), which in turn provide the skeleton of a person's attachment style (characteristic thoughts, feelings, and behaviors in close relationships). As we explained in Chapter 1, Bowlby took cues from earlier psychoanalytic theorists who used terms such as "internalization," "imago," and "object representation," and he updated these concepts by relying on what were, at the time he was writing, the current theories of cognition and cognitive development (e.g., Piaget, 1953). This is an important aspect of attachment theory, because the theory emphasizes cognitive processes when other kinds of theoretical constructs might have been accentuated instead: for example, behavioral patterns induced by imitation (as discussed by social learning theorists such as Bandura, 1977); Skinnerian "reinforcement" processes (Skinner, 1953); or experientially induced changes in the brain's limbic system (e.g., LeDoux, 1996).

Bowlby's emphasis on the cognitive underpinnings of attachment orientations coexisted comfortably with the cognitive emphasis in experimental social psychology when Hazan and Shaver (1987) first proposed using attachment theory as a framework for studying adolescent and adult romantic love. In their first studies of "romantic attachment," Hazan and Shaver (1987, 1990) included preliminary questionnaire measures of internal working models of self and romantic relationships, and found—in line with attachment theory—that self-reported attachment styles were predictably related to beliefs about self and relationships. For example, anxiously attached adults believed it is easy to fall in love and that this happens often, whereas avoidant adults doubted that romantic love even exists in real life. In one of the early elaborations of Hazan and Shaver's (1987) ideas, Bartholomew (1990; Bartholomew & Horowitz, 1991) reconceptualized adolescent and adult attachment styles in terms of positive and negative working models of self and relationship partners. Thus, the notion of working models or mental representations—whatever one chooses to call the cognitive elements of attachment style—became important to social and personality psychologists who study attachment.

In our own theoretical and empirical work, we have repeatedly discovered associations between individual differences in attachment-system functioning and people's perceptions of others (e.g., what one thinks about the availability, supportiveness, personal traits, and intentions of a relationship partner) and the self (what one thinks about one's own value to relationship partners, "lovability," and ability to handle challenges and threats). In this chapter, we focus on these cognitive aspects of attachment-system dynamics and review evidence concerning how adolescents and adults with different attachment styles appraise themselves, relationship partners, social groups, and humanity in general.

We begin with self-representations or models of self, then, in the second half of the chapter, consider representations or models of relationship partners and social groups. Because dreams provide what Freud (1911/1994) famously called the "royal road" to understanding the unconscious mind, we illustrate some of our points with excerpts from people's dreams. As we show, working models of self and others are evident even in a person's most private, idiosyncratic, and unintentional mental creations.

ATTACHMENT AND SELF-REPRESENTATIONS

In our model of the attachment behavioral system in adulthood (Chapter 2), the broaden-and-build cycle of attachment security initiated by repeated interactions with available, sensitive, and supportive attachment figures includes positive representations of self as worthy and competent. During these interactions, people find it easy to perceive themselves as valuable, lovable, and special, thanks to being valued, loved, and regarded as special by caring attachment figures. Moreover, they learn to view themselves as active, strong, and competent, because they can effectively mobilize an attachment figure's support and restore emotional equanimity, while turning their attention to exploration and learning (thanks to the "secure base" provided by one or more attachment figures). In this way, interactions with security-enhancing attachment figures become natural building blocks of what Carl Rogers (1961) called the "real self." These building blocks are genuine, nondefensive, positive self-perceptions derived from one's own accomplishments, approvingly mirrored by attachment figures, and from receipt of others' love and encouragement over the course of development. In Chapter 3, we reviewed evidence linking experiences of attachment figure availability to positive changes in self-esteem. In this chapter, we focus on associations between the chronic sense of attachment security (i.e., having a secure attachment style) and judgments of self-worth and competence.

In a study of attachment styles and dreams, Avihou (2006) asked university students, who completed the ECR attachment scales, to recall their dreams each morning for 30 consecutive days and to write a brief account of each one. Each dream was carefully coded. Two coders, who were blind to participants' ECR attachment scores, read each dream narrative and used the "core conflictual relationship themes" method (CCRT; Luborsky & Crits-Christoph, 1998) to characterize how participants represented themselves and their relationship partners. We say more later in this chapter about the results of the study, but here and elsewhere, we use sample dreams as examples of secure and insecure models of self and others.

Dreams show, simultaneously, that mental representations are associated with attachment style in a theoretically predictable way at an abstract (i.e., systematically coded) level, and yet are highly unusual and idiosyncratic at a detailed level. We believe that everyone's underlying attachment-related memories and cognitive–affective mental representations are likely to be theoretically interpretable yet idiographically unique in this same way. Dreams just happen to provide one "royal road" to gaining access to a person's attachment-related representations, without his or her disguising them by conscious distortion. This is why they have often been used clinically and in research.

In the following dream, recorded by a young woman who scored low on both the Anxious and Avoidant scales of the ECR (and was therefore classified as securely attached), we see an example of secure self-representations:

> "I was sitting in my elementary school library reading a book, and it seemed very natural [to be there] even though I haven't been there for years. I spoke with friends and teachers, and the place was just as it used to be (low ceiling and shelves full of kids' books, books that I read as a child). The principal came in and started yelling at us, saying we were barbaric children. I thought at first we might have been noisy and deserved this rebuke, but I immediately told him that, despite whatever bad behavior we engaged in, we didn't deserve such treatment and he had overlooked my many good qualities. I felt that despite being a little girl, I had enough self-esteem and self-respect to tell him he was wrong. So I got up and told him I was not a barbarian and I came to the library to read books that I like. He then apologized. I felt very proud of myself. At that instant, my mom appeared, hugged me, and said I was okay and she was very proud of me. (I don't know how my mom got there.) She then took me to some fun place; I don't know where. I just remember that we laughed a lot and bought some silly things—maybe in a mall."

Notice that although the dreamer was criticized by an authority figure and at first entertained the possibility that she might deserve criticism, she decided that in fact she did not deserve it and should stand up for herself. When she expressed her views, the authority figure apologized, and the dreamer's mother suddenly appeared to support her daughter's judgment and assertiveness. The dream ended happily, in a way that endorsed and perhaps reinforced the dreamer's self-esteem and autonomous assertiveness. This is a beautiful example of a point we make throughout this book: Being supported by attachment figures and becoming autonomous and assertive are interrelated, not mutually exclusive, processes. As Bowlby (1969/1982) insisted, contrary to previous notions of "childish dependency," healthy dependency on early attachment figures (having a safe haven and secure base) is the cradle of subsequent healthy independence and self-confidence.

Despite the seemingly reasonable and straightforward association between being loved and esteemed by others and having a strong sense of one's own personal value, some authors have suspected that interactions with security-enhancing attachment figures might result in overdependence on others for assistance in times of need, at the expense of autonomy and self-reliance (e.g., Kirkpatrick, 1998a). If so, securely attached people might represent themselves as vulnerable and dependent, and despite feeling valuable and lovable, their self-worth might depend precariously on other people's constant approval and affection. This is an adult version of what traditional members of modern societies call "spoiling" a child—a concept that Bowlby completely rejected. (In fact, behavior that traditionalists think stems from meeting a child's needs too readily is characteristic of anxiously attached children whose parents' have responded inconsistently, at times being neglectful and at other times trying to make up for it by being overindulgent.) The dream we quoted shows how support from a primary attachment figure and the ability, later, to fend for oneself go hand in hand.

Attachment research on infants indicates that a sense of attachment security during the first year of life allows children to cry less later on, whine and plead less, and distance themselves more easily from attachment figures to explore the world and learn about it and themselves. This kind of learning enriches competencies and strengthens self-regulatory skills, allowing secure individuals to do things on their own without excessive or continuous help from others (e.g., Sroufe, Fox, & Pancake, 1983). This kind of confident exploration of the environment is a crucial step in the development of an independent, competent self. (The child's early progress from being more or less continuously supported to becoming increasingly independent has been the focus of most of the attachment research in child developmental psychology; for reviews see Thompson, 1999, and Weinfield, Sroufe, Egeland, & Carlson, 1999.)

In middle childhood, the sense of attachment security allows children to engage effectively in affiliative play with peers (K. H. Rubin, Bukowski, & Parker, 1998; Hazan & Zeifman, 1999), which provides an increasing range of social options for exploring personal interests, developing skills, and broadening one's sense of self-worth and efficacy (Berlin & Cassidy, 1999). During adolescence and adulthood, secure individuals are able to form reciprocal and mutually satisfying relationships with special peers, relationships in which they not only provide comfort to their partners but also receive support and act as co-regulators of their own and their partners' occasional distress (see Chapters 10 and 11, this volume). These abilities strengthen a secure person's sense of value and mastery, and bolster confidence in being able to form satisfying relationships and provide comfort to others when needed.

This developmental analysis fits well with the contention of social psychologists Pelham and Swann (1989) that a person's core sense of self-worth develops in infancy from diffuse experiences of positive emotion, then contributes to and supports later childhood cognitive self-evaluations of domain-specific abilities. (See also Bylsma, Cozzarelli, & Sumer, 1997, who explored the same idea in a study of college students.) According to attachment theory, interactions with security-enhancing attachment figures during infancy and early childhood are important generators of positive emotion (Bowlby, 1969/1982), including an appropriate sense of pride in oneself that remains fairly stable throughout life despite inevitable setbacks and hardships. This does not mean that secure people hold positive self-views in every domain from social relations to nuclear physics, which would be unrealistic, but that they have more opportunities than less secure people to learn about their actual abilities in many domains and develop generally optimistic expectations about their competence.

The link between secure attachment and a positive sense of self is also sustained by including representations of supportive attachment figures in one's self-image. According to attachment theory, one cognitive consequence of close relationships is the inclusion of attachment figures' traits and capacities within mental representations of self and subsequent relationship partners. Through security-enhancing interactions with sensitive and responsive attachment figures, a child develops implicit beliefs that he or she embodies the goodness, strength, and wisdom provided originally by what Bowlby (1969/1982) called "stronger and wiser" others. Moreover, a well-treated child incorporates the protecting, soothing, approving, encouraging, and coaching functions originally performed by a security-enhancing attachment figure into his or her own mental processes, allowing the child to perform these functions autonomously, in relation to both self and others. As a result, secure individuals tend to think and feel that they can regulate their emotions and actions without always having to depend on other people's assistance or approval, and they are generally good at supporting and encouraging other people as well.

We (Mikulincer & Shaver, 2004) proposed that this process of identification with attachment figures and incorporation into the self-concept of these figures' qualities and responses causes people to treat themselves the way attachment figures treated them (see also Bollas, 1987; Winnicott, 1965; Chapter 2, this volume). In the case of people who have generally received sensitive and responsive treatment from significant others, the process of identification (and, to use a psychoanalytic term, "introjection") makes them relatively immune to harsh self-criticism, and they can—more easily than their insecure peers—retain a sense of self-worth, while recognizing their normal human mistakes, weaknesses, and shortcomings. This is partly a matter of internal composure and ability to self-soothe, but it is sustained by a person's previously validated belief that others will value and accept one despite the mistakes or faults that, of course, apply to everyone.

Borrowing from Kohut's (1971, 1977, 1984) self psychology, we can say that attachment security facilitates "healthy narcissism," which allows a person to establish a cohesive and comfortable self-structure. The sense of self-cohesion—the feeling that one's many qualities and experiences reside within a single, well-integrated self-structure—provides a subjective feeling of solidity, stability, and permanence, and allows a person to feel coherent, consistent, and clear-minded even under threatening or unpredictable conditions. Moreover, self-coherence provides a sense of resilience, calms a person in times of stress, and repairs wounds to self-esteem inflicted by inevitable disappointments and difficulties. Healthy narcissism promotes the development of a stable set of ambitions, ideals, and values, and a motivating but realistic set of self-standards (which Higgins, Bond, Klein, & Strauman [1986] called the "ideal-self" and the "ought-self"). These qualities and standards help a person pursue and attain important goals, which supply feelings of success, achievement, and growth, and move a person steadily, although by necessity not quickly, toward what Maslow (1954, 1971) called self-actualization.

Lack of parental availability, sensitivity, and responsiveness contributes to disorders of the self, characterized by a lack of self-cohesion, doubts about one's coherence and continuity over time, and vulnerable or unstable self-esteem (Kohut & Wolf, 1978). This is the condition of insecurely attached people, whose frustrating, frightening, and disappointing interactions with unavailable, inconsistent, or rejecting attachment figures raised doubts about the degree to which they are esteemed and loved by these important people. Insecure people's self-esteem is likely to be overly contingent on other people's approval, the experience of temporary successes and failures, or defensive mental processes that distort reality. During their many demoralizing interactions with attachment figures, insecure people gradually incorporate (or introject) dismissing, degrading, and disapproving messages, which makes it likely that they will regard and treat themselves and others with disapproval and disdain. Thus, insecure people are likely to suffer from self-criticism and painful self-doubts, or to erect distorting defenses to counter feelings of worthlessness and hopelessness.

Although both anxious and avoidant people have difficulty constructing an authentic, cohesive, and stable sense of self-worth, their reliance on different secondary attachment strategies (see Chapter 2, this volume) results in different self-configurations and disorders of the self. Anxious, hyperactivating strategies intensify doubts about self-worth and self-efficacy, and intensify a person's sense of vulnerability to rejection or abandonment. Avoidant, deactivating strategies, in contrast, are a person's attempts to suppress such doubts, while working to convince the self and others that one is self-sufficient and invincible.

Below is an example, in the form of a dream, from a male university student who scored high on the ECR Anxious Attachment scale. Notice that he portrays himself in very negative terms, then, unlike the secure student whose dream we quoted earlier, represents his father as suddenly appearing and brutally endorsing a negative self-image:

> "I am arguing with friends about who teaches a particular course. While arguing, I start running toward the city and see a bank robbery in progress. Suddenly I realize that I am the bank robber! I'm debating with myself about whether I should break into the bank or not, and I decide that I should. I get into the bank and yell, 'Give me the money!' The teller stoops down below the counter, gets the money, and hands it to me, and I run away. While exiting the bank, I shoot three times in the air and then run down the street with the weapon wrapped in a quilt. While running, I suddenly think about what I've done and what a bad person I am: 'Maybe I hit someone while shooting in the air.' I'm debating with myself about where to run and I suddenly notice that the money has disappeared. I think, 'Why can't I do something right for once in my life?' I want to cry. Suddenly the cops arrive to take me to jail. I say, 'Take me. Maybe it's for the best that I go to jail. No one actually cares about me anyhow.' I feel really ashamed of what I did. Suddenly my dad appears and yells at me: 'How dare you do such a foolish thing! You deserve to go to jail. You're worthless.' It hurts, but I know that what he says is true."

Consistent with the anxious stance depicted in the dream, it is common for an attachment-anxious person, who hopes to gain a partner's love, esteem, and protection, to take some of the blame for a partner's unreliable care ("Something is wrong with me; I don't have what it takes to gain my partner's reliable attention and regard"). It is also common for such a person to ruminate about why he or she is so worthless that others do not want to provide the love and approval that is so strongly desired. These thought processes heighten and reinforce the cognitive accessibility of negative self-representations and doubts about one's social value. Moreover, anxious overdependence on attachment figures interferes with the development of self-efficacy. Anxiously attached people generally prefer to rely on their partner rather than engage in challenging activities alone, thereby preventing them from exploring and learning new information and skills. In addition, deliberate but awkward or desperate attempts to gain proximity to an attachment figure reinforce a negative self-image, because anxious people often present themselves in degrading, incompetent, childish, or excessively needy ways in an effort to elicit compassion and support.

In the case of avoidant attachment, it is common to prop up one's self-image through unconscious defenses and narcissistic behavior (defensive self-enhancement). Avoidant people learn not to focus on or care about threats and not to seek support from attachment figures. These defensive efforts are accompanied by attempts to deny vulnerability, negative self-aspects, and memories of personal failures, while trying to focus on and display traits and feelings compatible with self-sufficiency. Avoidant people often entertain fantasies of perfection and power, exaggerate their achievements and talents, and avoid situations that challenge their defenses and threaten their grandiosity. They can become quite annoyed, however, when someone asks them to alter their behavior, be more considerate, soften their defenses, or admit their mistakes. Below is an example from an avoidant female university student's dream. In this dream, her prickliness is symbolically represented by wire spikes growing out of the dreamer's head and hair.

> "I'm at home, hearing my mom talking on the phone. Suddenly I realize she is talking with someone and making all kinds of arrangements for me that I had intended to make myself. I'm irritated and tell her to quit intruding: 'I don't deserve it, and I need more privacy and space at home.' I tell her she doesn't understand me or know me and should leave me alone. 'I'm strong enough to be on my own and make decisions for myself.' I go to a different room to get away from her, and suddenly I'm in some kind of military unit. I'm in a wooden barracks, looking around, and suddenly men in uniform arrive. One is looking at me angrily, wondering why I'm not saluting him. I don't have a clue who he is, and I think he has a lot of gall expecting me to salute him. He continues to tell me all kinds of things, presumably about my life. I ask him to stop talking, because it's all bullshit. I'm angry about what he says, and I leave the room. I touch my hair and find that it is full of metal wires braided into it. I start pulling them out of my hair, but there are more and more."

With these theoretical ideas and dream samples in mind, we now turn to more rigorous empirical tests. In the sections that immediately follow we review evidence concerning attachment style differences in feelings of self-worth and self-competence, as well as defensive self-enhancement. In addition, we review research on psychological processes that sustain insecure people's self-related vulnerabilities.

Appraisals of Self-Worth and Self-Competence

More than 60 studies have examined associations between attachment style and global self-esteem (Table 6.1 contains a summary of methods and findings). All studies that assessed secure attachment to parents or peers, without exception, found that attachment security is associated with higher self-esteem. In addition, almost of all the studies found that (1) anxious (preoccupied or fearful) participants have lower self-esteem than their secure counterparts, and (2) attachment anxiety is associated with lower self-esteem. In a study using the Rosenberg Self-Esteem Scale in 53 nations, Schmitt and Allik (2005) found a significant negative association between attachment anxiety and self-esteem in 49 countries. This is strong evidence that anxiously attached people have low self-esteem. This is to be expected, theoretically, because attachment anxiety is defined in terms of fear of rejection and abandonment, and that kind of fear goes hand in hand with being uncertain or doubtful of one's own value.

The findings are less consistent with respect to avoidant attachment. About half of the reviewed studies provide no evidence of explicit self-esteem deficits in avoidant people, which might be expected given that they, especially the dismissing ones, try defensively to maintain high self-esteem. Nevertheless, many studies have found a significant negative correlation between avoidant attachment and self-esteem, suggesting either that some measures of avoidance are different enough from others to produce different associations with self-esteem, or that some avoidant individuals (probably the fearfully avoidant ones), regardless of the measure used, really do experience low self-esteem. Although attachment theory does not necessarily predict self-esteem deficits in avoidant individuals, because of their defensive tendency to exclude thoughts of vulnerability and deficiency from consciousness, research suggests that these defenses are not always suc-

TABLE 6.1. A Summary of Findings Linking Attachment Orientations with Self-Esteem

Study	Attachment scale	Self-esteem scale	Main findings
Studies assessing secure attachment to parents or peers			
Armsden & Greenberg (1987)	IPPA	TSCS	Security (+)
Cotterell (1992)	IPPA	Rosenberg	Security (+)
Papini & Roggman (1992)	IPPA	SPP	Security (+)
Kenny et al. (1993)	PAQ	SPP	Security (+)
Paterson et al. (1995)	IPPA	Rosenberg	Security (+)
Davila et al. (1996)	IPPA	SPP	Security (+)
McCurdy & Scherman (1996)	PAQ	Rosenberg	Security (+)
K. A. Black & McCartney (1997)	IPPA	SPP	Security (+)
O'Koon (1997)	IPPA	Offer scale	Security (+)
Kenny et al. (1998)*	PAQ	SPP	Security (+)
Sharpe et al. (1998)	HS types	Single item	Secure > Insecure
Volling et al. (1998, couple study)	HS types	Rosenberg	Two partners secure > Two partners insecure
Noom et al. (1999)	IPPA	Rosenberg	Security (+)
Leondari & Kiosseoglou (2000)	IPPA	Rosenberg	Security (+)
Engels-Rutger et al. (2001)	IPPA	Rosenberg	Security (+)
Fass & Tubman (2002)	IPPA	Rosenberg	Security (+)
Cassidy et al. (2003, Study 1)	SS-mother	SPP	Security (+)
Cassidy et al. (2003, Study 2)	ECR-peer	SPP	Security (+)
Neyer & Voigt (2004)	6 items-peer	5-item scale	Security (+)
Rice & Lopez (2004)	AAQ-peer	Rosenberg	Security (+)
Scharf et al. (2004)	AAI	WAI	Security (ns)
Treboux et al. (2004, Study 2)	AAI, CRI	MSEI	Security (+) only for lovability but not for global self-esteem and likeability
Kenny et al. (2005)	PAQ	Offer scale	Security (+)
Studies assessing attachment types			
J. A. Feeney & Noller (1990)	HS types	Coopersmith	Secure > Anxious, Avoidant
Zeanah et al. (1993)	AAI	MSEI	No significant differences
McCormick & Kennedy (1994)	HS-parent	Coopersmith	Secure > Anxious, Avoidant
Salzman (1996)	Interview	Rosenberg	Secure > Anxious
Brennan & Morris (1997)	RQ	Rosenberg	Secure > Avoidant > Anxious, Fearful
Buunk (1997)	HS types	DPQ	Secure > Anxious, Avoidant
Bylsma et al. (1997)	RQ	Rosenberg	Secure > Anxious, Fearful
Pietromonaco & Barrett (1997)	RQ	Rosenberg	Secure > Anxious, Fearful
Brennan & Bossom (1998)	RQ	Rosenberg	Secure > Anxious, Fearful
Gittleman et al. (1998)	RQ-parent	Rosenberg	Secure > Anxious
Man & Hamid (1998)	RQ	Rosenberg	Secure > Avoidant > Anxious, Fearful
Meyers (1998)	HS types	Rosenberg	Secure > Anxious, Avoidant
McCarthy (1999)	HS types	Rosenberg	Secure > Anxious
Bifulco, Moran, Ball, & Lillie (2002)	Interview	SESSI	Secure > Anxious, Avoidant, Fearful
Huntsinger & Luecken (2004)	RQ	Rosenberg	Secure > Avoidant > Anxious, Fearful
L. E. Park et al. (2004)	RQ	Rosenberg	Secure > Anxious, Fearful

(cont.)

TABLE 6.1. *(cont.)*

Study	Attachment scale	Self-esteem scale	Main findings
Studies based on attachment-style ratings			
Bartholomew & Horowitz (1991)	RQ	Rosenberg	Secure (+), Anxious (−), Avoidant (+), Fearful (−)
Mickelson et al. (1997)	HS ratings	Rosenberg	Secure (+), Anxious (−), Avoidant (−),
Carranza & Kilmann (2000)	RSQ	TSCS	Secure (+), Anx (ns), Avo (ns), Fearful (ns)
Sheehan & Noller (2002)	ASQ	Coopersmith	Secure (+), Anxious (−), Avoidant (−)
Cyranowski et al. (2002)	RQ	TSCS	Secure (+), Anxious (−), Avoidant (ns), Fearful (−)
Davila et al. (2004)	RQ	SPP	Secure (+), Anxious (−), Avoidant (ns), Fearful (−)
Onishi et al. (2001)	ECR prototypes	Q-sort task	Secure (+), Anxious (−), Avoidant (ns), Fearful (−)
Hofstra et al. (2005, Study 1)	ASQ	Rosenberg	Secure (+), Anxious (−), Avoidant (ns), Fearful (−)
Hofstra et al. (2005, Study 2)	ASQ	SPP	Secure (+), Anxious (−), Avoidant (ns), Fearful (−)
Studies based on attachment dimensions			
Collins & Read (1990)	AAS	Rosenberg	Anxiety (−), Avoidance (ns)
Griffin & Bartholomew (1994b)	RQ	Rosenberg	Anxiety (−), Avoidance (ns)
Davila et al. (1996)	AAS	SPP	Anxiety (−), Avoidance (−)
Jones & Cunningham (1996)	AAS	Rosenberg	Anxiety (−), Avoidance (−) for W Anxiety (−), Avoidance (ns) for M
J. E. Roberts et al. (1996)*	AAS	Rosenberg	Anxiety (−), Avoidance (−)
Shaver, Papalia, et al. (1996)	RQ	Rosenberg	Anxiety (−), Avoidance (ns)
Cozzarelli et al. (1998)	RQ	Rosenberg	Anxiety (−), Avoidance (ns)
McCarthy & Taylor (1999)	HS ratings	Rosenberg	Anxiety (−), Avoidance (−)
Cozzarelli et al. (2000)	RQ-global RQ-specific	Rosenberg	Anxiety (ns), Avoidance (ns) Anxiety (−), Avoidance (ns)
Muller & Lemieux (2000)	RSQ	Rosenberg	Anxiety (−), Avoidance (ns)
R. Alexander et al. (2001)	ASQ	Coopersmith	Anxiety (−), Avoidance (−)
Davila & Bradbury (2001)	AAS	Rosenberg	Anxiety (−), Avoidance (−)
McGowan (2002)	RQ	SSE	Anxiety (−), Avoidance (ns)
Taubman Ben-Ari et al. (2002)	HS ratings	Rosenberg	Anxiety (−), Avoidance (−)
Ciesla et al. (2004)	RQ	Rosenberg	Anxiety (−), Avoidance (ns)
Gentzler & Kerns (2004)	ECR	Rosenberg	Anxiety (−), Avoidance (−)
Luke et al. (2004)	RQ, ECR	Rosenberg SRRS	Anxiety (−), Avoidance (ns) Anxiety (−), Avoidance (−)
Pereg & Mikulincer (2004, Study 1)	HS ratings	Rosenberg	Anxiety (−), Avoidance (ns)
Treboux et al. (2004, Study 2)	ECR	MSEI	Anxiety (−), Avoidance (−)
Doyle & Markiewicz (2005)*	RC-parents	SDQ	Anxiety (−), Avoidance (−)
Gamble & Roberts (2005)	AAS	Rosenberg	Anxiety (−), Avoidance (ns)
Hankin et al. (2005, Study 2)*	AAS	Rosenberg	Anxiety (−), Avoidance (−)
Klohnen et al. (2005)	RQ	Rosenberg	Anxiety (−), Avoidance (ns)
Schmitt & Allik (2005)	RQ	Rosenberg	Anxiety (−), Avoidance (ns)
Wearden et al. (2005)	RQ	Rosenberg	Anxiety (−), Avoidance (ns)

Note. *, longitudinal design; (−), significant inverse correlation; (+), significant positive correlation; (ns), nonsignificant effects; M, men; W, women; DPQ, Dutch Personality Questionnaire; HS, Hazan and Shaver; MSEI, Multidimensional Self-Esteem Inventory; SDQ, Self-Description Questionnaire; SESSI, Self-Evaluation and Social Support Interview; SPP, Self-Perception Profile; SRRS, Self-Rating Revised Scale; SS, Security Scale; SSE, State Self-Esteem; TSCS, Tennessee Self-Concept Scale; WAI, Weinberger Adjustment Inventory.

cessful in preventing self-doubts and mental pain (see Chapter 7, this volume, for additional evidence concerning the fragility of avoidant defenses). In fact, Schmitt and Allik (2005) found a significant negative correlation between avoidance and self-esteem in 18 of the 53 countries they sampled.

There is also evidence concerning attachment-related variations in kinds of self-evaluation other than self-esteem. For example, Salzman (1996) asked undergraduate women how strongly they identified with positive and negative aspects of their mothers, and found that more anxious women reported fewer positive identifications and more negative identifications with their mothers. Interestingly, avoidant women reported fewer positive identifications but not more negative identifications, perhaps reflecting an inability to identify with their mothers, combined with a defense against admissions of sharing a parent's negative qualities. In another example, Mikulincer (1995, Study 1) found that attachment-anxious adolescents selected fewer positive and more negative adjectives to describe themselves than did less anxious adolescents. Moreover, attachment-anxious adolescents displayed a negative memory bias, recalling more negative than positive self-attributes in a subsequent memory task. Avoidant adolescents had a more positive self-view than their anxious counterparts, perhaps reflecting their tendency to suppress negative self-attributes. (Throughout this and subsequent chapters we demonstrate that avoidant individuals' claims of high self-esteem and absence of negative self-attributes should be interpreted as a result of defensiveness.)

Using the CCRT method for coding open-ended narratives (Luborsky & Crits-Christoph, 1998), two studies (Avihou, 2006; Raz, 2002) provided further evidence concerning attachment style differences in self-views. In Raz's study, participants were asked to recall problematic interactions with a romantic partner and to describe in each case what happened, including what they and their partners said and did. In Avihou's (2006) study, as already mentioned, participants were asked to recall their dreams for 30 consecutive days. The findings were consistent across the two studies. Stories or dreams reported by attachment-anxious individuals included more representations of the self as anxious, weak, helpless, and unloved than stories or dreams reported by less anxiously attached individuals. Attachment avoidance was associated with representations of the self as unreceptive (distant, uncooperative, emotionally unexpressive, or angry). In other words, insecure people's self-related vulnerabilities were evident in memories of problematic interactions and in dreams.

Several studies examined correlations between attachment measures and scales measuring self-efficacy (Table 6.2 summarizes the methods and findings). The results are consistent in showing that attachment security is associated with greater self-assessed competence or efficacy, and that attachment anxiety is associated with relatively negative evaluations of competence across all life domains studied. Unlike anxious individuals' broad and undifferentiated negative self-views, the self-views of avoidant individuals seem to depend on the specific domain in which competence is assessed. Avoidant individuals exhibited little self-criticism in nonsocial domains, but they consistently appraised themselves unfavorably in social and interpersonal domains (see Table 6.2); that is, avoidant people seemed to know, or believe, that they are not very competent in social settings. We should keep in mind, however, that they also tend to dismiss the importance of this domain, and try to avoid interdependence and intimacy (see Chapter 9, this volume). So it is not yet clear whether their negative self-views in this domain imply that they feel unhappy or upset about it. Their declarations of incompetence might be like our own admission that we are not very good at karaoke singing: We're not, but on most days this doesn't bother us much.

Most of the studies summarized so far relied on cross-sectional designs from which

TABLE 6.2. A Summary of Findings Linking Attachment Orientations with Rated Self-Competence

Study	Attachment scale	Competence domain	Main findings
Studies assessing secure attachment to parents or peers			
Kenny (1990)	PAQ	Academic	Security (+)
		Social	Security (+)
Kenny & Donaldson (1991)	PAQ	Social	Security (+)
Nada-Raja et al. (1992)	IPPA	Personal	Security (+)
Papini & Roggman (1992)	IPPA	Physical	Security (+)
		Social	Security (+)
Kenny et al. (1993)*	PAQ	Academic	Security (+)
		Social	Security (+)
Kenny (1994)	PAQ	Social	Security (+)
Paterson et al. (1994)	IPPA	Social	Security (+)
Schultheiss & Blustein (1994)	IPPA	Academic	Security (+) for W
		Social	Security (+) for W
Rice et al. (1995)*	IPPA	Academic	Security (+)
O'Brien (1996)	IPPA	Academic	Security (+)
N. E. Ryan et al. (1996)	IPPA	Academic	Security (+)
Schneider & Younger (1996)	IPPA	Social	Security (+)
K. A. Black & McCartney (19967)	IPPA	Academic	Security (+)
Noom et al. (1999)	IPPA	Academic	Security (+)
		Social	Security (+)
Engels-Rutger et al. (2001)	IPPA	Social	Security (+)
Kenny & Gallagher (2002)	IPPA	Academic	Security (+)
		Social	Security (+)
Lopez & Gormley (2002)*	RQ	Social	Security (+)
		Physical	Security (+)
Kenny et al. (2005)	PAQ	Global	Security (+)
		Social	Security (+)
Studies assessing attachment types			
Kobak & Sceery (1988)	AAI	Social	Secure > Anxious
Bringle & Bagby (1992)	HS types	Achievement	Secure > Anxious
		Social	Secure > Avoidant
Pietromonaco & Carnelley (1994)	AAS	Social	Secure > Anxious, Avoidant
Brennan & Morris (1997)	RQ	Global	Secure > Anxious, Fearful
Bylsma et al. (1997)	RQ	Academic	Ns differences
		Social	Secure > Anxious, Fearful
		Athletic	Secure > Anxious, Fearful
Allen et al. (1998)	AAI	Social	Secure > Anxious, Avoidant
Brennan & Bosson (1998)	RQ	Global	Secure > Anxious, Fearful
Meyers (1998)	HS types	Global	Secure > Anxious, Avoidant
Moreira et al. (1998)	HS types	Social	Secure > Anxious, Avoidant
Cooper et al. (1998)	HS types	Academic	Secure > Anxious > Avoidant
		Social	Secure > Anxious > Avoidant
		Athletic	Secure > Anxious, Avoidant
Allen et al. (2002)*	AAI	Social	Secure > Anxious, Avoidant
Studies assessing attachment dimensions			
Collins & Read (1990)	AAS	Social	Anxiety (−), Avoidance (−)
Cozzarelli et al. (1998)*	RQ	Global	Anxiety (−), Avoidance (ns)
Corcoran & Mallinckrodt (2000)	ASQ	Social	Anxiety (−), Avoidance (−)
Taubman Ben-Ari et al. (2002, Study 2)	HS ratings	Social	Anxiety (−), Avoidance (ns)
Taubman Ben-Ari et al. (2002, Study 3)	HS ratings	Social	Anxiety (−), Avoidance (−)
Strodl & Noller (2003)	ASQ	Global	Anxiety (−), Avoidance (−)
Cash et al. (2004)	RSQ, ECR	Physical	Anxiety (−), Avoidance (ns)
Mallincrodt & Wei (2005)	ECR	Social	Anxiety (−), Avoidance (−)
Wei, Russell, & Zakalik (2005)	ECR	Social	Anxiety (−), Avoidance (−)

Note. *, longitudinal design; (−), significant inverse correlation; (+), significant positive correlation; (ns), nonsignificant effects; W, women; HS, Hazan and Shaver.

causal interpretations could not be derived. Fortunately, however, some studies that were prospective and longitudinal in nature found that insecure attachment is a significant predictor of subsequent deficits in self-esteem and self-efficacy, with the time span between assessments varying from 6 weeks to 2 years (see Tables 6.1 and 6.2). In a further attempt to overcome the deficiencies of cross-sectional designs, Pietromonaco and Barrett (1997) examined whether college students' attachment orientations could predict daily self-evaluations over the course of a week. For every interpersonal interaction that lasted 10 minutes or longer during the week, participants rated how worthy they felt during that interaction. Anxiously attached students reported more negative self-evaluations after everyday social interactions, and avoidant students' ratings fell between those of the anxious and secure students (based on a three-category self-report measure of attachment style). Interestingly, anxious participants' negative self-views were evident even following nonconflictual interactions, implying that their vulnerability to negative self-evaluations was chronic and pervasive.

Overall, there is excellent evidence for self-related vulnerabilities associated with attachment insecurity in general and anxious attachment in particular. Across different nations and assessment methods, anxiously attached adolescents and adults are consistently found to hold negative beliefs about their self-worth and self-efficacy. The self-image of avoidant persons tends to be more positive and sometimes to resemble that of securely attached persons, but it seems unlikely that this positive self-view reflects an authentic, solid, stable sense of self-worth. Most likely it is a result of defensive self-enhancement, as we show in the following section.

Defensive Self-Enhancement

According to attachment theory, defensive self-enhancement indicates that a person has been forced by frustrating social experiences to cope with life's difficulties without adequate mental representations of attachment security and has had to struggle to maintain a sense of self-worth (Mikulincer & Shaver, 2005). This is the fate of avoidant individuals (particularly those with what Bartholomew and Horowitz [1991] called a dismissingly avoidant attachment style), whose compulsive self-reliance and reluctance to rely on other people encourages them to inflate their positive self-views and deny or suppress negative information about themselves. In contrast, secure individuals do not usually need to rely on defensive self-enhancement, because their core feelings of being loved, accepted, and valued by attachment figures support a stable sense of self-worth.

Attachment research provides strong support for interpreting avoidant persons' self-esteem as defensive in nature. For example, Gjerde, Onishi, and Carlson (2004) found that people classified as avoidant in the Romantic Attachment Interview (which is similar to the AAI and CRI, described in Chapter 4, this volume) scored higher than secure people on the California Adult Q-Set (CAQ) index of self-enhancement. (Avoidant people's descriptions of their traits were more favorable than descriptions of the same people provided by trained observers.) Moreover, avoidant individuals scored lower than their secure counterparts on the CAQ index of self-insight (the correlation between a participant's self-description and raters' descriptions of him or her). Avoidant people's lack of self-insight has also been documented in another study that found positive correlations between avoidant attachment and scales measuring poor self-clarity (Davila & Cobb, 2003). Avoidant people seem not only to possess an unrealistically positive view of themselves but also a rather unclear, incoherent sense of self.

These positively biased self-conceptions were also noted by Mikulincer (1995), who measured the cognitive accessibility of self-relevant traits in a Stroop task (see Chapter 3, this volume, for a description of the task). He also measured the level of integration of different self-aspects (participants' ratings of mutual influence, trade-offs, and joint interactions between different self-aspects). Whereas secure participants demonstrated ready access to both positive and negative self-attributes in the Stroop task and scored relatively high on a measure of self-integration, avoidant participants exhibited defensive organizations of self-attributes. They had quick access to positive, but not to negative, self-attributes and their different self-aspects were poorly integrated. Their lack of self-integration has also been documented with scales that measure "splitting" defenses (i.e., attempts to protect desirable aspects of oneself by detaching them from undesirable aspects; Lopez, 2001; Lopez, Fuendeling, Thomas, & Sagula, 1997).

In a further attempt to examine the poor integration of avoidant people's self-representations, Kim (2005) used Donahue, Robins, Roberts, and John's (1993) operationalization of self-fragmentation (low correlations among self-attributes across different social roles) and asked participants to rate themselves on a list of traits for each of five social roles (e.g., student, friend). Although avoidant attachment was not directly related to self-fragmentation, Kim (2005) found an indirect link mediated by what she called "authentic self" (a mixture of self-determination, self-knowledge, and vitality). Specifically, avoidant attachment was associated with lower ratings on choice, authenticity, and vitality, which in turn contributed to higher fragmentation of the self across different social roles. It seems that avoidant people's problems in integrating different self-aspects may be due to poor self-understanding and a desire to avoid taking responsibility for their choices and actions.

There is also evidence that avoidant people react to threatening events with defensive self-inflation (Mikulincer, 1998a; Hart, Shaver, & Goldenberg, 2005, Study 2). Participants in several experiments were exposed to various kinds of threatening or neutral information, and self-appraisals were recorded on self-report scales and also assessed by subtler techniques, such as reaction time (RT) for trait recognition. Whereas Mikulincer (1998a) exposed participants to failure vs. neutral feedback in an ego-involving cognitive task, Hart et al. (2005) asked people to think about an attachment threat (separation from a close relationship partner) or a neutral topic (watching TV). Despite these methodological differences, both sets of studies found that avoidant people appraised themselves more positively (according to both explicit and implicit measures) following threatening compared with neutral manipulations. Interestingly, secure individuals' self-appraisals did not differ much across neutral and threatening conditions; that is, secure people made relatively stable and unbiased self-appraisals even when coping with threats.

Mikulincer (1998a), using procedures that discourage defensive self-enhancement (the presence of a knowledgeable friend or a "bogus pipeline" device that purportedly measures "true feelings about things"), also found that surveillance had no effect on secure people's self-appraisals. However, these goads to tell the truth diminished avoidant individuals' otherwise positively distorted self-views under threatening conditions. In addition, Mikulincer found that avoidant individuals' tendency to report more positive self-views under threatening conditions was inhibited by a message that broke the link between a positive self-view and self-reliance ("Empirical findings show that people who hold a balanced self-view and acknowledge both strong and weak self-aspects are better equipped to perform cognitive task alone and have been found to succeed in these tasks without the help of supervisors," p. 430). This finding implies that avoidant people's positive self-appraisals are strategic attempts to convince others of their admirable (and perhaps enviable) qualities.

Attachment-related individual differences in self-enhancement were also noted in studies of the effects of self-relevant feedback from a romantic partner (Brennan & Bosson, 1998). Securely attached people sought their partner's feedback and generally appreciated and accepted it; that is, they were open to their partner's feedback and tended to use it to adjust their self-appraisals and create a more accurate self-image. Once again, however, avoidant people (dismissing or fearful) reacted defensively and were averse to partner feedback, preferring partners who did not know them well, and reacting to feedback dismissively or with indifference.

Adult attachment researchers have suggested ways in which securely attached people maintain a stable sense of self-worth without relying on defensive self-enhancement. For example, Mikulincer (1998a) found that secure people recalled more self-attributes, both positive and negative, in threatening than in neutral situations, suggesting a self-affirmation process in which the secure person's self-representations serve as an inner anchor for dealing with threats. Instead of distorting and inflating their self-image, secure individuals seemed to affirm a stable and accurate self-view by keeping more self-attributes active in memory, whether the attributes were positive or negative. (This tendency is similar to the secure pattern of responding in the AAI, which is marked by realistic, convincing, and balanced descriptions of one's parents and of childhood relationships with them. Secure people do not generally look at themselves or their parents through distorted, one-sided, or rose-colored glasses.)

We (Mikulincer & Shaver, 2004) tested the possibility, discussed earlier in this chapter and also mentioned in Chapter 2, that security-based self-representations underlie the maintenance of a positive sense of self in times of stress. In two studies, we asked people to generate a list of traits that described either how one of their most security-providing attachment figures acted in relation to them when they sought support from him or her, or how they felt when interacting with this person. In a second session of each study (weeks after the first), we exposed each person either to failure or to neutral feedback during a frustrating series of cognitive tasks, noted the accessibility of various kinds of traits in their self-descriptions, and assessed their emotional and cognitive states.

As predicted, secure participants reacted to failure with heightened access to security-based self-representations: They rated qualities they had previously used to describe an attachment figure or feelings they had experienced when being comforted by this person as more self-descriptive when they were undergoing stress. No such heightened access to security-based self-representations was observed among insecure people. We also found that the more accessible the positive a person's self-representations were, the less negative was his or her current emotional state, despite the frustrating failure experience. Thus, it appears that secure individuals can mobilize caring qualities within themselves, qualities modeled on those of their attachment figures, as well as representations of being loved and valued by such figures, and these representations provide genuine comfort and relief during times of stress.

In all of the studies mentioned here, anxiously attached individuals did not exhibit defensive self-enhancement. Rather, they tended to suffer from negative and chaotic self-representations and to exaggerate their already negative self-views. For example, Mikulincer (1995) found that attachment-anxious people had ready mental access to negative self-attributes, scored low on the differentiation and integration of self-attributes, and evinced pervasive negative affect when sorting through these attributes. Similarly, Pietromonaco and Barrett (1997) noted that anxious individuals scored relatively high on measures of self-confusion and lack of self-knowledge. Moreover, anxiously attached people tended to make more negative self-appraisals in threatening compared with neutral conditions (Mikulincer, 1998a). Of great interest, Mikulincer showed that this tendency was reduced by a message that broke the likely connection between self-devaluation and others' supportive responses ("Findings show that people who hold a balanced self-view and can acknowledge both strong and weak self-aspects tend to elicit others' affection and support"; p. 430), implying that anxious people devalue themselves overtly at least partly to gain other people's sympathy, approval, and support. Such self-devaluation has also been noted in anxiously attached people's admittedly self-derogating, Woody Allenlike forms of humor; for example, "I will often try to make people like or accept me more by saying something funny about my own weaknesses or faults" (Kazarian & Martin, 2004; Saroglou & Scariot, 2002).

Interestingly, although avoidant people's defensive self-enhancement maneuvers and anxious people's self-derogating tendencies result in antithetical self-evaluations (positive in one case, negative in the other), both forms of insecurity are associated with pathological forms of narcissism (e.g., Dickinson & Pincus, 2003; Pistole, 1995a). In particular, avoidance is thought to predispose a person to, or to accompany, *overt* narcissism or grandiosity, which includes both self-praise and denial of weaknesses (Gabbard, 1998; Wink, 1991). Attachment anxiety, in contrast, seems to predispose a person to, or to accompany, *covert* narcissism, which is characterized by self-focused attention, hypersensitivity to other people's attention to or evaluation of oneself, and appraisal of oneself in terms of inherently unrealistic expectations and a sense of entitlement (Hendin & Cheek, 1997; Wink, 1991).

In one empirical exploration of these theoretical ideas, Dickinson and Pincus (2003) classified people according to the two kinds of narcissism (based on the Narcissistic Personality Inventory) and found an overrepresentation of dismissingly avoidant people in the overt, grandiosely narcissistic group and an overrepresentation of fearfully avoidant people in the covertly narcissistic group. Recently, Otway and Vignoles (2006) and Smolewska and Dion (2005) found that attachment anxiety was associated with covert narcissism. Smolewska and Dion also found that this form of narcissism is strongly related to fearful avoidance. However, these two studies found no evidence for dismissingly avoidant people's overt, grandiose narcissistic tendencies (as measured with the Narcissistic Personality Inventory). More research into this matter is needed.

Psychological Processes That Sustain Insecure People's Self-Related Vulnerabilities

Adult attachment researchers have identified psychological processes that sustain and exacerbate insecure people's self-related vulnerabilities. Studies have focused on insecure people's interpretation of negative life events; their search for negative information about the self; their reliance on unstable, external sources of self-worth; and their tendency to suffer from painful self-criticism and perfectionism. In the following sections we review evidence concerning attachment-related variations in these self-destructive processes.

Hopeless Cognitive Style

One way to validate and aggravate doubts about self-worth and self-efficacy is to employ what Abramson, Metalsky, and Alloy (1989) called a "hopeless" pattern of attributions, which includes taking responsibility for achievement-related failures and interpersonal rejections, and attributing these unpleasant experiences to a stable lack of ability, skill, or personal value. According to Abramson et al., this self-defeating attributional style reinforces self-blame, hopelessness, passivity, and helplessness, because its possessor sees him- or herself as not having the abilities and skills needed to alter unpleasant experiences. As a result, this hopeless cognitive style is a major risk factor for depression.

Adult attachment researchers have shown that attachment insecurities, especially attachment anxiety, are associated with a hopeless cognitive style. For example, two studies (Armsden et al., 1990; Greenberger & McLaughlin, 1998) assessed attachment security with parents and found that less secure adolescents were more likely to attribute academic and interpersonal problems or failures to lack of ability. Seven studies that assessed people's attachment orientations in close relationships found that attachment anxiety was associated with self-defeating, hopelessness-fostering attributions (Gamble & Roberts, 2005; Kennedy, 1999; Kogot, 2004; Man & Hamid, 1998; Safford, Alloy, Crossfield, Morocco, & Wang, 2004; Sumer & Cozzarelli, 2004; Williams & Riskind, 2004). With regard to avoidant attachment, two of these studies found that avoidant individuals displayed a "hopeless" cognitive style (Gamble & Roberts, 2005; N. Sumer & Cozzarelli, 2004), but two other studies found that avoidant people displayed a more defensive pattern of attributions (Kogot, 2004; Man & Hamid, 1998). (As always, these differences might be due in part to different measures of avoidance or the differences between dismissing and fearful forms of avoidance.) In these studies, avoidant people were less likely than secure ones to attribute negative events to lack of ability, suggesting that they could not bear the discomfort of self-blame.

Studies assessing beliefs about personal control have also documented anxious individuals' propensity to adopt a hopeless cognitive style (Fass & Tubman, 2002; J. A. Feeney, 1995b; Hexel, 2003; Marsa et al., 2004; Mickelson, Kessler, & Shaver, 1997). All of these studies found that attachment-anxious people tended to believe that luck and powerful others had more control over life events than their own actions did—a typical indication of helplessness (Mikulincer, 1994). Only one of these studies turned up evidence for an external locus of control in avoidant individuals (Mickelson et al., 1997), and it was still less pronounced than the external locus endorsed by anxious people. Also compatible with our analysis, Stober (2003) found a positive association between attachment anxiety and "self-pity," which Stober defined as feeling sorry for oneself because of suffering and helplessness.

Patterns of Feedback Seeking

According to Swann's (1990) self-verification hypothesis, people seek feedback to support and validate their knowledge about themselves and other people to navigate through life and predict others' behavior with some degree of certainty. In the case of people with low self-esteem, self-verification motives cause them to seek, and to be more open to receiving, negative information about the self. Such negative feedback, though offering the solace of belief validation, is still a cause of mental pain and suffering, and can aggravate doubts about self-worth and self-competence. In our view, this is common among anxiously attached people, whose core sense of unlovability and weakness often leads them to seek confirmatory negative information about themselves.

In an attempt to examine attachment-related variations in patterns of feedback seeking, Brennan and Morris (1997) asked people to imagine their romantic partner being asked questions about them in a number of different domains, then to rate the extent to which they would prefer questions evoking positive or negative information about themselves in each domain. In the relationship domain, for example, partners could be asked:

"Why do you think your partner might have difficulty maintaining an intimate relationship?" (negative information) or "Why do you think your partner is especially good at maintaining an intimate relationship?" (positive information). Insecure people, either anxious or avoidant, were more likely than secure ones to prefer negative feedback. This finding was replicated in subsequent studies (Brennan & Bosson, 1998; Cassidy, Ziv, Mehta, & Feeney, 2003). Only one study (Carnelley, Ruscher, & Shaw, 1999) found no association between attachment and feedback seeking. However, it focused on hypothetical rather than real partners and scenarios, which may have reduced self-verification strivings.

The link between avoidant attachment and preference for negative feedback deserves more attention. Whereas anxious people's openness to negative feedback is congruent with their negative self-views, avoidant people's dismissal of positive feedback does not match their reportedly high self-esteem. Brennan and Morris (1997) offered two explanations for this dissonant finding. Based on their negative models of others (discussed in later sections of this chapter), avoidant individuals may dismiss the importance of a romantic partner's feedback. Alternatively, avoidant people may be less certain about their positive self-views, and this uncertainty may inhibit the search for self-verifying feedback (Pelham & Swann, 1994). This alternative fits with the findings we reviewed earlier, indicating that avoidant individuals' self-representations lack clarity, coherence, and integration.

Bases of Self-Esteem

Adult attachment researchers have identified an additional process that can sustain attachment-anxious people's sense of worthlessness: their tendency to base self-appraisals on unstable, conditional sources of self-worth (e.g., others' approval). As we explained in Chapter 2, anxious people place great importance on receiving comfort and protection from close relationship partners and tend to perceive partners as their major source of value and esteem. Whereas this makes sense for a healthy but helpless infant, it becomes maladaptive for adolescents and adults who can base self-worth on inner standards of value and competence. This infantile stance causes the anxiously attached person to become dependent on continual validation from a relationship partner and overly susceptible to the partner's reactions—feeling good about oneself when the partner offers praise and affection; feeling bad about oneself when the partner is critical or rejecting. As a result, such people are unable to maintain a stable sense of self-esteem, because relationship partners cannot always be ideal attachment figures. Moreover, even minimal signs of a partner's disapproval, criticism, or disinterest can remind anxious people of their worthlessness, thereby validating and strengthening their low self-esteem.

There is correlational evidence that anxious people's self-worth is especially dependent on others' approval (Andersson & Perris, 2000; L. E. Park, Crocker, & Mickelson, 2004). In contrast, secure individuals are more likely to base their self-worth on domains that do not require constant external validation, such as long-term family support, that are less likely to be conditional. Interestingly, avoidant individuals are less dependent on interpersonal sources of self-esteem, at least in some studies, in line with their preference for self-reliance (L. E. Park et al., 2004). (See Chapter 12, this volume, however, for evidence that avoidant people, more than other people, may act in ways that will impress peers [e.g., about sexual exploits], which is another form of reliance on social approval for self-validation. Avoidant people may care more about their general public image than about close relationship partners' approval of them.)

Anxious people's tendency to derive self-worth from others' reactions has been further documented in naturalistic and experimental settings. In a study by Srivastava and Beer (2005), for example, participants took part in four weekly small-group meetings and, following each group session, rated their own likeability and the extent to which they liked each other person in the group. Participants who were more liked by others (based on the average of the other members' liking ratings) at the end of a particular group session reported more positive self-evaluations at a later session. However, this dependence on others' liking was mainly found among participants scoring high on attachment anxiety. For more securely attached group members, self-evaluations were quite high and relatively unaffected by what other members of the group thought.

Conceptually similar findings were reported by Broemer and Blumle (2003) based on two laboratory experiments. They assessed participants' attachment anxiety (Study 1) or primed representations of attachment anxiety (Study 2), exposed them to positive or negative self-relevant information, then asked them for their appraisals of themselves as relationship partners. In both studies, attachment-anxious participants or those primed with representations of attachment anxiety provided less positive self-evaluations following negative compared with positive information. In contrast, secure participants held equally positive self-views in positive and negative information conditions.

A recent set of two experimental studies suggests that the self-esteem of avoidant individuals may also rely on external sources of validation (Carvallo & Gabriel, 2006). In these studies, participants either were led to believe that they were accepted by others (Study 1) or were provided with information about their prospects of future success in interpersonal or achievement domains (Study 2). Their postfeedback self-esteem was then compared with that of study participants who received no feedback. In both studies, dismissingly avoidant people reported higher state self-esteem after receiving positive feedback than after no feedback. As usual, the self-esteem of more secure participants was not significantly affected by the experimental feedback.

M. A. Maier, Bernier, Pekrun, Zimmermann, and Grossmann (2004) extended the study of contingencies of self-worth to implicit responses to subliminal priming of rejection-related thoughts. Study participants were subliminally primed with a rejection message ("My mother rejects me") or a neutral message, and their RTs for endorsing positive sentences about self-worth or self-efficacy were assessed. Avoidant individuals (assessed with the AAI) reacted with longer RTs after being primed with a rejection message, implying that rejection-related primes blocked access to positive self-representations. Anxious participants also showed the same pattern of reaction, but RT differences did not reach statistical significance due to insufficient numbers of anxious participants. Overall, the reviewed findings indicate that insecurely attached people's susceptibility to others' reactions is evident in both explicit and implicit measures of self-esteem.

Self-Standards, Self-Criticism, and Perfectionism

Adult attachment researchers have also considered the negative effects that self-criticism and highly demanding self-standards have on insecure people's self-representations. Whereas adopting a critical attitude toward oneself can aggravate an anxious person's low self-esteem, overly demanding self-standards can help avoidant people defensively maintain a sense of superiority.

Self-criticism and demanding self-standards can come about through two interrelated processes. First, insecure people can incorporate their attachment figures' negative qualities into their own self-representations, then evaluate and treat themselves in the same critical and disapproving manner in which they were treated by inadequate attachment figures. Second, they can set overly demanding, unrealistic self-standards and strive for perfection as a way of coping with their insecurity. Whereas anxious people's hyperactivating strategies can drive them to attempt to be "perfect" and to pursue high self-ideals to gain others' love and esteem, avoidant people's deactivating strategies can incline them toward perfectionism as a way to hide imperfections, to self-enhance, and to justify self-reliance.

In support of this rather complex theoretical reasoning, Mikulincer (1995) found that anxious and avoidant people had relatively large discrepancies between their self-image and their self-standards (ideal-self and ought-self) compared with secure persons. In addition, Thompson and Zuroff (1999) found that adolescents who were less securely attached to their parents were more self-critical, and 11 other studies yielded positive associations between attachment anxiety and self-criticism (Batgos & Leadbeater, 1994; Besser & Priel, 2003, 2005; Carranza & Kilmann, 2000; Davila, 2001; Irons, Gilbert, Baldwin, Baccus, & Palmer, 2006; Murphy & Bates, 1997; Thompson & Zuroff, 2004; Whiffen, Aube, Thompson, & Campbell, 2000; Wiseman, Mayseless, & Sharabany, 2005; Zuroff & Fitzpatrick, 1995). Importantly, five of these studies (Batgos & Leadbeater, 1994; Davila, 2001; Murphy & Bates, 1997; Wiseman et al., 2005; Zuroff & Fitzpatrick, 1995) also found higher self-criticism among avoidant people.

There is also evidence linking attachment insecurity with perfectionism. Rice and Mirzadeh (2000) reported that secure attachment to parents was associated with adaptive forms of goal-setting (maintenance of demanding but achievable personal standards), but insecure attachment to parents was associated with less adaptive, more perfectionistic forms of goal setting (having unrealistically high standards, ruminating about mistakes, feeling pressured by others to be perfect, and perceiving large discrepancies between personal standards and performance). Similarly, ratings of attachment anxiety and avoidance were positively associated with measures of maladaptive perfectionism (Andersson & Perris, 2000; Gamble & Roberts, 2005; Rice, Lopez, & Vergara, 2005; Wei, Heppner, Russell, & Young, 2006). Interestingly, Rice and Lopez (2004) found that maladaptive perfectionism had a negative effect on self-esteem, but this association was reduced in people who scored high on attachment security; that is, secure people tended to have a stable sense of self-worth regardless of whether they held high performance standards.

In a finer-grained analysis of the link between attachment insecurities and maladaptive perfectionism, Rice et al. (2005) uncovered sources of insecure people's vulnerabilities. Appraisals of parental criticism about performance were associated with avoidant attachment, suggesting that internalization of a "critical parent" is a determinant of avoidant individuals' sense of self. Moreover, attachment anxiety was associated with a combination of appraisals of high parental criticism and low parental expectations. It seems that internalization of parental criticism that is not accompanied by high parental investment is particularly detrimental to anxious people's fragile sense of self.

A Model of Insecure People's Self-Vulnerabilities

Overall, for both anxious and avoidant people, a history of painful and frustrating interactions with unavailable, inconsistent, cold, or rejecting attachment figures interferes with the formation of a solid, stable sense of personal value and pride in oneself. Anxious people's desire to gain a partner's love, esteem, and protection keeps them from "owning" their anger toward this person and causes them to take responsibility for the frustration and pain, thereby reinforcing their sense of worthlessness and weakness. This negative self-view is then sustained and aggravated by a hopeless cognitive style, openness to negative information about the self, reliance on others' approval as a source of self-worth, self-criticism, and the endorsement of unrealistically high self-standards. These processes also encourage attachment-system hyperactivation, because a helpless person cannot live without constant care, love, and protection provided by other people. This is a self-exacerbating cycle in which attachment-system hyperactivation and lack of self-esteem reinforce each other.

Avoidant people's commitment to self-reliance leads them to push negative self-representations out of awareness and defensively inflate their self-image. As a result, they often report high levels of explicit self-esteem and describe themselves in positive terms. However, their positive models of self seem to be less healthy, stable, and authentic than the positive self-models of secure individuals. Avoidant people's self-enhancement is accompanied by unrealistically high self-standards, a need to be invincible, exceptional, and nearly perfect, which leads to reliance on external sources of validation combined with self-criticism, perfectionism, and a renewal of self-doubts. These dynamic processes create a self-exacerbating cycle in which self-criticism and defensive self-inflation reinforce each other. Moreover, as reviewed in Chapter 7, this volume, when a high cognitive or emotional load interferes with the avoidant defenses, otherwise suppressed negative self-conceptions tend to erupt into avoidant people's consciousness. Given these findings, we believe that "dismissing" people, who are high on avoidance but low on self-reported anxious attachment, do not have a solid sense of self-worth and should not be characterized by researchers as having positive working models of self.

ATTACHMENT AND MENTAL REPRESENTATIONS OF OTHERS

According to Bowlby (1973), beginning in infancy, social experiences with attachment figures provide the foundation of working models of relationship partners (i.e., beliefs about their availability, goodwill, supportiveness, and trustworthiness). As we explained in Chapter 1, these cognitive products can be generalized across recurrent interactions with an attachment figure and eventually be generalized across relationships via transference processes (Andersen & Glassman, 1996); that is, the models can be projected onto new partners, causing adolescents and adults to treat new partners the way they related to past attachment figures (Brumbaugh & Fraley, 2006). In adolescent and adult minds are many representations of other people, ranging from specific memories and partner-specific schemas to very general representations of other people. These can be conceptualized as hierarchically arranged in memory and activated differentially depending on circumstances. New relationships probably call at first on fairly general working models of others, but particular partners, or particular "button-pushing" behaviors on the part of particular partners, may evoke more specific representations, along with the fears and defenses associated with them.

Bowlby's reasoning about the formation of working models of others fits with our conceptualization of the broaden-and-build cycle of attachment security. As we explained in Chapter 2, this cycle is organized around positive mental representations of relationship partners and optimistic expectations concerning others' love, supportiveness, and trustworthiness. For securely attached persons, recurrent interactions with a sensitive and responsive primary attachment figure favor the formation of positive mental representations of this partner, which, when transferred to new partners, promotes positive views of other people. The secure individual tends to see other people in general as well-intentioned providers of protection, comfort, and security. This gives them a degree of confidence about relationship and interaction partners' dependability and generosity that is hard for less secure people to match. This means we can expect secure people to entertain benevolent, forgiving explanations of other people's negative behavior and attribute their positive actions to favorable traits and good intentions. In addition, secure people's stable and authentic sense of self-worth should allow them to accept others without defensively devaluing them or needing them to provide constant approval or admiration.

Here is an example of a secure female university student's dream, which reveals an underlying sense of trust and confidence even under potentially anxiety-provoking conditions (being separated temporarily from a relative and crossing a bridge alone into an unknown territory):

> "I'm on a train with one of my family members, and I don't know where he and I are going, but the whole situation is very real and vivid. We're sitting in the train, and I look out the window every once in a while and enjoy the ride. I ask him where we're going, and he tells me to wait and see, and I trust him. He sits on the seat opposite me (I'm facing toward the front of the train and he, opposite me, is facing the back of the train.) I can see that the train is about to cross a bridge spanning a body of water, and I tell him we are about to cross it, but he says I will cross it alone, and he prepares to get off the train. He says we will meet again after the bridge. He gives me a kiss, and the train stops, and he gets off. I stay on my own and still don't know why I'm on the train, but I trust my gut feeling that everything will be okay."

In line with Erikson's (1950/1993) well-known construct "basic trust," which is similar to Bowlby's (1969/1982) concept of security, the dreamer's sense of trust seems to extend beyond people to life conditions in general. Even though she is proceeding along an unknown path, she trusts both her companion and her fate.

Of course, the theoretical analysis that gives us our understanding of security implies that insecure people can be expected to hold more negative beliefs about others' intentions and traits. This does not mean, however, that anxious and avoidant people have the same negative models of others. In the case of avoidant people, deactivating strategies encourage negative views of others and preserve them in the face of disconfirming evidence. We attribute these biases to two psychological processes. First, deactivating strategies divert attention away from attachment-related information, including information about others' positive traits, intentions, and relational behavior. As a result, genuine signals of a partner's support and love can be missed and, even when noted, can be processed only shallowly, be easily forgotten, and remain inaccessible when later appraisals of relationship partners are made. This dismissal of positive information about relationship partners sustains avoidant people's negative and critical images of others.

Second, as discussed earlier in this chapter, deactivating strategies involve defensive self-enhancement, which includes suppression of negative self-aspects and placing undue emphasis on one's own uniqueness, value, and strength. These maneuvers, coupled with avoidant people's preference for emotional and cognitive distance from others, encourage projection of the suppressed material onto relationship partners (in a process that Freud [1915/1957] called "defensive projection"), thereby further reinforcing one's own uniqueness and value compared with the ordinariness of other people. This defensive projection exacerbates avoidant people's negative views of others. Here is an example from an avoidant female university student's dream:

> "My parents wanted me to go with them to my grandma's house, and a discussion ensued about whether it was worth going and if she would or wouldn't have food for us. I said I didn't want to go, and I went into the backyard alone. There was a 'cat party' going on, and many disgusting, filthy black cats were sitting in a circle, facing out, with their backs toward each other. Every cat screamed, one at a time, and if the cat opposite to the one that screamed correctly identified the screamer, that cat won. I sat in the corner with my computer and was afraid to move because of the cats. I thought, 'Why didn't they run away when they saw me?' I realized that because there were so many of them, they knew they had power over me and could easily wipe me out. Suddenly, my computer fell and landed close to the cats. I had to save it, so I got closer to them, but when I did, they jumped on the computer and threatened me with aggressive expressions and horrible screams. They started to sing, 'If you don't go home, you'll have to tell us who is a nice cat.' I had to answer them with a song saying that all of the cats were nice. They then let me have my computer. I wanted to wipe them out one by one, but instead I went inside with the computer. I woke up in terror."

The dream is interesting for several reasons. It shows how an avoidant person perceives others and represents social relationships: "If Grandma isn't going to give us food, there's no reason to visit her." In the backyard, the only companions available to the dreamer, as an alternative to working alone on a computer, are dirty, ugly, and scary, and their idea of a good time is to sit facing opposite directions and scream at each other. The dreamer thinks about the power the cats have to "wipe me out," and near the end thinks of "wiping them out one by one." When not being vicious and hostile, the cats require the dreamer to say they are nice, when in fact the dreamer finds them repulsive. The dreamer cannot get what she needs (her computer) without telling socially acceptable lies (which is similar to going to her grandma's house to get food while presumably having to act civilly toward her). Underlying the dreamer's anger and belligerence, she is actually terrified.

The avoidant bias against viewing others positively can backfire, because viewing oneself as having so many unsavory and inadequate relatives, friends, and romantic partners might be indicative of one's own imperfections and faults. As a result, some avoidant people may attempt to replace this view of others with a defensively idealized representation of at least some of them (e.g., parents; Hesse, 1999). But this defensive idealization, like other reality-distorting defenses, creates additional problems for avoidant people, because it conflicts with their desire for distance and blocks defensive projection of their own flaws onto other people. Strategically speaking, this trap can be avoided by targeting and confining idealization to specific figures in specific contexts, while maintaining a more generally negative view of most other people.

In a very different constellation of strategies, anxious individuals' hyperactivating tendencies lead to complex, ambivalent appraisals of others. Although attachment-anxious people presumably have a history of negative interactions with unreliable attachment figures, they still believe that if they intensify their proximity-seeking efforts, they may gain a partner's attention, esteem, and protection (as may have actually been the case with an inconsistent, self-preoccupied parent). As a result, they cannot form a simple, univalent negative view of others, because this would imply that proximity seeking is hopeless (the avoidant person's view). Rather, the anxious person, although often frightened, worried, or angry, takes some of the blame for frustrated proximity-seeking bids and continues to perceive relationship partners as potentially "stronger and wiser" figures who might be cajoled or coerced into providing support and care. These mental gyrations generate ambivalent views of others, which include conflicting appraisals of their potential value and their frequent unavailability, unreliability, or infidelity. In short, attachment-anxious people sustain both hope for love and protection and doubts about their ability to attain them. Here is an example from Avihou's (2006) study of dreams:

> "I was at a female friend's parents' house, together with a mixed-sex group of other friends, and at some point I went to the bathroom to blow my nose and I tossed the used toilet paper into the toilet. My friend's mom saw me doing it and yelled at me, saying I should throw it in the wastebasket, not in the toilet. She looked very powerful to me, and I was afraid of her. So I went and threw the toilet paper in the wastebasket. When I approached the wastebasket, she smiled at me and looked as if she liked and accepted me. I felt that I was doing the right thing and was foolish to have thrown the toilet paper into the toilet initially. But surprisingly, even when I tossed it into the wastebasket, my friend's mom yelled at me again, and I felt very hurt. I didn't understand what I had done wrong, and I ran away and never spoke to that friend again."

Notice how the dreamer moves back and forth between feeling attacked, wanting to be accepted, seeming briefly to be accepted, then suddenly finding that she is still unacceptable. Her rejection seems unwarranted and unintelligible, but rather than assert herself, like the secure person whose library dream we quoted earlier in this chapter, the anxious person runs away and forgoes a friendship.

Three additional cognitive processes strengthen the negative side of the anxious person's ambivalence. First, as we explained in Chapter 2, anxious, hyperactivating strategies intensify fears of rejection and abandonment, and make people more vigilant and sensitive about relationship partners' signals of unavailability, disinterest, or criticism. Hence, the likelihood of holding negative views of partners is increased, because real-life relationship partners cannot always be available, responsive, and at one's beck and call. Second, hyperactivating strategies involve rumination on real or imagined signs of a partner's lack of immediate responsiveness, which heightens the cognitive availability of negative views of a partner and causes these views to be more accessible in social perception. Third, hyperactivating strategies intensify the desire for close proximity to and fusion with relationship partners, which in turn encourages anxious people to project their negative self-views onto relationship partners, thereby creating an illusory sense of similarity and union. Thus, paradoxically, a negative view of others is guided partly by the anxious person's negative self-views combined with an intense longing for "twinship" (Kohut, 1984) and connectedness.

In subsequent sections, we review evidence concerning attachment-related individual differences in mental representations of others. The evidence comes from studies that have examined whether and how attachment patterns (assessed by the AAI or self-report attachment scales) relate to (1) adults' cognitive representations of their parents' attitudes and behaviors toward them during childhood; (2) their appraisals of relationship partners; (3) their perceptions of other people's supportiveness; (4) their expectations, appraisals, and explanations of others' behaviors; (5) their perceptions of self–other similarity and their use of projection as a defense; and (6) their perceptions of outgroup members.

Parental Representations

In their early study of adult romantic attachment, Hazan and Shaver (1987) provided preliminary evidence concerning attachment style differences in the ways adults remember and cognitively represent parents' attitudes and behaviors toward them during childhood. In both a newspaper survey of community members and a more typical study of college students, secure participants described their mothers and fathers as more respectful, responsive, caring, accepting, and undemanding than did anxiously attached participants, and reported warmer relationships between their parents. The findings also provided a preliminary hint concerning avoidant defensiveness: Whereas avoidant participants in the newspaper survey described their mothers and fathers in more negative terms than did secure participants, avoidant college students provided more positive descriptions of their parents. Hazan and Shaver interpreted this difference as indicating that avoidant college students tend to idealize their parents as a way of evading distressing memories, but that maturity, perspective, and distance from parents allows older adults to acknowledge unfavorable aspects of their childhood relationships with parents. Indeed, Hazan and Shaver found that the link between avoidance and negative parental representations was stronger among older than among younger adults in their community (newspaper) sample.

In the subsequent two decades, more than 50 studies have followed up Hazan and Shaver's (1987) findings by examining attachment-related variations in parental representations (Table 6.3 summarizes the methods and findings). These studies have consistently found that ratings of secure attachment to parents or the endorsement of a secure style in close relationships is associated with more positive representations of parents as caring, loving, and accepting (see Table 6.3). With regard to specific attachment insecurities, the findings yield no clear difference between anxiety and avoidance. More than two-thirds of the studies yielded significant associations between higher anxiety or avoidance scores and more negative descriptions of parents (see Table 6.3). Most of these studies assessed attachment patterns in close relationships in general or romantic relationships in particular, supporting the notion that negative parental representations are part of global or general working models.

Two of the studies summarized in Table 6.3 (K. N. Levy et al., 1998; Priel & Besser, 2001) assessed the contents and structure of participants' open-ended descriptions of parents with a scoring procedure developed by Blatt et al. (1992). In line with attachment theory, people scoring higher on anxiety or avoidance tended to view their parents as less benevolent and more punitive, and to describe them in more ambivalent terms. In addition, their narratives were scored as less conceptually complex than those of more secure people; that is, attachment-style measures were able to predict theoretically significant variations in the way people represented their parents in their own words.

Beyond assessing parental representations, some attachment studies have explored young adults' descriptions of the relational patterns in their family of origin. For example, Bell (1998) found that avoidant people (identified by the AAI) described family members as expressing fewer positive reactions (e.g., "praising someone for good work") than did secure people, whereas anxiously attached people described family members as expressing more negative reactions (e.g., "showing contempt for another's actions"). Similarly, attachment insecurities were associated with descriptions of the family as conflict-ridden, less cohesive, less emotionally expressive, and less encouraging of personal growth (Harvey & Byrd, 2000; Mallinckrodt, McCreary, & Robertson, 1995).

TABLE 6.3. A Summary of Findings Linking Attachment Orientations with Recalled Parental Behaviors

Study	Attachment scale	Parental scale	Target	Main findings for positive recollections of parental behavior
Studies assessing secure attachment to parents or peers				
Larose & Boivin (1997)	IPPA	MFP	M, F	Security (+)
Manassis et al. (1999)	AAI	PBI	M	Security (+)
Tavecchio & Thomeer (1999)	RQ	PBI	M, F	Security (+)
Thompson & Zuroff (1999)	IPPA	PBI	M	Security (+)
Landolt et al. (2004)	IPPA	EMBU	M, F	Security (+)
Studies assessing attachment types				
Hazan & Shaver (1987, Study 1)	HS types	HS items	M, F	Secure > Anxious, Avoidant
Hazan & Shaver (1987, Study 2)	HS types	HS items	M	Secure > Avoidant > Anxious
			F	Secure > Anxious, Avoidant
J. A. Feeney & Noller (1990)	HS types	HS items	M, F	Secure > Anxious, Avoidant
Mikulincer et al. (1990)	HS types	HS items	M	Secure > Avoidant
			F	Secure > Anxious, Avoidant
Bringle & Bagby (1992)	HS types	PFP	Ps	Secure > Avoidant
Zeanah et al. (1993)	AAI	MFP	Ps	Secure > Avoidant
J. A. Feeney & Ryan (1994)	HS types	New scale	Ps	Secure > Anxious, Avoidant
de Haas et al. (1994)	AAI	MMB	M	No significant differences
Gerlsma et al. (1996)	HS types	HS items	M	No significant differences
			F	Secure > Anxious, Avoidant
Brennan & Shaver (1998)	RQ	MFP	M, F	Secure > Anxious, Avoidant, Fearful
K. N. Levy et al. (1998)	HS types	Blatt scales	M, F	Secure > Anxious, Avoidant
Gittleman et al. (1998)	RQ	PBI	M, F	Secure > Fearful
Crowell, Treboux, & Waters (1999)	AAI, RQ	MFP	M	No significant differences
Priel & Besser (2000)	RQ	PBI	M	Secure > Anxious, Avoidant, Fearful
Priel & Besser (2001)	RQ	Blatt scales	M	Secure > Anxious, Avoidant, Fearful
Muris et al. (2003)	HS types	EMBU	M, F	Secure > Anxious, Avoidant
Bernier et al. (2005)	AAI	MFP	M, F	Secure > Anxious
Muris et al. (2004)	HS types	EMBU	M, F	Secure > Anxious, Avoidant
Studies based on attachment style ratings				
Carnelley & Janoff-Bulman (1992)	HS ratings	MFP	M	Secure (+), Anxious (−), Avoidant (−)
			F	Secure (ns), Anxious (ns), Avoidant (ns)
Mickelson et al. (1997)	HS ratings	PBI	M, F	Secure (+), Anxious (−), Avoidant (−)
Kennedy (1999)	RQ	MFP	Ps	Secure (+), Anxious (−), Avoidant (ns), Fearful (−)
Gerlsma & Luteijn (2000)	RQ	Interview	Ps	Secure (+), Anxious (ns), Avoidant (ns), Fearful (−)
Harvey & Byrd (2000)	AAS	FES	Ps	Secure (+), Anxious (−), Avoidant (−)
Magai et al. (2000)	AAI	New scale	Ps	Secure (+), Anxious (ns), Avoidant (ns), Fearful (−)
Sharabany et al. (2001)	RQ	WHOTO	M	Secure (+), Anxious (ns), Avoidant (ns), Fearful (−)
			F	Secure (ns), Anxious (ns), Avoidant (ns), Fearful (−)
Kelley et al. (2005)	RQ, ECR	CRPBI	M	Anxious (−), Avoidant (ns), Fearful (ns)
			F	Anxious (−), Avoidant (−), Fearful (−)
Wiseman et al. (2005)	HS ratings	PBI	Ps	Secure (+), Anxious (−), Avoidant (ns)
Irons et al. (2006)	RQ	EMBU	Ps	Secure (+), Anxious (−), Avoidant (ns), Fearful (−)

(cont.)

TABLE 6.3. *(cont.)*

Study	Attachment scale	Parental scale	Target	Main findings for positive recollections of parental behavior
Studies assessing attachment dimensions				
Collins & Read (1990, Study 1)	AAS	HS items	M, F	Anxiety (–), Avoidance (–)
Carnelley et al. (1994, Study 1)	RQ	PBI, MFP	M, F	Anxiety (–), Avoidance (–)
Carnelley et al. (1994, Study 2)	RQ	PBI, MFP	M	Anxiety (ns), Avoidance (–)
			F	Anxiety (ns), Avoidance (ns)
Glachan & Ney (1995)	AAS	HS items	Ps	Anxiety (ns), Avoidance (–)
Mallinckrodt, Coble, et al. (1995)	AAS	PBI	M, F	Anxiety (–), Avoidance (–)
J. A. Feeney (1996)	ASQ	PBI	M, F	Anxiety (ns), Avoidance (–)
Frazier et al. (1996, Study 3)	AAS	HS items	M, F	Anxiety (–), Avoidance (–)
Lopez, Gover, et al. (1997)	RQ	PBI	Ps	Anxiety (–), Avoidance (–)
Carranza & Kilmann (2000)	RSQ	PCQ	Ps	Anxiety (–), Avoidance (–)
Lopez et al. (2000)—Intact families sample	AAQ	PBI	M, F	Anxiety (–), Avoidance (–)
Lopez et al. (2000)—Divorced families sample	AAQ	PBI	M	Anxiety (–), Avoidance (ns)
			F	Anxiety (–), Avoidance (–)
Oliver & Whiffen (2000)	AAS	PCQ	M	Anxiety (–), Avoidance (–)
			F	Anxiety (ns), Avoidance (ns)
Perris & Andersson (2000)	RQ, ASQ	EMBU	M, F	Anxiety (–), Avoidance (–)
Swanson & Mallinckrodt (2001)	ECR	LWS, FES	Ps	Anxiety (ns), Avoidance (–)
DiFilippo & Overholser (2002)	ECR	PBI	SSP	Anxiety (ns), Avoidance (ns)
			OSP	Anxiety (ns), Avoidance (–)
Sheehan & Noller (2002)	ASQ	SIDE	M, F	Anxiety (–), Avoidance (–)
J. A. Feeney (2003)	RQ, ASQ	PBI	M	Anxiety (ns), Avoidance (–)
			F	Anxiety (–), Avoidance (ns)
Mohr & Fassinger (2003)	AAS	HS items	M	Anxiety (ns), Avoidance (–)
			F	Anxiety (–), Avoidance (ns)
Heinonen et al. (2004)	AAS	PBI, LIS	M	Anxiety (ns), Avoidance (–)
			F	Anxiety (–), Avoidance (–)
Luke et al. (2004, Study 2)	RQ	PTQ	M, F	Anxiety (–), Avoidance (–)
Doyle & Markiewicz (2005)	RQ	8 items	Ps	Anxiety (–), Avoidance (–)
Gamble & Roberts (2005)	AAS	CPI	Ps	Anxiety (–), Avoidance (–)

Note. (–), significant inverse correlation; (+), significant positive correlation; (ns), nonsignificant effects; F, Father; M, Mother; OSP, opposite-sex parent; Ps, parents; SSP, same-sex parent; CPI, Critical Parenting Inventory; CRPBI, Children's Report of Parent Behavior Inventory; EMBU, Recollection of Early Experiences Interview; FES, Family Environment Scale; HS, Hazan and Shaver; LIS, Love Inconsistency Scale; LWS, Love Withdrawal Scale; MFP, Mother–Father–Peer Scale; MMB, Memories of Maternal Behavior; PBI, Parental Bonding Inventory; PCQ, Parental Characteristic Questionnaire; PFP, Perceived Family Problems; PTQ, Parental Treatment Questionnaire; SIDE, Sibling Inventory of Differential Experience.

Of course, the studies summarized in Table 6.3 do not provide direct information about whether insecure people's negative parental representations are accurate (see Chapter 5, this volume) rather than being memory distortions based on secondary attachment strategies. For example, secondary attachment strategies can be manifested in avoidant people's idealization of their parents. Although findings summarized in Table 6.3 indicate that avoidant people possess negative representations of their parents, we should note that these studies were not designed to examine defensive idealization. In fact, using a better self-report scale, Brennan and Shaver (1998) found that avoidant people described their mothers and fathers as less accepting, yet at the same time defensively idealized them (e.g., saying that [mother/father] "had no single fault that I can think of").

A still better operationalization of parental idealization is offered by Hesse (1999) in his description of the AAI coding rules. He defined "idealization" as the discrepancy between the positivity of the traits a participant generates to describe his or her parents during the participant's childhood and the positivity of remembered experiences that were meant to illustrate or justify the choice of those traits. Following up this idea in a self-report attachment study, we (Shaver & Mikulincer, 2004) asked participants to name five traits or qualities that described their relationship with their mothers during childhood and to retrieve memories of experiences that exemplified those traits. We then asked judges to rate the positivity of these adjectives and memories independently. (The judges did not know which adjectives went with which memories.) We found that attachment anxiety, but not avoidance (measured with self-report scales), was associated with the generation of less positive adjectives describing the childhood relationship with the mother, but both anxiety and avoidance ratings were associated with retrieval of less positive memories of this relationship. As a result, the higher the avoidance scores, the larger the discrepancy between adjectival and narrative descriptions of the mother, a pattern that Hesse interpreted as indicating avoidant adults' defensive idealization of their childhood relationship with the mother.

Appraisals of Relationship Partners

There is extensive evidence that insecure people tend to describe specific friends and romantic partners in negative terms and also to hold negative views of humanity in general. In one of the first systematic studies of attachment style differences in mental representations of others, Collins and Read (1990) reported that anxiously attached people were more likely to believe that they have little control over their lives, and that others are difficult to understand. These authors also found that avoidant individuals were less likely than other people to believe that human beings are altruistic, willing to stand up for their beliefs, or able to control their lives. Subsequent studies have found that these negative views are also manifested in insecure people's lack of esteem for and acceptance of others (Cyranowski et al., 2002; Luke, Maio, & Carnelley, 2004; Shaver, Papalia, et al., 1996; Steiner-Pappalardo & Gurung, 2002), doubts about other people's trustworthiness (Carranza & Kilmann, 2000; Cozzarelli et al., 2000; Hofstra, van Oudenhoven, & Buunk, 2005), and disrespect for relationship partners (Frei & Shaver, 2002). Moreover, studies based on coding personal narratives or dream reports using the CCRT method (see the details presented earlier and examples scattered throughout this chapter) found that attachment anxiety and avoidance are associated with representations of others as more disgusting, hurtful, disapproving, or rejecting (Avihou, 2006; Raz, 2002).

Attachment studies have also found that anxiety and avoidance are associated with lower ratings of romantic partners' predictability, dependability, and faithfulness (Collins & Read, 1990; J. A. Feeney & Noller, 1992; Fuller & Fincham, 1995; Holtzworth-Munroe et al., 1997; Keelan, Dion, & Dion, 1994; Mikulincer, 1998b; Simpson, 1990). Moreover, Mikulincer (1998b) found that insecure people have faster access to memories of painful trust betrayals on the part of their relationship partners and report themselves to have fewer daily experiences in which their partner behaved in a trustworthy manner. In their 31-year longitudinal study, Klohnen and Bera (1998) found that 52-year-old women with a self-reported secure attachment had rated others as more trustworthy and dependable at ages 27 and 43, and still did so at age 52, compared with women with an insecure attachment style.

Insecure people's negative representations of others are also evident in their interpretations of others' facial expressions. B. Meyer, Pilkonis, and Beevers (2004) exposed study participants to a set of 10 photographs of people whose faces were shown in a "neutral" emotional condition, then asked them to say what the facial expressions indicated about each person. Higher attachment anxiety (on a self-report scale) was associated with seeing fewer positive traits and feelings in the target faces, and both anxiety and avoidance were associated with seeing more negative traits and feelings.

Recently, Zayas and Shoda (2005) assessed insecure people's negative appraisals of relationship partners using a cognitive task that tapped implicit mental processes, the Implicit Association Task (IAT; Greenwald, McGhee, & Schwartz, 1998). This categorization task was designed to measure the strength of automatic associations between a target concept (e.g., romantic partner) and an attribute (e.g., trustworthiness). In this task, a strong automatic association between a target concept and an attribute implies that activation of the target concept automatically and effortlessly activates the attribute (as indicated by a faster response to the attribute in the presence of the target concept than in the presence of a different concept). Zayas and Shoda (2005) found that self-reports of attachment anxiety and avoidance were related to stronger automatic associations (faster responses) between two target concepts—either a current romantic partner or one's mother—and negative personal attributes; that is, for insecure people, exposure to the name of a romantic partner or the name of one's mother automatically activated associations with negative traits, implying the existence of implicit negative representations of relationship partners in an associative memory network.

We also know that insecurely attached people tend to have poorly developed, undifferentiated, and confused representations of others (Davila & Cobb, 2003; Stalker & Davies, 1998; Steiner-Pappalardo & Gurung, 2002). Using the Social Cognition and Object Relation Scales (SCORS; Westen, 1991) for coding Thematic Apperception Test (TAT) stories, Gilad (2002) found that the stories generated by avoidant individuals in response to TAT cards did not take other people's emotions and concerns into account. Moreover, anxious people's narratives were marked by undifferentiated representations of others, and distorted and egocentric causal attributions for others' behavior. Calabrese, Farber, and Westen (2005) also used the SCORS for coding narratives of interactions with parents, friends, and romantic partners, and found that more insecurely attached people were less able to recognize and show genuine concern for others' needs and less able to read social situations accurately. These findings show that attachment insecurities are associated with less complex mental representations of others, which in turn are likely to interfere with accurate understanding of other people's emotions, concerns, and actions.

Although insecure people tend to hold generalized and stable negative images of others, some studies have identified systematic fluctuations in these negative views that probably reflect the biasing action of secondary attachment strategies. For example, A. M. Young and Acitelli (1998) found that anxiously attached people's negative appraisals of a romantic partner were stronger in married than in dating couples, and J. A. Feeney (2002a) found that these negative views increase with length of marriage. In the early stages of a couple relationship, anxious individuals may be influenced by an urgent wish for security and strong fear of rejection, which cause them to view their dating partner as the long-awaited "savior" who will love and understand them. However, with marriage (presumably viewed as a long-lasting, committed relationship), fear of rejection declines somewhat, defensive idealization is no longer needed, and anxious people's generally negative models of others may begin to dominate the way they appraise a spouse's traits and behaviors. Alternatively, as J. A. Feeney noted, "It is possible that insecure spouses become less optimistic about their relationships across the marital life-cycle and more attuned to potential signs of negativity and rejection" (p. 51).

Pietromonaco and Barrett's (1997) diary study of interpersonal interactions yields additional information about daily fluctuations in insecure people's appraisals of others. Whereas secure and insecure people did not differ in appraising their partners across many daily interactions, anxiously attached individuals made more positive appraisals and avoidant participants made more negative appraisals during highly discordant interactions. For anxious people, these interactions may seem to be ones in which the other person at least paid attention, therefore seeming to "care" (Bartholomew & Allison, 2006). For avoidant people, such clashes may not only increase the sense that other people are frustrating and discouraging but also raise questions about one's own value ("She clearly thinks I'm wrong, stupid, disgusting"). Avoidant people may attempt to restore autonomy and self-esteem by devaluing their partner's position and projecting onto him or her one's own negative traits (we expand on this idea about defensive projection in a later section). Interestingly, and in line with theory, secure participants in Pietromonaco and Barrett's (1997) diary study exhibited no notable difference in appraisals of their partners following disagreements compared with neutral interactions, implying that they can maintain stable appraisals despite temporary conflicts and tensions.

However, anxious individuals' approval of partners seems to evaporate when contentious interactions occur over major relationship problems. Simpson et al. (1996) asked dating couples jointly to identify a minor or a major unresolved problem in their relationship, then to discuss and resolve it. After the discussion, each person reported his or her appraisals of the other. These appraisals became more negative when attachment-anxious individuals discussed a major rather than a minor problem. In contrast, secure people's appraisals of their partners improved after discussing a major problem, and these effects were not explained by the quality of the discussion or the distress experienced during the interaction. Taken together, the findings suggest that anxious people overvalue their partners early in a relationship and following conflicts, but devalue them over time and in response to major disagreements. This complex pattern of reactions provides a good example of anxious people's ambivalent and fluctuating appraisals of relationship partners (for similar examples, see Pietromonaco & Barrett, 1997, 2000). These erratic appraisals call into question the wisdom of conceptualizing anxious individuals as having a "positive model of others" (Bartholomew & Horowitz, 1991). They may have a "hopeful," pro-relationship model of others when they are alone and desperately need attention and reassurance; they may have an ecstatic or still-hopeful model during the first flush of romantic excitement, but in general they are often distrusting and disapproving of others—a negative, combative stance that can eventually destroy a relationship.

Attachment-anxious individuals' fluctuating appraisals of relationship partners were further documented in Zhang and Hazan's (2002) study of person perception. Participants received a list of positive and negative traits, and were asked to estimate the number of behavioral instances they would need to confirm or disconfirm the existence of each trait in a hypothetical romantic partner or classmate. More anxious participants required less evidence to confirm the presence of both positive and negative traits and to disconfirm the possession of negative traits; that is, anxious individuals tended to make positive and negative judgments about others relatively quickly, and without much behavioral evidence. Although their desire for attention and security may make them quick to idealize others, their fear of rejection may heighten vigilance concerning a partner's negative behavior, and lead to quick and overly negative appraisals when circumstances seem to warrant them (Zhang & Hazan, 2002). Avoidant study participants requested more behavioral evidence before concluding that others possessed positive traits and/or that their possession of negative traits was disconfirmed. This finding suggests that avoidance encourages hard to refute, negative appraisals of others' traits. Moreover, it implies that avoidant people's negative views of others may be more stable and pervasive than those of anxiously attached people, who tend to be more receptive to others' positive behaviors.

Perceptions of Others' Supportiveness

Attachment-related differences in mental representations of other people have obvious implications for perceiving others' supportiveness. In fact, Sarason, Pierce, and Sarason (1990) equated attachment security with the perception of social support, defining *perceived social support* as "feelings that you are loved, valued, and unconditionally accepted" (p. 110). More than 40 independent studies have provided strong empirical support for this definition (see Table 6.4 for methods and findings), indicating that attachment security is associated with perceptions of support availability, greater confidence in the supportiveness of specific relationship partners, and greater satisfaction with support received. Moreover, most of these studies found that insecure adults, both anxious and avoidant, reported less available support and were less satisfied with the support they received (see Table 6.4). Fortunately, of these studies, the several that were based on prospective, longitudinal designs also found that attachment orientations assessed at a particular time predicted subsequent changes in perceived support across periods ranging from 1 month to 4 years (see Table 6.4).

In an effort to overcome the limitations of correlational studies and to assess the cognitive biases associated with attachment insecurities, Collins and Feeney (2004, Study 1) experimentally manipulated partner supportiveness and assessed attachment-style differences in perceptions of partner support. Dating couples were brought into the lab; one member of the couple was informed that he or she would perform a stressful task (giving a videotaped speech); the couple was then unobtrusively observed for 5 minutes, so that the researchers could record spontaneously emitted supportive behaviors. Next, couple members were separated, and support was manipulated by having the non-speech-making partner copy either two clearly supportive notes (e.g., "Don't worry—just say how you feel and what you think and you'll do great") or two ambiguously supportive notes (e.g., "Try not to say anything too embarrassing—especially since so many people will be watching your tape") to send to the partner who had to give a speech. The speech giver then read the notes and rated both their supportiveness and the partner's behaviors during the prior interaction.

Although there was no significant attachment style difference in appraisals of clearly supportive notes, insecure study participants rated the ambiguous notes as less supportive and more upsetting, and inferred more negative intent than did secure participants. More important, after receiving the ambiguous notes, participants scoring higher on attachment anxiety or avoidance rated their prior interaction as less supportive than would be expected on the basis of judges' ratings of the interactions. It seems that ambiguously supportive notes reactivated attachment-related worries and heightened access to negative working models of others, which in turn negatively biased insecure people's appraisals of the note and led them to reconstrue negatively their partner's supportiveness during the prior interaction.

Collins and Feeney (2004, Study 1) also found that secure individuals were not very vulnerable to the ambiguous notes or to the evocation of attachment-related worries.

TABLE 6.4. A Summary of Findings Linking Attachment Orientations with Appraisals of Social Support

Study	Attachment scale	Support scale	Support figure	Main findings for positive perceptions of social support
Studies assessing secure attachment to parents or peers				
Cotterell (1992)	IPPA (within-relationship)	SSQ	Family	Security (+)
			Friends	Security (+)
			Teachers	Security (+)
DeKlyen (1996)	AAI	QSS	Family	Security (ns)
			Friends	Security (ns)
			Partner	Security (+)
Larose & Boivin (1997)	IPPA parents	ISEL, SNI MPSS	Mother	Security (+)
			Father	Security (+)
			Friends	Security (ns)
Trinke & Bartholomew (1997)	RQ	SSQ	Global	Security (+)
Larose & Boivin (1998)*	IPPA parents	ISEL, MPSS	Global	Security (+)
			Friends	Security (+)
Herzberg et al. (1999)*	IPPA	SSQ	Global	Security (+)
Mullis et al. (1999)	PAQ	RFSS	Global	Security (+)
La Guardia et al. (2000, Study 1)	IPPA	15 items	Global	Security (+)
Asendorpf & Wilpers (2000)*	RQ (within-relationship)	Single item	Parents	Security (+)
			Friends	Security (+)
Elizur & Mintzer (2001)	HS ratings	PSSS	Family	Security (+)
			Friends	Security (+)
Larose et al. (2001)*	IPPA parents	ACBS	Counselor	Security (+)
Larose et al. (2002)*	IPPA parents	SNI	Global	Security (+)
Elizur & Mintzer (2003)	HS ratings	PSSS	Family	Security (ns)
			Friends	Security (+)
Scharf et al. (2004)	AAI	SSQ	Parents	Security (+)
Tarabulsy et al. (2005)	AAI	SSQ	Mother	Security (ns)
			Partner	Security (ns)
Studies assessing attachment types				
Kobak & Sceery (1988)*	AAI	PSSS	Family	Secure > Avoidant
			Friends	Ns differences
Blain et al. (1993)	RQ	PSSS	Family	Secure > Anxious, Avoidant, Fearful
			Friends	Secure > Anxious, Avoidant, Fearful
J. L. Wallace & Vaux (1993)	HS types	NOS	Global	Secure > Anxious, Avoidant
Zeanah et al. (1993)	AAI	MSSI	Global	Ns differences
Florian et al. (1995)	HS types	PSSS	Parents	Secure > Anxious, Avoidant
			Friends	Secure > Anxious, Avoidant
Priel & Shamai (1995)	HS types	SSQ	Global	Secure > Anxious, Avoidant
M. H. Davis et al. (1998)	HS types	SPS, SPC	Global	Secure > Anxious, Avoidant
			Family	Secure > Anxious, Avoidant
			Friend	Secure > Anxious, Avoidant
			Partner	Secure > Anxious, Avoidant
Volling et al. (1998)	HS types	SPS	Global	Both partners secure > Both partners insecure (married couples)
Freeman & Brown (2001)	SAT	ASI	Mother	Secure > Anxious, Avoidant
			Father	Secure > Anxious, Avoidant
			Friend	No significant differences
Bifulco, Moran, Ball, & Lillie (2002)	Interview	SESSI	Partner	Secure > Anxious, Avoidant, Fearful

(cont.)

TABLE 6.4. *(cont.)*

Study	Attachment scale	Support scale	Support figure	Main findings for positive perceptions of social support
Studies based on attachment-style ratings				
Amir et al. (1999)	HS ratings	PSSS	Family	Secure (ns), Anxious (ns), Avoidant (–)
			Peers	Secure (ns), Anxious (ns), Avoidant (ns)
Granqvist et al. (2001)	AAS	FSS	Family	Secure (ns), Anxious (–), Avoidant (–)
Meyers & Landsberger (2002)	HS ratings	PSSS	Global	Secure (+), Anxious (ns), Avoidant (–)
Studies assessing attachment dimensions				
Markiewicz et al. (1997)	AAQ	8 items	Global	Anxiety (–), Avoidance (ns)
Bell (1998)	AAI	PSSS	Family	Anxiety (ns), Avoidance (ns)
Cozzarelli et al. (1998)*	RQ	SPS	Partner	Anxiety (–), Avoidance (ns)
Ognibene & Collins (1998)	RSQ	PSSS	Family	Anxiety (–), Avoidance (–)
			Friend	Anxiety (–), Avoidance (–)
Anders & Tucker (2000)	ECR	SSQ	Global	Anxiety (–), Avoidance (–)
La Guardia et al. (2000, Studies 2–3)	RQ	15 items	Parents	Anxiety (–), Avoidance (–)
			Friends	Anxiety (–), Avoidance (–)
Muller & Lemieux (2000)	RSQ	NSSQ	Global	Anxiety (–), Avoidance (ns)
Rankin et al. (2000)	ASQ	PRQ-85	Global	Anxiety (–), Avoidance (–)
Alexander et al. (2001)	ASQ	SBI	Global	Anxiety (–), Avoidance (–)
Gallo & Smith (2001)	AAS	QRI	Partner	Anxiety (ns), Avoidance (–) for M Anxiety (–), Avoidance (–) for W
Larose & Bernier (2001)*	AAI	MPSS	Global	Anxiety (–), Avoidance (–)
Larose et al. (2001)*	ASQ	ACBS	Counselor	Anxiety (–), Avoidance (ns)
Rholes et al. (2001)*	AAQ	SPS	Partner	Anxiety (–), Avoidance (–)
Besser et al. (2002)*	RQ	SEI	Partner	Anxiety (–), Avoidance (–)
Moreira et al. (2003)	RSQ	SPS	Global	Anxiety (–), Avoidance (–)
J. A. Feeney (2002b)	RQ, ASQ	SSI	Family	Anxiety (ns), Avoidance (–)
			Friends	Anxiety (ns), Avoidance (–)
J. A. Feeney et al. (2003)	ASQ	SBI	Global	Anxiety (–), Avoidance (–)
Gallo et al. (2003)	AAS	ISEL	Global	Anxiety (–), Avoidance (–)
Moller et al. (2003)	ASQ	PSSS	Family	Anxiety (–), Avoidance (–)
			Friends	Anxiety (–), Avoidance (–)
Collins & Feeney (2004)	ECR	QRI	Partner	Anxiety (–), Avoidance (–)
Mallinckrodt & Wei (2005)	ECR	SPS	Global	Anxiety (–), Avoidance (–)
Vogel & Wei (2005)	ECR	SPS	Global	Anxiety (–), Avoidance (–)

Note. *, longitudinal design; M, men; W, women; (–), significant inverse correlation; (+) significant positive correlation; (ns), nonsignificant effects; ACBS, Academic Counseling Behavior Scale; ASI, Attachment Support Inventory; FSS, Family Support Scale; HS, Hazan and Shaver; ISEL, Interpersonal Support Evaluation List; MPSS, Measure of Perceived Social Support; MSSI, Modified Social Support Interview; NOS, Network Orientation Scale; NSSQ, Norbeck Social Support Questionnaire; PRQ-85, Personal Resources Questionnaire; PSSS, Perceived Social Support Scale; QRI, Quality of Relationship Inventory; QSS, Questionnaire of Social Support; RFSS, Relative and Friend Support Scale; SAT, Separation Anxiety Test; SBI, Support Behaviors Inventory; SEI, Support Expectation Index; SESSI, Self-Evaluation and Social Support Interview; SNI, Social Network Inventory; SPC, Support Provisions Checklist; SPS, Social Provisions Scale; SSI, Social Support Inventory; SSQ, Social Support Questionnaire.

Although secure participants evaluated the ambiguous notes as less supportive than the clearly supportive notes, they did not negatively reconstrue their partner's behaviors during the prior interaction. These findings were replicated in a second study (Collins & Feeney, 2004, Study 2) in which partners were allowed to write authentic notes. Compared with secure individuals, insecure ones rated the notes as less supportive mainly when the notes were ambiguous (as rated by independent judges). Taken together, the two studies indicate that insecurely attached people are predisposed to perceive and remember a partner's helpful behavior as less supportive mainly when the behavior is ambiguous, open to subjective construal, and able to reactivate insecure people's worries about their partners' availability and supportiveness.

Recently, Campbell, Simpson, Boldry, and Kashy (2005) documented another kind of cognitive bias in insecure people's interpretation of partners' everyday helpful behavior. Both members of dating couples completed a questionnaire each evening for 14 consecutive days. Each day, they were asked to think about a partner's supportive behavior (if any) that day, and rate the positivity of this experience and its implications for the stability of the relationship. Although both anxious and avoidant people believed that their partners' support was not very available in general, they differed substantially in their evaluations of daily supportive events. Avoidant people were less likely to say that they experienced supportive events positively, perhaps because those events tended to challenge their desire for interpersonal distance and self-reliance. In contrast, anxious study participants viewed daily supportive events as having stronger and more positive implications for relationship stability, probably because their unmet needs for security were temporarily assuaged. We think this means that anxiously attached people place high importance on their partners' supportive behavior, but this may sometimes exacerbate their frustration, pain, and dissatisfaction when their partner is not immediately available and responsive to their needs.

Although there is some evidence that insecure people's negative appraisals of support stem from biased perception of partner behavior, the appraisals may still reflect actual nonsupportive behavior on the partner's part; that is, partners of insecure people may actually be less supportive than partners of secure people. Rholes, Simpson, Campbell, and Grich (2001) proposed that, beyond choosing less supportive partners, insecurely attached people may actively interfere with partners' supportive behavior, thus confirming and strengthening their doubts about other people's supportiveness. Rholes et al. suggested two processes by which attachment insecurity might discourage a partner's support. First, insecure people's disbelief in others' support may cause them to be more suspicious about their relationship partner's helpful actions, which in turn might lead the partner to withdraw support over time. Second, insecure people may repeatedly claim that their partner is unsupportive, until the partner accepts this view and begins to withdraw and behave nonsupportively. In line with this possibility, Magai and Cohen (1998) found that attachment insecurities among older patients with dementia were associated with their caregivers' reports that the patients were a caregiving burden.

The involvement of both cognitive biases and a partner's actual behavior in determining an insecure person's perception of support was documented by Rholes et al. (2001) in their study of the transition to parenthood. Married women described both their attachment orientation and the spousal support they perceived themselves as receiving approximately 6 weeks prior to the birth of their first child and again 6 months after delivery. In addition, husbands provided information about how supportively they actually behaved toward their wives. The more attachment-anxious wives perceived their spouses as less supportive at both time points than the husbands claimed to be. This association could not be explained by husbands' reports of the support they offered their wives. However, findings also provided some evidence for the accuracy of anxious women's negative appraisals: Men married to more anxiously attached women reported being less supportive than men married to less anxious women. Taken together, these findings suggest that although anxious women's hyperactivating strategies may negatively bias their memories of a partner's helpful behavior and cause them to complain about lack of support during the transition to parenthood, there is at least some degree of accuracy in their complaints about their husbands' lack of support. We cannot tell yet, based on existing studies, which came first: the women's anxiety or the husbands' lack of support.

Attachment studies of marital processes provide further information about the role of partners' actual characteristics in influencing perceptions of support. Volling, Notaro, and Larsen (1998) and Gallo and Smith (2001) asked both spouses to report on their attachment patterns and perceptions of spousal support. They found that doubly secure couples (i.e., in which both partners were securely attached) were more confident about the availability of their spouse's support than doubly insecure couples (i.e., in which both spouses had insecure attachment styles). No significant difference was found among secure couples and mixed couples (in which only one partner was secure), implying that the negative perceptions of the insecure partner can sometimes be mitigated by the attachment security of the other partner (see Chapter 10, this volume, for a review of studies of the effects of couples' attachment patterns on relationship functioning). Moreover, because secure spouses tend actually to be more sensitive, responsive, and supportive than insecure spouses (see Chapter 11, this volume), this finding suggests that an insecure person's perceived support from a spouse can be positively affected by the spouse's truly supportive behaviors.

Overall, the research so far supports the prediction that insecurely attached people tend to appraise their partners' supportiveness somewhat negatively. The findings also indicate that the negative appraisals stem from both intrapsychic processes (negative biases in interpretation and memory of a partner's helpful behavior) and dyadic processes (actual partner unavailability and unresponsiveness). However, more research is needed on the dynamic interplay of these two processes, that is, the ways in which they reinforce each other and create an amplifying cycle of attachment worries and lack of partner support. We also need to understand better how this cycle can be broken by either changes in partner supportiveness or other therapeutic interventions by a couple counselor (S. M. Johnson, 2003).

Expectations and Explanations of Partner Behaviors

According to social cognition researchers (e.g., Baldwin, 1992; Fiske & Taylor, 1991), mental representations of others organize our perceptions of their behavior, shaping expectations about future behavior and affecting the way we explain and understand their behavior. From an attachment perspective, we can extend this claim to insecure individuals' negative mental representations of others, which cause them to have negative expectations about relationship partners' behavior along dimensions such as attention, caring, and trustworthiness. Moreover, insecure people's negative characterization of others' personalities can cause them to attribute instances of negative partner behavior to partners' negative personality traits rather than to less stable contextual factors. In this way, they perpetuate their negative appraisals of others.

In one of the first studies designed to examine attachment style differences in expectations concerning a relationship partner's behavior, Baldwin et al. (1993, Study 1) constructed self-report scales to assess "if–then" relational expectations regarding trust, dependency, and closeness-seeking, and asked people to rate the likelihood of a romantic partner's positive and negative behaviors. Study participants received specific relational context sentences (e.g., "You want to spend more time with your partner"), and after each context sentence they read one positive and one negative partner behavior (e.g., "He or she accepts you" and "He or she rejects you"). For each context, participants were asked to imagine being in the situation and to rate each behavior according to how often their partners would respond in that way. Participants with an insecure attachment style had more negative expectations and fewer positive expectations about partner behavior than those with a secure style. The findings have been conceptually replicated in subsequent studies (Baldwin et al., 1996; Mikulincer & Arad, 1999; Rowe & Carnelley, 2003; You & Malley-Morrison, 2000; Whiffen, 2005).

Insecure people's negative expectations have also been revealed by measures of implicit mental processes. For example, Baldwin et al. (1993, Study 2) used a lexical decision task in which participants read sentences that established either an attachment-related interpersonal context ("If I depend on my partner, then my partner will . . . ") or an attachment-unrelated context ("If I wash the dishes, then my partner will . . . "), and were presented with target strings of letters that designated positive partner behaviors (*support*), negative partner behaviors (*leave*), or neutral behaviors (*read*), or were not words at all (*scpprot*). Participants were asked to determine as quickly as possible whether each target string of letters was a word. RTs provided a measure of the accessibility of thoughts related to the target words. In this study, secure people reacted with shorter decision times to words naming positive interpersonal behaviors than to words referring to negative behaviors. In contrast, insecurely attached people responded faster to words implying negative behaviors than to words implying positive behaviors. That is, whereas secure people seemed to have ready mental access to positive expectations, insecure people had easier access to pessimistic expectations.

There is also evidence for attachment style differences in explanations of others' negative behavior. For example, Collins (1996) presented study participants with six hypothetical vignettes about a romantic partner's negative behavior (e.g., "Your partner didn't comfort you when you were feeling down") and asked them to write an open-ended explanation of each event and to complete an attribution questionnaire assessing the extent to which the behavior was attributed to internal, stable, controllable, and intentional causes. Insecure individuals' explanations emphasized the partner's bad intentions and negative traits. Specifically, more anxious and avoidant people were more likely to believe that their partners' negative behaviors were caused by partners' lack of love, to attribute these behaviors to stable and global causes, and to view them as negatively motivated. The findings have been conceptually replicated several times (Collins, Ford, Guichard, & Allard, 2006; Heene, Buysse, & Van Oost, 2005; Gallo & Smith, 2001; McCarthy & Taylor, 1999; N. Sumer & Cozzarelli, 2004; Whisman & Allan, 1996).

Although insecure people tend to be predisposed to offer pessimistic explanations of other people's behavior, two studies show that this tendency can be moderated by contextual forces. Pereg and Mikulincer (2004) exposed study participants to a negative-mood or neutral-mood induction and found that anxious people's pessimistic attributions were strengthened by the negative-mood induction. Collins et al. (2006) found that anxious people's tendency to offer pessimistic attributions was attenuated for those involved in a satisfying relationship. In both studies, avoidant people's pessimistic explanations remained the same regardless of variations in mood or relationship satisfaction; that is, whereas anxious people's negative cognitive biases seemed to be responsive to fluctuations in mood and relationship-specific factors, avoidant people's biases were stable and likely to yield pessimistic inferences even when a satisfactory relationship encouraged more benign attributions.

Projection and Self–Other Differentiation

Attachment insecurities are likely to bias the appraisal of self–other similarities. In the case of avoidant individuals, who want to maintain distance from others and view themselves as superior, if not actually perfect, their perceptions are likely to be biased toward distinctiveness, uniqueness, and devaluation of others. In contrast, in the case of anxious individuals, who want to be loved and accepted, perception is likely to be biased toward similarity, connectedness, and false consensus. Attachment security can attenuate both false-uniqueness and false-consensus biases, thereby allowing people to make more accurate interpretations of social reality. With regard to false uniqueness, attachment security increases confidence that one possesses unique and special internal qualities (lovable qualities, prosocial motives) that render unnecessary any defensive efforts to portray oneself as especially unique. With regard to false consensus, given that security establishes a sense of connectedness and support from others, secure people should not need to amplify their symbolic connections with others by imagining false self–other similarities. It is mainly people who lack security who need to compensate by defensively biasing social perception to bolster a false sense of uniqueness or consensus.

In a series of six studies, Mikulincer, Orbach, and Iavnieli (1998) in fact found that secure people were more accurate than insecure people in assessing self–other similarity. These authors also discovered that avoidant individuals were more likely than secure ones to perceive others as dissimilar to themselves and to exhibit a false-distinctiveness bias. Anxious individuals were more likely than their secure counterparts to perceive others as similar to themselves and to show a false-consensus bias in both trait and opinion descriptions. Pietromonaco and Barrett (1997) and Lopez (2001) found similar associations between attachment anxiety and lack of self–other differentiation, and Gabriel, Carvallo, Dean, Tippin, and Renaud (2005) reported that avoidant people (compared with nonavoidant ones) were more likely to exaggerate dissimilarities between themselves and a specific friend after being asked to think about the friend.

Mikulincer, Orbach, et al. (1998) also found that insecure people were likely to handle threats by defensively biasing self–other boundaries. Attachment-anxious individuals reacted to threats by generating a self-description that was more similar to a partner's description and by recalling more partner traits that they shared. In contrast, avoidant individuals reacted to the same threats by generating a self-description that was more dissimilar to a partner's description and by forgetting more of the traits they shared with the partner. Secure individuals' self-descriptions and their memories of their partners' traits were not affected by threats, indicating that they could handle threats effectively without distorting social reality.

Following up these experiments, Mikulincer and Horesh (1999) examined the projective mechanisms that might underlie insecure people's perceptions of others. Specifically, they examined (1) avoidant individuals' tendency to project unwanted traits of the self onto others defensively, which increases self–other differentiation and, by comparison, enhances their sense of self-worth, and (2) anxious individuals' tendency to project their actual-self traits onto others, which increases self–other similarity and the sense of closeness. These tendencies were examined in three two-session studies. In the first session, participants generated actual-self traits and unwanted-self traits. In the second session, they described their impressions of hypothetical people, their ability to retrieve memories of actual familiar people was assessed, and they made inferences about the features of hypothetical people.

As expected, avoidant people projected unwanted self-traits onto others; that is, they tended to perceive in others the very traits they had listed as ones they did not like in themselves, they easily retrieved examples of known individuals whose traits resembled those of their unwanted selves, and they made faulty inferences that their own unwanted traits were among the features of a target person who was described as being similar to them in other respects. It seems, therefore, that avoidant individuals' attempts to exclude negative information about themselves from awareness and to maintain interpersonal distance from others dominate their perceptions of others. This fits the clinical definition of "defensive projection" (Freud, 1915/1957).

The findings also demonstrated quite clearly that anxious people projected their actual-self traits onto others. They perceived in an unfamiliar person traits that defined their actual self, easily retrieved an example of a known person whose traits resembled their actual-self traits, and made faulty inferences that their own actual-self traits were among the features of a target person who was described as resembling them in other respects. It therefore seems that anxious people's intense desire for closeness causes them to engage in what Klein (1940) called "projective identification"—projection of self-traits as a means of blurring self–other boundaries and defending against threats of distinctness, separation, and loss.

Mikulincer and Horesh (1999) also found that secure people's representations of others were relatively unbiased by projective mechanisms. This suggests that secure individuals perceive others as what object relations psychoanalysts call "whole objects," not as "part objects" that exist solely to satisfy the perceiver's egocentric needs. Whereas projective mechanisms reflect little real concern for others and are aimed at avoiding the perceiver's own discomfort, regardless of the potential costs to the "object" (Joseph, 1989), secure people's perceptions of others seem to be guided by a genuine interest in knowing and understanding others' attributes, beliefs, and preferences, perhaps because this information is relevant to forming mature and satisfying relationships.

Intergroup Biases

Secure people's genuine interest in others may extend even to those who do not belong to their own social group. They may be less prone to intergroup bias—the tendency to perceive one's own social group (ingroup) as better than others (e.g., Allport, 1954; Devine, 1995). This tendency has been documented in numerous studies of ingroup favoritism, derogation of members of other groups (outgroup members), and prejudice toward people who are different from oneself. This destructive human tendency seems to serve a self-protective function, maintenance of self-esteem: "We, including I, are better than they are" (Tajfel & Turner, 1986). Unfortunately, this method of maintaining self-esteem depends on emphasizing real or imagined differences between ingroups and outgroups, especially ways in which the ingroup can be perceived as better (Tajfel & Turner, 1986).

We thought it likely that intergroup biases would be especially characteristic of insecure people. A secure person, who maintains a sense of value based on other people's affection and support, should have less need to fear and disparage outgroup members. In his account of human behavioral systems, Bowlby (1969/1982) stated that activation of the attachment system is closely related to innate fear of strangers, and that attachment figure availability mitigates this innate reaction and fosters a more tolerant attitude toward unfamiliarity and novelty.

In a series of five studies involving secular Israeli Jewish students, we (Mikulincer & Shaver, 2001) examined secure and insecure people's intergroup biases, and found that the higher a participant's attachment anxiety, the more negative and hostile his or her appraisals of Israeli Arabs, ultra-Orthodox Jews, Russian immigrants, and homosexuals.

This association was mediated by threat appraisal: More anxiously attached participants were more likely to appraise these outgroup members as threatening, and this appraisal was closely associated with hostile and derogating reactions to outgroups. In addition, as already shown in Chapter 3, this volume, experimental priming of representations of security-enhancing attachment figures eliminated negative appraisals of outgroups. This elimination of bias occurred even when study participants were led to believe they had failed on a cognitive task or their national group had been insulted by an outgroup member. In other words, dispositional or experimentally augmented security minimized the tendency to derogate outgroup members, even when derogation would have been an understandable reaction.

These findings should not be interpreted as implying that securely attached people fail to identify with their own group. That interpretation would contradict Bowlby's (1988) portrayal of attachment security as promoting a sense of togetherness, as well as E. R. Smith, Murphy, and Coats's (1999) discovery of a positive association between secure attachment and identification with social groups (see Chapter 15, this volume). Brewer (1999) has challenged the assumed connection between ingroup love and outgroup hatred, showing that attachment to one's ingroup does not require hostility toward outgroups. We agree that securely attached people can love their own group without experiencing outgroup hostility.

CONCLUDING REMARKS

The notion that attachment styles are based on, or comprise, internal working models of self and others was one of Bowlby's (1969/1982) most important theoretical ideas. As we mentioned at the outset of this chapter, it also happened to mesh well with cognitive–social psychology around the time that Hazan and Shaver (1987) extended Bowlby's theory to the realm of adolescent and adult romantic relationships. Moreover, the dominance of cognitive theories in psychology generally during the past few decades, along with the invention and refinement of cognitive assessment procedures (e.g., computer-administered subliminal primes, Stroop tasks, and lexical decision tasks), has allowed researchers, including ourselves, to test psychodynamic ideas central to attachment theory using methods that earlier psychodynamic researchers could only dream about. This has tightened the links and increased the affinities among cognitive, social, and psychodynamic perspectives.

Twenty years of research on adult attachment has yielded extensive evidence regarding insecure people's shaky self-concepts and negative views of others. Moreover, the research reviewed in this chapter sheds light on the dynamics and complexities of insecure people's mental representations and goes against theoretical formulations that equate avoidant attachments with positive models of self and anxious attachment with positive models of others (e.g., Bartholomew & Horowitz, 1991). Although dismissingly avoidant people do hold explicit positive views of self, these views are based on defensive self-enhancement and involve harsh self-criticism and perfectionist self-standards that can sometimes provoke self-doubts and demoralization. Moreover, even though anxious people hope to gain a partner's love and esteem, and tend to view their partner, at first, as a badly needed personal "savior," they still hold both explicit and implicit negative views of relationship partners in particular, and humanity in general, and this negativity, combined with vigilance and sometimes false accusations, can eventually erode a relationship partner's good intentions and supportive behavior. Although a large amount of very creative and illuminating research has already been conducted to examine internal working models of self and others, there is more to learn about the complex dynamics of secondary attachment strategies, the way dyadic processes interact with intrapsychic processes, and the way the initiation of a broaden-and-build cycle of attachment security can counteract the negative cognitive biases of insecurely attached persons. These topics are extremely important not only for the domain of dyadic relationships but also for understanding group dynamics and intergroup relations, as we explain in later chapters.

CHAPTER 7

■ ■ ■

Attachment Processes
and Emotion Regulation

In this chapter we focus on the role of the attachment system in emotion regulation. Although Bowlby did not devote a great deal of attention to the nature of emotions per se (only a single brief chapter in Volume 1 of *Attachment and Loss* [1969/1982]), the subtitles of Volumes 2 and 3—*Separation: Anxiety and Anger* (1973) and *Loss: Sadness and Depression* (1980)—make clear that emotions were a primary concern. He was interested in the causes and consequences of emotions aroused by attachment (e.g., love, joy), separation (anxiety, anger), and loss (grief, sadness, despair). And his theory is an attempt to explain how secure attachments help a person survive temporary bouts of negative emotion and reestablish hope, optimism, and equanimity, and how different forms of insecurity interfere with emotion regulation, social adjustment, and mental health. Research inspired by the theory, including research about attachment processes and attachment styles in adulthood, is the basis for the model we presented in Chapter 2, which outlines the regulatory function of the attachment system and helps explain individual differences in emotion and emotion regulation.

In thinking about the implications of the attachment system for emotion regulation, we were guided by an updated version of Shaver, Schwartz, Kirson, and O'Connor's (1987) model of the emotion process (Figure 7.1), based on both theoretical considerations (e.g., Frijda, 1986; Lazarus, 1991) and ordinary people's accounts of emotional experiences (e.g., Shaver et al., 1987; C. A. Smith & Ellsworth, 1987). It has been used to conceptualize both emotions and emotional development (e.g., K. W. Fischer, Shaver, & Carnochan, 1990). In the model, emotions, considered to be biologically functional, organized systems of evaluative thoughts and action tendencies supported by physiological changes, are generated by the appraisal of internal and external events in relation to

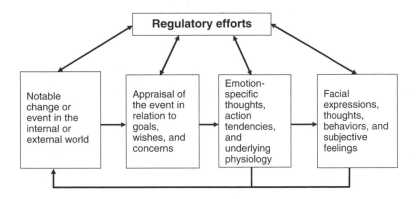

FIGURE 7.1. Flowchart model of the emotion process.

goals and concerns. The emotions that arise in conjunction with appraisals are experienced and expressed through changes in thoughts, available memories, action tendencies, behaviors, and subjective feelings (Oatley & Jenkins, 1996). The subjectively experienced aspects of emotions are obviously associated with physiological changes, some of which have perceptible consequences (e.g., speeded heart rate, blushing, gasping for air). Both the generation and the expression of emotions are affected by regulatory efforts, which can alter, obstruct, or suppress appraisals, concerns, action tendencies, and subjective feelings.

According to Shaver et al. (1987) and Oatley and Jenkins (1996), the onset of emotion depends on a perceived change in the internal or external environment, especially an unexpected, surprising, or personally significant change. These changes are automatically, and often unconsciously, appraised in relation to needs, goals, and concerns. If the perceived changes are favorable to goal attainment, the resulting emotions are generally positive (i.e., hedonically positive in valence). If the changes are unfavorable, the resulting emotions are generally negative. The particular emotion that arises depends on the specific pattern of concerns and appraisals that get activated. When a specific appraisal pattern occurs, a corresponding emotion, including its evolutionarily functional action tendencies and physiological substrates (e.g., changes in attention, blood pressure, and muscle tension), follows automatically. These consequences can be manifested in thoughts, feelings, vocalizations, and actions; expressed both verbally and nonverbally; and measured in numerous ways.

Shaver et al. (1987) claimed that regulatory efforts can alter the emotion process. If there is no reason to postpone, dampen, redirect, or deny an emerging emotion, its action tendencies are automatically expressed in congruent thoughts, feelings, words, and actions. However, when other goals are in play (e.g., social norms, personal standards, self-protective defenses) that make the experience, enactment, or expression of an emotion undesirable, regulatory efforts are exerted to alter, obstruct, or suppress the emotion and bring about a more desirable state—or, at least, the outward appearance of a more desirable state. In this model, regulatory efforts can be directed at various parts of the emotion process, altering appraisals, concerns, action tendencies, arousal level, thoughts, facial expressions, and actions. As a result, the person doing the regulating thinks, feels, and acts in accordance with the altered emotional state.

ATTACHMENT PATTERNS AND EMOTION REGULATION: THEORETICAL BACKGROUND

With Figure 7.1 in mind, it is possible to chart the effects of the attachment system on emotion regulation. As we discussed in Chapter 3, the attachment system is, in itself, an emotion regulation device. Perceived threats automatically activate the system, which in turn causes the threatened individual to seek proximity to protective others (or to evoke mental representations of them) as a means of managing the threat and restoring emotional balance. Attachment-system activation and proximity seeking are integral parts of a person's regulatory efforts, and they play an important role in shaping his or her emotional responses. They are inborn, commonly used methods of altering undesirable emotional states and promoting more goal-congruent, positive states.

In Chapter 3 we also discussed the emotional effects of attachment figure availability. An available and responsive attachment figure facilitates coping with threats and attaining states of positive emotion, whereas the unavailability of such a figure disrupts coping, and increases the frequency and intensity of distress. In addition, an available attachment figure enables a person to fulfill the main goal of the attachment system—proximity maintenance (as a way of attaining protection and coping with threats and distress). In contrast, attachment figure unavailability is a goal-incongruent state, blocking the attainment of proximity and protection, thereby generating and amplifying negative emotions.

Beyond these normative links between attachment processes and emotion regulation, individual differences in attachment-system functioning affect how people appraise emotion-eliciting events and regulate the generation, experience, and expression of emotions in thoughts, feelings, action tendencies, and behavior. According to our model, achieving a continuing sense of attachment security promotes the development of healthy, flexible, and reality-attuned regulatory processes that allow emotions to be experienced and expressed without defensive distortion. In contrast, attachment insecurities contribute to distortion or denial of emotional experience, unconscious suppression of potentially functional emotions, dysfunctional rumination on threats, and poor coping skills. For this reason, Bowlby (1988) viewed attachment insecurity as a risk factor for clinically significant emotional problems and poor adjustment (see Chapter 13, this volume). In this chapter, we consider attachment style differences in the emotion-regulation process. In Chapter 13, we discuss implications of research on attachment and emotion regulation for psychopathology.

Attachment Security and Constructive Emotion Regulation

We begin with a theoretical overview, which we then flesh out with specific evidence from published studies. When regulating emotions (Figure 7.1), a secure person is able to direct most of his or her effort to the emotion-*generation* process—changing the emotion-eliciting event (e.g., by resolving a conflict or solving a problem) or reappraising it constructively—and can therefore sidestep or short-circuit many painful experiences. Specifically, when a secure person encounters internal or external stimuli or events that might provoke undesirable emotions, he or she can engage in problem solving, planning, and cognitive reappraisal; place the negative event in perspective, making it seem less overwhelming; and mobilize support from people with additional resources or perspectives for solving the problem or reducing its stressful effects. The secure person is also more likely to have developed self-soothing skills, calming him- or herself with implicit and explicit emotion-regulation techniques learned from security-providing attachment figures. He or she can maintain attention on constructive alternatives rather than becoming a victim of rumination or catastrophizing. These beneficial regulatory efforts are what Epstein and Meier (1989) called "constructive ways of coping" and J. J. Gross (1999) called "antecedent-focused emotion regulation" (as distinct from suppressing an emotion after its antecedents have already had their full effect).

Theoretically, secure people's constructive approach to emotion regulation is a result of repeated interactions with attachment figures who are (or were) sensitive and responsive to bids for protection and support. During such interactions, secure people learned that support seeking usually results in protection, comfort, and relief. They came away with heightened confidence that turning to others is an effective way to cope. Moreover, such interactions heighten a secure person's positive expectations about the availability of social support (see Chapter 6, this volume), which makes it easy to ask for coping assistance when needed.

Supportive interactions with security-enhancing attachment figures also facilitate problem solving. Part of effective problem solving is recognizing that one's previous course of action was unsuccessful and must be changed if the problem is to be solved. Experiencing, or having experienced, attachment figures as loving and supportive allows secure people to revise erroneous beliefs and strategies without excessive self-doubt or self-criticism (see Chapter 6, this volume). In addition, secure people's self-confidence allows them to open their minds to new information and adjust their plans flexibly to deal realistically with whatever is happening at the moment (see Chapter 8, this volume). Believing that support will be available if needed, secure people can creatively explore a challenging situation, while tolerating ambiguity and uncertainty.

Secure people can also reappraise situations, construe events in relatively benign terms, symbolically transform threats into challenges, maintain an optimistic sense of self-efficacy, and attribute undesirable events to controllable, temporary, or context-dependent causes. This foundation for constructive appraisals is sustained by deeply ingrained positive beliefs about self and world (see Chapter 6, this volume). While interacting with available and supportive attachment figures, secure individuals learn that distress is manageable and external obstacles surmountable.

Having managed emotion-eliciting events or reappraised them in benign terms, secure people do not often have to alter or suppress other parts of the emotion process. They make what Lazarus (1991) called a "short circuit of threat," sidestepping the interfering and dysfunctional aspects of emotions, while benefiting from their functional, adaptive qualities. They can remain open to their emotions, express and communicate feelings freely and accurately to others, and experience them fully without distortion. They can expect emotional expression to result in beneficial responses from others. For example, a secure person can experience and acknowledge anger as a signal that a partner's behavior should be reconsidered and altered. The anger can be expressed in a regulated way, with the person keeping attention on the need to redress a wrong rather than attempting to punish or injure the partner. A secure person generally expects wrongs to be righted, but without damaging a relationship. Bowlby (1973) called this the "anger of hope," because it targets a specific problem and is intended to repair a damaged relationship. "Hope" refers to the positive expectation that a relationship partner, seeing that the securely attached person has been wronged, will be willing to discuss the matter and change accordingly.

Secure people can also attend to their own distress without fear of losing control or becoming overwhelmed. For individuals whose attachment figures have been available and responsive, expression of negative emotions has usually led to distress-alleviating support and guidance. A person with supportive attachment figures learns that distress can be expressed honestly, without the relationship being at risk, and this fosters an increasingly balanced way of experiencing and expressing emotions—with a sensible goal in mind and without undue hostility, vengeance, or anxiety about losing control or being abandoned. According to Cassidy (1994), "The experience of security is based not on the denial of negative affect but on the ability to tolerate negative affects temporarily in order to achieve mastery over threatening or frustrating situations" (p. 233). In other words, for relatively secure individuals, "emotion regulation" does not require avoidance, suppression, or denial of emotions.

This openness to emotional experiences is manifested in what Fonagy, Steele, Steele, Moran, et al. (1991) called self-reflective capacity—the ability to notice, think about, and understand mental states. Interactions with available and supportive attachment figures provide secure people with the capacity to understand and articulate their emotional experiences and to integrate these experiences into their self-concept. Fonagy, Steele, Steele, Moran, et al. described the security-enhancing caregiver of an infant as able "to reflect on the infant's mental experience and re-present it to the infant translated into the language of actions the infant can understand. The baby is, thus, [encouraged to feel that] the process of reflection was performed within its own mental boundaries" (p. 207). This process has been studied with the help of the AAI (see Chapter 4, this volume) and Fonagy, Target, Steele, and Steele's (1998) measure of "mentalization" or "reflective functioning." It has been emphasized in recent analyses of "intersubjectivity" (Hennighausen & Lyons-Ruth, 2005), which is a key part of close relationships and of children's developing abilities to understand their own and other people's minds.

Avoidant Attachment and the Inhibition or Suppression of Emotional Experience

People with an avoidant attachment style cannot risk allowing emotion to flow freely and be acknowledged consciously. Avoidant defenses are largely designed to inhibit emotional states that are incongruent with the goal of keeping the attachment system deactivated (Main & Weston, 1982). Defensive inhibition is directed mainly at fear, anxiety, anger, sadness, shame, guilt, and distress, because these emotions are triggered by threats and can cause unwanted activation of the attachment system. In addition, anger implies emotional involvement in a relationship, and such involvement may undermine an avoidant person's commitment to self-reliance (Cassidy, 1994). Moreover, fear, anxiety, sadness, shame, and guilt can be interpreted as signs of weakness or vulnerability, which contradict an avoidant person's sense of strength and independence. Avoidant individuals may even feel uncomfortable with joy and happiness, because they promote interpersonal closeness and may be interpreted by a relationship partner as indications of investment in the relationship (Cassidy, 1994).

Avoidant individuals also attempt to block emotional reactions to the potential or actual unavailability of attachment figures (rejection, separation, loss), because such reactions imply neediness and dependence. Like secure people, avoidant ones attempt to down-regulate threat-related emotions. But whereas secure people's regulatory efforts usually promote communication, compromise, and relationship maintenance or repair, avoidant people's efforts are aimed at minimizing closeness and interdependence, regardless of the deleterious effects on a relationship.

The avoidant approach to emotion regulation often interferes with support seeking, problem solving, and reappraisal. For avoidant people, who stress interpersonal distance and self-reliance, support seeking in times of need is perceived as risky and uncomfortable. Moreover, they may have difficulty with problem solving or reappraisal, because these coping techniques require recognizing threats and errors that avoidant people prefer to deny. Problem solving can also be blocked if it hints at the possibility of failure or requires a person to admit that some problems are unsolvable, which does not sit well with an avoidant person's sense of, or wish for, autonomy and superiority.

Inability or unwillingness to deal directly with the causes of painful emotions often leaves avoidant people with only one regulatory option: suppressing emotion or dissociating themselves from its effects on experience and behavior (by using what Lazarus & Folkman [1984] called "distancing coping" and Gross [1999] called "response-focused emotion regulation"). These regulatory attempts consist of denial or suppression of emotion-related thoughts and memories, diversion of attention away from emotion-related material, suppression of emotion-related action tendencies, and inhibition or masking of verbal and nonverbal expressions of emotion. By preventing the conscious experience and expression of emotions, avoidant individuals make it less likely that emotional experiences will be integrated into their memories or that they will use these experiences effectively in information processing and social behavior. For them, emotions are best hidden and suppressed rather than used flexibly in behavior regulation, presumably because they have learned during many painful interactions with cool, rejecting attachment figures that expressing distress or vulnerability invites punishment or rejection (Cassidy, 1994).

Attachment Anxiety and the Intensification of Undesirable Emotions

Unlike secure and avoidant people, who tend to view negative emotions as goal-incongruent states that should either be managed effectively or suppressed, anxiously attached individuals often perceive these emotions as congruent with attachment goals and, therefore, as worth sustaining or even exaggerating. Anxiously attached people are guided by an unfulfilled wish to get attachment figures to pay attention and provide more reliable protection, which causes them to intensify emotions that call for attention and care, such as jealousy and anger, or emotions that implicitly emphasize vulnerability and neediness, such as sadness, anxiety, fear, and shame. Anxious hyperactivation is also manifested in attempts to sustain and intensify emotions that activate the attachment system, such as fear, worries about abandonment, and doubts about self-efficacy. This kind of emotional expression runs counter to most discussions of emotion regulation, because "regulation" usually means *down*-regulation. In the case of anxiously attached persons, however, "regulation" can also include intensification.

According to Cassidy (1994), an anxious person's intensification of emotion is a way to capture a caregiver's attention.

> The negative emotionality of the insecure/ambivalent child may be exaggerated and chronic because the child recognizes that to relax and allow herself to be soothed by the presence of an attachment figure is to run the risk of then losing contact with the inconsistently available parent. One reasonable strategy involves fearfulness in response to relatively benign stimuli. Through exaggerated fearfulness, the infant increases the likelihood of gaining the attention of a frequently unavailable caregiver should true danger arise. (p. 241)

Hyperactivation of negative emotions sometimes renders problem solving irrelevant. In fact, problem solving may thwart an anxious person's wish to perpetuate problematic situations and continue expressing needs and dissatisfactions. Moreover, problem solving works against the anxious person's self-construal as helpless and incompetent (see Chapter 6, this volume): Demonstrations of competence might result in the loss of an attachment figure's attention (Cassidy & Berlin, 1994). Anxious people may also have problems with support seeking. Although their intense wish for security and protection often intensifies support-seeking efforts, their doubts about support availability (see Chapter 6, this volume), coupled with fear of rejection, may make them hesitant at times to ask directly for assistance. As a result, they may be ambivalent about support seeking and may express their need for protection in indirect ways that seem less likely to provoke rejection (e.g., exaggerating facial expressions of sadness, without directly asking for help).

How is anxious hyperactivation sustained? Several possible methods include making catastrophic appraisals, amplifying the threatening aspects of even minor troubles, maintaining pessimistic beliefs about one's inability to manage distress, and attributing threatening events to uncontrollable causes and global personal inadequacies (Chapter 6, this volume, contains a review of findings regarding this self-defeating attribution pattern). Another approach is to pay close attention to internal signs of insecurity, anxiety, or distress (engaging in what Lazarus & Folkman [1984] called "emotion-focused coping"). This involves hypervigilant attention to the physiological changes associated with emotion, heightened recall of threat-related feelings, and rumination on actual and potential threats. A paradoxical strategy is to intensify negative emotions by adopting a counterphobic stance toward threats or making self-defeating decisions and taking ineffective courses of action that end in lamentable failure. All of these strategies create a self-amplifying cycle of distress, which is maintained by ruminative thoughts even after a threat subsides. As a result, anxious individuals experience many negative emotions, their cognitive processes are often burdened and disrupted by distress, and their stream of consciousness is overflowing with threat-related thoughts and feelings. Main (1990) described this "state of mind with respect to attachment" (as seen in the AAI) as involving high levels of anxiety, preoccupation, confusion, ambivalence, unresolved anger, and incoherence.

Interestingly, although hyperactivating and deactivating strategies lead to opposite patterns of emotional expression (intensification vs. suppression), both result in dysfunctional emotions. Avoidant people miss the adaptive aspects of emotional experiences by blocking conscious access to them, and anxious people miss adaptive possibilities by riveting their attention on disruptive rather than potentially functional aspects of emotional experience. As a result, anxious individuals perceive themselves as helpless to control the self-amplifying flow of painful thoughts and feelings, even though they contribute to it.

EMPIRICAL EVIDENCE FOR ATTACHMENT-RELATED DIFFERENCES IN EMOTION REGULATION

A large body of evidence supports the forgoing theoretical analysis. In subsequent sections we review evidence concerning attachment style differences in (1) use of the primary attachment strategy (support seeking); (2) appraisal, reappraisal, and other aspects of coping with stress (problem solving, emotion-focused strategies, distancing); (3) management of attachment-related threats; (4) experience and management of specific emotional states; and (5) mental access to emotional memories and experiences.

Thoughts and Behaviors Related to the Primary Attachment Strategy, Support Seeking

According to attachment theory, support seeking is the attachment system's primary strategy. As we explained in Chapter 2, activation of the attachment system includes both heightened access to attachment-related cognitions and memories (preconscious activation) and enactment of support-seeking mental strategies and actual behaviors. For secure people, threat appraisals actually increase mental access to comforting thoughts about positive interactions with attachment figures (thoughts of proximity, support, and relief), which in turn sustain support seeking. For insecure people, however, painful attachment experiences have created associative links in memory between proximity seeking and worries about separation or rejection, causing overly easy access to these worries whenever an urge to seek proximity is aroused. As a result, threat appraisals can arouse attachment-related worries, which then interfere with effective support seeking.

Preconscious Activation of Attachment Cognitions

The studies we reviewed in Chapter 3 (Mikulincer et al., 2000; Mikulincer, Gillath, & Shaver, 2002) offered initial evidence for attachment style differences in preconscious activation of attachment-related thoughts. In those studies, secure people reacted to subliminal threats (compared with neutral subliminal primes) with heightened access to thoughts of proximity and relief, and to the names of security-providing attachment figures. Secure individuals displayed relatively slow access to words related to separation and rejection. In contrast, anxious individuals had ready access to attachment-related mental contents following either a threatening or a neutral prime and also access to words associated with separation and rejection. We attribute these findings to anxious individuals' hyperactivating strategies, which keep rejection-related thoughts available in working memory even under nonthreatening conditions.

For avoidant individuals, worries about rejection and separation seemed generally to be mentally inaccessible. However, such worries *did* become accessible in response to threat primes if a "cognitive load" was added to a lexical decision task (Mikulincer et al., 2000). Social cognition research has shown that addition of a cognitive load increases the accessibility of material that a person is trying to suppress (e.g., Wegner, Erber, & Zanakos, 1993). Thus, our results support the theoretical proposition that avoidant people suppress attachment-related worries but have trouble doing so when a cognitive load is added. In addition, when the word "separation" was used as a subliminal threat prime, avoidant individuals were slower to activate the names of their attachment figures (Mikulincer, Gillath, & Shaver, 2002), making it seem that their attachment system was preconsciously *deactivated* when the issue of separation was raised. This may reflect prior experiences in which expressions of need for help and support, especially when an attachment figure was leaving or threatening to leave, were punished (Main & Weston, 1982).

Support-Seeking Tendencies

Several studies have confirmed the predicted link between attachment security and self-reported support seeking (Table 7.1 contains a summary of methods and findings). For example, Florian, Mikulincer, and Bucholtz (1995) found that secure individuals (compared with their insecure counterparts) reported a stronger tendency to seek instrumental and emotional support from parents, close friends, and a romantic partner. Similarly, Larose, Bernier, Souey, and Duchesne (1999) found that attachment security favors the

TABLE 7.1. A Summary of Findings Concerning Attachment Orientations and Support-Seeking Tendencies

Study	Attachment scale	Support scale	Target	Main findings for the tendency to seek support
Studies assessing secure attachment to parents or peers				
Greenberger & McLaughlin (1998)	HS ratings	COPE	Global	Security (+)
Torquati & Vazsonyi (1999)	AAS	CAPSI	Global	Security (+)
Larose et al. (2001)*	IPPA	ACBS	Counselor	Security (+)
Paley et al. (2002)*	AAI	Interview	Spouse	Security (+) (only for husbands)
Studies assessing attachment types				
J. A. Feeney & Ryan (1994)	HS ratings	1 item	Professional	Secure > Avoidant
Florian et al. (1995)	HS types	SSS	Parents, peers	Secure > Anxious, Avoidant
Mikulincer et al. (1993)	HS types	WOCS	Global	Secure > Anxious, Avoidant
Mikulincer & Florian (1995)*	HS types	WOCS	Global	Secure > Avoidant
Birnbaum et al. (1997)	HS types	WOCS	Global	No significant differences
Mikulincer & Florian (1998)	HS types	WOCS	Global	Secure > Anxious, Avoidant
Ognibene & Collins (1998)	RSQ	WOCS	Global	Secure > Avoidant, Fearful
Priel et al. (1998)	RQ	1 item	Friends	Secure > Avoidant
Kemp & Neimeyer (1999)	RQ	WOCS	Global	No significant differences
Mikulincer & Florian (1999c)	HS types	WOCS	Global	Secure > Anxious, Avoidant
Berant et al. (2001a)	HS ratings	WOCS	Global	Secure > Anxious, Avoidant
R. DeFronzo et al. (2001)	RSQ	SSFQ	Global	Secure > Avoidant
Schmidt et al. (2002)	New scale	BCM	Global	Secure > Avoidant
Seiffge-Krenke & Beyers (2005)*	AAI	CASQ	Global	Secure > Avoidant, Anxious
Studies based on attachment ratings or dimensions				
Radecki-Bush et al. (1993)	HS ratings	WOCS	Global	Avoidance (–)
Kotler et al. (1994)	HS ratings	WOCS	Global	Anxiety (ns), Avoidance (–)
Glachan & Ney (1995)	AAS	Narrative	Global	Anxiety (ns), Avoidance (ns)
J. A. Feeney (1998)	ASQ	Narrative	Global	Anxiety (–), Avoidance (–)
Lopez et al. (1998)	RQ model of other	ATSPPH WSCS	Professional Counselor	Avoidance (ns) Avoidance (–)
Pierce & Lydon (1998)	AAS	6 items	Global	Anxiety (ns), Avoidance (–)
Larose et al. (1999, Study 1)	ASQ	SHTS	Teacher	Anxiety (–), Avoidance (–)
Larose et al. (1999, Study 2)*	ASQ	SHTS	Mentor	Anxiety (ns), Avoidance (–)
Harvey & Byrd (2000)	AAS	FCOPES	Global	Secure (+), Anxious (–), Avoidant (–)
Alexander et al. (2001)	ASQ	WOCS	Global	Anxiety (ns), Avoidance (–)
Berant et al. (2001b)*	HS ratings	WOCS	Global	Anxiety (+), Avoidance (–)
Horppu & Ikonen-Varila (2001)	RQ	14 items	Global	Secure (ns), Anxious (ns), Avoidant (–)
Larose et al. (2001)*	ASQ	ACBS	Counselor	Anxiety (–), Avoidance (–)
Larose & Bernier (2001)*	AAI	TRAC	Teacher	Anxiety (–), Avoidance (–)
Howard & Medway (2004)	RSQ	COPE	Global	Anxiety (–), Avoidance (–)
Jerome & Liss (2005)	ECR	COPE	Global	Anxiety (+), Avoidance (–)
Vogel & Wei (2005)	ECR	ISCI	Counselor	Anxiety (+), Avoidance (–)

Note. *, longitudinal design; (–), significant inverse correlation; (+), significant positive correlation; (ns), nonsignificant effects; ACBS, Academic Counseling Behavior Scale; ATSPPH, Attitude toward Seeking Professional Psychological Help; BCM, Bernese Coping Modes; CAPSI, Child and Adolescent Problem-Solving Inventory; CASQ, Coping across Situations Questionnaire; FCOPES, Family Crises–Oriented Personal Evaluation Scale; HS, Hazan and Shaver; ISCI, Intentions to Seek Counseling Inventory; SHTS, Seeking Help from Teacher Scale; SSFQ, Stress and Social Feedback Questionnaire; SSS, Support-Seeking Scale; TRAC, Test of Reactions and Adaptation to College; WSCS, Willingness to Seek Counseling Scale; WOCS, Ways of Coping Scale.

seeking of assistance from professional sources, such as teachers, academic mentors, and counselors (see Table 7.1). Such findings were also obtained in a 7-year longitudinal study examining "state of mind" differences (assessed with the AAI) in coping trajectories from early adolescence to young adulthood (Seiffge-Krenke & Beyers, 2005).

The link between attachment security and support seeking was also noticed in retrospective accounts by Israeli ex-prisoners (ex-POWs) of the Yom Kippur War, collected 18 years after the war (Z. Solomon, Ginzburg, Mikulincer, Neria, & Ohry, 1998). A content analysis of these accounts revealed that compared with insecure ex-POWs, securely attached ex-POWs were more likely to report having dealt with captivity by recruiting positive memories or creating positive imaginary encounters with loved ones. In other words, they coped by seeking symbolic proximity to, and comfort from, internalized attachment figures.

Secure people's reliance on support seeking was also documented in three experiments examining proximity seeking to symbolic attachment figures, such as God, in times of need (Birgegard & Granqvist, 2004). Swedish undergraduates were subliminally exposed to attachment-related threats ("Mother is gone," "God has abandoned me") or neutral statements (e.g., "People are walking"), then completed a measure of seeking proximity to God (e.g., "I turn to God when I am in pain," "I strive to maintain closeness to God"). In all three studies, secure individuals reacted to the subliminal separation prime (compared to a neutral prime) with a heightened effort to get close to God. Less secure participants evinced less seeking of proximity to God following the separation prime.

In line with theory, a series of studies found that secure people are more likely than their insecure counterparts to benefit from supportive interactions when coping with stress, and even from mere proximity to a close relationship partner. For example, Mikulincer and Florian (1997) reported that, for secure people, after anticipating handling a snake, both an emotionally supportive conversation (talking about the emotions elicited by the snake) and an instrumentally supportive conversation (talking about how to deal with the snake) were effective in restoring emotional equanimity. However, these conversations failed to improve the affective states of insecure people; in fact the emotionally supportive conversation worsened avoidant individuals' reactions, and the instrumentally supportive conversation worsened the affective reactions of anxious individuals.

E. M. Carpenter and Kirkpatrick (1996) and B. C. Feeney and Kirkpatrick (1996) examined attachment-style differences in physiological stress responses when a relationship partner was either present or absent. In two laboratory studies, women's physiological responses (heart rate and blood pressure) to stressful events (e.g., performing a stressful arithmetic task) were assessed in either the presence or the absence of their romantic partner. Secure women had milder physiological stress responses than avoidant or anxiously attached women in both experimental conditions (whether or not their romantic partner was present). More important, the physiological stress responses of avoidant and anxiously attached women were exacerbated rather than mitigated by the presence of their romantic partner (compared to the partner-absent condition). According to B. C. Feeney and Kirkpatrick, a partner's presence had no effect on secure women's responses, possibly because they were able to regulate their emotions with or without the partner's presence. For insecure women, their partner's presence seemed to add to their distress, possibly because the partner had been perceived as overly critical or inadequately supportive in the past. Although these studies failed to reveal a calming effect of a relationship partner's presence, they did indicate that partner presence can be a source of distress rather than comfort for insecure people.

Other research has shown that symbolic proximity to a relationship partner in times of need has beneficial effects on secure individuals. McGowan (2002) asked people to think about a significant other or a mere acquaintance while waiting to take part in a stressful task. Thinking about a significant other lowered distress and heightened self-esteem among secure people, but insecure ones reported heightened distress after thinking about a significant other rather than an acquaintance.

With regard to avoidant attachment, studies consistently show that avoidance is associated with weaker tendencies to seek support (see Table 7.1). For example, Priel, Mitrany, and Shahar (1998) found that adolescents scoring higher on avoidance perceived themselves and were perceived by peers as less likely to seek support. Larose et al. (2001) found that avoidant attachment predicted less support seeking across a 10-session counseling program, and Lopez, Melendez, Sauer, Berger, and Wyssmann (1998) noted that the inhibiting effects of avoidance on support seeking were most notable when participants had many problems (and, therefore, needed more help).

The link between avoidant attachment and inhibition of support seeking has also been noted following experimentally induced symbolic threats to cultural worldviews or self-esteem (Hart et al., 2005, Studies 3–4). In these studies, American undergraduates read either a negative (hostile) or neutral essay about America, or were exposed to failure feedback or no feedback in an ego-involving cognitive task. Following the manipulations, participants rated their desire for closeness in romantic relationships. They were asked to imagine their ideal romantic relationship and rate how close they would like the relationship to be, and how much they would hope to be able to rely on their partner for sympathy and support. Both studies indicated that avoidant people (either dismissing or fearful) reported less desire for closeness than nonavoidant people, even in neutral conditions (neutral essay, no feedback). More important, dismissingly avoidant individuals (but not people with other attachment styles) exhibited a further decrease in desire for closeness after reading an anti-American essay or failing on a cognitive task. Thus, it seems that avoidant people, especially those with low attachment anxiety, inhibit proximity seeking when defending themselves from threats to their worldviews or self-esteem.

Findings regarding attachment anxiety are less consistent. Although around half of the studies summarized in Table 7.1 indicate that attachment anxiety is associated with lower levels of support seeking, the remaining studies failed to find a significant association. These inconsistent results may reflect anxious people's ambivalent approach to support seeking (intense wishes for security, coupled with doubts about support availability). Indeed, Vogel and Wei (2005) found two opposing causal pathways by which attachment anxiety affected support seeking. In one, attachment anxiety was associated with greater psychological distress, which in turn heightened support seeking. In the other, attachment anxiety was linked with negative perceptions of others' supportiveness, which led to reduced support seeking. This inhibiting effect of negative perceptions of support availability was also observed in Rholes et al.'s (2001) study of the transition to parenthood. Attachment-anxious pregnant women who perceived their husbands to be unsupportive 6 weeks before delivery sought less support from them 6 months postpartum. However, when anxious women perceived their husbands to be supportive, their wish for care and protection resulted in a significant increase in support seeking after delivery (compared with less anxious women). There were also differences in postpartum depression, which was most common among anxiously attached women who were dissatisfied with the degree of support provided by their husbands during pregnancy (Simpson & Rholes, 2004).

Actual Support-Seeking Behavior

Attachment style differences have also been noted in observational studies of the actual seeking of support from dating and marital partners. In two studies, Simpson et al. told one member of a dating couple (women in Simpson et al., 1992; men in Simpson et al., 2002) that she or he would undergo a painful laboratory procedure after waiting with a partner for 5 minutes. During this period, participants' behavior was unobtrusively videotaped, and raters later coded the extent to which each participant sought the partner's support. A comparison of results from the two studies revealed an interesting gender difference in the link between attachment style and support seeking. For women, avoidance inhibited support seeking mainly when their level of distress was high. In such cases, avoidant women often attempted to distract themselves by reading magazines instead of asking for support. For men, however, there was no association between attachment and support seeking. Simpson et al. (2002) attributed this lack of association to social norms that inhibit men's seeking of support from women or to men's tendency to perceive the experimental tasks as less threatening.

Based on Ainsworth et al.'s (1978) analyses of secure base interactions between infants and parents, Crowell, Treboux, et al. (2002) coded the support-seeking behaviors of both members of dating couples while they discussed a problem in their relationship. The researchers created a Secure Base Scoring System to assess the extent to which one partner signaled his or her needs to the other in a clear and consistent manner and approached the partner for help or support during the conversation. Men and women who were classified as secure by the AAI more frequently sought support compared with their insecure counterparts.

Two other observational studies provide additional evidence for avoidant and anxious people's different attitudes toward support seeking (Collins & Feeney, 2000; Fraley & Shaver, 1998). Fraley and Shaver unobtrusively coded expressions of desire for proximity and support when romantic or marital partners were about to separate from each other at a metropolitan airport, and Collins and Feeney (2000) coded support-seeking behavior while members of seriously dating couples talked about a personal problem in the laboratory. In both studies, avoidance was associated with less frequent seeking of proximity or support. In addition, although attachment anxiety did not affect direct requests for partner proximity and support, it was associated with indirect methods of support seeking, such as conveying a need for help through nonverbal distress signals (crying, pouting, or sulking).

Overall, research indicates that attachment security fosters support seeking, generally in constructive and effective ways, whereas attachment insecurities inhibit or interfere with effective support seeking. Avoidant individuals react to threats with preconscious activation of the attachment system, but their deactivating strategies inhibit behavioral expressions of need for care or support. Anxious individuals also show strong evidence of preconscious activation of attachment-related thoughts, but for them the associated preconscious activation of worries about rejection and abandonment seems to disorganize their efforts to seek support. These worries, coupled with doubts about others' supportiveness, can sometimes inhibit direct requests for help and channel support-seeking efforts toward nonverbal expressions of helplessness and distress.

Appraisal Patterns and Ways of Coping with Stressful Events

The emotion-regulatory aspects of attachment strategies have been studied with respect to a wide variety of both attachment-related (i.e., social-relational) threats, such as divorce or the transition to parenthood, and attachment-unrelated threats, such as missile attacks and chronic pain (Table 7.2 summarizes the studies). Such events commonly evoke negative emotions and emotion-regulatory efforts. Not surprisingly, attachment strategies are evident in the ways people appraise, cope, and react emotionally to stressful events.

Appraisal Patterns

Attachment orientations are related to people's beliefs and expectations about being able to resist stress or to cope effectively with it. In addition to studies reviewed in Chapter 6, this volume, concerning secure individuals' sense of self-efficacy, research has shown that attachment security is associated with ego-resiliency (Gjerde et al., 2004; Kerns & Stevens, 1996; Klohnen et al., 2005; Kobak & Sceery, 1988) and perceived coping resources (Brack, Gay, & Matheny, 1993; Buelow, Lyddon, & Johnson, 2002; Koopman et al., 2000; Myers & Vetere, 2002). Secure attachment is also associated with more positive expectations regarding the regulation of negative moods (Creasey, 2002b; Creasey, Kershaw, & Boston, 1999; Creasey & Ladd, 2004; Moller, McCarthy, & Fouladi, 2002), greater confidence in one's ability to solve life problems (Wei, Heppner, & Mallinckrodt, 2003), more optimistic and hopeful attitudes toward life (Heinonen, Raikkonen, Keltikangas-Jarvinen, & Strandberg, 2004; Shorey Snyder, Yang, & Lewin, 2003), and hardier, more stress-resistant attitudes (Mayseless, 2004; Neria et al., 2001). In contrast, anxiety and avoidance have been associated with lower levels of ego-resiliency and hardiness, and more pessimistic and hopeless attitudes.

Several studies have shown that attachment style contributes to people's threat appraisals and ability to cope (e.g., Berant, Mikulincer, & Florian, 2001a, 2001b; Birnbaum et al., 1997; Cozzarelli, Sumer, & Major, 1998; Mikulincer & Florian, 1995, 1998; Moller, Fouladi, McCarthy, & Hatch, 2003). The findings are consistent regarding secure and anxious attachment. Attachment security is associated with distress-alleviating appraisals—that is, appraising stressful events in less threatening ways and appraising oneself as being able to cope effectively. In contrast, attachment anxiety is associated with distress-intensifying appraisals—appraising threats as extreme and coping resources as deficient.

For avoidant individuals the findings are less consistent. With regard to the appraisal of one's own coping abilities, most studies have found that avoidant people's appraisals are similar to those of secure people (appraising coping resources as adequate). With regard to threat appraisals, however, most studies have found that avoidant attachment, like attachment anxiety, is associated with appraising stressful events as highly threatening. Such appraisals were noted, for example, when avoidant people confronted undeniable and prolonged stressful events, such as 6 months of intensive combat training (Mikulincer & Florian, 1995), divorce (Birnbaum et al., 1997), or caring for a child with a congenital heart defect (Berant et al., 2001a, 2001b). In addition, Williams and Riskind (2004) found that both attachment anxiety and avoidance were associated with appraising potential threats as rapidly rising in risk and progressively worsening, an appraisal pattern associated with anxiety disorders. Such findings can be cautiously interpreted as implying causality, because Berant et al. (2001b) found, in their prospective longitudinal study, that avoidance predicted increasingly pessimistic appraisals of stressful events over a 1-year period.

Coping Strategies

Some of the studies summarized in Table 7.2 included assessments of participants' use of particular coping strategies (problem solving, emotion-focused coping, distancing cop-

TABLE 7.2. Studies Linking Attachment Orientations with Patterns of Coping with Stressful Events

Study	Attachment scale	Coping scale	Type of stressful event
Mikulincer et al. (1993)	HS types	WOCS	Missile attack
Radecki-Bush et al. (1993)	HS ratings	WOCS	Partner infidelity
Kotler et al. (1994)	HS ratings	WOCS	College transition
J. A. Feeney (1995b)	ASQ	MBS	Recent major stressors
Glachan & Ney (1995)	AAS	Narrative	Infant's distress
Mikulincer & Florian (1995)*	HS types	WOCS	Combat training
Birnbaum et al. (1997)	HS types	WOCS	Divorce
Lopez (1996)	ASQ	GCTS	Recent major stressors
Lussier et al. (1997)	HS ratings	CISS	Relation conflicts
Greenberger & McLaughlin (1998)	HS ratings	COPE	Recent major stressors
J. A. Feeney (1998)	ASQ	Narrative	Separation
Meyers (1998)	HS types	DMI	Recent major stressors
Mikulincer & Florian (1998)	HS types	WOCS	Chronic pain
Mikulincer & Florian (1998)	HS types	WOCS	Parenthood
Mikulincer & Florian (1998)	HS types	WOCS	Caring for a mentally ill adolescent
Ognibene & Collins (1998)	RSQ	WOCS	Recent major stressors
Raskin et al. (1998)	HS types	CSI	Work load
Z. Solomon et al. (1998)	HS types	Narrative	Captivity
Kemp & Neimeyer (1999)	RQ	WOCS	Recent major stressors
Mikulincer & Florian (1999c)	HS types	WOCS	Pregnancy
Shapiro & Levendosky (1999)	AAS	COPE	Relationship conflicts
Torquati & Vazsonyi (1999)	AAS	CAPSI	Relationship conflicts
Harvey & Byrd (2000)	AAS	FCOPES	Family problems
Marshall et al. (2000)	HS ratings	CISS	Recent major stressors
Alexander et al. (2001)	ASQ	WOCS	Parenthood
Berant et al. (2001a)	HS ratings	WOCS	Parenthood
Berant et al. (2001a)	HS ratings	WOCS	Caring for an infant with CHD
Berant et al. (2001b)*	HS ratings	WOCS	Caring for an infant with CHD
J. A. Feeney & Hohaus (2001)	RQ	Narrative	Caregiving-related stress
Horppu & Ikonen-Varila (2001)	RQ	14 items	College exam
Lopez et al. (2001)	ECR	PF-SOC	Recent major stressors
Lopez et al. (2002)	ECR	PF-SOC	Recent major stressors
Lopez & Gormley (2002)*	RQ	PF-SOC	College transition
Schmidt et al. (2002)	AAPR	BCM	Health problems
Williamson et al. (2002)	RQ	WOCS	Caring for a child with chronic pain
Turan et al. (2003)	RSQ	DCM	Diabetes
Wei et al. (2003)	AAS	PF-SOC	Recent major stressors
Howard & Medway (2004)	RSQ	COPE	Recent major stressors
Scharf et al. (2004)*	AAI	WOCS	Combat training
Jerome & Liss (2005)	ECR	COPE	Recent major stressors
Seiffge-Krenke & Beyers (2005)*	AAI	CASQ	Recent major stressors

Note. *, longitudinal design; AAPR, Adult Attachment Prototype Rating; BCM, Bernese Coping Modes; CAPSI, Child and Adolescent Problem-Solving Inventory; CASQ, Coping across Situations Questionnaire; CISS, Coping Inventory for Stressful Situations; CSI, Coping Style Inventory; DCM, Diabetes Coping Measure; DMI, Defense Mechanism Inventory; FCOPES, Family Crises–Oriented Personal Evaluation Scale; GCTS, Global Constructive Thinking Scale; HS, Hazan and Shaver; MBS, Monitor Blunting Scale; PF-SOC, Problem-Focused Styles of Coping; WOCS, Ways of Coping Scale.

ing). Some researchers who assessed problem-focused coping found that secure people are more likely than insecure ones to use this strategy (e.g., Lussier, Sabourin, & Turgeon, 1997; Mikulincer & Florian, 1998; Raskin, Kummel, & Bannister, 1998), but other studies found no significant association between attachment style and problem solving (e.g., Berant et al., 2001a; Mikulincer & Florian, 1995; Mikulincer, Florian, & Weller, 1993). Some of the latter studies focused on stressful events for which people received extensive problem-solving instructions, such as media information about what to do in case of missile attacks, officers' instructions about how to solve problems during combat training, and counselors' instructions about how to care for an infant with a congenital heart defect. This may have caused most study participants, regardless of attachment style, to deal with the stressful events in a problem-focused way.

Several of the studies summarized in Table 7.2 found links between avoidant attachment and reliance on distancing coping strategies, such as stress denial, diversion of attention, and behavioral or cognitive disengagement (e.g., J. A. Feeney, 1998; Lopez, Mauricio, Gormley, Simko, & Berger, 2001; Marshall Serran, & Cortoni, 2000; Shapiro & Levendosky, 1999). Also compatible with theory, avoidance was associated with repression (e.g., Gjerde et al., 2004; Mikulincer & Orbach, 1995; Vetere & Myers, 2002) and behavioral blunting (using distraction to avoid having to confront stressors; J. A. Feeney, 1995b). Turan, Osar, Turan, Ilkova, and Damci (2003) found that diabetics scoring higher on avoidance relied more on cognitive distancing and passive resignation as coping strategies, which in turn were associated with poor adherence to medical regimens.

Relations between attachment style and distancing coping were also examined in two longitudinal studies. In a 31-year study, Klohnen and Bera (1998) found that women with a secure attachment style at age 52 had scored lower on repressive defensiveness at ages 21 and 43 than women who endorsed an avoidant style at age 52. Similarly, Zhang and Labouvie-Vief (2004), in a 6-year longitudinal study of people ranging in age from late adolescence to late adulthood, found that although attachment style was relatively stable over the 6-year period, there was some fluidity associated with variations in coping strategies and mental health. An increase in attachment security over the 6-year period covaried with decreased use of distancing coping and increased use of constructive, flexible, and reality-oriented coping strategies. These findings fit with the theoretical notion that felt security is a resiliency resource that helps people maintain emotional balance without the use of avoidant defenses.

In only one study (Berant et al., 2001a) were secure individuals more likely than their avoidant peers to rely on distancing coping. Secure mothers of both healthy infants and infants with a mild coronary heart defect (CHD) relied on support seeking and problem solving, but secure mothers of infants with a severe CHD tended to rely on distancing strategies. This implies that secure mothers can employ distancing coping when thoughts about the stressful condition might impair effective functioning. Suppression of painful thoughts about their infants' illness might have allowed secure women to maintain a positive appraisal of motherhood. As a result, the overwhelming demands of the infant's illness might not have been so discouraging, allowing the mother to mobilize internal and external resources for taking caring of a vulnerable baby. Consistent with this reasoning, Schmidt, Nachtigall, Wuethrich-Martone, and Strauss (2002) found that attachment security is associated with greater coping flexibility.

Researchers who assessed emotion-focused coping (e.g., wishful thinking, self-blame, rumination) consistently found that it is associated with attachment anxiety (see Table 7.2). With the exception of three studies (Berant et al., 2001b; Kotler, Buzwell, Romeo, &

Bowland, 1994; Scharf, Mayseless, & Kivenson-Baron, 2004), attachment-anxious adults were more likely than secure adults to use emotion-focused coping. They tend to direct their attention toward their own distress rather than focusing on possible solutions to the problem at hand. This distress-focused coping strategy was also noted by Mikulincer and Florian (1998), who assessed worrying and rumination during laboratory failure experiences. Failure evoked more frequent bursts of task-related worries mainly among people who scored high on attachment anxiety.

Interestingly and unexpectedly, some of the studies summarized in Table 7.2 revealed associations between avoidant attachment and emotion-focused coping (e.g., Birnbaum et al., 1997; Lussier et al., 1997; Shapiro & Levendosky, 1999). These findings may help to identify limits on deactivating strategies. For example, Berant et al. (2001a, 2001b) found that avoidant mothers of newborns tended to rely on distancing coping if their infant was born healthy or with only a mild CHD, but they used emotion-focused coping if their infant was diagnosed with a life-threatening CHD, and they showed a notable increase in the use of this coping strategy a year after the diagnosis. Thus, avoidant defenses, which may be sufficient for dealing with minor stressors, may fail when people encounter severe and persistent stressors. This conclusion is consistent with Bowlby's (1980) idea that avoidant people's segregated mental systems cannot be hidden from conscious awareness indefinitely, and that traumatic events can resurrect distress that had been sealed off from consciousness.

Overall, the research summarized in Table 7.2 supports hypothesized links between attachment styles and coping strategies. Attachment security is associated with problem solving (and distancing, when a problem cannot be solved), anxious attachment is associated mainly with emotion-focused coping strategies, and avoidant attachment is associated with distancing strategies (and emotion-focused strategies, when stressors are severe and persistent).

Emotional Reactions to Stressful Events

In addition to examining attachment-related coping strategies, several of the studies summarized in Table 7.2 included participants' reports of psychological distress, negative affectivity (anxiety, depression, anger), and psychological well-being during stressful events. Attachment security was associated with lower levels of distress and higher levels of psychological well-being, whereas attachment insecurities—anxiety, avoidance, or both—were associated with heightened distress and deteriorated well-being (e.g., Birnbaum et al., 1997; Mikulincer & Florian, 1998, 1999c; Mikulincer et al., 1993); that is, even avoidance was associated with negative emotional reactions to stressful events. In fact, Berant et al. (2001b) and Berant, Mikulincer, and Shaver (in press) found that avoidant attachment among mothers of infants with severe forms of CHD (measured immediately following the CHD diagnosis) was a stronger predictor of deteriorated mental health than attachment anxiety 1 and 7 years later. Under chronic, demanding, stressful conditions, such as caring for a child with a life-threatening illness, deactivating strategies seem to collapse, causing avoidant people to have even higher levels of distress than anxious people. This is reminiscent of laboratory studies showing that avoidant defenses collapse under a cognitive load (Mikulincer et al., 2004).

Avoidant people's heightened stress reactivity has also been noticed in studies examining physiological reactions to stressors. Two studies found that avoidant people had high levels of physiological arousal (heightened electrodermal activity) when coping with painful childhood memories aroused by the AAI (Dozier & Kobak, 1992; Roisman, Tsai,

& Chiang, 2004). In three recent experiments (L. M. Diamond, Hicks, & Otter-Henderson, 2006; Kim, 2006; Maunder, Lancee, Nolan, Hunter, & Tannenbaum, 2006), people were exposed to various laboratory stressors (e.g., recalling a stressful situation, performing demanding math tasks, watching a film clip depicting relationship distress, discussing relationship problems with a dating partner). Avoidant attachment (measured with self-report scales) was associated with heightened physiological reactivity: decreased heart rate variability (Maunder et al., 2006), increased skin conductance (Diamond et al., 2006), and heightened diastolic blood pressure (Kim, 2006). In addition, Kim found that avoidance was associated with a decrease in rate pressure product (pulse rate multiplied by systolic blood pressure) during a couple discussion (compared to baseline), indicating an inability to supply oxygen to cardiac muscles while coping with stress. According to Kim, "These findings suggest that individuals scoring high on the avoidance attachment dimension are vulnerable to hypertension and other cardiovascular diseases due to such dysfunctional physiological patterns, particularly when they face relationship conflicts" (p. 111).

Interestingly, Maunder et al. (2006) found that attachment-*anxious* people's responsiveness to stressors was manifested in higher levels of reported distress, but not in heart rate measures, again suggesting that anxious people exaggerate their distress. In Kim's (2006) study, anxious participants' physiological reactivity (heightened diastolic blood pressure) was observed only when they also reported high levels of distress. This tendency contrasts with avoidant individuals' dissociation between subjective reports of lack of distress and heightened physiological reactivity. (Later we review findings related to this psychobiological dissociation.)

Some of the studies summarized in Table 7.2 compared the emotional reactions of people undergoing stressful experiences with those of controls, thereby revealing an additional benefit of attachment security (e.g., Berant et al., 2001a; Birnbaum et al., 1997; Z. Solomon et al., 1998; Mikulincer & Florian, 1998). Stressful events arouse negative emotions mainly among insecurely attached people. For secure people, there is often no notable difference in emotion between neutral and stressful conditions. Similar findings were obtained by researchers (Amir, Horesh, & Lin-Stein, 1999; Mikulincer et al., 1993) who studied the association between psychological distress and objective characteristics of stressors (e.g., physical distance from the areas in Israel hit by Iraqi Scud missiles, severity of infertility problems). Insecure people were measurably affected by objective characteristics of stressors, but secure people seemed to be relatively calm even under stressful conditions, another indication that felt security is an effective stress buffer.

Overall, data support the hypothesis that secure people's optimistic appraisals and reliance on constructive ways of coping mitigate distress and maintain mental health during periods of stress. They also indicate that anxious or avoidant attachment can interfere with effective coping and increase the intensity of distress. In the long run, this means that attachment insecurities increase the risk for developing serious emotional problems, as shown in Chapter 13, this volume.

Management of Attachment-Related Threats

Attachment strategies are also evident in the way people deal with separation from a close relationship partner or the death of a spouse. As we explained in Chapter 3, these attachment-related threats, which were among Bowlby's (1980) major concerns, are potent triggers of negative emotions and attachment strategies aimed at regulating emotions.

Reactions to Actual Separations and Relationship Breakups

Two of the studies summarized in Table 7.2 examined attachment-related differences in coping with divorce (Birnbaum et al., 1997) and temporary separations from a dating partner (J. A. Feeney, 1998). Attachment-anxious individuals were more likely to rely on emotion-focused coping strategies, and avoidant individuals, on distancing strategies. Similar coping strategies were noted by D. Davis, Shaver, and Vernon (2003) in a survey of more that 5,000 Internet respondents who described romantic relationship breakups. Avoidant respondents were less likely to seek support and more likely to cope with the breakup alone, while avoiding new romantic involvements. Anxious respondents reacted with angry protests, heightened sexual attraction to the former partner, intense preoccupation with the lost partner, a lost sense of identity, and interference with school and work activities. These reactions are compatible with our idea that anxiously attached people attempt to reestablish proximity to a lost partner and overemphasize the importance of the lost partner as an element of the self. Both anxious and avoidant individuals used alcohol and drugs as a means of coping with separation, which is not generally an effective coping strategy.

Several studies have demonstrated theoretically predicted attachment-related differences in the intensity and duration of distress following a romantic relationship breakup (D. Davis et al., 2003; J. A. Feeney & Noller, 1992; Moller et al., 2002, 2003; Pistole, 1995b; Sbarra, 2006; Sbarra & Emery, 2005; Simpson, 1990; Sprecher, Felmlee, Metta, Fehr, & Vanni, 1998), divorce (Birnbaum et al., 1997), wartime separations from marital partners (Cafferty et al., 1994; Medway et al., 1995), temporary separations from romantic partners (J. A. Feeney, 1998; Fraley & Shaver, 1998), and parasocial separation from favorite television characters (J. Cohen, 2004). In all of these studies, distress intensification was a common response of anxiously attached people. In contrast, attachment security was associated with faster emotional recovery and adjustment. For example, Sbarra (2006), who collected daily emotion data for 4 weeks from young adults who had recently experienced a romantic relationship breakup, found that attachment security was associated with faster recovery from sadness and anger, an association mediated by acceptance of the separation; that is, relatively secure people were more likely to accept the loss, which facilitated recovery.

For avoidant individuals, the findings depended on the nature of the separation. Avoidance was associated with higher levels of distress following divorce and wartime separations but lower levels of distress and greater relief following temporary separations from, or permanent breakups with, dating partners. We therefore conclude that avoidant people, who can handle the distress of brief separations or the dissolution of casual bonds, are less successful in dealing with major separations requiring reorganization of relational routines, goals, and plans. This fits with other data, including evidence from experiments (e.g., Mikulincer et al., 2004), that avoidant defenses collapse under pressure.

Reactions to Separation-Related Thoughts

Studies that induced thoughts about hypothetical or actual separations also provide important information about attachment-related differences in emotion regulation. Two studies examined associations between responses to imagined separations in the projective Separation Anxiety Test and either self-reports of romantic attachment (Mayseless, Danieli, & Sharabany, 1996) or AAI state of mind with respect to attachment to parents

(Scharf, 2001). Both studies indicated that secure people cope more effectively with both mild and severe separations, and benefit from a balance between self-reliance and reliance on others for support. Mayseless et al. (1996) also found that whereas avoidant people refrained from dealing with the threat, anxious people reacted to separation with strong self-blame and intense distress. Similarly, B. Meyer, Olivier, and Roth (2005) asked young women to imagine that their romantic partner planned to spend time with a highly attractive woman, and found that avoidant attachment was associated with distancing responses, such as ending the relationship or avoiding contact with the partner. Attachment anxiety was associated with more intense distress and more attempts to persuade the partner to change his mind.

In a series of three studies, Mikulincer, Florian, Birnbaum, and Malishkevich (2002) examined another reaction to separation. Participants were asked to imagine being separated from a loved partner, then to perform a word completion task that measured the accessibility of death-related thoughts (see Chapter 3, this volume). Participants who scored higher on attachment anxiety reacted to separation reminders with more death-related thoughts. This tendency was particularly strong when the imagined separation was long-lasting or final. In other words, for anxious individuals, separation evoked thoughts of death, which might partially explain why attachment-anxious people tend to experience intense distress and despair following separation.

This mental equation of separation and death was also noted by Hart et al. (2005), who examined defensive reactions to separation and reminders of death. Undergraduates were asked to think about their own death, separation from a close relationship partner, or a control theme, then to report their attitudes toward the writer of a pro-American essay. People who scored relatively high on attachment anxiety or avoidance rated the pro-American writer more favorably in the death reminders than in the control condition—the typical defensive reaction to mortality salience (discussed later in this chapter). However, anxious individuals, but not avoidant ones, also reacted more favorably to the pro-American writer in the separation condition. In other words, anxious people showed the same defensive reaction to reminders of death and separation.

For avoidant people, the main method of dealing with separation-related thoughts is to suppress them. In a pair of experimental studies, Fraley and Shaver (1997) used Wegner's (1994) thought suppression paradigm and obtained evidence of avoidant suppression. Participants wrote about whatever thoughts and feelings they experienced while being asked to suppress thoughts about a romantic partner leaving them for someone else. In the first study, the ability to suppress these thoughts was assessed by the number of times the thoughts appeared in participants' stream of consciousness following the suppression period. In the second study, this ability was assessed by the level of physiological arousal (skin conductance) during the suppression task: The lower the arousal, the greater the presumed ability to suppress the troubling thoughts.

The findings fit with what we have been saying about attachment-related emotion regulation strategies. Anxious people were less able to suppress separation-related thoughts, as indicated by more frequent thoughts of loss following the suppression task and higher skin conductance during the task. In contrast, avoidant people were able to suppress separation-related thoughts, as indicated by less frequent thoughts of loss following the suppression task and lower skin conductance during the task. A recent fMRI study (Gillath, Bunge, Shaver, Wendelken, & Mikulincer, 2005) went further and documented attachment-related differences in patterns of brain activation when people were thinking about breakups and losses or attempting to suppress such thoughts.

Mikulincer et al. (2004) replicated and extended Fraley and Shaver's (1997) findings while assessing, in a Stroop color-naming task, the cognitive activation of previously suppressed thoughts about a painful separation. Avoidant individuals were able to suppress thoughts related to the breakup; for them, such thoughts were relatively inaccessible, and their own positive self-traits became even more accessible than usual (presumably for defensive reasons). However, their ability to maintain this defensive stance was disrupted when a cognitive load—remembering a 7-digit number—was added to the experimental task. Under high cognitive load, avoidant individuals suddenly evinced high availability of thoughts of separation and *negative* self-traits; that is, the suppressed material resurfaced in experience and behavior when a high cognitive demand was imposed. We suspect that a similar resurfacing occurs when a high emotional demand is imposed, as in the studies we mentioned earlier that dealt with the strain of caring for a child with a congenital heart defect (Berant et al., 2001a, 2001b, in press).

While probing further into the regulatory mechanisms underlying avoidant defenses, Fraley, Gardner, and Shaver (2000) asked whether they function in a *preemptive* manner (e.g., by directing attention away from, or encoding in a shallow way, attachment-related information) or in a *postemptive manner*(repressing material that has already been encoded). Participants listened to an interview about the loss of a close relationship partner and were asked later to recall details of the interview, either soon after hearing them (Study 1) or after various delays ranging from half an hour to 21 days (Study 2). An analysis of forgetting curves revealed that (1) avoidant people initially encoded less information about the interview, and (2) people with different attachment styles forgot encoded information at the same rate. Thus, avoidant defenses sometimes act preemptively by blocking threatening material from awareness before it is encoded.

This implies that avoidant people should be vigilant to attachment-related information so that they can block its encoding. M. A. Maier et al.'s (2005) experimental study of perceptual thresholds to social and nonsocial pictures provided support for this idea. Participants were exposed to a series of pictures for 15 milliseconds each, and exposure time was gradually increased, until a participant could accurately describe the content of the picture. Avoidance (assessed with the AAI) was associated with lower identification thresholds (less exposure time needed to identify a picture) for pictures depicting affect-laden human faces and social interactions. This association was not significant for pictures of neutral faces, natural scenes, or inanimate objects. Thus, avoidant defenses seem to demand perceptual vigilance to emotional and social stimuli to keep them from being processed further. We suspect that this is the default avoidant defense. Postemptive strategies (e.g., thought suppression) are called upon only if the preemptive approach fails or the defenses are attacked from behind (or from underneath), so to speak (e.g., when a threatening memory is aroused by association).

Reactions to the Death of a Close Relationship Partner

As we explained in Chapter 3, Bowlby (1980) drew a distinction between two atypical forms of mourning—chronic mourning and prolonged absence of conscious grieving—and associated each of these reactions with a different kind of insecure attachment. Anxiously attached people's tendency to intensify distress and ruminate about losses encourages chronic mourning, whereas avoidant people's tendency to suppress negative emotions encourages an absence of conscious grieving (Fraley & Shaver, 1999; Mikulincer & Shaver, in press). In addition, anxious individuals' overdependence on relationship partners can lead to a larger than usual emotional investment in the deceased partner and the lost relationship. In contrast, avoidant individuals' lower commitment to partners and extreme self-reliance may make them less vulnerable to prolonged grieving: They are less likely to feel that something crucial has been lost, and their senses of identity and well-being are less likely to be jeopardized by the loss (Fraley & Shaver, 1999).

Secure attachment allows a person to steer clear of both insecure forms of mourning (Mikulincer & Shaver, in press). Securely attached people can recall and think about a lost partner without extreme difficulty, and can discuss the loss coherently in the same way they are able in the AAI to discuss memories of their childhood relationships with parents (Hesse, 1999; Shaver & Tancredy, 2001). Moreover, their constructive coping strategies allow them to experience and express grief, anger, and distress without feeling overwhelmed by emotion, and without total disruption of normal functioning (Parkes, 2001; M. Stroebe et al., 2005). In addition, their positive models of self and others facilitate flexible, balanced alternations between continuing attachment and gradual detachment from the deceased partner (Shaver & Tancredy, 2001). Secure individuals' positive models of a lost partner allow them to continue to think positively about the deceased, whereas their positive models of self allow them to cope with the loss and begin to form new relationships (Mikulincer & Shaver, in press).

Few studies have directly examined the attachment–bereavement association, but their findings generally support the idea that secure attachment facilitates emotional adjustment during bereavement. For example, Van Doorn et al. (1998) interviewed adults while they were caring for their terminally ill spouses and found that global attachment security in romantic relationships and specific attachment security in the marriage were both associated with less intense grief reactions to the critical illness of their spouse. Similarly, Fraley and Bonanno (2004) found that people classified as securely attached 4 months after the loss of a spouse reported relatively low levels of bereavement-related anxiety, grief, depression, and posttraumatic distress 4 and 18 months after the loss. Conceptually similar findings were reported by Wayment and Vierthaler (2002) and Waskowic and Chartier (2003).

There is also evidence of anxiously attached people's intensification of grief reactions (Field & Sundin, 2001; Fraley & Bonanno, 2004; Wayment & Vierthaler, 2002). For example, Field and Sundin (2001) found that anxious attachment, assessed 10 months after the death of a spouse, predicted higher levels of psychological distress 14, 25, and 60 months after the loss. In an unpublished study, Parkes (2003) collected retrospective accounts of attachment patterns in childhood in a sample of 181 individuals referred for psychiatric help with bereavement complications and found that attachment anxiety was associated with having had a conflicted and clinging relationship with the lost partner and higher levels of protracted grief.

With regard to avoidance, studies have generally found no significant association between this attachment dimension and depression, grief, or distress (Field & Sundin, 2001; Fraley & Bonanno, 2004; Wayment & Vierthaler, 2002). However, Wayment and Vierthaler found that avoidance was associated with higher levels of somatic symptoms, implying that avoidant defenses might block conscious access to anxiety and depression, but without preventing the subtler and less conscious somatic reactions to loss (see findings reviewed earlier in this chapter concerning avoidant people's heightened physiological reactivity to stress, and Chapter 13, this volume, for evidence of similar reactions to other kinds of trauma). Parkes (2003) found that avoidant attachment was associated with more severe problems in expressing affection and grief during bereavement. Both Fraley and Bonanno (2004) and Parkes (2003) found that combinations of avoidance and attachment anxiety (the pattern Bartholomew & Horowitz [1991] called "fearful avoidance," which in Chapter 2 we speculatively linked with disorganized or unresolved attachment) produced the most severe mourning complications (the highest levels of anxiety, depression, grief, trauma-related symptoms, and alcohol consumption).

There is also some evidence concerning individual differences in continuing attachment to and detachment from a lost partner. Field and Sundin (2001) found, for example, that people who scored higher on avoidance reported more negative thoughts about their lost spouse 14 months after the loss, perhaps reflecting a distancing, derogating attitude toward the deceased. In contrast, attachment anxiety was associated with more positive thoughts about the lost spouse, probably reflecting a continuing emotional investment in an idealized figure. This kind of idealization was also evident in Nager and De Vries's (2004) content analysis of memorial websites created by adult daughters for their deceased mothers. Comments about missing the deceased and idealized descriptions of mothers (e.g., "You were the most beautiful, strongest, determined, smartest, fascinating woman in the world") were more frequently found on websites created by anxiously attached daughters than by secure or avoidant daughters. Using the Continuing Bonds Scale, Waskowic and Chartier (2003) found that secure people maintained an adaptive, flexible attitude toward a lost partner. Although they scored lower than insecure people on rumination about and preoccupation with a lost spouse, they still scored higher on positive reminiscences and symbolic exchanges with the spouse.

Experiencing and Managing Death Anxiety

Adult attachment studies have also explored whether attachment styles are associated with the experience and management of particular emotional states. For example, a number of studies conducted in Mikulincer's laboratory have focused on attachment style differences in the strength of death anxiety, assessed in terms of overt fear of death (Florian & Mikulincer, 1998; Mikulincer et al., 1990), unconscious expressions of this fear (responses to projective TAT cards; Mikulincer et al., 1990), or the accessibility of death-related thoughts (the number of death-related words produced in a word completion task; Mikulincer & Florian, 2000; Mikulincer, Florian, Birnbaum, et al., 2002).

Anxious individuals intensify death concerns and keep death-related thoughts active in working memory; that is, attachment anxiety is associated with heightened fear of death at both conscious and unconscious levels, as well as heightened accessibility of death-related thoughts, even when no death reminder is present. Avoidant individuals suppress death concerns and exhibit dissociation between their conscious claims and unconscious dynamics. Avoidance is related to both low levels of self-reported fear of death and heightened death-related anxiety assessed with a projective measure.

Attachment style differences have also been found in people's construal of death anxiety (Florian & Mikulincer, 1998; Mikulincer et al., 1990). Anxiously attached people tend to attribute this fear to the loss of social identity after death (e.g., "People will forget me"), whereas avoidant people tend to attribute it to the unknown nature of the hereafter (e.g., uncertainty about what to expect). These findings are compatible with secondary attachment strategies. Anxious people hyperactivate worries about rejection and abandonment, viewing death as yet another relational setting in which they can be abandoned or forgotten. Avoidant people work to sustain self-reliance and strong personal control, which leads to fear of the uncertain and unknown aspects of death—threats to perceived control.

A related line of research examined attachment style differences in the way people manage anxiety aroused by death reminders. According to terror management theory (J. Greenberg et al., 1997), human beings' knowledge that they are destined to die, coexisting with strong wishes to perceive themselves as special, important, and immortal, makes it necessary for them to engage in self-promotion, to defend their cultural worldviews, and to deny their animal nature. Many studies have shown that experimentally induced death reminders lead to more negative reactions to the human body, to moral (i.e., worldview) transgressors, and to members of outgroups (see J. Greenberg et al., 1997, for a review).

Although worldview validation has been assumed to be a normative defense against universal existential threats (J. Greenberg et al., 1997), Mikulincer and colleagues (Caspi-Berkowitz, 2003; Mikulincer & Florian, 2000) found that this response is more characteristic of insecure than of secure people. For example, experimentally induced death reminders produced more severe judgments and punishments of moral transgressors, and greater willingness to die for a cause only among insecurely attached people, either anxious or avoidant (Caspi-Berkowitz, 2003; Mikulincer & Florian, 2000). Securely attached people were not affected by death reminders, did not recommend harsher punishments for transgressors following a mortality salience induction, and were generally averse to endangering people's lives to protect cultural values.

Some of the studies reveal ways in which securely attached adults react to death reminders. Mikulincer and Florian (2000) found that secure people react to mortality salience with an increased sense of symbolic immortality—a constructive, transformational strategy that, while not solving the unsolvable problem of death, leads people to invest in their children's care and to engage in creative, growth-oriented activities whose products live on after death. Secure people also react to mortality salience with heightened attachment needs—a more intense desire for intimacy in close relationships (Mikulincer & Florian, 2000) and greater willingness to engage in social interactions (Taubman Ben-Ari, Findler, & Mikulincer, 2002). Caspi-Berkowitz (2003) also found that secure people reacted to death reminders by strengthening their desire to care for others. In her study, people read hypothetical scenarios in which a relationship partner (e.g., spouse) was in danger of death; participants were then asked about their willingness to endanger their own lives to save their partners' lives. Securely attached people reacted to death reminders with heightened willingness to sacrifice themselves. Insecure people were generally averse to self-sacrifice and reacted to death reminders with less willingness to save others' lives. It is notable that insecure individuals, who seem more ready than secure ones to die for their self-enhancing cultural worldviews, are more reluctant to sacrifice themselves for a particular other person. (See our related discussion of attachment and altruism in Chapter 11, this volume.)

These studies imply that even when faced with their biological finitude, securely attached people maintain felt security. They pursue the primary attachment strategy (seeking proximity to others) even when coping with the threat of death; they heighten their sense of social connectedness and symbolically transform the threat of death into an opportunity to contribute to others and to grow personally. This makes it seem that being part of a loving, accepting human world—having strong emotional and caring bonds with others—is a pathway to self-transcendence (being part of a larger entity that transcends one's biological self). It promotes a sense of symbolic immortality, making it less necessary to validate one's worldview and promote oneself and one's own group. This suggests to us that fostering attachment security might contribute to world peace, whereas making people feel insecure, either dispositionally (in families) or contextually (in political speeches), may contribute to perpetual conflict and premature death. (See Chapter 16, this volume, for further thoughts on this important matter.)

Defensive, distorting reactions to mortality seem to result from recurrent failures of attachment figures to accomplish their protective, supportive, anxiety-buffering functions. As a result, insecure people lack a sense of continuity with and connection to the world, and are unable to rely on a solid psychological foundation that sustains vitality even in the face of mortality. Instead, they cling to particular cultural worldviews and derogate alternative views in an attempt to enhance their impoverished self-concepts and achieve a stronger sense of value and meaning. For avoidant individuals, these strategies seem to be effective in buffering existential fears at a conscious level. However, they are ineffective in decreasing the unconscious fear of death, and they leave avoidant individuals bothered by the uncertainty and uncontrollability of death. For anxiously attached individuals, adherence to cultural worldviews is ineffective in buffering death anxiety, perhaps because it is not an adequate antidote to hyperactivated fears, ruminations, and needs for protection, support, and love.

Experiencing and Managing Anger

Adult attachment researchers have also studied the experience and management of anger. In Bowlby's (1973) analysis of emotional reactions to separation, he viewed anger as a functional response to separation from an attachment figure, if it succeeded in gaining an unreliable figure's attention or caused him or her to become more reliably available. Anger is functional to the degree that it is not intended to hurt or destroy the attachment figure but only to discourage his or her frustrating or frightening behavior and to reestablish a warm and satisfying relationship. However, Bowlby (1973, 1988) also noted that anger can become so intense that it alienates the partner or becomes vengeful rather than corrective. In particular, Bowlby (1988) discussed how some cases of family violence can be understood as exaggerated forms of otherwise functional behavior. For example, he characterized certain coercive behaviors within close relationships (including battering) as strategies for controlling the other and keeping him or her from departing. He realized, of course, that although violent and uncontrollable anger might have evolutionarily functional roots (i.e., be "designed" to discourage a partner's frightening or frustrating behavior), it is dysfunctional when extreme and has the potential to destroy the partner and the relationship that one fears losing.

Bowlby's analysis of the complex, multifaceted nature of anger is consistent with other theoretical perspectives on this emotion, which note that it can be motivated by either constructive or destructive goals, be expressed in functional or dysfunctional ways, result in positive or negative relational behaviors, elicit positive or negative responses from a relationship partner, and have positive or negative effects on a relationship (e.g., Averill, 1982; Tangney et al., 1996). Functional forms of anger are motivated by constructive goals (e.g., maintaining a relationship, bringing about a beneficial change in a partner's behavior), are typically expressed in the form of focused complaints and problem-solving discussions, and do not entail animosity, hostility, or hatred. In contrast, dysfunctional forms of anger include resentment toward one's partner, deliberately injuring the partner emotionally or physically, and seeking revenge, which can easily result in lasting "attachment injuries" (S. M. Johnson, Makinen, & Millikin, 2001) and weaken emotional bonds (Tangney et al., 1996).

Attachment Security and Anger

Functional experiences and expressions of anger are typical of secure individuals. For example, Mikulincer (1998b) found that when confronted with anger-eliciting events, secure people held optimistic expectations about their partners' subsequent behavior (e.g., "He or she will accept me") and made well-differentiated, reality-attuned appraisals of their partners' intentions. Only when there were clear indications, provided by the experimenter, that a partner actually had acted with hostile intent did a secure person attribute hostility to the partner and react with anger. Moreover, secure people's accounts of anger-eliciting events were characterized by the constructive goals of repairing the relationship, engaging in adaptive problem solving, and experiencing positive affect following the temporary period of discord. Barrett and Holmes (2001) also found that greater security in one's relationships with parents or romantic partners is associated with more constructive, prosocial, and less aggressive responses to hypothetical anger-eliciting provocations, and Meesters and Muris (2002) found inverse associations between attachment security and self-reports of aggression and hostility.

The constructive nature of secure people's anger was also demonstrated in a recent study by Zimmermann, Maier, Winter, and Grossmann (2001). Adolescents performed a difficult, frustrating cognitive task with the help of a friend, and the researchers assessed disappointment and anger during the task, as well as negative behaviors toward the friend (e.g., rejecting the friend's suggestions without discussion). Disappointment and anger were associated with more frequent disruptive behavior only among insecure adolescents (identified with the AAI). Among those classified as secure on the AAI, these emotions were associated with less rather than more disruptive behavior. Therefore, secure people's anger seemed to be well regulated and channeled in useful directions.

Avoidant Attachment and Anger

Theoretically, avoidant individuals' attempts to sidestep negative emotions should cause them to suppress anger, but the anger might still be expressed in unconscious or unintended ways, or take the form of otherwise unexplained hostility or hatred for a partner (which Mikulincer [1998b] labeled "dissociated anger"). In support of this view, Mikulincer found that avoidant individuals did not *report* intense anger in response to another person's negative behavior, but they nevertheless displayed intense physiological arousal. They also reported using distancing strategies to cope with anger-eliciting events and attributed hostility to partners even when there were clear indications (provided by the experimenter) of partners' nonhostile intent. Similarly, Hudson and Ward (1997) reported an association between avoidance and self-reports of anger suppression in a sample of violent incarcerated men (whose violence suggested that they were actually quite angry).

There is also evidence that avoidant people are more hostile and aggressive than secure ones (e.g., Calamari & Pini, 2003; Magai, Hunziker, Mesias, & Culver, 2000; Mikulincer, 1998b; Troisi & D'Argenio, 2004; Zimmermann, 2004), and are perceived by their friends to be hostile (Kerns & Stevens, 1996; Kobak & Sceery, 1988). These dysfunctional responses are evident both behaviorally and cognitively. Kobak et al. (1993) found that avoidant teens (identified with the AAI) displayed more dysfunctional anger than secure teens toward their mothers and engaged in less cooperative dialogue during a problem-solving interaction. Kirsh (1996) found that avoidant individuals had better memory than secure ones for figural depictions of anger.

The dysfunctional nature of avoidant individuals' anger has also been documented in a study of support seeking (Rholes et al., 1999). Women were told they would engage in an anxiety-provoking task and were asked to wait for 5 minutes with their dating partner before it began. Women's avoidance (assessed with the AAQ) was associated with more intense (and observable) anger toward their partner during the 5-minute waiting period, and this was especially so when the women were more distressed and received less support from their partners. It therefore seems that avoidant women's lack of confidence in their partners' support might have caused them to become angry when they were seeking support.

Anxious Attachment and Anger

Anxiously attached individuals' intensification of negative emotions and rumination on threats and slights may fuel intense and prolonged bouts of anger. However, their fear of separation and desperate desire for others' love may hold their resentment and anger in check, and redirect it toward themselves. As a result, anxious people's anger can include a complex mixture of resentment, hostility, self-criticism, fear, sadness, and depression.

Mikulincer (1998b) provided evidence for this characterization of anxiously attached people's anger. Their recollections of anger-provoking experiences included an uncontrollable flood of angry feelings, persistent rumination on these feelings, and sadness and despair following conflicts. Mikulincer also found that anxious people held more negative expectations about others' responses during anger episodes and tended to make more undifferentiated, negatively biased appraisals of relationship partners' intentions. They attributed hostility to their partner and reacted in kind, even when there were only ambiguous cues concerning hostile intent. There is also evidence, cited earlier, that attachment anxiety is associated with anger, aggression, and hostility (e.g., Buunk, 1997; Calamari & Pini, 2003; Dutton, Saunders, Starzomski, & Bartholomew, 1994; Magai et al., 2000; Mikulincer, 1998b; Troisi & D'Argenio, 2004; Zimmermann, 2004). Using an uncommon method, Woike et al. (1996) found that attachment anxiety is associated with writing more violent projective stories in response to TAT pictures. Attachment anxiety is also associated with relationship violence, as explained and documented in Chapter 10, this volume.

The dysfunctional nature of anxious people's anger has been observed in dyadic interactions. Simpson et al. (1996) found that attachment anxiety is associated with displaying and reporting more anger and hostility while discussing an unresolved problem with a dating partner. And in a previously mentioned study of support seeking, although Rholes et al. (1999) found no association between attachment anxiety and anger toward a male dating partner while women waited to undertake an anxiety-provoking task, after they were told they would not really have to perform the task, their attachment anxiety was associated with anger toward their partners. This was particularly true for women who had been more upset during the waiting period and had sought more support from their partners. Thus, it seems that anxious women's strong need for reassurance counteracted, or encouraged suppression of, anger expressions during support seeking, but their anger surfaced when support was no longer necessary.

Anxious people's problems in managing anger have also been studied with physiological measures. L. M. Diamond and Hicks (2005) exposed young men to two anger-provoking experimental inductions (performance of serial subtraction accompanied by discouraging feedback from the experimenter; recollection of a recent anger-eliciting event) and measured reports of anxiety and anger during and after the inductions. They also recorded participants' vagal tone (indexed by resting levels of respiration-related variability in heart rate), a common index of parasympathetic down-regulation of negative emotion, and found that attachment anxiety was associated with lower vagal tone—a sign that the parasympathetic nervous system responded less quickly and flexibly to the stressful tasks and that attachment-anxious individuals recovered poorly from frustration and anger. In addition, attachment anxiety was associated with self-reported distress and anger during and after the tasks, and vagal tone mediated the association between attachment anxiety and heightened anger.

Cognitive Access and the Architecture of Emotional Experiences

Theoretically, attachment strategies should influence the access a person has to emotion-related information and the way he or she encodes and organizes this information in an associative memory network (Mikulincer & Shaver, 2003). In an experimental study of emotional memories, Mikulincer and Orbach (1995) obtained support for this expectation. Participants were asked to recall early childhood experiences of anger, sadness, anxiety, or happiness, and their memory retrieval latencies were recorded as indicators of cognitive accessibility or inaccessibility. Participants also rated the intensity of focal and nonfocal emotions in each recalled event. In the memory task, avoidant people exhibited the poorest access (longest recall latencies) to sad and anxious memories; anxious people had the quickest access to such memories, and secure people fell in between. Moreover, whereas secure individuals took more time to retrieve negative than positive emotional memories, anxious ones took longer to retrieve positive than negative memories. In the emotion-rating task, avoidant individuals rated focal emotions (e.g., sadness when instructed to retrieve a sad memory) and nonfocal emotions (e.g., anger when instructed to retrieve a sad memory) as less intense than did secure individuals, whereas anxious individuals reported experiencing very intense focal *and* nonfocal emotions when asked to remember instances of anxiety, sadness, and anger. In contrast, secure people rated focal emotions as much more intense than nonfocal emotions.

The findings provide additional support for the idea that securely attached people rely on constructive and generally effective emotion regulation strategies. They acknowledge distress, retain access to negative memories, and process these experiences fully. However, they also have better access to positive memories and tend not to suffer from a spread of activation from one negative memory to another. Van Emmichoven, van IJzendoorn, de Ruiter, and Brosschot (2003) noted secure people's open attitude toward distress-eliciting information even in a sample of patients with anxiety disorders. Secure participants (assessed with the AAI), as compared with insecure (mostly avoidant) ones, showed a larger Stroop interference effect for threatening words (longer RTs for naming the color in which threatening words were printed) and better recall of threatening words in a free recall task. Both results indicate secure people's easy access to threat-related thoughts, which other studies suggest can occur without causing an overload of negative emotion.

Mikulincer and Orbach's (1995) findings also provide insight into avoidant emotion regulation strategies. Avoidant people displayed reduced access to negative emotional memories, and the ones they recalled were fairly shallow. This unavailability of negative memories was also documented in Edelstein et al.'s (2005) study of long-term memories for child sexual abuse (CSA). In a sample of 102 documented CSA victims whose cases were referred for prosecution, self-reports of avoidant attachment were negatively associated with memory accuracy for specific, well documented, severe CSA incidents that had occurred approximately 14 years earlier. Interestingly, these memory problems were reduced among people who reported relatively high levels of maternal support after the abuse, highlighting the buffering effect of security-enhancing interactions with supportive attachment figures.

In Mikulincer and Orbach's (1995) study, attachment anxiety was associated with ready access to negative emotional memories and impaired control of the spread of activation from one negative memory to others. These findings fit with the theoretical portrayal of anxious people as having an undifferentiated, chaotic emotional architecture, which makes emergence from negative emotional spirals difficult. They also fit with Roisman et al.'s (2004) findings about people's facial expressions during the AAI. Whereas securely attached individuals' facial expressions were highly congruent with the valence of the childhood events they were describing, anxiously attached individuals showed marked discrepancies between the quality of the childhood experiences they described and their facial expressions (e.g., facial expressions of sadness or anger when speaking about neutral or positive childhood experiences). According to Roisman et al., these discrepancies reflect anxious individuals' confusion and emotional dysregulation when being asked to talk about emotionally charged experiences.

Pereg and Mikulincer's (2004) studies of the cognitive effects of induced negative mood provide further evidence of anxious people's lack of control of the spread of activation among negative emotional memories and of avoidant people's lack of access to negative emotion and emotional memories. In two studies, participants were assigned to a negative mood condition (reading an article about a car accident) or to a control condition (reading about a hobby kit), after which incidental recall or causal attributions were assessed. In Study 1, participants read a booklet with positive and negative headlines, then, without warning, were asked to recall as many of the headlines as possible. In Study 2, participants were asked to list the causes of a hypothetical negative relationship event ("Your partner disclosed something you asked him to keep secret").

The induction of a negative mood, as compared with a control condition, led secure participants to recall more positive headlines and fewer negative headlines, and to attribute a negative event to less global and stables causes. This is a mood-incongruent pattern of cognition (Forgas, 1995), which is likely to inhibit the spread of negative affect and to activate competing positive cognitions (positive headlines, attributions that maintain a positive view of the partner). As a result, secure people are able to work against the pervasive effects of negative affect and maintain or restore emotional equanimity. In contrast, more attachment-anxious participants react to the induced negative mood with heightened recall of negative headlines and an increased tendency to attribute a negative event to more global and stables causes. This is a mood-congruent pattern of cognition (Forgas, 1995), which favors the spread of negative affect in memory and heightens access to distress-eliciting thoughts. These negative cognitions can exacerbate anxious people's chronic negative mood, negative views of others, and fears of rejection and abandonment, thus contributing to continued activation of the attachment system.

Pereg and Mikulincer's (2004) studies also indicated that the memories and causal attribution patterns of avoidant people were not significantly affected by induced negative mood. Avoidant people seemed to exclude negative affect from awareness and were therefore less likely to use it in cognitive processing. This is similar to the preemptive exclusion of negative, attachment-related information we discussed earlier in connection with Fraley, Garner, and Shaver's (2000) memory studies.

Avoidant Attachment and Lack of Psychobiological Coherence

Avoidant people's reduced access to emotions and emotion-eliciting thoughts is also evident in studies examining the coherence between self-reports of emotional experience and less conscious, more automatic indicators of these experiences. (We assume that higher concordance between these measures implies greater access to emotional experience.) As we already mentioned, Mikulincer et al. (1990) found that avoidant individuals scored relatively low on explicit fear of death but implicitly revealed fear of death in stories written about TAT pictures. Mikulincer (1998b) reported that avoidant people, compared with secure ones, reacted to anger-eliciting episodes with lower levels of self-reported anger and increased levels of physiological arousal (heart rate). Three related studies examining access to emotions during the AAI all found that avoidant people verbally express few negative feelings during the interview but exhibit high levels of physiological arousal (heightened electrodermal activity; Dozier & Kobak, 1992; Roisman et al., 2004) and more intense facial expressions of anger, sadness, and negative surprise (Zimmermann, Wulf, & Grossmann, 1997) while speaking about their relationships with parents.

Spangler and Zimmermann (1999) examined attachment style differences (based on the AAI) in the coherence of facial muscle reactions (measured with electromyography of the smile and frown muscles) and subjective reactions (pleasantness ratings) to 24 film fragments. For each study participant, they computed the correlation between muscular and subjective reactions across the 24 scenes, with higher positive correlations reflecting higher psychobiological coherence. Attachment security was positively associated with psychobiological coherence, but avoidance was associated with less accurate awareness of physiological states. Zimmermann et al. (2001) extended these findings to the experience of emotions during a problem-solving task: Avoidant people (identified with the AAI) were characterized by a greater discrepancy between self-reported anger and sadness, and congruent facial expressions.

This pattern of physiological responses resembles the way avoidant infants react in the Strange Situation. Although outwardly they appear to be less distressed than secure infants when separated from their mothers (Ainsworth et al., 1978), Sroufe and Waters (1977a) and Zelenko et al. (2005) found that they displayed the same level of tachycardia as secure infants. Moreover, Sroufe and Waters (1977a) reported that avoidant infants did not show heart rate deceleration after reunion with their mothers, unlike secure infants (but Zelenko et al. [2005] failed to replicate this finding). These results suggest that avoidant individuals, whether infants or adults, hide their emotional reactions behaviorally while still reacting physiologically.

Sonnby-Borgstrom and Jonsson (2004) provided further evidence of avoidant individuals' lack of psychobiological coherence when undergoing negative emotions. In their study, people were exposed to pictures of happy and angry faces at three different exposure times (17, 56, and 2,350 milliseconds), and their facial muscle reactions were continuously assessed. When the pictures were presented subliminally and participants could not recognize the faces (at exposure times of 17 or 53 milliseconds), both avoidant and secure individuals activated muscles involved in negative emotional displays (corrugator or "frowning" muscles) when they were presented with angry faces. However, when participants were able to recognize the faces (at an exposure time of 2,350 milliseconds), avoidant participants showed lower levels of corrugator activity and increased zygomaticus muscle responses (a "smiling" reaction) when exposed to angry faces. In contrast, secure people reacted to these pictures by mimicking them (heightened corrugator activity). According to Sonnby-Borgstrom and Jonsson, avoidant people's heightened corrugator reaction to subliminal exposure to angry faces indicated that these pictures had automatically elicited negative emotions. Therefore, the avoidant participants' tendency to smile when they consciously saw the angry faces (at 2,350 milliseconds) suggests a defensive attempt to block cognitive access to and visible expression of negative emotions.

Insecure People's Problems in Attending to Emotions: The Case of Alexithymia

Studies of attachment style and alexithymia (having difficulty identifying and describing feelings) also confirm avoidant people's lack of conscious access to emotions. Avoidant attachment (assessed with either self-report scales or the AAI) is related to inattention to feelings (Kim, 2005; Searle & Meara, 1999), less awareness of fear and sadness in the Meta-Emotion Interview (DeOliveira, Moran, & Pederson, 2005), and alexithymia (e.g., Hexel, 2003; Mallinckrodt & Wei, 2005; Montebarocci, Codispoti, Baldaro, & Rossi, 2004; Picardi, Toni, & Caroppo, 2005; Troisi, D'Argenio, Peracchio, & Petti, 2001; Wearden, Lamberton, Crook, & Walsh, 2005). Moreover, McNamara, Andresen, Clark, Zborowski, and Duffy (2001) found that avoidant people recalled fewer dreams than secure people, and Bucheim and Mergenthaler (2000) found that avoidant people (measured with the AAI) scored lower on "emotion abstraction" (the ability to reflect on emotional themes) while speaking about their childhood experiences in the AAI.

Using the Mayer–Salovey–Caruso Emotional Intelligence Test (MSCEIT V2.0), Kafetsios obtained an unexpected finding. Avoidant individuals scored higher on emotion understanding (the ability to label emotions and group emotional terms appropriately). Kafetsios (2004) attempted to integrate this finding with all of the evidence on avoidant people's tendency to block access to emotions, and speculated that emotional suppression may reduce the intensity of emotional experiences, which in turn may facilitate cognitive understanding of emotions. Alternatively, Kafetsios's finding might indicate that avoidant people's well-documented lack of access to emotion results from a defensive emotion regulation strategy rather than from deficits in understanding emotions. It is even possible that monitoring emotions to suppress them requires special understanding of them. Thus, avoidant people may be quite adept at describing how anger develops into rage (one of the MSCEIT V2.0 items), while simultaneously ignoring, suppressing, or denying their own anger and rage.

Interestingly, most of the studies that have examined attachment-related differences in alexithymia reveal that anxiously attached people also have difficulty identifying and describing their feelings (e.g., Hexel, 2003; Mallinckrodt & Wei, 2005; Montebarocci et al., 2004; Picardi, Toni, & Caroppo, 2005; Wearden et al., 2005). According to Mallinckrodt and Wei (2005), higher alexithymia scores reflect not only lack of awareness of one's feelings but also difficulties in differentiating global emotional arousal into more specific emotional states and communicating the specific feelings to others. It seems possible, therefore, that anxious strategies, which impair control of the spread of emotion-related activation across an associative memory network and create an undifferentiated, chaotic emotional architecture, also create difficulties in differentiating and identifying specific feelings.

Attachment-anxious individuals' problems in differentiating and identifying specific feelings may also be a result of the intensity of their reactions to threatening events. Several studies have found that people who score high on attachment anxiety also score high on measures of emotional reactivity or intensity (e.g., Pietromonaco & Barrett, 1997; Searle & Meara, 1999; Wei, Vogel, Ku, & Zakalik, 2005). Similarly, J. A. Feeney (1999a) reported correlations between attachment anxiety and the intensity of anger, sadness, and anxiety during daily social interactions. Some of these studies (J. A. Feeney, 1999a; Pietromonaco & Barrett, 1997) also found that avoidant attachment was associated with lower emotional reactivity or intensity. Interestingly, these attachment style differences have been found in the intensity and expression of positive emotions, such as love, pride

(J. A. Feeney, 1999a), as well as negative emotions, such as anger and sadness. This fits with our idea that even positive emotions play a role in strengthening attachment bonds—something that anxious people wish to do and avoidant people wish not to do.

CONCLUDING REMARKS

Because emotion regulation is so important in so many different areas of psychological research (Gross, 2007), including clinical, developmental, and social psychology, as well as affective neuroscience, attachment researchers have conducted many studies on the topic. Although there are still methods to be tried, ideas to be explored, and loose ends to be tied, the literature already indicates that attachment style is an important construct for researchers and clinicians interested in individual differences in emotion regulation. Secure adults, most of whom have enjoyed favorable treatment by attachment figures, are able to experience, express, and acknowledge emotions with minimal distortion, and without becoming overwhelmed by feelings. They are able not only to regulate emotions autonomously but also to seek emotional and social support when desired. They can remember emotional experiences, including ones that occurred years ago, without defensive distortion, and without being knocked off their secure foundation by a flood of negative memories. Anxiously attached people are vigilant with respect to possible injuries, slights, and threats, and tend to amplify their negative reactions to threats. They have trouble remaining mentally organized when encountering threats or recalling psychological injuries, and they are ambivalent about seeking support. They want to be loved, soothed, and attended to, but they fear displeasing their relationship partners and being rejected. Avoidant individuals, in contrast, downplay threats and vulnerabilities, deny negative emotions, and suppress or repress negative memories. But there are many indications that they cannot always maintain this defensive stance in the face of major or prolonged stressors. Their defenses collapse under strain.

The same differences can be seen in people's reactions to breakups and losses, with secure individuals maintaining emotional bonds with lost loved ones, while effectively pursuing new relationships. They can reorganize their attachment hierarchies without defensively quarantining past experiences. Anxious individuals overreact to breakups and losses, and seem unable to get beyond them. Avoidant individuals seem relatively unperturbed by breakups and losses, but the cost of maintaining psychological distance may be high both for them and for their subsequent relationship partners.

The research literature on attachment styles and emotion regulation should prove useful to both clinicians and laypeople. It touches on many of the classic issues in psychodynamic psychology but does so in terms that most people can understand, and with a degree of clarity and empirical support never achieved by clinical writers who lacked today's probing research methods. Much more thought is still needed regarding how to apply research on attachment and emotion regulation clinically. Some suggestions and early evaluation studies are discussed in Chapter 14, this volume.

CHAPTER 8

Attachment Orientations, Behavioral Self-Regulation, and Personal Growth

One of the novel features of Bowlby's (1969/1982) attachment theory when he first proposed it was the inclusion of ideas from the relatively new field of cybernetics, an approach to conceptualizing goal-directed behavior that ushered in the era of flowchart models, computer simulation, computer-guided industrial technologies, and "smart bombs." Bowlby was also influenced by Piaget's (1953) theory of cognitive development, an approach to conceptualizing human development that was unavailable when Freud created the first psychodynamic theory of psychosexual development. In attempting to improve upon and supersede Freud's drive theory, Bowlby emphasized cognitive processes (e.g., "set-goals" and "internal working models") and cognitively guided "behavioral systems" (see Chapter 1, this volume). The same emphasis now characterizes much of psychology, including the field of social cognition, which provided many of the research techniques we use in our own experimental studies of attachment.

In this chapter we focus on behavioral self-regulation and personal growth. We begin with Carver and Scheier's (1981, 1998) feedback-control theory, an example of cybernetics-inspired theories in the contemporary social/personality field, and an example that Bowlby probably would have found congenial if it had existed when he was writing. We then examine links between individual differences in attachment style and the components and outcomes of behavioral self-regulation: choosing and organizing personal goals, remaining open to new information concerning progress or lack of progress in achieving goals, and disengaging from unproductive goals. We also consider major life tasks requiring self-regulation, such as constructing a social identity, performing well academically, choosing and managing a career, and maintaining good health. At the end of the chapter we consider the role of attachment processes in developing mature religiosity or spirituality.

FEEDBACK-CONTROL THEORY

Our analysis of the deliberate, or intentional, regulation of attachment-related feelings and behaviors is based on Carver and Scheier's (1981, 1990, 1998) feedback-control theory, according to which the organization of intentional behavior requires effective means–end plans for attaining a goal. It also requires self-regulation, or what W. T. Powers (1973) called feedback-control processes, by which people assess progress toward a goal, make corrective adjustments in their efforts to attain the goal, and decide whether to persist or to disengage from goal pursuit when difficulties arise. When successful, these self-regulatory efforts allow people to accomplish what psychologists call "personal projects" (Little, 1989) or "life tasks" (Cantor & Kihlstrom, 1987), and achieve greater life satisfaction and personal growth, reaching all the way to what humanistic psychologists of a previous generation (e.g., Maslow, 1968; C. R. Rogers, 1961) called "self-actualization." In contrast, self-regulatory failures disrupt intentional behavior, create problems in social and emotional adjustment, and block the path to self-actualization.

The first step in organizing intentional behavior is goal setting. According to Carver and Scheier (1998), there are two major kinds of goals, approach and avoidance (see also the Higgins's [1998] discussion of promotion and prevention goals). Approach goals are desirable conditions that people wish to attain (e.g., getting an "A" on an exam, achieving or maintaining good health, developing a successful career). Avoidance goals (sometimes called anti-goals) are undesirable conditions that people wish to evade (e.g., being fired from a job, being rejected by a friend, experiencing what Erikson [1959] called "identity confusion" or "role diffusion"). Whereas approach goals motivate self-regulatory efforts to reduce the discrepancy between a current state and a desired end state, avoidance goals motivate efforts to enlarge the discrepancy between the current state and an aversive end state. Beyond drawing this distinction, Carver and Scheier (1981, 1998) explained that goals differ in their level of abstraction or breadth, from overarching goals related to personal identity and major developmental tasks at the abstract extreme, to very narrow and concrete goals that are subsumed by more abstract goals. That is, goals coexist in a hierarchy, with higher-level goals determining lower-level goals and lower-level goals contributing to the attainment of higher-level goals.

Goal setting is followed by the formulation of means–ends plans and the initiation of goal-directed actions. These steps are accompanied from the start by cognitive processes that assess action effectiveness, correct means–ends plans, and adjust specific behaviors until the goal is attained or abandoned. People collect, encode, and analyze information about what is currently happening in the environment and within themselves (information that Carver and Scheier called the "input function"), compare this with the desired goal state (the "reference value"), and make behavioral corrections based on the comparison (the "output function"). These behavioral corrections may in turn alter the environment, which generates new information that has to be analyzed and compared against the goal. Through successive input-goal comparisons and behavioral accommodations, people usually make progress toward goal attainment until they either reach the desired end state or decide to disengage.

Beyond describing the simple feedback loop underlying progress toward goal attainment, Carver and Scheier (1981, 1998) introduced a sequence of behavioral interruption and expectancy assessments that occurs when an external or internal obstacle to goal attainment is encountered. In such cases, a person is likely to interrupt the behavioral flow momentarily and assess the likelihood of attaining the goal. If the conclusion is favorable, the person reactivates the behavioral flow and the feedback process, and continues to pursue the goal. If the conclusion is negative, for example, because the person believes he or she lacks the necessary skills, energy, or response options, he or she is likely to withdraw mentally and behaviorally from goal pursuit. In Carver and Scheier's (1998) model, adaptive self-regulation results from accurate assessments of the opportunities for, and constraints on, goal attainment in a given situation. If a person is regularly pursuing a sensible strategy, he or she will rarely miss an opportunity to reach attainable goals but will avoid recurrent failures. All of these considerations come into play in the special case of attachment behavior, which Bowlby (1969/1982) explicitly conceptualized as behavior aimed at attaining the "set-goal" of proximity and, indirectly, of safety.

Effective self-regulation involves a variety of cognitive skills that facilitate information processing and adjustment of behavioral plans and actions. Optimal functioning of the input and comparator functions requires a positive and open attitude toward seeking and processing new information about oneself and the environment, even if this information is discrepant from existing knowledge and temporarily results in ambiguity or confusion. Moreover, optimal functioning requires attention to environmental and personal changes, as well as a clear and well-organized goal hierarchy against which a person can assess behavioral effectiveness. The output function requires cognitive flexibility, diverse problem-solving abilities, and considerable creativity. Beyond these cognitive skills, effective self-regulation requires a calm, confident, and secure state of mind, which facilitates behavioral reorganization in the face of internal or external obstacles. This is where attachment security comes into play.

Adopting Carver and Scheier's feedback-control theory, we view the behavioral systems postulated by Bowlby (1969/1982) as regulatory devices that organize intentional behavior and use input–goal comparisons and behavioral accommodations to achieve desired end states. Behavioral system activation transforms what were originally neutral person–environment transactions into either desired "goal states" that facilitate need satisfaction or aversive "anti-goal states" that interfere with or hinder need satisfaction. The resulting goals then motivate approach tendencies that move a person toward desired goal states or avoidance tendencies that move the person away from aversive anti-goal states. In the case of the attachment system, its activation transforms proximity maintenance and the attainment of security, comfort, and protection into major goal states, and rejection, separation, and attachment figure unavailability into aversive anti-goal states. It also directs a person's cognitive processes and actions toward the attainment of proximity and security, and away from certain situations such as separations from attachment figures that disrupt "felt security" (Sroufe & Waters, 1977b).

Behavioral systems include evaluations of progress toward their primary goal, and these evaluations induce strategic adjustments that make goal attainment more likely (see Chapter 1, this volume). One of Bowlby's most important observations, which increased his confidence in the notion of goal-corrected rather than merely habitual behavior, is that behavioral sequences get altered, if necessary, to put a person, even an infant, back on the track to goal attainment. In the case of the attachment system, this goal-corrected behavioral adjustment involves monitoring and appraising inner and outer sources of stress and distress, an attachment figure's responses to one's proximity-seeking efforts, and the effectiveness of one's proximity-seeking bids in a given situation. If one mode of behavior (e.g., calling, signaling to be picked up) fails to attain the goal, another route to the same goal (e.g., crying, tugging, or clinging) may be attempted.

Our model of attachment-system functioning (see Chapter 2, this volume) includes self-regulatory processes that shape the course of proximity seeking when a person finds that he or she is too distant from an external or internalized (symbolically represented) attachment figure. In such cases, the person explicitly or implicitly assesses the likelihood of attaining security, as well as the viability of proximity-seeking efforts, then decides whether to persist in or disengage from proximity seeking. In other words, the person makes a conscious or unconscious choice between what we have been calling "hyperactivating" and "deactivating" strategies.

Beyond these normative self-regulatory aspects of the attachment system, individual differences in attachment style also have important effects on self-regulation and, hence, on the accomplishment of personal projects and life tasks. A strong sense of attachment security allows a person to maintain a calm, coherent, and confident state of mind while dealing with threats and challenges, and to devote cognitive resources to important projects and tasks. In contrast, attachment insecurities motivate defensive distortions of perception, helpless or unrealistically confident stances toward problem solving, and feelings of being threatened or endangered that interfere with realistic planning and effective action. Over time, these insecurities impair self-regulation and interfere with close relationships, important life projects, and personal growth.

In the rest of this chapter, we consider effects of individual differences in attachment style on components of the self-regulation process (goal setting, the input–comparator–output feedback loop, and the process of disengaging from a goal). We also consider the effects of attachment style on personal growth in various domains of adult life. In Chapters 9 through 12, this volume, we focus on the interpersonal implications of these individual differences.

ATTACHMENT-SYSTEM FUNCTIONING AND THE PROCESS OF SELF-REGULATION

Goal Setting

People differ in the motives and goals that guide their intentional behavior and their appraisals of progress in various life domains (e.g., J. W. Atkinson, 1957; Elliot & Church, 1997; Emmons, 1992). We are especially interested in how attachment style differences affect goal setting and goal organization.

Approach versus Avoidance Goals

Evidence reviewed in previous chapters suggests that anxiously attached individuals are unusually sensitive to anti-goal states (rejection, separation, loss, and the many failures that cause a person to wish for support, while not being certain of its availability). When a person's motives are organized in this way, avoiding aversive states becomes the main source of satisfaction, which is not as gratifying as attaining positive goals, a difference reflected in the separate terms "relief" and "joy" (Roseman & Evdokas, 2004).

Avoidant people tend to be detached from both approach goals and aversive states. Avoidant defenses sometimes discourage personal investment or involvement in demanding and challenging activities, because these activities can lead to frustration and humiliation, which naturally tend to reactivate the attachment system. These self-protective strategies sometimes cause avoidant people to restrict their pursuit of challenging goals, which, if not attained, might bring on strong feelings of failure and loss of control. Avoidant people are therefore likely to choose activities that do not seem diagnostic of their abilities (e.g., tasks that are either very easy or very difficult). In many cases, such people are likely to be unaware of pursuing a safe strategy; focusing on the dangers of aversive states might work against their general attempt to avoid feeling threatened, needy, or vulnerable (see Chapter 7, this volume). But always playing it safe may lead to boredom and result in missed opportunities for personal growth.

These theoretical ideas have been supported in four studies of achievement motivation (Elliot & Reis, 2003; Kogot, 2004; Learner & Kruger, 1997; Lopez, 1997), in which approach or appetitive motivation was conceptualized as a need for achievement, which results in feelings of pride following success and a desire for even greater challenge and mastery. The anti-goal state in achievement situations is failure, along with the shame it evokes, and the motivation to avoid this state is fear of failure (Elliot & McGregor, 2001). The four studies conducted on this topic show, as expected, that attachment security (with respect to parents, teachers, or a romantic partner) is associated with stronger need for achievement and with endorsement of mastery goals, as well as weaker fear of failure and reduced likelihood of adopting avoidance goals.

Elliot and Reis (2003) and Kogot (2004) also found that avoidant attachment is associated with weaker need for achievement and less frequent adoption of mastery goals, whereas attachment anxiety is associated with stronger fear of failure and an emphasis on anti-goals (i.e., striving to avoid failure). In addition, Elliot and Reis (2003) found that avoidant individuals' lack of endorsement of mastery goals was based on a tendency to dismiss the excitement and challenges involved in achievement activities. Anxious individuals' emphasis on anti-goals included an exaggeration of achievement-related threats. Interestingly, Elliot and Reis found that avoidant individuals were also prone to give up easily, thereby displaying a passive fear of failure ("I can't do that"). They tended to disengage prematurely from challenging activities if they encountered even relatively minor difficulties.

Although these findings seem to be at odds with the dismissingly avoidant view that relationships are secondary to achievement (see Bartholomew & Horowitz, 1991; Chapters 4 and 9, this volume) and with Hazan and Shaver's (1990) finding that avoidant employees use work to evade social involvements, avoidant people evidently use work as an excuse for retreating from social relationships, yet are simultaneously less than fully invested in work. Their jobs seem to serve as an excuse for social avoidance and a facade of self-reliance, importance, and control. This is reminiscent of Ainsworth et al.'s (1978) comment that avoidance in infancy "protects the baby from reexperiencing the rebuff that he has come to expect when he seeks close contact with his mother. It thus somewhat lowers his level of anxiety (arousal). It also leads him to turn to the neutral world of things, even though displacement exploratory behavior is devoid of the true interest that is inherent in nonanxious exploration" (p. 320).

A conceptually similar pattern of findings was reported by Meyer et al. (2005), who examined attachment-related individual differences in J. A. Gray's (1982) two major motivational systems: the behavioral approach system (BAS, a neural system that specializes in processing reward-related information and triggering approach behavior) and the behavioral inhibition system (BIS, a neural system specialized in processing threat-related information and triggering escape or avoidance behaviors). Avoidant attachment was associated with reduced approach activity (lower scores on Carver and White's [1994] BAS scale), whereas attachment anxiety was associated with higher scores on the BIS scale. We recently replicated these correlations in a new sample of 324 Americans and 125 Israelis (see Table 8.1). The findings fit well with the frequently observed associations between attachment anxiety and the personality trait of neuroticism, which can be interpreted as high BIS sensitivity (see Table 13.1 for a summary of findings), and between avoidant attachment

TABLE 8.1. Pearson Correlations between Attachment Dimensions
and BIS/BAS Scores

BIS/BAS scores	ECR anxiety	ECR avoidance
American sample (N = 324)		
Behavioral inhibition	.37**	−.07
Behavioral activation	.04	−.29**
Israeli sample (N = 125)		
Behavioral inhibition	.40**	−.10
Behavioral activation	.07	−.38**

**$p < .01$.

and low scores on the personality trait of extraversion, which implies that avoidant individuals are characterized by low BAS activity (see Table 9.1 for a summary of findings).

The Construal and Organization of Personal Goals

In his theory of "personal strivings," Emmons (1992, 1997) specified four dimensions along which people vary in construing their personal goals. The first dimension is degree of commitment—the value and importance placed on personal goals, and the effort invested in pursuing them. The second dimension concerns the anticipated outcome of goal pursuit—the expectation of success and personal control in attaining one's habitual goals. The third dimension is appraisal of threats and demands in goal pursuit—the difficulties, obstacles, and problems people anticipate as they strive toward goals. The fourth dimension, level of abstraction, concerns the extent to which people frame their central goals in broad and abstract terms ("being a psychologist") versus narrow and concrete terms ("getting an A in this psychology course").

Emmons (1997) also discussed three dimensions along which people vary when organizing their strivings within a goal system. The first dimension is level of intergoal conflict, the extent to which people think pursuit or attainment of one goal interferes with pursuit or attainment of another. The second dimension, goal differentiation, concerns the extent to which people perceive their goals as distinct, dissimilar, and unrelated to each other. The third dimension is goal integration, the extent to which people possess superordinate goal categories that connect different subordinate goals, without eliminating their uniqueness and contradictions. Highly integrated people can compare different goals, evaluate trade-offs, and view specific goals as alternative means of attaining superordinate goals or supporting personal meaning structures. Less integrated people have fragmented goal systems in which different goals are not coherently linked to an overarching, unifying goal, or set of goals.

Anxiously attached people's sense of themselves as relatively vulnerable, helpless, weak, and incompetent (see Chapter 6, this volume) should cause them to appraise threats and problems during goal pursuit in inflated terms and thereby have pessimistic expectations about their ability to attain their goals. Moreover, because they are so focused on unmet attachment needs, they may perceive attachment-unrelated activities as interfering with the pursuit of attachment security. As a result, they may experience conflict among their goals and have difficulty forming a coherent, integrated goal system.

Avoidant people's defensive withdrawal from challenging, demanding activities may cause them to reduce their degree of commitment to and investment in goal pursuit. Moreover, they may frame their strivings in more concrete and narrow terms, because broader and more abstract strivings generally entail greater risk and more investment, opening avoidant people to the possibility of frustration, disappointment, and embarrassment (Little, 1989). In addition, avoidant people's tendency to exclude attachment-related needs and goals from awareness (see Chapter 7, this volume) may cause them to form fragmented, unintegrated goal systems.

We recently conducted a study examining attachment-related differences in the construal and organization of personal goals (Mikulincer & Shaver, 2007), in which participants generated a list of six personal goals and rated each one along the commitment, anticipated outcome, and difficulty dimensions. They also compared each pair of goals and provided ratings of intergoal conflict ("how much being successful in one area of striving has a harmful effect on the other striving domain"), goal differentiation ("how dissimilar the two strivings are"), and goal integration ("how much the two strivings are perceived as being part of a single broader purpose in life"). In addition, two independent judges coded the goals generated by each participant according to his or her level of breadth and abstraction.

The findings were consistent with our reasoning and hypotheses. Attachment anxiety was associated with pessimistic appraisal of goal pursuit (lower ratings of success and higher ratings of difficulty in goal pursuit) and relatively high conflict among goals. Avoidant attachment was associated with low commitment to goal pursuit and lower levels of abstraction in framing personal goals. Moreover, both forms of insecure attachment were associated with lower goal integration. These associations between attachment dimensions and features of people's goal systems could not be explained by alternative variables such as trait anxiety and self-esteem.

Exploration and Cognitive Openness

Effective goal pursuit often requires exploration, openness to new information, and the learning of new means–end associations and stimulus–response contingencies. According to Bowlby (1969/1982), these activities are governed by an exploration, or exploratory, behavioral system—an innate system aimed at investigating, manipulating, and mastering the environment. This behavioral system is activated whenever people encounter novel or unexpected stimuli, or conditions that challenge their knowledge, beliefs, or actions. Under cognitively challenging conditions, the exploration system motivates people to learn more about a situation, to remain open and receptive to new information, and to accommodate existing knowledge structures to incoming evidence until a new cognitive integration is achieved. (This aspect of Bowlby's theory was influenced by Piaget [1953] who conceptualized cognitive development in terms of mental structures that "assimilate" information and "accommodate," or self-correct, if necessary, to incorporate new information.) Optimal functioning of the exploration system facilitates behavioral self-regulation, sustains adaptation and growth, and increases a person's sense of competence and mastery—states that White (1965) called the " joy in being a cause" (p. 203).

As we explained in Chapter 3, Bowlby (1973) and Ainsworth (1991) assumed that attachment security would enhance curiosity, encourage relaxed exploration of new, unusual information and phenomena, and favor the formation of open and flexible cognitive structures. Being confident in their ability to deal with distress (see Chapter 7, this volume), secure individuals should be able to incorporate new information at the expense of temporary perplexity or confusion. Cognitive ambiguity should not generally threaten their sense of competence, lovability, and control. They should realize that perplexity, like other challenging experiences, is short-lived and can lead to greater mastery and broaden their sense of coherence and meaning.

In contrast, lack of attachment security is likely to be associated with fragile views of self and world (see Chapter 6, this volume), which make new information seem threatening and destabilizing. Because insecure people lack a sense of mastery in dealing with distress (see Chapter 7, this volume), they may experience confusion as highly threatening, causing them to block the intake of new information. They may mistake cognitive stability for security, even if faulty knowledge leads to poor decisions and regrettable actions. In addition, anxious individuals' tendency to intensify distress and worries (see Chapter 7, this volume) can interfere with and overwhelm the calm and steady state of mind necessary for open, curious exploration of novel stimuli and conditions. Avoidant defenses can also interfere with the incorporation of new evidence and unusual thoughts, because relaxed exploration and "loosening" of cognitive operations open the door to threats and dangers that might reactivate the attachment system.

These ideas have received strong support in studies of infants and children. For example, Ainsworth, Bell, and Stayton (1973) found that a secure infant could "move away from his mother, even out of sight into another room. He is by no means oblivious to his mother, but he keeps track of her whereabouts" (p. 1156). In contrast, anxious infants in Ainsworth et al.'s studies clung to their mothers and were afraid of novel stimuli. Avoidant infants diverted their attention to new objects, apparently (as mentioned earlier) as a defense against unpleasant contact with their mothers, but they did not display joy or interest in exploration. These kinds of findings were subsequently obtained by other investigators in studies of diverse exploratory behaviors, including those of older children (e.g., Arend, Gove, & Sroufe, 1979; Hazen & Durrett, 1982; Sroufe, 1979).

With respect to adults, several lines of research have examined the hypothesized link between attachment and exploration. One line focuses on the five-factor model of personality (McCrae & Costa, 1990) and examines attachment-related differences in openness to experience (see Table 8.2 for a summary of methods and findings). Although some of the summarized studies yielded evidence of the expected association between attachment insecurities and lower levels of openness, most of them found no significant association. Before reaching any conclusion about this, however, we should note that the superordinate trait of openness in most personality questionnaires includes some facets that are less relevant to behavioral self-regulation, such as aesthetic interests, reliance on sensations, and hypnotic susceptibility, and these might not be much affected by attachment insecurities (McCrae & Costa, 1990). As we explain below, studies focusing on specific facets of openness that are more relevant to exploration and self-regulation (e.g., curiosity, tolerance of ambiguity, and creative problem solving) have consistently yielded evidence for the hypothesized attachment–exploration link.

Adult attachment studies have found that avoidant people score lower on self-report measures of novelty seeking (Carnelley & Ruscher, 2000; Chotai, Jonasson, Hagglof, & Adolfsson, 2005), trait curiosity (Mikulincer, 1997), and exploratory interest (Aspelmeier & Kerns, 2003; Green & Campbell, 2000; Johnston, 1999; Reich & Siegel, 2002), and they have more negative attitudes toward curiosity itself (Mikulincer, 1997). With regard to attachment anxiety, only two studies have found that anxious people report fewer exploratory interests (Aspelmeier & Kerns, 2003; J. D. Green & Campbell, 2000). However, Mikulincer (1997) found that although anxious individuals did not score lower than secure ones on trait curiosity, they did report less curiosity-related benefits (e.g., personal growth), more curiosity-related threats (e.g., discovering painful things, jeopardizing relationships, hurting other people), and less joy and excitement during exploration. In addition, J. D. Green and Campbell (2000) and Reich and Siegel (2002) found that, compared with secure people, attachment-anxious people engaged in exploratory activities for what we consider "anti-goal" reasons, such as distracting oneself from a negative mood or seeking others' love and approval so as to avoid rejection and isolation.

TABLE 8.2. A Summary of Findings on Attachment Orientations and the Big-Five Traits of Openness and Conscientiousness

Study	Attachment measure	Personality measure	Openness		Conscientiousness	
			Anxiety	Avoidance	Anxiety	Avoidance
Shaver & Brennan (1992)	HS ratings	NEO-PI	(ns)	(ns)	(−)	(−)
Griffin & Bartholomew (1994a)	RQ	NEO-PI	(ns)	(ns)	(−)	(ns)
Griffin & Bartholomew (1994a)	RSQ	NEO-PI	(ns)	(ns)	(−)	(ns)
Becker et al. (1997)	New scale	BFM	(−)	(ns)	(ns)	(−)
Carver (1997, Study 3)	MAQ	NEO-FFI	(ns)	(ns)	(ns)	(ns)
Carver (1997, Study 4)	MAQ	NEO-FFI	(ns)	(−)	(ns)	(−)
Carver (1997, Study 4)	RQ	NEO-FFI	(ns)	(ns)	(−)	(ns)
Markiewicz et al. (1997)	AAQ	NEO-PI			(ns)	(ns)
Mickelson et al. (1997)	HS ratings	BFM	(−)	(−)		
Backstrom & Holmes (2001)	RSQ	NEO-PI	(ns)	(−)	(ns)	(ns)
Shafer (2001)	ASQ	BBM	(ns)	(ns)	(−)	(ns)
Gallo et al. (2003)	AAS	BFA	(ns)	(ns)	(−)	(−)
Edelstein et al. (2004)	RSQ	NEO-PI	(ns)	(ns)	(ns)	(ns)
Heaven et al. (2004)	AAS	IPIP	(ns)	(−)	(−)	(−)
Picardi, Toni, et al. (2005)	ECR	BFQ	(−)	(−)	(ns)	(ns)
Noftle & Shaver (2006, Study 1)	ECR	BFI	(−)	(−)	(−)	(−)
Noftle & Shaver (2006, Study 2)	ECR	NEO-PI-R	(ns)	(−)	(−)	(−)

Note. (−), significant inverse correlation; (ns), nonsignificant correlation; BBM, Brief Bipolar Markers; BFA, Big Five Adjectives; BFI, Big Five Inventory; BFM, Big Five Markers; BFQ, Big Five Questionnaire; HS, Hazan and Shaver; IPIP, International Personality Item Pool; MAQ, Multidimensional Attachment Questionnaire; NEO-FFI, NEO Five-Factor Inventory; NEO-PI, NEO Personality Inventory; NEO-PI-R, NEO Personality Inventory—Revised.

Beyond measuring attachment-related differences in self-reported information searches, Aspelmeier and Kerns (2003) found similar differences in exploratory behavior. At the beginning of an experimental session, undergraduates were unobtrusively videotaped (for 5 minutes) while waiting alone for the experimenter in a testing room containing five puzzle games. (Participants were told that the room was also used for parent–child play sessions, and the games had apparently been left there accidentally.) The amount of time participants spent manipulating the puzzles served as an index of behavioral exploration. Following the 5-minute waiting period, participants were asked to imagine that they had a chance to go on a blind date with one of three people. Each of these people had written 20 self-descriptive statements, each on an index card. The participants were asked to examine each deck, viewing as many cards as necessary to decide whether they wanted to date that person. The number of cards a participant examined served as an index of social information search. More avoidant people devoted less time to the puzzles and were less likely to engage in social information search. (The puzzle time effect was significant only for the men, probably because the women were generally reluctant to handle the "children's" puzzles.) Although these findings fit with avoidant people's hypothesized reluctance to engage in exploratory activities, their lower engagement in the social information search might also reflect anti-relational tendencies or having simpler, quicker ways to categorize and judge people.

Studies have also shown that attachment insecurities induce what Kruglanski (1989) called "epistemic freezing"—cognitive closure, dogmatic thinking, intolerance of ambiguity, and rejection of information that challenges the validity of one's beliefs (Gjerde et al., 2004; Green-Hennessy & Reis, 1998; Mikulincer, 1997). For example, Mikulincer and Green-Hennessy and Reis (1998) studied the well-known "primacy effect"—the tendency to make judgments based on early information and to ignore later data—and found that insecurely attached people were more likely than secure ones to rate a target person based on the first information received. In another study, Mikulincer (1997) examined stereotype-based judgments (i.e., judging a member of a group based on a generalized notion about the group rather than on exploration of specific information about the member). Anxious and avoidant individuals tended to evaluate the quality of an essay based on the supposed ethnicity of the writer. The more positive the stereotype of the writer's ethnic group, the higher the grade assigned to the essay. In contrast, secure individuals were relatively unaffected by ethnic stereotypes.

Based on these findings, Mikulincer and Arad (1999) examined attachment style differences in revising knowledge about a relationship partner following behavior on the part of the partner that seemed inconsistent with prior conceptions. Compared to secure people, both anxious and avoidant people displayed fewer changes in their perception of the partner after being exposed to expectation-incongruent information about the partner's behavior. This finding was replicated when relationship-specific attachment orientations were assessed. The higher the attachment anxiety or avoidance with respect to a particular partner, the fewer the revisions people made in their perception of this partner after receiving expectation-incongruent information (Mikulincer & Arad, 1999, Study 2).

Interestingly, insecurely attached people's cognitive closure can be observed even in contexts that facilitate relaxed exploration, such as ones that increase the level of positive emotion. In a series of three experiments, Mikulincer and Sheffi (2000) exposed people to positive experiences (retrieving a happy memory or watching a brief comedy film) or to a neutral condition, and assessed creative problem solving. The previously documented beneficial effects of positive affect on cognitive functioning were observed only among people with a secure attachment style, who reacted to a positive induction by performing better on a creative problem-solving task. In contrast, avoidant individuals were not affected by positive affect inductions, and anxious ones actually reacted to positive inductions with *impaired* creativity (the opposite of what occurred with secure individuals and the same as what happened in previous studies following negative rather than positive mood inductions).

We interpret these results as indicating that secure people's openness to emotional experience (see Chapter 7, this volume) allows them to treat positive affect as information to be cognitively processed (viewing it as a signal that all is going well), which allows them to "loosen" their cognitive control and explore unusual associations. Avoidant people seem to dismiss affective signals of safety, perhaps in an effort to prevent the loosening of cognitive control, which might increase uncertainty, confusion, or loss of control. Interestingly, anxious people somehow turned a signal of safety into a harbinger of trouble. We interpret this result as indicating that anxious people's tendency to mix positive with negative reactions and associations (see Chapter 7, this volume) can occur even following a clearly positive message. Perhaps they initially experienced a positive state, as intended by the experimenter, but were then reminded of the downside of previous experiences that began positively and ended painfully. Once attuned to these negative memories, the anxious mind may suffer from a spread of negative associations that interferes with exploration and creativity. (This is similar to activation of both positive and negative aspects of attachment, such as love and loss, in people threatened subliminally in the experiments by Mikulincer et al., 2000; see Chapter 7, this volume.)

Behavioral Organization, Conscientiousness, and Self-Control

The self-regulatory deficiencies of insecurely attached people can also be seen in the organization and enactment of plans—the "output function" of Carver and Scheier's feedback model. Well-organized and carefully executed plans require a certain amount of self-discipline, orderliness, responsibility, persistence in the face of temporary obstacles; concentration on the task at hand; engagement in deliberate, nonimpulsive actions; and prioritization of self-regulation and goal attainment over other, competing wishes and demands (e.g., gaining immediate release from a negative mood). Well-regulated goal seeking also requires considerable self-control—"the ability to override or change one's inner responses, as well as to interrupt undesirable behavioral tendencies (such as impulses) and refrain from acting on them" (Tangney, Baumeister, & Boone, 2004, p. 274). These regulatory capacities, which resemble the facets of the superordinate trait of conscientiousness in the five-factor model of personality (McCrae & Costa, 1990), allow a person to stay on the path of goal attainment, thereby facilitating the accomplishment of important personal projects and life tasks.

We suspect that the depleted psychological resources of anxiously attached people jeopardize goal organization and full engagement in goal-oriented behavior. The deficiencies can be exacerbated by anxious individuals' prioritization of attachment goals over other life tasks, their sense of helplessness and self-defeating attitudes and beliefs, and their lack of control over the spread of activation from one distress-eliciting thought or memory to another. Avoidant people can also suffer from organizational deficiencies caused by a tendency to prioritize defensive self-enhancement over task engagement. Such people prefer not to acknowledge that their beliefs, decisions, and plans are mistaken and need to be revised.

There is some evidence concerning the link between attachment orientations and organizational capacities. Around half of the studies that assessed attachment-related differences in conscientiousness (see Table 8.2 for a summary of methods and findings) found that attachment insecurity, either anxiety or avoidance, is associated with lower conscientiousness. The remaining studies, however, did not yield significant associations, and the reasons for the mixed results are unclear.

In other studies, Tangney et al. (2004) reported that more anxious or avoidant people scored lower on a scale measuring self-control, even after controlling for social desirability. Learner and Kruger (1997) found that people who scored lower on a measure of secure attachment to parents reported less planning and poorer organization of academic activities. In a qualitative analysis of adolescents' descriptions of how they dealt with school-related demands and activities, Soares, Lemos, and Almeida (2005) found that less secure adolescents (based on the Separation Anxiety Test [SAT]) were less likely to rely on constructive strategies (e.g., evaluation of alternatives, definition of priorities, and inhibition of distracting tendencies). Rather, they tended to jump from one goal to another, never completing a course of action, and their behavior appeared to be disorganized, confused, and impulsive.

In a new study of 118 Israeli undergraduates, reported for the first time here, participants completed the ECR attachment scales, together with scales tapping (1) the extent to which they engaged in effective mental preparation (problem analysis and plan rehearsal rather that stagnant deliberation) before tackling a problem (Mental Anticipatory Processes Scale; Feldman & Hayes, 2005); (2) task concentration, goal prioritizing, task persistence, and behavioral reorganization (Selective Optimization with Compensation Scale; Bajor & Baltes, 2003); (3) difficulties in decision making (Judgmental Self-Doubt Scale; Mirels, Greblo, & Dean, 2002); and (4) the tendency to delay and intentionally put off tasks that needed to be done (General Procrastination Scale; Lay, 1988). As can be seen in Table 8.3, more anxious and avoidant people than secure people scored lower on problem analysis, plan rehearsal, task concentration, task persistence, and behavioral reorganization, and they got higher scores on procrastination. Moreover, attachment anxiety, but not avoidance, was significantly associated with "stagnant [fruitless] deliberation" and more difficulties in concentrating, goal prioritizing, and decision making, perhaps reflecting a tendency to devote time and attention to attachment worries.

Beyond these correlational findings, some of the participants ($n = 75$) were invited for a second experimental session, in which we contextually primed representations of attachment security (visualizing a supportive, caring relationship partner), representations of attachment insecurity (visualizing a rejecting, nonsupportive relationship partner), or neutral representations (visualizing a drugstore clerk). All participants were then told they would perform a series of complex reasoning tasks and were asked to complete the task persistence/concentration items of the Selective Optimization with Compensation Scale to show how they planned to deal with these tasks. As can be seen in Figure 8.1, compared to participants in the neutral priming condition, participants in the security priming condition planned to concentrate harder and to be more persistent on the tasks. In contrast, insecure attachment primes (compared to neutral primes) reduced participants' task concentration and persistence. Interestingly, the beneficial effects of security priming were observed even in chronically anxious and avoidant people (all betas > .39, all ps < .01). However, the impairments produced by the insecure primes were observed mainly among chronically insecure people (all betas > .43, all ps < .01). The relatively secure participants were not much affected by insecure primes (all betas < .08).

Although some researchers might interpret the correlational findings in the opposite causal direction—that is, as indicating that self-control and conscientiousness contribute to better relational outcomes and thus promote attachment security (Tangney et al., 2004)—our experimental findings support the claim that attachment security is a cause of improved organization of goal-oriented behaviors. Our findings also highlight the impairments produced by contextual activation of attachment insecurities and the resilient self-regulation of chronically secure people.

Goal Disengagement

Attachment-related worries and defenses can cause people to make poor decisions about goal persistence and disengagement. As we explained earlier, the deactivating strategies

TABLE 8.3. Pearson Correlations and Standardized Regression Coefficients (β) Showing Associations between Attachment Dimensions and Behavioral Self-Regulation Variables

	ECR anxiety		ECR avoidance	
Behavioral self-regulation	r	β	r	β
Mental anticipatory processes				
Problem analysis	−.40**	−.44**	−.32**	−.36**
Plan rehearsal	−.41**	−.45**	−.30**	−.35**
Stagnant deliberation	.40**	.41**	.04	.08
Selective optimization processes				
Task concentration	−.24**	−.28**	−.30**	−.33**
Goal prioritizing	−.21	−.22	−.08	−.10
Task persistence	−.28**	−.32**	−.33**	−.37**
Behavioral reorganization	−.24**	−.27**	−.28**	−.32**
Judgmental self-doubt scale	.35**	.37**	.13	.17
Procrastination scale	.47**	.52**	.33**	.39**

Note. N = 118.
**p < .01.

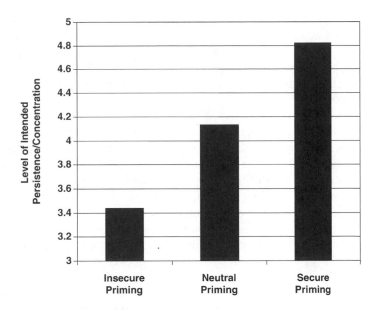

FIGURE 8.1. Mean intention regarding task concentration/persistence as a function of priming condition.

favored by avoidant individuals reduce commitment to and investment in goal strivings. The inclination to withdraw prematurely from goal pursuit may be further exacerbated when an avoidant person encounters difficulties and impediments that threaten highly valued senses of self-efficacy and self-reliance. Theoretically, we expect avoidant individuals to react to obstacles defensively, by withdrawing commitment and suspending effort. Although this may help them avoid failures, it also results in missed opportunities and an accumulation of overly cautious choices to engage in ultimately unchallenging, boring activities.

In contrast, anxiously attached individuals are predisposed to continue pursuing unattainable goals. After all, their prototypical striving is for reassurance and commitment in a relationship that they perceive to be inadequately supportive and reliable. This often produces a long chain of self-fulfilling prophecies and "Oh woe is me" experiences in troubled love relationships (see Chapter 10, this volume). The payoff for this strategy, if there is one, is to continue to feel that one has suffered unduly and deserves more sympathy and support. It fits well with low and unstable self-esteem, and sustains a sense of vulnerability and need.

Although adult attachment researchers have not yet systematically documented attachment-style differences in goal disengagement, there is some preliminary evidence for the hypothesized effects of attachment insecurities. In a series of studies of investment escalation behavior, Jayson (2004) assessed patterns of goal disengagement in non-attachment settings. In the first study, participants read about hypothetical scenarios in which they were asked to imagine they were the research and development (R&D) manager of a pharmaceutical firm that had invested money in a new anticancer drug. They were then told that development of the drug was not going well, and in fact was causing the firm to lose money. The participants were given an amount of money to invest in R&D and asked to divide it between further development of the questionable drug and creation of an alternative product. The amount the participants chose to invest in the as yet unsuccessful drug was interpreted as indicating continued commitment to the original investment. In two subsequent studies, Jayson used similar scenarios to see what would happen if he experimentally manipulated participants' personal responsibility for the initial investment (high, low) and expectations of success in further developing the questionable drug (low, high).

Jayson (2004) observed the expected inverse association between avoidant attachment and goal persistence: The higher a person's avoidance score, the less money he or she decided to allocate to the troubled project. However, this association was not significant in experimental conditions that minimized the participant's personal responsibility for the initial investment, a result that supports our idea that avoidant individuals' disengagement from frustrating activities is a defensive maneuver aimed at preventing further damage to a fragile sense of self-worth. Other findings supported our ideas concerning the difficulty anxiously attached people experience when they need to abandon unattainable goals. When expectations about continuing to develop the original drug were experimentally manipulated to be favorable, attachment anxiety was not significantly associated with the amount of money invested in further development of the drug. However, when participants were led to believe that the goal of successful development might be unattainable (they received pessimistic messages about the drug's prospects), attachment anxiety was associated with a paradoxical escalation in the amount of money participants allocated to the losing investment; that is, anxiously attached people seemed to find it difficult to withdraw commitment to an unattainable goal.

Following this line of research, we (Mikulincer & Shaver, 2007) conducted a correlational study in which participants twice completed Wrosch, Scheier, Miller, Schultz, and Carver's (2003) four-item Goal-Disengagement Scale (e.g., "It's easy for me to stop thinking about a goal and let it go"). In one condition they were asked about goal disengagement after experiencing some unexpected problems that could be solved by investing further effort. In the other condition, participants were asked about goal disengagement after experiencing recurrent failure over an extended period of time. We observed a positive association between avoidant attachment and goal disengagement when the goal was attainable, but not in the unattainable goal condition. Everyone, regardless of degree of avoidance, disengaged in the unattainable goal condition. However, only avoidant participants disengaged from goal pursuit when there were still opportunities to achieve the goal (a case of premature disengagement). As expected theoretically, attachment anxiety was inversely associated with goal disengagement when the goal was unattainable, but not when it was attainable. In a conceptual replication of Jayson's (2004) findings, attachment anxiety interfered with disengagement from an unattainable goal.

LIFE TASKS AND PERSONAL GROWTH DURING ADOLESCENCE AND ADULTHOOD

So far we have focused on fairly specific goals and goal pursuits. We now turn to the much broader goals that developmental psychologists call "major life tasks," such as identity formation and career development. Theoretically, we expect the attachment-related differences in self-regulation we have already discussed to be manifested as well in the pursuit of adolescent and adult life tasks. In this section, we focus on some of the

most important life tasks encountered in adolescence and adulthood: (1) identity formation, (2) career development, (3) school and academic performance, (4) performance on
the job, (5) health maintenance, and (6) attaining and maintaining a meaningful religious,
philosophical, or spiritual approach to life.

Identity Formation

One of the tasks of adolescence and young adulthood is to establish a stable identity—a
coherent set of personal goals, values, and beliefs that provides an inner sense of same-
ness and continuity (Erikson, 1968; Marcia, 1980). In his lifespan theory of psychosocial
development, Erikson (1968) considered the process of identity formation (and overcoming role confusion and identity diffusion) to be the central task of adolescence. However,
although personal identity reaches its initial resolution during adolescence, identity
exploration and identity concerns continue throughout adulthood (Marcia, 1980), and
many people attain a more mature personal identity later in life (Josselson, 1987). Successful resolution of this task is closely associated with personal adjustment and subjective well-being, and is an important step on the road to maturity (Marcia, 1980).

According to Marcia (1980), identity formation involves two cognitive processes:
exploration and commitment. "Exploration," as used in this context, is an active quest
for personal meaning that involves a search for information about alternative lifestyles,
beliefs, and values. Commitment is based on integrating the different possibilities, deciding which fits better with one's unique personality, and implementing this decision in a
variety of personal projects. In other words, identity formation is a self-regulation task
that involves information search, comparison of alternatives, correction of one's values
and beliefs, and implementation of decisions in the pursuit of meaningful personal
strivings. Stated in these terms, it is clear that identity formation is the kind of self-
regulatory task we would expect to be associated with attachment style.

We know from developmental research that there are important individual differences in identity formation. Not everyone is willing or able to undertake a vigorous
search for identity. Some people never experience the need for a personal identity, and
others hold fast to values and beliefs supplied ready-made by their family or culture.
Moreover, not everyone is able to achieve a stable identity: Some become anxious and
confused by the exploration process, and others feel they cannot commit to a particular
identity, which leaves them in a chronic state of self-scrutiny and indecision. Marcia
(1980) organized these measurable individual differences into a taxonomy of four identity statuses. Individuals characterized by *identity diffusion* exhibit no strong commitment to any value, goal, or belief, and do not conduct an organized evaluation of alternatives. *Foreclosure* is marked by an early personal commitment that is achieved with little
or no exploration. *Moratorium* is a state in which a person is still exploring personal
identity, without having reached a decision about values, goals, or beliefs. Individuals in
the *achievement* category engage in active exploration among alternatives and are able to
overcome the moratorium state and make a commitment to a unique identity. Viewed
from the perspective of optimal adult development, identity diffusion is the least adaptive
status, and identity achievement represents a successful outcome to the identity formation
task.

Attachment security should contribute to identity formation (Marcia, 1980). As
shown earlier, securely attached people feel confident when examining alternatives and
exploring opportunities, and they generally have sufficient resources and abilities to organize new information and effectively pursue personal goals. Secure individuals feel loved,

valued, and accepted by others even if they question familial or cultural worldviews and do not automatically incorporate these worldviews into their identity. Moreover, their positive self-regard, rooted in prior unconditional support and acceptance by caregivers, confers upon secure individuals a strong sense of self-directedness and autonomy (see Chapter 6, this volume). This psychological bedrock makes it easier to commit to a chosen ideology, role, career, or occupation without feeling shame, guilt, or remorse for having violated other people's expectations. In contrast, insecure people tend to experience problems in exploration generally, and in the search for a personal identity in particular, which can result in identity diffusion or foreclosure.

We now know quite a bit about links between attachment security and identity formation. Several studies have shown, for example, that adolescents' secure attachment to parents (as assessed with the IPPA) is associated with higher scores on identity achievement and lower scores on identity diffusion (e.g., M. J. Benson, Harris, & Rogers, 1992; Meeus, Oosterwegel, & Vollebergh, 2002; Schultheiss & Blustein, 1994). These findings have been replicated with other measures of parental attachment, such as the Family Attachment Interview and the AAI (e.g., MacKinnon & Marcia, 2002; Samuolis, Layburn, & Schiaffino, 2001; Zimmermann & Becker-Stoll, 2002). In three studies that employed self-report measures of attachment style (Hoegh & Bourgeois, 2002; Kennedy, 1999; Reich & Siegel, 2002), secure individuals scored higher than their less secure peers on identity achievement, but differences between anxious and avoidant forms of attachment insecurity were not consistent.

As always, we have to be concerned that the vast majority of studies were cross-sectional rather than longitudinal or experimental in nature (but see Zimmermann & Becker-Stoll [2002] for a 2-year longitudinal study). Moreover, the findings are somewhat discrepant concerning sex differences and the relative importance of maternal and paternal attachment. Whereas Samuolis et al. (2001) and Schultheiss and Blustein (1994) found the beneficial effects of attachment security on identity achievement to be more pronounced among women than among men, other studies have failed to replicate this sex difference. In addition, M. J. Benson et al. (1992) found that secure attachment to the mother was more strongly associated with identity achievement than secure attachment to the father, regardless of gender. But other studies failed to replicate this finding. Thus, more research is needed on the links, across developmental periods, between attachment patterns and identity status.

Attachment style is related to another important component of identity—gender role identity or one's basic sense of femininity or masculinity. According to Bem (1981), one important developmental task of adolescence is to explore femininity (expressive, communion-oriented traits) and masculinity (agentic, instrumental traits), and to integrate them in a mature, flexible, and adaptive gender role identity while resisting rigid, sexist, or restrictive gender roles that may be encouraged by family or culture. The successful resolution of this task should result in a unique, personalized mixture of femininity and masculinity—an androgynous gender role identity that allows a person to engage flexibly in expressive or instrumental behavior when it is situationally appropriate. Androgyny, like attachment security, is viewed as a desirable mixture of self-confidence, autonomy, and healthy capacity for intimate relationships (e.g., Bem, 1981).

From an attachment perspective, we expect insecure individuals' cognitive closure and reliance on stereotypical thinking to favor endorsement of traditional gender roles, thereby preventing exploration of less conventional ideologies and the development of psychological androgyny. Moreover, specific attachment insecurities may interfere in particular ways with the integration of masculinity and femininity. Whereas anxious people's doubts about their self-efficacy and mastery might interfere with the development of masculine, agentic traits, avoidant people's preference for interpersonal distance and their tendency to suppress emotions might prevent the exploration of feminine, expressive traits.

In support of this reasoning, more secure attachment to parents has been found to correlate with higher levels of psychological androgyny, as assessed with the Bem Sex Role Inventory in both adolescent boys and girls (Fass & Tubman, 2002; Haigler, Day, & Marshall, 1995; Kenny & Gallagher, 2002). Moreover, in three studies, Shaver, Papalia, et al. (1996) found that people who were secure in romantic relationships scored higher than anxious or avoidant people on psychological androgyny (as assessed with the Personal Attributes Questionnaire). Moreover, attachment anxiety is associated with lower scores on measures of masculinity, whereas avoidance is associated with lower scores on femininity (e.g., Alonso-Arbiol, Shaver, & Yarnoz, 2002; Collins & Read, 1990; Shaver, Papalia, et al., 1996).

Additional studies have found that men's insecure attachments to parents, as well as ratings of anxiety or avoidance in close relationships, are associated with stronger conflicts regarding the "feminine" trait of emotional expressiveness (Blazina & Watkins, 2000; DeFranc & Mahalik, 2002; A. R. Fischer & Good, 1998; Mahalik, Aldarondo, Gilbert-Gokhale, & Shore, 2005; Schwartz, Waldo, & Higgins, 2004). In all of these studies, insecure men were more likely than secure men to feel stressed by failing to live up to masculine ideals. Hence, it seems that attachment insecurities can influence men to overidentify with traditional, rigid masculine ideologies; to fear appearing feminine; and to form negative attitudes toward women that sometimes contribute to relational violence and abuse (see Chapter 10, this volume).

The beneficial effects of attachment security on identity formation have also been documented in stigmatized social groups, such as gay, lesbian, and transgendered individuals. Such people are subjected to strong external pressures to suppress parts of their authentic selves when constructing an identity, and to accept cultural norms and roles that do not fit their own wishes, inclinations, beliefs, and values. As a result, they often have difficulty accepting their sexual orientation, reaching the identity achievement status, and integrating private and public aspects of their identity (e.g., Mohr, 1999). For them, feelings of unconditional love, being valued, and being accepted by others, as well as the sense of possessing something worthy within themselves—the core components of secure attachment—are crucial for resisting external pressures; exploring, accepting, and disclosing their unconventional sexual orientation; and integrating it within a stable sense of personal identity.

Studies of gay and lesbian individuals consistently find that attachment security is associated with disclosure of sexual orientation to others, and at an earlier age (e.g., Elizur & Mintzer, 2003; Jellison & McConnell, 2003; Mohr & Fassinger, 2003). In addition, Ridge and Feeney (1998) found that although people with different attachment styles did not differ in retrospective reports of relationship quality with their mother before "coming out" (i.e., declaring their sexual orientation), secure lesbian women reported more positive relationships with their mothers after coming out (compared with their insecure counterparts); that is, attachment security not only facilitates early disclosure to parents but also contributes to maintaining healthy relationships with parents after disclosure. In this case, it seems likely that the ultimate independent variable is parental acceptance and support in the offspring's early years, which contributes to a child's secure attachment, and in turn helps the child later in life to achieve an authentic and positive identity.

There is also evidence that more secure gay and lesbian individuals hold more positive attitudes toward their homosexuality (e.g., Elizur & Mintzer, 2003; Jellison & McConnell, 2003; Mohr & Fassinger, 2003). In two samples of lesbian women, Wells (2003) and Wells and Hansen (2003) found that ratings of secure attachment were associated with less internalized shame and higher integration of private and public aspects of lesbian identity. In contrast, high ratings of either anxiety or avoidance were associated with higher levels of shame and more diffusion of lesbian identity.

Career Development

Another life task for adolescents and young adults is selecting and undertaking a career (Erikson, 1968). Like identity formation, this task involves exploring one's skills, abilities, preferences, and external opportunities and constraints, as well as committing oneself to specific career goals and plans (e.g., Super, Savickas, & Super, 1996). Effective resolution of the exploration and commitment tasks results in effective, reality-attuned career plans, formulation of coherent career goals that are well integrated with an emerging sense of personal identity, and the choice of a satisfying and productive career (Super et al., 1996). In contrast, premature commitment to a career without sufficient exploration, engaging in endless exploration, or remaining undecided about a career interfere with optimal career development and have negative consequences for the transition from adolescence to adulthood. Given the centrality of exploration and commitment in formulating and implementing a career plan, several researchers (e.g., Blustein, 1997; O'Brien, 1996) have targeted attachment security as a factor that might facilitate career development. In fact, the same psychological processes that underlie secure people's achievement of a stable sense of identity (cognitive openness, unconditional positive self-regard, self-confidence) are also likely to foster successful career development.

Research strongly supports a link between attachment security and career exploration. For example, adolescents who are more securely attached to their parents tend to report higher levels of exploration of career alternatives and self-focused exploration of their own career-related skills (Felsman & Blustein, 1999; Ketterson & Blustein, 1997; H. Y. Lee & Hughey, 2001). Another example is that more secure adolescents are more likely to read career brochures (Vignoli, Croity Belz, Chapeland, de Fillipis, & Garcia, 2005). Security of attachment to parents is associated with greater self-reported self-efficacy in career exploration (N.E. Ryan, Solberg, & Brown, 1996), more frequent engagement in thinking about and planning a career (Kenny, 1990; H. Y. Lee & Hughey, 2001), and less inclination to commit to a particular career without sufficient exploration (Blustein, Wallbridge, Friedlander, & Palladino, 1991; D. J. Scott & Church, 2001).

There is also evidence that attachment security facilitates career commitment and more effective performance in a chosen career. Adolescents who are more securely attached to parents make more progress in committing to particular career goals, and in being more aware of potential career-related obstacles and more willing to overcome these obstacles (Blustein et al., 1991; Felsman & Blustein, 1999; D. J. Scott & Church, 2001). They also report greater self-efficacy in career decision making, more often aspire to leadership positions within their career field, and make more realistic career choices that coincide with their abilities (O'Brien, 1996; O'Brien & Fassinger, 1993; O'Brien, Friedman, Tipton, & Linn, 2000; Rainey & Borders, 1997). In addition, Tokar, Withrow, Hall, and Moradi (2003) and Roney, Meredith, and Strong (2004) found that attachment anxiety or avoidance in close relationships is associated with indecisiveness about a career path and less satisfaction with one's choice.

Although this research provides consistent support for the idea that attachment security contributes to career development, the vast majority of studies published to date were based on cross-sectional designs and self-report measures. However, in a longitudinal study O'Brien et al. (2000) found that secure attachment to parents during adolescence contributed to greater self-efficacy in career decision making and higher career aspirations 5 years later. More remarkably, Roisman, Bahadur, and Oster (2000) found that attachment security in infancy (assessed with the Attachment Behavior Q-Sort; E. Waters, 1994) and current attachment security in relation to the mother (less maternal idealization and less maternal derogation in the AAI) significantly and uniquely contributed to higher levels of career exploration and planning during adolescence. These findings indicate that security (or something associated with it) is an important antecedent of favorable career development.

Academic Adjustment

Attachment-related differences in self-regulation should also affect academic performance and adjustment to school—important developmental tasks for adolescents and young adults in modern societies. Academic success requires a host of cognitive and social competencies and complex behavior-regulation skills. It requires cognitive openness, self-control, positive attitudes toward learning and problem solving, optimistic expectancies of academic success, and constructive ways of coping with frustrations and failures. A competent student is willing and able to learn new material and master increasingly complex cognitive problems, finds academic tasks enjoyable and rewarding, appraises academic tasks as challenges rather than threats, displays self-discipline and responsibility in completing assignments, persists in the face of academic obstacles, concentrates on academic tasks, and inhibits impulses that impair academic performance. As discussed earlier, attachment security supports such self-regulatory skills and should therefore contribute to academic success.

In fact, developmental studies of children and adolescents consistently show that secure attachment in infancy (assessed in the Strange Situation) contributes to academic skills, attitudes, and achievement later on. Specifically, attachment security in infancy is associated with more frequent spontaneous reading (Bus & van IJzendoorn, 1988), more enthusiastic engagement in challenging tasks (Matas, Arend, & Sroufe, 1978), and more efficient problem solving (Grossmann, Grossmann, & Zimmermann, 1999) during preschool. Moreover, Aviezer, Sagi, Resnick, and Gini (2002) found that secure infants were rated by their teachers at age 10 or 11 as having superior scholastic attitudes (motivation, persistence, and attention) and skills (oral and writing skills), even after controlling for intelligence and perceived competence.

Similar effects have been found when attachment security in relation to parents was assessed during elementary school. For example, Moss and St. Laurent (2001) assessed attachment behavior at age 6 and found that securely attached children got higher grades in school than their insecure counterparts at age 8. Jacobsen, Edelstein, and Hofmann (1994) found that attachment security at age 7 was an important predictor of superior concrete and formal operational reasoning between ages 7 and 15, and of superior formal deductive reasoning between ages 9 and 17 (even after controlling for intelligence and attention problems). Moreover, Jacobsen and Hofmann (1997) found that children who were securely attached at age 7 got higher teacher ratings on attention and participation in class, and superior school grades at ages 9, 12, and 15.

Several studies have also found positive associations between security of attachment to parents during late adolescence (using the IPPA or PAQ) and adjustment to college (Kenny & Donaldson, 1992; Lapsley, Rice, & Fitzgerald, 1990; Rice & Whaley, 1994; Vivona, 2000). Unfortunately, all of these studies used cross-sectional designs and exclusively relied on a single self-report measure of adaptation to the educational demands of college—the Student Adaptation to College Questionnaire (SACQ; R. W. Baker & Siryk, 1984). However, the link between secure attachment to parents and better academic adjustment to college has also been documented with other measures of academic adjustment (Cotterell, 1992) and replicated in a 2-year longitudinal study (Burge et al., 1997; Rice, Fitzgerald, Whaley, & Gibbs, 1995).

There is also evidence that attachment style in adolescent and adult close relationships is associated with academic adjustment. For example, Lapsley and Edgerton (2002) found that anxiously attached adolescents (assessed with the RQ) reported poorer college adjustment than did secure adolescents. In addition, Aspelmeier and Kerns (2003) found in two different samples that higher scores on attachment anxiety or avoidance (based on the AAQ) were associated with more problems in maintaining attention and concentration in academic tasks. Kogot (2004) found that more avoidant and anxious undergraduates (assessed with the ECR) reported lower self-efficacy in dealing with academic tasks.

Studies based on prospective or longitudinal designs also find connections between adolescents' attachment style, measured in various ways, and academic adjustment. A. L. Miller, Notaro, and Zimmermann (2002) assessed attachment security to friends twice in 2 years during adolescence and found that adolescents with a stably secure attachment orientation across the two waves of measurement had a more positive attitude toward school and higher academic self-efficacy than did adolescents who were stably insecure. Burge et al. (1997) found that greater security of attachment in close relationships during late adolescence (assessed with the AAS) was associated with self-reports of better school performance 2 years later (greater school satisfaction, fewer problems with deadlines). Furthermore, Doyle and Markiewicz (2005) found that more anxiously attached adolescents at age 13 exhibited a decline in school grades over the next 3 years (after controlling for social desirability).

The role played by attachment style in academic settings may be especially important during the transition to college. College students are expected to be more autonomous in managing their lives and to rely on self-regulatory skills when dealing with academic tasks (Larose, Bernier, & Tarabulsy, 2005). For example, they need to navigate and master a new environment and take more responsibility than ever for keeping themselves on track (registering, selecting courses, and getting to classes and examinations on time). They need greater self-discipline and have to resist more temptations than when they attended high school and lived at home. Moreover, the transition to college often involves separation from attachment figures (parents, friends, boyfriend or girlfriend), which activates attachment needs and creates emotional turmoil that can interfere with academic performance (Kenny, 1987b). Whereas anxiously attached students may be overwhelmed by the emotional turmoil of separation and the increasing demands for autonomous self-regulation, avoidant students' defensiveness may inhibit effective engagement and persistence in challenging and demanding academic activities.

These ideas were examined in Larose et al.'s (2005) longitudinal study of the transition to college. Students completed the Test of Reaction and Adaptation to College (TRAC) at the end of high school and again at the end of the first semester in college. They also completed the AAI during the second wave of measurement. In addition, academic grades were recorded at the end of high school, and at the end of each of the first three semesters in college. Both anxious and avoidant students reported poorer preparation for examinations and poorer attention to academic tasks at both points of measurement (compared with secure students). Moreover, anxiously attached students reported an increase in fear of academic failure and a decrease in the priority they assigned to studies during the college transition. Avoidance was associated with a decrease in quality of attention and exam preparation during the college transition, and lower grades after each of the first three semesters of college (even after Larose et al. controlled for high school grades). In contrast, secure students did not show a decrement in academic achievement during the transition to college, suggesting that they dealt effectively with the transition. Bernier, Larose, Boivin, and Soucy (2004) also found that insecure attachment (assessed with the AAI) was related to a drop in school grades during the transition from high school to college.

Attachment and Work

Freud has often been described as saying that the ability to work effectively is one of two main criteria for mental health and personal adjustment (the other being the ability to love). In fact, working effectively is a major life task from young adulthood to retirement age and an important contributor to life satisfaction, self-esteem, and social prestige, whereas not working effectively (and experiencing overload, burnout, dismissal, or unemployment) can be extremely stressful and cause serious emotional and physical maladies. Accomplishing the major life task of working effectively involves some of the same self-regulatory skills required for effective academic performance. One has to explore alternatives, develop and refine skills, adjust to changes in task and role demands, and practice conscientiousness and self-control. In most jobs and careers, there is also a high need for interpersonal communication, negotiation, and adaptation. Hence, various aspects of work are likely to be affected by individual differences in attachment style.

In their pioneering study of "love and work" viewed from an attachment-theoretical perspective, Hazan and Shaver (1990) accepted Bowlby's (1973) premise that secure attachment facilitates exploration, and argued that work is an adult form of exploration. As they explained,

> Adult work activity can be viewed as functionally parallel to what Bowlby calls exploration: For adults, work (like early childhood play and exploration) is a major source of actual and perceived competence. Adults' tendencies to seek and maintain proximity to an attachment figure and to move away from that figure in order to interact and master the environment are expressed, among other ways, in romantic love relationships and in productive work. (Hazan & Shaver, 1990, p. 271)

To test the validity of this idea, Hazan and Shaver assessed work attitudes and orientations in a large, self-selected sample of adult newspaper readers and found that securely attached people had more positive attitudes toward work and fewer work-related problems; they were more satisfied with their work activities and less likely than their insecure peers to allow work to interfere with relationships.

Hazan and Shaver (1990) also discovered that anxious people's work experiences were affected by their chronic hyperactivation of attachment needs and goal strivings. They perceived work as not only an additional opportunity for social acceptance but also a potential source of disapproval and rejection based on poor performance. They tended to be so preoccupied with attachment-related worries at work that they had trouble meeting job requirements (e.g., deadlines). This seemed to account for their lower than average salaries, even when gender and education were statistically controlled. Avoidant individuals tended to use work to evade social involvements and seemed not to balance work, social relations, and refreshing leisure effectively.

Building on Hazan and Shaver's (1990) study, Hardy and Barkham (1994) examined the influence of attachment style on job performance in a sample of adults referred for psychological treatment due to work-related distress. The results provided a conceptual replication of Hazan and Shaver's (1990) findings: More anxious or avoidant adults reported lower levels of work satisfaction. Moreover, anxiously attached people reported more concerns over their job performance, and avoidant people reported more conflicts with coworkers. Other cross-sectional studies have also found that higher levels of attachment anxiety and avoidance are associated with job dissatisfaction, work-related distress, and burnout (e.g., Krausz, Bizman, & Braslavsky, 2001; Pines, 2004; Schirmer & Lopez, 2001). These associations have also been corroborated in two longitudinal studies. Burge et al. (1997) found that attachment insecurities in parent–child or romantic relationships predicted decreases in adolescent women's work functioning 2 years later, and Vasquez, Durik, and Hyde (2002) found that insecure attachment in a sample of parents 1 year after the birth of their child predicted a greater feeling of work overload 3.5 years later. Of special importance, most of these associations persisted even when other psychological problems (e.g., depression) were statistically controlled. Taken together, these studies indicate that attachment insecurities contribute to poor adjustment in the workplace.

There is also evidence that attachment style contributes to the interaction of work and family dynamics. It is well known that family demands can divert mental resources away from work, and that family-related distress can spill over into the workplace (e.g., Zedeck, 1992). H. Sumer and Knight (2001) found that greater attachment security (assessed with the RQ) was associated with positive affect from family relations "spilling over" into the workplace, and with lower levels of spillover from family-related distress. Significantly, this adaptive regulation of positive and negative spillover from family to workplace was associated with secure people's higher job and life satisfaction.

H. Sumer and Knight (2001) also found that insecurely attached workers either missed the beneficial effects of family-related happiness or were overwhelmed by family-related distresses. Participants scoring higher on avoidant attachment reported more segmentation of work and family domains, and lower levels of spillover of family-related happiness into the workplace (perhaps another case of the tendency to deflect or suppress emotion, even when it is positive; see Chapter 7, this volume). Participants scoring higher on attachment anxiety reported greater spillover of family-related distress into the workplace (perhaps another case of their failure to control the automatic spread of distress-related thoughts and feelings from one mental or life domain to another; see Chapter 7, this volume). Anxious adults' maladaptive responses to family and work stresses were also documented by Raskin et al. (1998), who found that attachment-anxious women said they would cope with hypothetical work–family conflicts by trying to please others rather than negotiating their roles and creating a better balance between family and work.

Attachment, Self-Regulation, and Health Maintenance

As they move from childhood through adolescence to adulthood, people are expected to take greater responsibility for their own physical health. This requires self-regulatory skills such as exploring and learning about diseases, symptoms, and treatments; behavioral organization and planning (e.g., consulting with appropriate health professionals, purchasing insurance, making health-related decisions); self-discipline (e.g., exercising regularly, adhering to medical treatment regimens); avoiding unhealthy behavior (e.g., overeating, exposing oneself to dangerous drugs or other hazards); and maintaining optimism while dealing with inevitable physical illnesses and painful treatments. As shown throughout this chapter, secure attachment strengthens these kinds of self-regulatory processes and should therefore contribute to health maintenance.

Bowlby's (1969/1982) analysis of the conditions that activate the attachment system reveals how closely attachment-system and health-related conditions are likely to be. As we explained in Chapter 1, the attachment system is automatically activated by three kinds of threats: dangerous conditions in the external environment (e.g., a predator, a malevolent stranger), actual or anticipated separation from an attachment figure (which implies greater vulnerability to threats), and distressing internal conditions (e.g., fatigue, pain, or sickness). This analysis implies that actual or anticipated physical discomfort, pain, or illness is likely to activate attachment concerns, which means that people with different attachment orientations should differ in their responses to physical problems. Whereas secure individuals should be able to regulate distress effectively and reorganize behavior to prevent more serious physical problems, insecure individuals are likely to experience difficulties in dealing with unusual and distressing physical symptoms. Anxious people should be more concerned with the distress itself and the wish for others' love than with the best way to deal with the physical problem. Avoidant people's reluctance to explore novel situations, seek help, and engage in difficult problem solving, as well as their tendency to suppress distressing thoughts and emotions rather than cope effectively with their causes, may interfere with effective health care.

This attachment-theoretical analysis jibes well with Mikail, Henderson, and Tasca's (1994) interpersonal model of chronic pain. According to this model, securely attached people should be less susceptible to chronic pain because of their willingness to consult with health professionals, comply with professional advice, and react adaptively to life changes and medical interventions. In contrast, anxiously attached people are likely to be overwhelmed by distressing physical pain, feel that health professionals provide insufficient assistance, and engage in self-blame for injuries and illnesses. Mikail et al. also predicted that avoidant individuals would be reluctant to seek professional help and hostile toward and distrusting of health professionals. As a result, insecure people, whether anxious, avoidant, or both (i.e., fearfully avoidant), were expected to suffer more from chronic and severe physical pain.

These ideas have received some attention from adult attachment researchers, although no systematic research program has been developed to probe relations between attachment-related individual differences in self- and emotion regulation on the one hand, and effective health maintenance on the other. Studies to date have focused on attachment-related variations in health-promoting behaviors, adherence to medical treatment, and health status, without systematically examining the underlying regulatory skills that might account for the findings. Moreover, most of the studies rely on cross-sectional designs and so cannot reject the alternative hypothesis that physical health problems evoke changes in the attachment system, including diminution of the sense of attachment security. Nevertheless, the initial studies are intriguing and strongly suggest links between attachment and health, and they invite more systematic research on the topic.

In the first comprehensive study of attachment and health, J. A. Feeney and Ryan (1994) found that avoidant attachment was related to fewer self-reported healthcare visits over the next 10 weeks, even after controlling for the severity of physical symptoms.

More anxiously attached individuals reported a greater need to lose weight, combined with a lower rate of physical exercise (even after J. A. Feeney and Ryan controlled for body mass); that is, although anxious individuals expressed greater concern about their weight (see Chapter 13, this volume, for a discussion of links between attachment insecurities and eating disorders), they failed to take the necessary steps to lose weight.

These findings have been replicated and extended in subsequent studies. For example, attachment security was associated with reports of engaging in more health-promoting behaviors, such as maintaining a healthy diet or engaging in exercise, and avoiding health-related risks, such as smoking, drinking, and drug abuse (Huntsinger & Luecken, 2004; Scharfe & Eldredge, 2001). (See Chapter 13, this volume, for a discussion of links between attachment insecurities and substance abuse.) Ciechanowski, Walker, Katon, and Russo (2002) assessed attachment style in a large sample of primary care patients and found that fearfully avoidant women were less likely than secure women to make health care visits over a 6-month period despite reporting higher symptom levels. According to Ciechanowski, Walker, et al., "It is very likely that individuals with fearful attachment report more physical symptoms as a result of their increased distress and focus on negative affect, yet because of their cognitive schema of attachment, they are also more likely to engage inconsistently in any one mode of health care" (p. 665).

There is also evidence that attachment insecurities interfere with the patient–physician relationship. For example, Ciechanowski et al. (2004a) found, in a study of diabetic patients, that avoidant attachment was associated with poorer patient–physician communication, and Noyes et al. (2003) found that anxious attachment was associated with lower satisfaction with medical care and with feeling less assured by physicians. In a recent study, Maunder et al. (2006) overcame methodological problems associated with patient self-reports and asked physicians (who were blind to patients' attachment scores) to rate the difficulty of their relationships with particular patients. The results indicated that insecure patients, whether anxious, avoidant, or both, had more troubled relationships with their physicians than did secure patients; that is, insecure patients' relational problems, which have been studied mainly in the domain of close personal relationships, were also evident in doctor–patient relationships.

Research has also shown that attachment insecurities interfere with adherence to medical regimens. Ciechanowski, Katon, Russo, and Walker (2001) examined self-management in patients with diabetes and found that, compared with other attachment groups, avoidant patients who reported poor communication with their physicians adhered less well to glucose monitoring, generated more interruptions in treatment, and had higher levels of HbA1c (a physiological indicator of poor glucose control). In addition, Ciechanowski et al. (2004a) found that avoidant diabetic patients engaged in less exercise, maintained a poorer diet, cared less well for their feet (an important part of diabetes treatment), and took their medication less regularly than their secure counterparts. Of special significance from a theoretical standpoint, avoidant patients' poorer self-care was mediated by the poor quality of their relationships with their doctors. These findings were replicated and extended by Turan et al. (2003) and O. Cohen et al. (2005) in Turkish and Israeli samples, respectively, of diabetes patients. Overall, avoidant patients' poor self-care increased the severity and life-threatening danger of a serious chronic illness.

Other studies have found that attachment anxiety is linked with more frequent somatic symptoms, physical complaints, and hypochondriacal concerns in samples of healthy (i.e., nonpatient) young adults (e.g., J. A. Feeney, 1995b; J. A. Feeney & Ryan, 1994; Kidd & Sheffield, 2005; Muris, Meesters, & van den Berg, 2003; Myers & Vetere, 2002; Wearden, Cook, & Vaughan-Jones, 2003). These findings remained significant even after controlling for neuroticism (Bakker, Van Oudenhoven, & Van Der Zee, 2004; Noyes et al., 2003), negative affectivity (J. A. Feeney & Ryan, 1994; Wearden et al., 2005), or ways of coping (J. A. Feeney, 1995b), implying that attachment-anxious individuals tend to experience more physical problems for reasons beyond general personality traits. This tendency is also reflected in attachment-anxious individuals' reports of troubled sleep (Carmichael & Reis, 2005; Scharfe & Eldredge, 2001), persistent physical pain (MacDonald & Kingsbury, 2006), higher threat appraisals of chronic pain (Meredith, Strong, & Feeney, 2005), and lower perceived efficacy to deal with chronic pain (Meredith, Strong, & Feeney, 2006b).

The observed associations between anxious attachment and physical complaints can, with due caution, be interpreted causally, because Meredith, Strong, and Feeney (2006a), in a study of reactions to experimentally induced pain, found that attachment anxiety is a vulnerability factor for chronic pain. Participants with no history of chronic pain completed the RQ and were then exposed to an acute (coldpressor) pain experience. More attachment-anxious participants had lower coldpressor thresholds (i.e., they took less time after immersing their hand in ice cold water to report pain), higher reports of catastrophizing ideation (e.g., "It was terrible and I felt it was never going to get any better") following the coldpressor task, and lower perceptions of control over pain and ability to decrease pain. In contrast, secure participants were less likely to catastrophize and more likely to believe they could control the pain.

With regard to avoidant attachment, studies have not revealed a strong and consistent link between this kind of insecurity and reports of physical health problems (e.g., J. A. Feeney, 1995b; Kidd & Sheffield, 2005; Muris et al., 2003; Myers & Vetere, 2002; Wearden et al., 2003). Because all of the studies relied on self-reports, the inconsistency may be due to avoidant people's reluctance to acknowledge life difficulties, or to disclose personal weaknesses or vulnerabilities. However, when researchers studied patients with diagnosed physical diseases, the negative influence of avoidance was clearer and more consistent. Compared to nonclinical control samples, women with breast cancer are relatively high on avoidant attachment (Tacon, Caldera, & Bell, 2001), as are patients diagnosed with somatoform diseases (Waller, Scheidt, & Hartmann, 2004) and those suffering from gastroesophageal reflux disease (Ercolani, Farinelli, Trombini, & Bortolotti, 2004). In addition, Picardi et al. (2003) and Picardi, Mazzotti, et al. (2005) found higher avoidance among patients suffering from vitiligo (a skin pigmentation disorder) or psoriasis (a chronic inflammatory skin disease) than among outpatients with skin conditions in which psychosomatic factors are negligible (even after controlling for stressful life events). In a sample of clinical tinnitus patients (who experience a ringing or buzzing in their ears in the absence of external sounds), Granqvist, Lantto, Ortiz, and Andersson (2001) found that both attachment anxiety and avoidance were associated with more severe tinnitus.

In a study of genetic markers of ulcerative colitis (UC), Maunder, Lancee, Greenberg, Hunter, and Fernandes (2000) found higher avoidance among patients with UC who had no genetic marker for developing the disorder than in patients with a UC genetic marker. This implies that avoidant attachment is involved in developing the disorder, rather than being a mere consequence of the disorder, because it would be difficult to explain why genetically unexplained UC produced more avoidance than genetically caused UC. This dramatic conclusion is reinforced by findings from studies showing that insecure attachment is more common in patients whose symptoms lacked an organic explanation than among patients with organically explicable physical symptoms, even after controlling for general mental health (Ciechanowski, Katon, Russo, & Dwight-Johnson, 2002; R. E. Taylor, Mann, White, & Goldberg, 2000).

Attachment Foundations of a Religious or Spiritual Approach to Life

Beyond contributing to physical survival and mastering various life tasks such as career development, academic performance, and health maintenance, attachment security may facilitate what the psychoanalyst Carl Jung (1958) viewed as an important indicator of psychological growth and maturity in adulthood: the development of a religious, spiritual, or philosophical approach to life. This often involves developing a faith that life goes beyond the biological realm and that one is part of a larger spiritual entity or enterprise ("God") that provides meaning to existence, transcends biological limitations, and expands the boundaries and capacities of the isolated self. It also typically involves endorsement of the humane values and ethical behavior encouraged by most religious denominations, such as benevolence, compassion, forgiveness, and generosity toward other human beings, if not "all sentient beings" (Dalai Lama, 2001). In terms of Jung's (1958) theory of psychological development, the attainment of a mature religious or spiritual approach to life is the heart of the individuation process by which people integrate personal and collective aspects of their personality, as well as biological and spiritual realms of existence. This component of individuation involves confronting the mysteries of life and death, achieving deep respect for other beings, and living a meaningful life.

How might attachment security contribute to a mature religious or spiritual perspective? Attachment theorists (e.g., Granqvist, 2005; Kirkpatrick, 2005) have noted that the relationship between a believer and his or her "God" often meets the three defining criteria of an attachment relationship—seeking and maintaining proximity (e.g., the Protestant hymn, "Nearer My God to Thee"), achieving a safe haven in times of distress ("Yea, though I walk through the valley of the shadow of death, I will fear no evil, for thou art with me"; Psalm 23:4), and using a "stronger and wiser" other as a secure base (e.g., "On the day I called, you answered me and made me bold with strength in my soul"; Psalm 138:3). Believers assume that God is omnipresent, therefore, always nearby, and that they can increase proximity and closeness through religious practices, such as praying, meditating, performing sacred rituals, and engaging in altruistic acts. It is also well known that people turn to God in times of stress and distress; countless prayers amount to asking for assistance, comfort, reassurance, and relief. Thus, it seems likely that people project their working models of human attachment figures onto God (a tenet that Kirkpatrick calls the "correspondence" hypothesis). In other words, secure adults are likely to be able to project positive working models onto God and feel comfortable seeking proximity to God, confident in God's supportiveness, and emotionally secure in opening themselves up to faith and spiritual transformation. Less secure individuals may have more difficulty imagining God as an always-available, highly responsive attachment figure.

Secure people's self-regulatory skills should contribute to more mature forms of spirituality. Their cognitive openness should allow them to explore spiritual possibilities and engage in what Batson (1976; Batson, Schoenrade, & Ventis, 1993) called a religious "quest"—exploration of core existential questions and development of an autonomous, individuated spirituality that includes tolerance of the ambiguity, uncertainty, and confusion inherent in an open-minded quest. In addition, their willingness to take responsibility for their decisions and actions may facilitate an understanding of the ways their actions promote or hinder the welfare of others. Beyond these self-regulatory skills, secure individuals' relative lack of fear, their sense of connection with others (see Chapter 9, this volume), and their caring and compassionate attitudes toward others' suffering (see Chapter 12, this volume) may help them adhere to the humanistic values (e.g., the Golden Rule) embodied in most world religions.

We do not mean to imply, of course, that insecurely attached people have no religious experiences or religious beliefs. In fact, Kirkpatrick (2005) assumed that insecure people can sometimes compensate (or, at least, attempt to compensate) for their frustrating human attachment experiences by directing their unmet attachment needs to God (the "compensation" hypothesis); that is, insecure people can turn to God as an alternative attachment figure whose beneficence may overcome fears associated with human attachment figures. However, their approach to religion can be expected to differ from that of more secure individuals. Whereas secure people's spirituality results, theoretically, from exploratory, growth, and self-expansion motives, insecure people's spirituality may include defensive efforts to overcome mundane frustrations and pains. Moreover, insecure people may project not only their need for a good attachment figure onto God but also the insecurities and negative working models acquired in other attachment relationships. They may view God, at least at times, as a harsh, rejecting figure; feel uncertain about God's love, care, and acceptance (in the case of anxious people); or try to maintain distance and independence from God (in the case of avoidant people). (One of our avoidant friends once said, jokingly, "I definitely have a relationship with God: I leave him alone and he leaves me alone.") In addition, cognitive closure motivated by insecurity may prevent a comfortable religious quest and interfere with the attainment of autonomous spirituality. Insecure people may be especially prone to dogmatic, fundamentalist beliefs that portray God as an angry, sometimes arbitrary, judgmental figure who needs to be obeyed and placated lest he explode in rage and violence.

In the first studies of attachment and religiosity, Kirkpatrick and Shaver (1990, 1992) found that people who reported being more securely attached to parents or romantic partners were also more likely to report having a personal relationship with God ("I feel that I have a relationship with God") and to believe in a personal God ("God is a living, personal being who is interested and involved in human lives and affairs"). These findings were replicated in subsequent cross-sectional studies (Granqvist, 1998; Granqvist & Hagekull, 1999, 2000; Kirkpatrick, 1998b) and extended to other measures of religiosity. Attachment security has been associated with a more intrinsic (autonomous) religious orientation (Diller, 2006; Kirkpatrick & Shaver, 1990), greater commitment to religious beliefs and practices (Byrd & Boe, 2001; Kirkpatrick & Shaver, 1990, 1992; Mickelson et al., 1997; Saroglou, Pichon, Trompette, Verschueren, & Dernelle, 2005), and higher scores on a measure of mature spirituality (TenElshof & Furrow, 2000). Although most of these studies focused on Christians in the United States and Sweden, some of the findings have been replicated in two studies of Israeli Jews (Diller, 2006; Gurwitz, 2004).

Several studies have found that the association between attachment security and religiosity is moderated by parental religiosity; that is, young adults who are securely attached to their parents tend to display higher levels of religiosity than their insecure counterparts, mainly when their parental attachment figures were also religious (Granqvist, 1998, 2002; Granqvist & Hagekull, 1999; Kirkpatrick & Shaver, 1990). In fact, Granqvist and Hagekull (1999; Granqvist, 2002) found that more secure people scored higher on a measure of socialization-based religiosity (the extent to which participants adopt their parents' religious standards). These findings led Granqvist (2005) to propose a two-level correspondence hypothesis, by which social learning of parental religiosity in the context of secure attachment has effects on an offspring's religiosity beyond the projection of positive working models onto God.

There are also interesting findings about the religiosity of insecurely attached adults. Kirkpatrick (1997) asked participants in Hazan and Shaver's (1987) early survey study of romantic attachment to complete a questionnaire on religiousness 4 years later. He found that insecure women, whether anxious or avoidant, were more likely than secure women to report having formed a new relationship with God during the preceding 4-year period. Anxiously attached women were also more likely to report increases in religious experiences, such as being "born again" and speaking in tongues (glossolalia). This association between attachment anxiety and increases in religiousness over time was also observed by Kirkpatrick (1998b) in a subsequent study over a shorter time period (4 months) and in both sexes.

Research has also linked attachment insecurities with sudden religious conversions, that is, increases in religiousness characterized by a sudden and intense personal experience (e.g., Kirkpatrick & Shaver, 1990; Granqvist, 1998, 2002; Granqvist & Hagekull, 1999, 2001). In a meta-analysis of all available data on this issue, encompassing around 1,500 research participants, Granqvist and Kirkpatrick (2004) concluded that people classified as insecure in their relationships with parents are more likely than secure people to experience a sudden religious conversion. There is also evidence that attachment insecurity, assessed either by self-report scales or the AAI, is associated with greater interest in New Age beliefs, spiritualism, and esotericism (Granqvist & Hagekull, 2001, 2005; Saroglou, Kempeneers, & Seynhaeve, 2003).

Given that both secure and insecure individuals can adopt a religious approach to life, it has been important to explore differences in secure and insecure forms of religiosity. The meta-analysis by Granqvist and Kirkpatrick (2004) revealed that whereas people who were securely attached to their parents report gradual changes in religiousness, the changes experienced by insecure people were more sudden and emotionally turbulent. In addition, secure people's increases in religiosity were characterized by themes of affiliation and correspondence with significant others' religious standards, such as becoming more religious in connection with close friendships with believers (Granqvist & Hagekull, 1999, 2001). In contrast, insecure people's religious changes were characterized by themes of compensation, such as becoming more religious in response to problematic close relationships, personal crises, and mental or physical illness (Granqvist, 2002; Granqvist & Hagekull, 1999, 2001). Furthermore, whereas secure people were more religious if their parents had been religious, insecure people were more religious mainly when parents displayed low levels of religiosity (Granqvist, 1998; Kirkpatrick & Shaver, 1990). Thus, insecure religiosity may be a defensive attempt to distance oneself from parents and compensate for insecurities and personal crises, rather than a gradual and positive identification with the values and beliefs held by parents and other close relationship partners.

In a prospective (15-month) study of changes in religiosity during adolescence, Granqvist and Hagekull (2003) found that secure people exhibited increases in religiosity over the 15-month period mainly when they had formed a new romantic relationship during this period. Thus, their sense of spirituality or religiosity seemed to be influenced by an intimate interpersonal relationship. In contrast, insecure adolescents showed an increase in religiosity mainly when a painful romantic relationship breakup occurred during the 15-month study. These findings suggest that religiosity is more "compensatory" for insecure adults. The same patterns occurred in a subsequent study that used the AAI as a measure of adult attachment orientation (Granqvist & Hagekull, 2005).

Secure and insecure adults also differ in the extent to which God and religious beliefs provide a sense of having a safe haven and secure base. For example, securely attached people score higher than their insecurely attached counterparts on scales tapping emotionally based religiosity—the use of God as a safe haven and secure base (Granqvist,

2002; Granqvist & Hagekull, 2000)—and react to subliminal primes of rejection and separation with heightened religiosity of this kind (Birgegard & Granqvist, 2004). In a conceptual replication of these findings among Jewish believers, Gurwitz (2004) found that more secure participants (those with lower scores on the ECR Anxiety and Avoidance dimensions) reacted to subliminal exposure to threat-related words such as "failure" or "death" (compared with neutral words) with higher mental activation of God-related concepts (indicated by shorter reaction times in a lexical decision task). Gurwitz also found that more secure participants reacted to subliminal exposure to religion-related pictures (compared with neutral pictures) with more positive affect (projected onto previously neutral stimuli). Together, these findings indicate that (1) secure people displayed higher automatic activation of religious mental representations during threatening conditions than insecure people, and (2) this activation had more beneficial affective consequences for secure than for insecure people. This suggests that attachment security supports effective use of religious concepts and images as a psychological "safe haven."

If God is truly used as an attachment figure, in the sense implied by Bowlby's (1969/1982) theory, secure and insecure people should appraise and relate to God somewhat differently. Using P. Benson and Spilka's (1973) Loving and Controlling God-Image Scales, several researchers have found that more securely attached people (assessed with either self-report measures or the AAI) are more likely to view God as a loving, approving, and caring figure (Gurwitz, 2004; Granqvist & Hagekull, 2005; Kirkpatrick, 1998b; Kirkpatrick & Shaver, 1990, 1992). This finding has been conceptually replicated in a study using a less explicit measure of God images. Gurwitz (2004) found that whereas secure participants reacted to subliminal exposure to the word "God" (compared to a neutral word) with faster reactions to positive trait terms (e.g., loving, caring) in a lexical decision task, insecure participants reacted faster to negative trait terms (e.g., rejecting, distant). This indicates, again, that attachment security is associated with greater cognitive access to positive mental representations of God, and that attachment working models forged in early human relationships get transferred onto God.

In an early attempt to probe attachment style differences in the way people (mostly Christians) relate to God, Kirkpatrick and Shaver (1992) constructed a self-report scale to measure attachment to God and found that insecure participants (in human relationships) were more likely to have an insecure relationship with God. This correspondence between human attachment style and style of attachment to God has been replicated by researchers using other measures of attachment to God (R. Beck & McDonald, 2004; McDonald, Beck, Allison, & Norsworthy, 2005; Rowatt & Kirkpatrick, 2002) and in Israeli Jewish samples (Diller, 2006; Gurwitz, 2004).

In a recent study of religious orientations among young-adult Israeli Jews, Diller (2006) found links between insecure attachment and difficulties with religious exploration: More avoidant individuals were less involved in a religious quest (assessed with Batson's Religion as Quest Scale), experienced more distress during periods of uncertainty and doubt about religious beliefs, and were more negative in their appraisals of a hypothetical person who was asking spiritual or existential questions. Although attachment anxiety was not associated in either direction with a questing orientation to religion, it was associated with greater emotional turmoil during periods of religious quest and more ambivalent feelings about a person who was engaged in a religious quest. Thus, insecure people were more disturbed than their secure peers by a questing approach to religion or spirituality. This supports our idea that attachment security provides a foundation for mature religiosity. We say this without endorsing any particular religion; so far, the findings seem to be theoretically consistent across the different religions studied. Thus, we interpret the findings in psychological, not theological, terms.

CONCLUDING REMARKS

We began this chapter by explaining that Bowlby's (1969/1982) attachment theory was innovative partly by virtue of taking seriously the cybernetic approach to conceptualizing goal-directed, and "goal-corrected" (Bowlby's term), behavior. This was in stark contrast to Freud's drive theory of motivation, which was understandably weak in its conceptualization of cognitive processes—a central aspect of mental life that had to await the arrival of digital computers and technologies that provide models of cognitive programming and behavioral self-regulation. Bowlby was influenced both by then-new military technology (he served in the British Navy during World War II) and Piaget's theory of cognitive development, which was as different from previous learning theories as cybernetics was from psychoanalysis. As a result of his emphasis on cognitive models and cognitive development, Bowlby was especially interested in cognitive aspects of both behavioral and emotional self-regulation.

Throughout this chapter we have shown that Bowlby's ideas provide fruitful guidelines for studying the role played by adult attachment style in self-regulation, in domains as different as daily personal strivings, success in college, balancing work–family pressures, maintaining good health, and achieving a mature spiritual perspective on life. Although many interesting findings have been obtained over the first 20 years of adult attachment research, most of the studies have been correlational and cross-sectional in design rather than longitudinal and experimental; many have involved only self-report measures; and only a few have measured both the primary independent and dependent variables and the proposed mediating variables. Few studies have included measures relevant to alternative explanations, such as common determination of independent and dependent variables by genetic or temperamental factors of the kind assessed indirectly by measures of the "Big Five" personality factors or common influences of states of mental health, such as depression. Fortunately, in cases when these potential confounds have been assessed and statistically controlled, the attachment-theoretical interpretations of the findings have been supported.

The prospects are therefore excellent for future research that explores mediating processes and evaluates the replicability and generalizability of existing findings to other societies and non-Western forms of religion, or to major philosophies of life that take the place of traditional religions. For example, we know almost nothing about the role of attachment processes in Buddhism or Taoism, where there is no personal God with whom one might establish a close relationship. Interestingly, a common Buddhist prayer encourages adherents to "take refuge in the Buddha, the Dharma, and the Sangha"—a mentally represented loving teacher, the scriptures flowing from his teachings, and the local religious community that disseminates the teachings and supports their practice (see Chapter 16, this volume). Combined with reverence for personal teachers and models, such as local monks and internationally known exemplars such as the Dalai Lama, these safe havens ("refuges") may serve some of the same psychological functions as the image of God the Father and Jesus Christ in Judaism and Christianity, respectively. Finding ways to retain these essential attachment-related aspects of religion, while deemphasizing dogmatic differences between sects, would be one good way to improve the chances of world peace and personal security of all kinds.

PART III

INTERPERSONAL MANIFESTATIONS OF ATTACHMENT-SYSTEM FUNCTIONING

CHAPTER 9

∎ ∎ ∎

An Attachment Perspective on Interpersonal Regulation

Although, as we have shown in previous chapters, attachment-system functioning can be studied productively at the intrapsychic level, where it can be characterized in terms of wishes, fears, defenses, and self-regulatory strategies, it also (1) shapes interpersonal behavior (e.g., proximity seeking, intimacy avoidance), (2) biases the operation of other behavioral systems (e.g., caregiving, sex), and (3) contributes to the quality of social interactions in general and close relationships in particular. Moreover, attachment-system functioning involves not only actual interpersonal behavior but also imagined interactions with actual (externally present) and internalized (symbolic) relationship partners. It is important to note that the causal processes relating attachment-system functioning with other people's social behavior are bidirectional; that is, the parameters of the attachment system are gradually shaped by relationship partners' responses to bids for proximity and emotional support, and these parameters in turn influence (and sometimes bias) people's feelings, thoughts, attitudes, and behaviors, which in turn influence relationship partners' reactions.

In this chapter we focus on *interpersonal regulation*—the processes that regulate a person's interactions with others. This is a special case of self-regulation (Chapter 8, this volume), in which people formulate, organize, and enact behavioral plans to get closer to a desired goal state or distance themselves from a feared or unwanted anti-goal state. The additional complexity in this chapter is that interpersonal regulation involves at least one other person (a relationship partner), and the goal and anti-goal states are desired and undesired forms of interactions and connections with the partner (e.g., becoming more intimate, controlling the partner's behavior, avoiding intimacy, avoiding the partner's influence or control). Whereas the pursuit of personal goals of the kind discussed in Chapter 8, this volume, depends largely on one's own intentions and ability to organize one's own behavior (e.g., studying effectively for an exam, conforming to a particular diet to get healthier, choosing a suitable career or social identity), pursuing interpersonal goals depends on a partner's intentions and actions, as well as one's own (e.g., on his or her responsiveness to one's bids for closeness or influence).

In interpersonal regulation, one's behavioral plans have to be oriented toward affecting a partner's views or responses, so that one can attain a desired interpersonal outcome. Thus, interpersonal regulation involves "interdependence" (Thibault & Kelley, 1959): One's own outcomes depend on a partner's choices and actions, and the partner's outcomes depend on one's own choices and actions. In attachment theory, interdependence is evident when the attachment system becomes activated and a person attempts to elicit care and support from an attachment figure. The outcome depends on both the first person's strategy for eliciting care and the attachment figure's response to this strategy.

These special features of interpersonal regulation make it complicated, and somewhat unpredictable and risky. Like other forms of self-regulation, it requires not only effective organization and execution of intentional behaviors, as well as inhibition of interfering motives and responses, but also effective communication; attentiveness to a partner's needs, intentions, preferences, and actions; and flexible adjustment of plans in accordance with a partner's reactions. Interpersonal regulation is somewhat like dancing with a partner; it requires well-timed, subtle communication and the coordination of complex, synchronized movements. When successful, this kind of "dancing" helps both partners satisfy their social needs and form a satisfying, long-lasting relationship. It can be exciting, demanding, and very rewarding. Although one person can sometimes get some of what he or she wants without being very cognizant or considerate of a partner's needs and preferences, in the long run neither coercion nor inattentiveness to the other's needs and wishes is likely to yield a stable, mutually rewarding relationship.

As in self-regulation, the first step in interpersonal regulation is goal setting, based on the kind of interaction a person desires at a particular time, and under a particular set of circumstances. This first step depends on context, because it often does not make sense to seek a goal that cannot possibly be attained in a particular situation. However, goal setting also reflects core wishes that a person generally wants to satisfy in interpersonal relations, as well as interpersonal dispositions (i.e., traits) that habitually structure the person's social interactions. Both core wishes and interpersonal dispositions make particular goals chronically salient and cause people to move toward them almost regardless of context. For example, attachment-anxious people who chronically yearn for love and affection often try to maximize closeness even when their partner is uninterested or temporarily occupied with another goal.

According to most theoretical accounts of interpersonal needs, traits, and behaviors (e.g., L. S. Benjamin, 1974, 1994; Kiesler, 1996; T. Leary, 1957; Wiggins, 1979), interpersonal goals are organized around two orthogonal dimensions: (1) *nurturance* or *affiliation*, which ranges from close, intimate, warm, and friendly interactions to distant, cold, and hostile interactions; and (2) *social dominance*, which ranges from submissive, unconfident behavior to assertive, commanding behavior. One's position along the nurturance dimension is determined by the amount of closeness or distance he or she wishes to maintain with respect to relationship partners. One's position along the dominance dimension reflects the amount of control or power he or she wants to exert over others. Different kinds of interpersonal goals can be represented conceptually by pairs of locations on the two dimensions, and the goals can be portrayed as arranged in a circular, or circumplex, pattern, as depicted in Figure 9.1. For example, obtaining support from a "stronger, wiser" partner in times of need is located in the close–submissive quadrant; providing care to a needy other is located in the close–dominant quadrant.

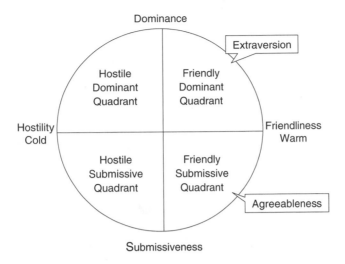

Dominance

FIGURE 9.1. The interpersonal circumplex.

The same circumplex can be used to characterize a person's interpersonal dispositions or traits. For example, extraverted behavior (or the underlying trait of extraversion) is located in the close–dominant quadrant of the circumplex; agreeable behavior (or the trait of agreeableness) is located in the close–submissive quadrant (McCrae & Costa, 1989). Several factor-analytic studies have shown that the circumplex model accounts for a large portion of the variance in people's interpersonal traits and behaviors (e.g., Conte & Plutchik, 1981; Wiggins, 1991).

Interpersonal regulation also depends on behavioral plans of the kind we discussed in Chapter 8, which involve assessment of action effectiveness and adjustment of interpersonal behavior based on feedback. Interpersonal regulation also involves behavioral interruptions and goal disengagement when the likelihood of altering a partner's behavior seems low and a person becomes convinced that he or she simply does not have the skills, persistence, or response options required for achieving the desired outcome, at least under present circumstances. In line with Carver and Scheier's (1981, 1998) model of self-regulation (described in Chapter 8, this volume), goal disengagement from one partner at a particular time allows a person to move flexibly among different interaction partners. Some partners are good support providers, for example, and others are not, although they may be good at something else. Flexibility and diversity increase the complexity of one's interpersonal world and prevent the accumulation of interpersonal tensions. In fact, behavioral rigidity and compulsive fixation on one interpersonal goal (e.g., extreme closeness or distance) create problems in a relationship and lead to poor outcomes.

Beyond the cognitive skills that facilitate individual-level goal setting, behavioral organization, and flexible deployment of intentional behavior (see Chapter 8, this volume), interpersonal regulation also depends on interpersonal competencies that allow a person to negotiate interpersonal exchanges—competencies such as expressiveness, sensitivity, and conflict management (e.g., Fincham & Beach, 1999; Riggio, 1986, 1993). "Expressiveness" is the ability to convey needs, intentions, emotions, and thoughts through verbal and nonverbal channels. Without this ability, people are unable to communicate effectively about what they need or want or feel, and their partners are likely to dismiss or misinterpret the poor communicators' interpersonal needs and actions (Riggio, 1986). Interpersonal "sensitivity" is the ability to perceive accurately and interpret a partner's verbal and nonverbal signals. Without this ability, people are unable to monitor and understand partners' responses and are therefore less likely to adjust their behavior to comply with partners' needs and signals (Riggio, 1986). "Conflict management" refers to the ability to handle interpersonal problems in ways that restore relationship harmony. This ability is crucial whenever partners hold incompatible goals, which is a common occurrence in any highly involved, long-term relationship (Fincham & Beach, 1999).

By definition, the attachment system is an interpersonal regulatory device. Perceived threats and dangers make salient the interpersonal goal of gaining proximity to and support from a security-providing attachment figure, and this encourages people to learn, organize, and implement behavioral plans aimed at attaining safety and support. As explained in earlier chapters, Bowlby (1969/1982) assumed that the attachment system operates in a "goal-corrected" manner; that is, a person evaluates the progress he or she is making toward achieving support and comfort from a partner and corrects intended actions, if necessary, to attain these goals. Effective functioning of the attachment system includes the use of partner-tailored proximity-seeking strategies that take into account a partner's needs and preferences (creating what Bowlby [1973] called a "goal-corrected partnership"). This facilitates satisfying, harmonious interactions that might otherwise devolve into intrusive, coercive, or angry exchanges rooted in coordination failures and mismatched needs and responses.

Attachment-system functioning, like all interpersonal regulation, involves competent expressiveness, sensitivity, and conflict management. To achieve the set-goal of security, children must express their needs for proximity and support, attend carefully to attachment figures' responses, be sensitive to verbal and nonverbal signals generated by attachment figures in response to proximity-seeking bids, and manage the occasional misalignment of cues or the goal conflicts that endanger support provision. Although the foundations of these competencies are assumed to be innate aspects of the attachment system, interactions with available attachment figures allow children to learn about the effectiveness of their interpersonal skills and provide opportunities to practice and refine them. In contrast, interactions with rejecting figures cast a pall over early efforts to be expressive, sensitive, and cooperative. Unresponsive attachment figures force a child to acquire interpersonal skills that may seem adaptive in their original context (e.g., inhibiting the expression of attachment needs when a parent is avoidant) but can cause trouble later on, when a person encounters new relationship partners, with different salient needs and preferences, who make different relational demands.

Our model of attachment-system functioning (Chapter 2, this volume) indicates that individual differences in attachment style learned in particular relationships can bias subsequent interpersonal goal setting. Attachment-anxious people overemphasize the need for protection and intimacy, and avoidant people overemphasize the need for autonomy and interpersonal distance. In addition, attachment insecurities can interfere with the graceful "dance" of coordinated intimacy, because an insecure person can be so wrapped up in worries and defenses that he or she is unable to attend to a partner's cues. In the following sections, we consider associations between attachment style and various aspects of interpersonal regulation.

ATTACHMENT-SYSTEM FUNCTIONING
AND THE PROCESS OF INTERPERSONAL REGULATION

Here we examine various components of interpersonal regulation. First, we deal with associations between attachment style and interpersonal wishes and goals. Second, we review evidence concerning attachment style differences in interpersonal dispositions. Third, we consider the adverse effects of attachment insecurities on the interpersonal competencies of expressiveness, sensitivity, and conflict management. Fourth, we present new findings concerning attachment style differences in the coordination of one's own and a partner's needs and actions.

Interpersonal Wishes and Goals

According to our model, each of the major organized attachment strategies—secure, anxious, and avoidant—involves particular wishes and fears about regulating security, closeness, dependency, and autonomy within relationships; that is, people with different attachment styles differ in the extent to which they are motivated to seek closeness, avoid rejection, and maintain autonomy. For example, secure individuals have learned that proximity seeking is rewarding and contributes to an authentic, autonomous sense of self-worth (Chapter 6, this volume). As a result, secure people do not view closeness and autonomy as antagonistic goals. Getting close to others does not threaten the sense of autonomy, and maintaining an autonomous stance does not induce worries about connectedness or lovability. In other words, secure individuals can flexibly move along the closeness–distance dimension of the circumplex without being afraid of losing autonomy or a partner's love.

In contrast, insecurely attached people are less able to balance or coordinate closeness and autonomy. They are compulsively driven to pursue goals that serve unmet attachment needs, reduce their fears, and allow them to maintain well-practiced defenses. Anxious people tend to select interpersonal goals compatible with their intense needs for closeness and security, which causes them to behave in a clingy, dependent, and vigilant manner aimed, often unsuccessfully, at gaining partners' reliable love. Avoidant people tend to organize their interactions around desires for optimal distance, self-reliance, and control. Whereas anxious people fear rejection and abandonment, avoidant ones are averse to closeness and interdependence.

Core Interpersonal Wishes

Using the Core conflictual relationship themes (CCRT) method for coding open-ended narratives (Luborsky & Crits-Christoph, 1998), three studies (Avihou, 2006; Raz, 2002; Waldinger et al., 2003) provide evidence of predictable links between attachment orientation and interpersonal wishes. In Raz's (2002) and Waldinger et al.'s (2003) studies, participants were asked to recall and describe interactions with close relationship partners. Judges read the narratives and used the CCRT coding scheme to infer the underlying wishes. Whereas Raz (2002) assessed attachment style with a self-report scale (the RQ), Waldinger et al. (2003) used the AAI. Despite the use of different measures, both studies found that avoidant attachment was associated with wishes, revealed in interpersonal narratives, for autonomy and distance (to assert oneself, to retain emotional distance). In addition, Raz (2002) found that attachment anxiety was associated with wishes to be loved and accepted by others. Waldinger et al. (2003) found no association between anxious attachment assessed with the AAI and any of the CCRT wish categories.

Avihou's (2006) study of dreams (described in Chapter 6, this volume) revealed that attachment-related interpersonal wishes are expressed in dreams. Using the CCRT coding scheme, judges analyzed dreams reported by study participants over a 30-day period and coded the interpersonal wishes evident in each one. People who scored high on attachment anxiety expressed more wishes to be loved and accepted by others in their dreams. In contrast, avoidant people expressed more wishes to assert themselves, to oppose and control others, and to remain distant while avoiding conflicts. Interestingly, these attachment-related differences were more notable in dreams occurring on nights when participants reported higher levels of negative emotion before falling asleep; that is, theoretically speaking, attachment-related wishes seem to be unconsciously aroused mainly when the attachment system is activated by distress.

In a recent study, Banai, Mikulincer, and Shaver (2005) constructed a self-report scale to assess Kohut's (1977, 1984) needs for mirroring, idealization, and twinship, and examined associations between these constructs and self-reports of attachment anxiety and avoidance. Attachment anxiety was correlated with "hunger for mirroring" (i.e., wishing to be admired for one's qualities and accomplishments), idealization (forming idealized images of significant others, then wishing to merge with them), and twinship (feeling similar to others and being accepted by them in close relationships). These correlations indicate, once again, in terms of a psychodynamic theory other than attachment theory (i.e., Kohut's self psychology), that anxious people suffer from unmet needs and wishes for love, closeness, and merger. In contrast, avoidant people shun or deny these three needs, indicating again that they prefer to distance themselves from others.

Interpersonal Goals

Research has also shown that attachment insecurities bias the kinds of goals people habitually pursue in interpersonal exchanges. For example, Collins, Guichard, Ford, and Feeney (2004) reported that, compared with secure young adults, anxiously attached adults tended to overemphasize the importance of a partner's love and support within couple relationships, and avoidant participants tended to dismiss these closeness-related goals. Similarly, J. A. Feeney (1999b), who asked dating couples to describe the conflicts occurring in their relationships, found that whereas avoidant men spontaneously mentioned more goal conflicts related to needs for self-reliance and control of the emotional climate of the relationship, anxious women mentioned more goal conflicts related to needs for closeness and merger.

Additional evidence comes from Mikulincer's (1998c) studies of goals related to establishing a sense of interpersonal trust. Attachment-anxious individuals' reactions reflected their characteristic pursuit of closeness and security. They reported trusting others as a means of gaining a partner's love and support, and displayed heightened access to thoughts about attachment security after being primed with sentences reflecting a partner's trustworthiness (faster lexical decision times for security-related words). For them, relationship episodes in which a partner behaved in a trustworthy manner were appraised as contributing to felt security, whereas betrayal of trust was appraised as damaging this feeling. Avoidant people's reactions reflected a desire for dominance and control. They viewed expressions of interpersonal trust as manipulative means to control others' behavior ("If I trust you, you should trust me and allow me to do what I want").

In a study of attachment and affiliation in adolescent friendships, Mikulincer and Selinger (2001) obtained evidence for secure adolescents' flexible goals and ability to integrate goals. These adolescents placed high value on both attachment-related goals (support and security) and affiliation-related goals (having fun together, working on joint projects). Moreover, they were able to alter their goals in accordance with contextual cues, for example, pursuing attachment goals in attachment-relevant contexts (disclosing a secret, dealing with a sad mood) and pursuing affiliation goals in less demanding, less intimate contexts (going to a party together, sharing a positive mood). In contrast, insecure adolescents were less flexible in pursuing their goals. Attachment-anxious adolescents were almost exclusively focused on gaining support and security even in nonintimate contexts. Avoidant adolescents dismissed both attachment and affiliation goals without regard to context; that is, avoidant adolescents not only dismissed security needs but also deemphasized goals associated with affiliation, thereby rejecting both nurturance and sociability.

Besides assessing attachment style differences in goals states, researchers have examined outcomes people try to avoid in interpersonal settings (anti-goal states). There is strong evidence that avoidant people are intimacy-averse. For example, avoidance is associated with higher scores on fear of intimacy (Doi & Thelen, 1993; Greenfield & Thelen, 1997; Hudson & Ward, 1997), a correlation that could not be explained by differences in trait anxiety (Doi & Thelen, 1993). Using a hierarchical relationship-mapping technique, Rowe and Carnelley (2005) found that avoidant people (based on the Experiences in Close Relationships scale, ECR) were more likely than secure people to place partners (family members, friends, romantic partners) at a greater distance from their "core self."

Avoidant people's aversion to intimacy was also noted by Kaitz, Bar-Haim, Lehrer, and Grossman (2004), who assessed the regulation of literal physical closeness. In one study, they used a stop distance paradigm, in which participants rated their level of discomfort as the experimenter moved toward them. In another study, they assessed the physical distance freely chosen by participants when seated facing the experimenter and talking about personal issues. These investigators found that people who scored higher on avoidance (in either its dismissing or fearful form) were less tolerant of physical proximity and expressed more discomfort when the experimenter moved into their personal space. Moreover, fearfully avoidant people sat significantly further away from the experimenter than did secure people.

There is also evidence that anxiously attached people view rejection as a major anti-goal state. They have higher than normal levels of rejection sensitivity—the measurable tendency to anticipate and overreact to rejection (Downey & Feldman, 1996; Taubman Ben-Ari et al., 2002)—and are quicker to recognize rejection-related words in lexical decision tasks (Baldwin & Kay, 2003; Baldwin & Meunier, 1999). Moreover, attachment-anxious people have difficulty inhibiting rejection-related thoughts (Baldwin & Kay, 2003; Baldwin & Meunier, 1999). For example, Baldwin and Kay (2003) exposed people to tones paired with rejecting (frowning) or accepting (smiling) faces, then administered a lexical decision task in which rejection-related words were paired with each of the tones. Secure people were slower to react to rejection-related words when they were paired with rejection tones (compared to a neutral tone), but anxious people reacted faster to these words even in the presence of the acceptance tone. This implies that anxious people are so hypervigilant to rejection that they are unable to dispense with rejection-related thoughts even in accepting interpersonal contexts. This seems similar to Mikulincer and Sheffi's (2000) finding that even a positive mood induction led attachment people to have an anxious, mind-constricting reaction (see Chapter 8, this volume).

Anxiously attached people's hypersensitivity to rejection has also been noted in studies of excessive reassurance seeking (ERS; Davila, 2001; Shaver, Schachner, & Mikulincer, 2005). In a target article summarizing studies of depression and relationship dissolution, Joiner, Metalsky, Katz, and Beach (1999) defined ERS as "the relatively stable tendency to excessively and persistently seek assurances from others that one is lovable and worthy, regardless of whether such assurance has already been provided" (p. 270). In a commentary on the target article, Brennan and Carnelley (1999) suggested that the tendency to engage in ERS originates in experiences with inconsistent attachment figures and is part of anxiously attached people's defensive attempts to reduce their fear of rejection ("If I can evoke assurances that my partner loves me, I don't need to worry as much about rejection"). In support of this view, Davila (2001) and Shaver et al. (2005) found that attachment-anxious people also had higher levels of ERS, as reported by both the people themselves and their relationship partners.

In a recent series of four studies, Vorauer, Cameron, Holmes, and Pearce (2003) showed that anxiously attached people tend to organize interpersonal communication so as to avoid experiencing rejection. Specifically, more anxious people were more likely to exhibit a "signal amplification bias"—optimistically appraising their messages to an interaction partner as having been received with greater interest than was actually the case—and to expect a partner to appreciate their effort and be less likely therefore to reject them. Vorauer et al. (2003) reasoned that this bias can attenuate anxious people's fear of rejection at a particular moment but still have maladaptive consequences over time, if it causes anxious people to misinterpret their interaction partners' feelings. The study is interesting because, as seen throughout this chapter, anxious individuals' perceptions and inferences about interactions are often negatively biased by fear of rejection. But the Vorauer et al. study suggests that perceptions can sometimes be colored by anxious hope. In both cases, however, the underlying motive is probably fear of rejection.

Researchers have also assessed the importance people assign to *interpersonal* goals relative to nonrelational goals. Whereas anxious people place greater weight on interpersonal goals, avoidant people assign greater importance to nonrelational goals (Brennan & Bosson, 1998; Brennan & Morris, 1997). In a laboratory experiment, Mikulincer (1997) showed that these goal preferences guided decisions about resource allocation in social and nonsocial settings. Participants were asked to report how much time they wanted to spend learning about a new product and were informed that the more time they spent on the task, the less time they would have for a second task (either a sensory task or a social interaction). Avoidant participants spent more time on the first task when the second one involved social interaction rather than a sensory test—a reflection of their desire to avoid social interchanges. In contrast, anxious people decided to spend less time on the first task when the second one involved a social interaction. Secure participants' decisions were not affected by the nature of the second task, suggesting that their allocation of resources was not biased by attempts to regulate proximity.

Attachment Anxiety and Ambivalence

In our model of attachment-system functioning (Chapter 2, this volume), the anxious mind is marked by ambivalence. This ambivalence has been documented in mental representations of relationship partners (see Chapter 6, this volume) and seems to be the cognitive–affective trademark of anxious people's interpersonal goals. On the one hand, as reviewed earlier, anxious people place strong emphasis on garnering attention, affection, and support, and tend compulsively to approach interaction partners with these needs in mind. On the other hand, they suffer from intense fear of rejection and harbor serious doubts about their ability to inspire partners' loyalty and love. This insecurity can cause them to inhibit approach tendencies and demands on their partners when they sense the possibility of disapproval or rejection. Being caught in an approach–avoidance conflict, they are likely to ruminate obsessively about how to react in social situations, thereby interfering with adaptive interpersonal regulation. They often make important mistakes, failing to initiate new relationships that might be rewarding or effusively expressing their desires to relationship partners, which can leave them vulnerable to abuse, unwanted sexual experiences, rejection, or hurt feelings (Chapter 10, this volume). This is less likely for avoidant individuals, who pursue goals located in the distance portion of the circumplex, and view closeness and intimacy as anti-goal states.

Although few studies have directly addressed the ambivalence issue, two provide preliminary evidence that anxiously attached undergraduates are more ambivalent (i.e., have stronger positive *and* negative attitudes) toward parents and romantic partners than their secure counterparts (Bar-On, 2005; Maio, Fincham, & Lycett, 2000). These associations were not explained by other properties of attitudes, such as valence and commitment (Maio et al., 2000), or by general, noninterpersonal ambivalence (Bar-On, 2005). In addition, D. Davis, Shaver, and Vernon (2004) found that anxious adults wanted both more sex *and* less sex under certain conditions—more when they thought about sex as a barometer of their partner's love and commitment, less when they thought about the unpleasantness of acceding to the partner's sexual demands as a way to avoid disapproval or rejection.

Bar-On (2005) also showed that the association between attachment anxiety and ambivalence is measurable at an implicit, unconscious level. In a procedure developed by M. Chen and Bargh (1999), participants in Bar-On's study were exposed to a set of positive and negative attachment-related words (e.g., "hug," "rejection") on a computer screen and asked either to pull a lever (move the lever toward them; an approach response) or push it away (an avoidance response) as soon as they identified the target word. This allowed the computation of an implicit ambivalence score: the ratio between the sum of the velocities of approach and avoidance responses for a target and the absolute difference between these two scores (the faster the approach and avoidance reactions to a given word, the higher the implicit ambivalence). Bar-On found that attachment-anxious people displayed greater implicit ambivalence toward both positive and negative attachment-related words. This association was not observed for attachment-irrelevant words, implying that anxious people's implicit ambivalence was specifically related to attachment issues.

In a series of three experimental studies, Bartz and Lydon (2006) creatively measured anxious people's ambivalence in "interdependence dilemmas" (Holmes, 1991) at the outset of a relationship—that is, juggling uncertainties about a new partner's responses and intentions while expressing interest and affection toward this partner. In Study 1, participants were given an opportunity to follow communal norms while interacting with an attractive, opposite-sex confederate in the laboratory (benefits could be given freely to the partner without expecting reciprocity). Attachment anxiety was associated with conformity to these norms, indicating anxious people's desire for closeness. In Studies 2 and 4, participants were divided into two conditions based on a confederate's expression of communal norms (yes, no) or overt expression of interest in working with the participant as a team (yes, no). The participants' feelings of interpersonal anxiety and ability to concentrate on an unrelated cognitive task were then assessed. Compared to control conditions, a confederate's adoption of communal norms or expressions of interest in the participant heightened attachment-anxious people's feelings of social anxiety and diminished their performance on the cognitive task. Less anxious (more secure) people reacted to the confederate's comments with less anxiety and improved cognitive performance; that is, whereas a partner's expression of interest lessened secure people's uncertainties, it exacerbated anxious people's doubts and worries.

This pattern of findings is compatible with the notion that attachment-anxious individuals are prone to ambivalence. Although they are highly interested in becoming close to a new partner, they become anxious and confused when the partner unexpectedly signals interest and affection. According to Bartz and Lydon (2006), their fear of rejection and negative working model of self make them anxious and uncertain about the "true" meaning of others' expressions of affection and interest (e.g., "Is this person really interested in me?"), thereby preventing them from taking a leap of faith into a potentially rewarding relationship. The mixture of desire for security and rejection sensitivity generates ambivalence and contributes to anxious people's confusion about what they and their partners really want in interpersonal situations.

Interpersonal Dispositions

Attachment style differences in interpersonal wishes can also be observed in the traits and behaviors people typically exhibit in interpersonal situations. Avoidant people are likely to display traits and behaviors in the distance region of the interpersonal circumplex (e.g., coldness, hostility); attachment-anxious people are likely to display traits and behaviors in the closeness portion of the circumplex (e.g., warmth, dependence). However, anxious individuals' ambivalence can cause them to express inconsistent traits, making their location in the circumplex unclear.

Several studies have examined how attachment style is related to the interpersonal dispositions arrayed in the circumplex model. Some have examined these associations using two traits in the five-factor model of personality (McCrae & Costa, 1989): extraversion and agreeableness. Others have relied on a measure called the structural analysis of social behavior (SASB; Benjamin, 1974, 1994). In each case, interpersonal dispositions have proven to be systematically related to attachment style.

Attachment, Extraversion, and Agreeableness

In the five-factor model of personality, two of the five superordinate traits (openness to experience, conscientiousness, extraversion, agreeableness, and neuroticism) are frequently involved in interpersonal relations: *extraversion* and *agreeableness*. Extraversion, which has been included in virtually all major taxonomies of personality traits, is defined by six "facets" (i.e., more specific constituent traits; McCrae & Costa, 1989): gregariousness, warmth, assertiveness/dominance, activity, excitement seeking, and positive emotions. In terms of the circumplex model of personality, high scores on the extraversion dimension reflect a combination of dominance and nurturance (McCrae & Costa, 1989). Agreeableness, in contrast, includes six different facets: interpersonal trust, straightforwardness/ingenuity, selflessness/altruism, compliance, cooperativeness, and tendermindedness. High scores on the agreeableness dimension reflect a blend of nurturance and moderate submissiveness.

Avoidant attachment undermines nurturance and interferes with or precludes extraversion and agreeableness in interpersonal exchanges. Avoidant individuals' preference for emotional distance and independence from others naturally runs counter to the gregariousness and warmth facets of extraversion, and the compliance and cooperativeness facets of agreeableness. Moreover, avoidant people tend to suppress or inhibit emotions (Chapter 7, this volume), thereby countering the emotional positivity and expressiveness of extraversion. In addition, avoidant individuals' negative internal working models of others (Chapter 6, this volume) run counter to the interpersonal trust facet of agreeableness.

Attachment anxiety can also distort or interfere with extraversion and agreeableness, but for different reasons. Anxious people tend to exaggerate the expression of negative emotions and to harbor serious doubts about self-efficacy (Chapters 6–7, this volume), which interfere with facets of extraversion such as positive emotions and self-confidence. Attachment-anxious people are also plagued by doubts about their partner's trustworthiness (Chapter 6, this volume) and remain vigilant for signs of a partner's unavailability or coolness, making it difficult for them to approach their partners in a relaxed, open, and agreeable manner.

To test these hypotheses, several researchers have examined correlations between self-report attachment measures and scales measuring extraversion and agreeableness (see Table 9.1 for a summary of methods and findings). With regard to avoidant attachment, the results are consistent and theoretically sensible. Higher scores on avoidance are associated with lower scores on extraversion and agreeableness. With regard to attachment anxiety, the results are theoretically reasonable but less consistent. Although significant negative correlations have been found between attachment anxiety on the one hand, and extraversion and agreeableness on the other, several studies have failed to turn up significant associations between these variables. In any case, most of the correlations between Big-Five traits and the two attachment-insecurity dimensions are only modest or moderate in size, implying that attachment orientations are not mere clones of extraversion or agreeableness.

In a finer-grained analysis of interpersonal dispositions, Noftle and Shaver (2006, Study 2) found that attachment anxiety and avoidance were related to different facets of extraversion and agreeableness. With regard to extraversion, avoidance was inversely associated with the facets of gregariousness, warmth, positive emotions, assertiveness, and activity, whereas attachment anxiety was associated negatively only with assertiveness and positive emotions; that is, whereas avoidance had negative links with both the nurturance and dominance aspects of extraversion, attachment anxiety was negatively associated only with the dominance aspect. With regard to agreeableness, both avoidance and anxiety were associated with lower interpersonal trust. However, avoidance was also associated with lower altruism, and anxiety was associated with lower straightforwardness.

Attachment and the SASB Model

Another line of attachment research has taken advantage of L. S. Benjamin's (1974, 1994) refinement of the interpersonal circumplex model, the SASB. In her SASB model, Benjamin distinguishes between behaviors a person directs toward others (called "transitive, active") and a person's responses to others' demands ("intransitive, reactive"). This distinction leads her to decompose the dominance dimension into two different axes. In the transitive domain, the dominance dimension runs from granting autonomy or independence to others at one end, to influencing and controlling others' intentions and actions at the other. In the intransitive domain, this dimension runs from submissiveness

TABLE 9.1. A Summary of Findings on Attachment Orientations and the Big-Five Traits of Extraversion and Agreeableness

Study	Attachment measure	Personality measure	Extraversion		Agreeableness	
			Anxiety	Avoidance	Anxiety	Avoidance
Shaver & Brennan (1992)	HS ratings	NEO-PI	(ns)	(–)	(–)	(–)
Griffin & Bartholomew (1994a)	RQ	NEO-PI	(–)	(–)	(–)	(–)
Griffin & Bartholomew (1994a)	RSQ	NEO-PI	(–)	(–)	(–)	(–)
Shaver, Papalia, et al. (1996)	RQ	NEO-PI	(–)	(–)		
Becker et al. (1997)	New scale	BFM	(–)	(–)	(ns)	(–)
Carver (1997, Study 2)	MAQ	EPI	(ns)	(–)		
Carver (1997, Study 3)	MAQ	NEO-FFI	(ns)	(–)	(ns)	(–)
Carver (1997, Study 4)	MAQ	NEO-FFI	(ns)	(–)	(ns)	(–)
Carver (1997, Study 4)	RQ	NEO-FFI	(ns)	(–)	(ns)	(–)
Markiewicz et al. (1997)	AAQ	NEO-PI	(ns)	(–)	(–)	(–)
Mickelson et al. (1997)	HS ratings	BFM	(–)	(–)		
Moreira et al. (1998)	HS types	EPI	(ns)	(–)		
Backstrom & Holmes (2001)	RSQ	NEO-PI	(–)	(–)	(–)	(–)
Shafer (2001)	ASQ	BBM	(–)	(–)	(ns)	(–)
Gallo et al. (2003)	AAS	BFA	(–)	(–)	(–)	(–)
Noyes et al. (2003)	RSQ	NEO-FFI	(+)	(–)		
Bakker et al. (2004)	ASQ	FFPQ	(–)	(–)	(–)	(ns)
Edelstein et al. (2004)	RSQ	NEO-PI	(ns)	(–)	(–)	(ns)
Heaven et al. (2004)	AAS	IPIP	(–)	(–)	(–)	(–)
Picardi, Toni, et al. (2005)	ECR	BFQ	(–)	(–)	(–)	(–)
Noftle & Shaver (2006, Study 1)	ECR	BFI	(–)	(–)	(–)	(–)
Noftle & Shaver (2006, Study 2)	ECR	NEO-PI	(–)	(–)	(ns)	(ns)

Note. (–), significant inverse correlation; (+), significant positive correlation; (ns), nonsignificant correlation; BBM, Brief Bipolar Markers; BFA, Big Five Adjectives; BFM, Big Five Markers; BFI, Big Five Inventory; BFQ, Big Five Questionnaire; EPI, Eysenck Personality Inventory; FFPQ, Five-Factors Personality Questionnaire; HS, Hazan and Shaver; IPIP, International Personality Item Pool; MAQ, Multidimensional Attachment Questionnaire; NEO-FFI, NEO Five-Factor Inventory; NEO-PI, NEO Personality Inventory.

to and compliance with others' demands to asserting autonomy and independence. Whereas high dominance scores in the transitive domain reflect a tendency to control others' behavior, high dominance scores in the intransitive domain reflect a tendency to assert autonomy.

The SASB model deepens our understanding of anxiously attached people's interpersonal dispositions. They are reluctant to grant autonomy to a partner, because it might free the partner to turn attention away and express affection to someone else. Moreover, anxious individuals have trouble asserting autonomy, because assertiveness might increase self–other differentiation and increase distance. This heightens anxious people's ambivalence and causes them to vacillate between an intrusive, controlling posture and a submissive, accommodating stance toward their partners' demands. Both of these seemingly incompatible strategies are attempts to maintain closeness and connectedness, while avoiding rejection and abandonment.

Avoidant individuals, especially the less consciously anxious ones that Bartholomew and Horowitz (1991) called "dismissing," are less likely to have problems asserting autonomy and resisting others' demands. They view themselves as strong and self-reliant and do not like to display signs of weakness or dependency (Chapter 6, this volume). However, they often have difficulty granting autonomy to a partner. They limit closeness and dependency while maintaining a degree of proximity and involvement, so as not to lose a partner's interest and risk either humiliation or complete isolation. They are reluctant to grant autonomy to a partner, because an autonomous partner might make unwanted bids for intimacy or decide to end a disappointing, frustratingly cool relationship. In other words, avoidance may generate simultaneous wishes to maintain a relationship and to control it in the interest of maintaining optimal distance. This kind of control is intended to quell fears of rejection, while defensively avoiding intimacy and vulnerability.

Four studies of attachment processes have used L. S. Benjamin's SASB model to assess interpersonal dispositions in relationships with friends, romantic partners, and parents (Gallo, Smith, & Ruiz, 2003; Morrison, Goodlin-Jones, & Urquiza, 1997; Morrison, Urquiza, & Goodlin-Jones, 1997; Pincus, Dickinson, Schut, Castonguay, & Bedics, 1999). Across the various kinds of relationships, all four studies found that both anxiety and avoidance are associated with relatively low nurturance in both the transitive and intransitive domains. In addition, both anxiety and avoidance are associated with controlling tendencies in the transitive domain; that is, both anxious and avoidant people tended to grant less autonomy and freedom to others. In the intransitive domain, only one study (Morrison, Goodlin-Jones, & Urquiza, 1997) found a significant association between attachment anxiety and lack of assertiveness.

Several studies have explored associations between attachment measures and other interpersonal dispositions. For example, some researchers have found that avoidance, but not anxiety, is associated with lack of sociability—a preference for being alone rather than affiliating with others (Bartholomew & Horowitz, 1991; Cyranowski et al., 2002; Duggan & Brennan, 1994; Griffin & Bartholomew, 1994b; Shaver, Papalia, et al., 1996). In addition, Duggan and Brennan (1994) found that attachment anxiety, but not avoidance, is associated with shyness. These findings suggest that avoidant people are relatively non-nurturant, because they are not very friendly or sociable, whereas anxious people are relatively non-nurturant, because they have doubts about their social value—a typical characteristic of shy people (Cheek & Buss, 1981).

Researchers have also explored attachment-related differences in interpersonal dependency. Anxiously attached people reported higher dependency in both emotional and instrumental contexts (Alonzo-Arbiol et al., 2002). Interestingly, although avoidance was not associated in either direction with emotional dependency, it was positively associated with instrumental dependency. According to Alonzo-Arbiol et al., this association may indicate that avoidant people can sometimes express dependency, but only in a rather unemotional, instrumental context: "Instrumental dependency may be a way of expressing insecurity (e.g., asking for advice and guidance) without opening oneself to rejection" (p. 487).

In the circumplex model, dependency falls in the close–submissive quadrant and, according to Pincus and Gurtman (1995), includes two forms: *loving* dependency (high nurturance, average dominance) and *submissive* dependency (average nurturance, low dominance). Operationalizing this distinction, Pincus and Wilson (2001) found that attachment security is associated with loving, nurturant dependency, but attachment anxiety and other indicators of pathologically anxious attachment (angry withdrawal and compulsive care seeking, as assessed by the Reciprocal Attachment Scale) are associated with submissive dependency. This is further evidence for anxiously attached people's submissive position in the interpersonal circumplex. In addition, there is evidence that anxiously attached people report having more difficulty asserting themselves, taking personal responsibility, and exerting autonomy in close relationships (Anders & Tucker, 2000; Batgos & Leadbeater, 1994; J. A. Feeney, Kelly, Gallois, Peterson, & Terry, 1999; Kobak & Sceery, 1988; Pietromonaco & Carnelley, 1994; Taubman Ben-Ari et al., 2002).

Overall, researchers have painted distinct portraits of different forms of insecure attachment as these are expressed in interpersonal dispositions. Both avoidant and anxious people adopt a controlling stance toward others, but they differ along the nurturance and dominance dimensions. Avoidant people are unwilling, or unable, to approach others in a warm, friendly, and agreeable manner. Attachment-anxious people are shy, dependent, and lacking in assertiveness.

Interpersonal Competencies

Beyond its biasing effects on goal setting, attachment style can also influence interpersonal skills. Smooth functioning of the attachment system implies that a person (1) has learned interpretable, efficacious ways of expressing inner states and eliciting support, (2) is sensitive to, and relatively accurate in interpreting, interaction partners' signals, and (3) is effective in managing minor misunderstandings and even significant conflicts. In contrast, recurrent failure to obtain support and security from attachment figures, and the consequent adoption of secondary attachment strategies (anxious hyperactivation or avoidant deactivation), can produce serious deficiencies in interpersonal skills.

Expressivity and Sensitivity

Secondary attachment strategies are defensive ways of relating to others that interfere with normal proximity seeking, and disrupt the sending and receiving of effective social signals. Hyperactivating strategies cause anxious people to focus on their own unsatisfied needs, weaknesses, and vulnerabilities. As a result, they often express distress, vulnerability, and neediness but may be unskilled at expressing positive mental states, such as satisfaction, happiness, and gratitude. With regard to interpersonal sensitivity, anxious individuals' excessive focus on attachment-related worries may draw mental resources away from accurate interpretation of others' social signals and needs. In addition, due to their negative self-representations (see Chapter 6, this volume), anxiously attached people may dismiss positive signals from others and misinterpret them as sarcastic expressions of negative feelings (Noller, 2005). They are also likely to be inaccurate in interpreting negative signals from others, because these signals reactivate their deeply entrenched attachment-related worries, intensify distress, and produce a chaotic state of mind that interferes with accurate social perception.

Avoidant individuals are not so likely to share personal thoughts and feelings with others, because self-disclosure encourages unwanted closeness, intimacy, or nurturance. Their lack of trust in others (Chapter 6, this volume) can also interfere with self-disclosure and emotional expressiveness. With regard to interpersonal sensitivity, avoidant people's lack of nurturance makes them less likely than other people to attend to relationship partners' verbal and nonverbal messages and signals; therefore they may be less accurate in decoding these signals (Schachner, Shaver, & Mikulincer, 2005). Their indifference and decoding inaccuracies are especially likely when relationship partners send signals of desire for proximity, closeness, or reassurance. These messages invite the kind of intimacy that avoidant people wish to deflect.

Several studies have examined attachment-related differences in self-reported expressiveness (see Table 9.2 for a summary of methods and findings), and the results are quite

TABLE 9.2. A Summary of Findings Concerning Attachment Orientations and Interpersonal Expressivity

Study	Attachment measure	Expressivity measure	Main findings for the tendency to express personal feelings
Studies assessing attachment types			
Mikulincer & Nachshon (1991)	HS types	SDI	Secure > Avoidant
Pistole (1993)	HS types	SDI	Secure > Avoidant
Batgos & Leadbeater (1994)	HS types	ICQ	Secure > Avoidant
Keelan et al. (1998)	RQ types	SDI	Secure > Avoidant, Fearful
		Opener scale	Secure > Avoidant, Fearful
Searle & Meara (1999)	RQ types	EES	Secure > Avoidant, Fearful
Grabill & Kerns (2000)	RQ	SDI	Secure > Avoidant, Anxious, Fearful
		Opener scale	Secure > Avoidant, Anxious, Fearful
Ducharme et al. (2002)	RQ mother	EES	Secure > Avoidant, Fearful
	RQ father	EES	No significant differences
Guerrero & Jones (2003)	RQ types	SSI—social	Secure > Avoidant, Fearful
		SSI—emotional	Secure > Avoidant, Fearful
Kerr et al. (2003)	HS types	EES	Secure > Anxious, Avoidant
		Emotion control	Secure < Anxious, Avoidant
Studies based on attachment style ratings			
Simpson (1990)	AAQ	SDI	Avoidant (−) Anxious (ns) Secure (+)
Collins et al. (2002)*	HS ratings	SDI	Avoidant (−) Anxious (ns) Secure (ns)
Vrij et al. (2003)	HS ratings	Secretiveness	Avoidant (+) Anxious (ns) Secure (−)
Studies assessing attachment dimensions			
Collins & Read (1990)	AAS	Opener scale	Avoidance (−) Anxiety (ns)
Kotler et al. (1994)	HS ratings	Emotion control	Avoidance (+) Anxiety (ns)
J. A. Feeney (1995a)	ASQ	Emotion control	Avoidance (+) Anxiety (ns)
J. A. Feeney (1999a)	ASQ	Emotion control	Avoidance (+) Anxiety (ns)
Tucker & Anders (1999)	AAQ	SDI	Avoidance (−) Anxiety (ns)
		EEQ	Avoidance (−) Anxiety (−)
Anders & Tucker (2000)	ECR	ICC	Avoidance (−) Anxiety (ns)
Lopez (2001)	ECR	Self-concealment	Avoidance (+) Anxiety (+)
Tacon et al. (2001)	AAQ avoidance	Emotion control	Avoidance (+)
S. A. Bradford et al. (2002)	ECR	SDI, RDI	Avoidance (−) Anxiety (ns)
		Opener scale	Avoidance (ns) Anxiety (ns)
Taubman Ben-Ari et al. (2002)	HS ratings	ICQ	Avoidance (−) Anxiety (ns)
DiTommaso et al. (2003)	RSQ	SSI—social	Avoidance (−) Anxiety (ns)
		SSI—emotional	Avoidance (−) Anxiety (ns)
Deniz et al. (2005)	RSQ	SSI—social	Avoidance (−) Anxiety (ns)
		SSI—emotional	Avoidance (−) Anxiety (ns)
Wei, Russell, & Zakalik (2005)	ECR	DDI	Avoidance (−) Anxiety (ns)

Note. *, longitudinal design; (−), significant inverse correlation; (+), significant positive correlation; (ns), nonsignificant effects; DDI, Distress Disclosure Index; EEQ, Emotional Expressivity Questionnaire; EES, Emotional Expressivity Scale; HS, Hazan and Shaver; ICC, Interpersonal Communication Competencies; ICQ, Interpersonal Competencies Questionnaire; RDI, Relationship Disclosure Index; SDI, Self-Disclosure Index; SSI, Social Skills Inventory.

consistent. The vast majority of studies yield no significant association between attachment anxiety and expressiveness, but all of them find evidence for the hypothesized expression deficits of avoidant people. Avoidant individuals (whether dismissing or fearful) report less inclination to disclose personal feelings to others or express emotions (either positive or negative) spontaneously. Moreover, they are less likely to elicit self-disclosures from other people. They are prone to secrecy and concealment of personal information. This has been noted in both cross-sectional and prospective longitudinal studies. For example, Collins, Cooper, Albino, and Allard (2002) found that avoidance (assessed during adolescence) significantly predicted inhibited self-disclosure 6 years later.

Studies assessing expressive behavior in the laboratory have also documented avoidant people's deficits. For example, Magai et al. (2000) videotaped participants during an emotion induction procedure and found that avoidant people expressed less joy (based on coding facial expressions). These results were replicated in a sample of patients with dementia (Magai, Cohen, Culver, Gomberg, & Malatesta, 1997). Spangler and Zimmermann (1999) exposed participants to emotional film clips and found that the more avoidant ones (based on the AAI) had restricted activity in both their smile and frown muscles (assessed with electromyography) even when the scene they were watching was highly distressing. Zimmermann, Wulf, et al. (1997) found that German participants classified as avoidant by the AAI displayed fewer facial expressions of interest and joy, and more facial expressions of anger, sadness, and negative surprise during the interview than secure participants, but Roisman et al. (2004) failed to replicate this finding in an American sample.

Researchers have also reported evidence of anxious people's negative biases in expressing mental states. Magai et al. (1997, 2000) found that attachment-anxious people were more expressive of negative emotions (again based on coding facial expressions) during an emotion induction procedure. Roisman et al. (2004) replicated this finding with emotional expressions displayed by attachment-anxious people during the AAI. A similar negative bias in facial expression was noted by Sonnby-Borgstrom and Jonsson (2003), who exposed people to pictures of happy and angry faces, and assessed the activity of smile and frown muscles. More attachment-anxious participants had more active "frown" muscles while watching either happy or angry faces, implying heightened tonic expression of negative emotions.

Attachment-related differences in expressiveness have also been noted during social interactions. For example, Becker-Stoll, Delius, and Scheitenberger (2001) found that avoidant adolescents, classified by the AAI, expressed less emotion (in a second-by-second analysis of their facial responses) than secure adolescents during a problem-solving discussion with their mothers. This inhibitory effect of avoidance on the expression of emotions was also documented in studies of nonverbal communication during interactions with a romantic partner (e.g., Guerrero, 1996). (We review these studies in more detail in Chapter 10, when we discuss dyadic communication in dating and married couples.)

With regard to possible links between attachment and interpersonal sensitivity, studies based on self-report scales have not yielded consistent findings (e.g., Anders & Tucker, 2000; Deniz, Hamarta, & Ari, 2005; DiTommaso, Brannen-McNulty, Ross, & Burgess, 2003; Guerrero & Jones, 2003). For example, Guerrero and Jones found that dismissingly avoidant people reported lower social sensitivity than secure ones and were perceived as insensitive by their romantic partners. However, the other studies found no significant association between avoidance and self-reported sensitivity. With regard to attachment anxiety, three studies unexpectedly yielded positive correlations between anxiety and the social sensitivity scale of the Social Skills Inventory (SSI; Deniz et al., 2005; DiTommaso et al., 2003; Guerrero & Jones, 2003). However, examination of the scale items reveals that higher scores tap "oversensitivity" to criticism and a strong need for external validation. Thus, the findings probably reflect anxious people's hypersensitivity to negative interpersonal outcomes rather than accuracy in decoding other people's verbal and nonverbal communications.

A more consistent and coherent pattern of findings arises from studies based on performance tests of ability to decode others' nonverbal expressions. Using Ekman and Friesen's (1975) facial action coding system (FACS), Magai, Distel, and Liker (1995; Magai et al., 2000) found that secure people were relatively accurate in decoding facial expressions of emotion, avoidant individuals were deficient in facial affect decoding, and anxious individuals were particularly inaccurate in decoding anger. Insecure people's sensitivity deficits have also been noted in two other studies (E. L. Cooley, 2005; Kafetsios, 2004), which employed MSCEIT or the Nowicki Diagnostic Analysis of Nonverbal Accuracy Test. These deficits have also been noted in studies assessing ability to accurately infer a romantic partner's feelings (see Chapter 10, this volume).

In another study of facial affect decoding, Niedenthal, Brauer, Robin, and Innes-Ker (2002) used a "morph" movie paradigm. Participants were shown computerized movies of faces in which a particular facial expression of emotion gradually changed to a neutral expression. Participants were instructed to stop the display when they perceived that the initial expression had disappeared from the face and the neutral expression was coming into view. Whereas fearful avoidant participants (those scoring high on both attachment anxiety and avoidance) perceived the offset of emotional expressions earlier than did secure participants, preoccupied participants (those high on anxiety but low on avoidance) tended to notice the offset of emotional expressions later than did secure adults. According to Niedenthal et al. these findings imply that fearful avoidance is associated with a tendency to minimize the encoding of emotional information, and that anxious attachment is associated with elevated emotional sensitivity. However, attachment-anxious people's tendency to see a negative emotional expression persisting can alternatively be interpreted as a sign of heightened vigilance to negative cues.

To deal with this interpretational ambiguity, Fraley, Niedenthal, Marks, Brumbaugh, and Vicary (2006) introduced two variations in the morph movie paradigm. First, they reversed the direction in which the morph movies were played: The movies began with a neutral facial expression that gradually changed into one of anger, happiness, or sadness. Second, they collected data on emotional sensitivity; once participants had made their judgment about the onset of an emotional expression, they judged which emotion the face was expressing (anger, happiness, or sadness). The authors found that more attachment-anxious individuals tended to perceive the onset of facial expressions of emotion earlier and to make more errors in judging the particular emotion the face was expressing. These results indicate that anxious people's early recognition of emotional expressions is a sign of heightened vigilance to emotional cues rather than a reflection of emotional sensitivity or decoding accuracy.

Fraley, Niedenthal, et al. (2006) believed that this heightened vigilance might lead attachment-anxious people "to jump to emotional conclusions, so to speak, ultimately undermining their ability to perceive emotions accurately" (p. 1179). Indeed, when anxious participants were required to watch the movies for the same length of time as more secure participants, there was no longer a significant association between attachment anxiety and accuracy in detecting the emotion a face expressed (Study 4). Thus, it seems that attachment-anxious people's inaccuracies in detecting particular emotional expressions do not reflect a true cognitive deficit (i.e., inability to evaluate others' emotional states). Rather, their problems in decoding emotions seem to result from heightened vigilance to emotional cues and the resulting tendency to make premature judgments.

Recently, Guterman (2006) provided further evidence for insecure people's difficulties in accurately decoding facial expressions of emotion (using the MSCEIT in one study and the Japanese and Caucasian Brief Affect Recognition Test in another), while examining the effects of security priming (subliminal exposure to the names of security providers). In both studies, attachment anxiety and avoidance were associated with poorer emotion decoding. In addition, security priming improved anxious people's interpersonal sensitivity, suggesting that their previously documented deficit was a consequence of anxiety about rejection or disapproval. However, security priming did not ameliorate avoidant individuals' decoding deficits. (For other studies in which avoidant individuals were unaffected by contextual security priming, see Chapter 13, this volume.)

Conflict Management

Attachment research has shed light on the ways people perceive, react to, and manage interpersonal conflicts. Secure individuals, who generally view others as "well intentioned and kindhearted" (Hazan & Shaver, 1987) and perceive themselves as capable of handling life's problems (see Chapters 6 and 7, this volume), are likely to emphasize the challenging rather than the threatening aspects of conflicts and believe they can deal effectively with them. Moreover, their constructive approach to emotion regulation (Chapter 7, this volume) may help them communicate openly but not threateningly during conflict, negotiate with a relationship partner in a collaborative manner, and apply effective conflict resolution strategies, such as compromising and integrating their own and their partners' positions. In so doing, secure individuals are likely to guide their relationships back from conflict to harmony.

Insecure people are likely to appraise interpersonal conflicts in more threatening terms and apply less effective conflict resolution strategies. For anxious people, conflicts threaten their wish to gain approval, support, and security, arousing fear of rejection and triggering hyperactivating emotion regulation strategies. They are likely to appraise conflict in catastrophic terms, display intense negative emotions, and ruminate obsessively; hence, they fail to attend to and understand what their partners are trying to tell to them. This egocentric, fearful stance is likely to interfere with calm, open communication, negotiation, and the use of compromising and integrative strategies that depend on keeping a partner's needs and perspective in mind. Anxious individuals are likely either to try to dominate the interaction (in an effort to get their own needs met) or to accede submissively to a partner's demands to avoid rejection.

Avoidant people are likely to view conflicts as aversive primarily because conflicts interfere with autonomy and call for expressions of love and care, or need and vulnerability. Avoidant people are likely to downplay the significance of conflict, while minimizing the importance of their partners' complaints; to distance themselves cognitively or emotionally from the conflict; or try to avoid interacting with their partners. When circumstances do not allow escape from conflict, avoidant people are likely to attempt to dominate their partners, in line with their need for control, their negative models of others, and high confidence in their own views (Chapter 6, this volume). This defensive stance is likely to interfere with negotiation and compromise.

Table 9.3 summarizes studies that have examined attachment-related differences in self-reported responses to conflict. (Studies that specifically examine conflicts within couple relationships, such as marriages, are reviewed in Chapter 10, this volume). The findings indicate that secure individuals appraise conflicts in less threatening terms, believe they are equipped to deal with conflicts, and report less conflict-related distress than do insecure people. Moreover, they report better conflict-management skills (e.g., understanding their partners' perspective), are more likely to rely on compromising and integrative strategies, and are less likely to behave in ways that escalate conflicts (coercion, fighting) or leave a conflict unresolved.

TABLE 9.3. A Summary of Findings on Attachment Orientations and Conflict Management Strategies

Study	Attachment measures	Conflict measures	Dependent variables	Main findings
Studies assessing attachment types				
Batgos & Leadbeater (1994)	HS types	ICQ	Management skills	Secure > Anxious, Avoidant
Torquati & Vazsonyi (1999)	AAS	Appraisal, emotion, and problem-solving items	Threat appraisal	Secure < Anxious, Avoidant
			Avoidance coping	Secure < Anxious, Avoidant
			Support seeking	Secure > Anxious, Avoidant
			Distress	Secure < Anxious
Bippus & Rollin (2003)	RQ	ROCI	Integrating	Secure > Insecure
Pistole & Arricale (2003)	RQ	Scales assessing feelings about conflict and conflict tactics	Threat appraisal	Secure < Anxious
			Closeness concerns	Secure < Anxious
			Avoidance coping	Secure < Avoidance
			Fighting	Secure < Fearful
			Problem solving	Secure > Insecure
Studies assessing attachment dimensions				
Levy & Davis (1988)	HS ratings	ROCI	Integrating	Anxiety (−) Avoidance (−)
			Compromising	Anxiety (−) Avoidance (−)
			Dominating	Anxiety (+) Avoidance (ns)
Pistole (1989)	HS ratings	ROCI	Integrating	Anxiety (−) Avoidance (−)
			Compromising	Anxiety (−) Avoidance (−)
			Obliging	Anxiety (+) Avoidance (ns)
Carnelley et al. (1994)	48 items	CSQ	Constructive style	Anxiety (ns) Avoidance (−)
Beinstein Miller (1996)	AAQ	New scale	Flexible strategies	Anxiety (−) Avoidance (ns)
Davila et al. (1996)	AAS	P-S scale	Negotiation	Anxiety (ns) Avoidance (−)
Lopez, Gover, et al. (1997)	RQ	CSQ	Constructive style	Anxiety (−) Avoidance (−)
Creasey et al. (1999)	RSQ	MADS	Positive tactics	Anxiety (−) Avoidance (−)
			Aggression	Anxiety (+) Avoidance (+)
			Conflict escalation	Anxiety (+) Avoidance (+)
			Withdrawal	Anxiety (+) Avoidance (+)
Corcoran & Mallinckrodt (2000)	ASQ	ROCI	Integrating	Anxiety (−) Avoidance (−)
			Compromising	Anxiety (−) Avoidance (−)
			Avoidant	Anxiety (+) Avoidance (+)
Creasey & Hesson-McInnis (2001)	RSQ	MADS	Positive tactics	Anxiety (−) Avoidance (−)
			Aggression	Anxiety (+) Avoidance (+)
			Conflict escalation	Anxiety (+) Avoidance (+)
			Withdrawal	Anxiety (ns) Avoidance (+)
			Distress	Anxiety (+) Avoidance (ns)
J. P. Allen et al. (2002)	AAI	P-S scale	Problem solving	Anxiety (−) Avoidance (−)
Taubman Ben-Ari et al. (2002)	HS ratings	ICQ	Management skills	Anxiety (−) Avoidance (−)
Reese-Weber & Marchand (2002)	AAS—anxiety	MADS	Positive strategies	Anxiety (−)
			Negative strategies	Anxiety (+)

Note. (−), significant inverse correlation; (+), significant positive correlation; (ns), nonsignificant effects; CSQ, Conflict Style Questionnaire; HS, Hazan and Shaver; ICQ, Interpersonal Competencies Questionnaire; MADS, Managing Affect and Differences Scale; P-S, Problem Solving; ROCI, Rahim Organizational Conflict Inventory.

Table 9.3 also highlights several similarities between anxious and avoidant people's reactions to conflict. Both groups appraise conflicts in threatening terms and report poorer conflict-management skills and stronger tendencies to escalate conflicts or withdraw from them. In addition, attachment-anxious people report high concern with closeness during conflicts (Pistole & Arricale, 2003) and strong conflict-related distress (Creasey & Hesson McInnis, 2001; Torquati & Vazsonyi, 1999), probably reflecting their fear that disagreement may provoke their partners' disapproval, rejection, or abandonment. In addition, anxious individuals react to the priming of rejection concerns with less flexibility in conflict management strategies (Beinstein Miller, 1996), suggesting that their fear of rejection, when heightened experimentally, interferes with constructive approaches to conflict resolution.

In general, the research to date provides strong support for hypothesized deficits in avoidant people's interpersonal expressivity, sensitivity, and conflict management. Attachment-anxious people also show marked deficits in decoding emotional expressions and managing interpersonal conflict, mostly because of hypersensitivity to disapproval and criticism.

Coordination of One's Own and a Partner's Needs and Behaviors

Insecure individuals' egocentric focus on their attachment-related worries and defenses can interfere with effective coordination of their own and their partners' needs and behaviors. They are so preoccupied with avoiding rejection (in the case of anxiously attached people) or preventing unwanted interdependence (in the case of avoidant people) that they lack the resources necessary to adjust their actions flexibly to their partners' behavior and to coordinate their own and their partners' actions. They are more likely to engage in self-focused or defensive monologues rather than constructive, dialogical interchanges.

This lack of flexibility was documented by Mikulincer and Nachshon (1991) in their study of self-disclosure. Whereas securely attached people reported disclosing more personal feelings to a close relationship partner than to a stranger, insecure people reported similar levels of self-disclosure to different kinds of partners. Anxiously attached people tended to report heightened self-disclosure even to a stranger, and avoidant people reported relatively low levels of self-disclosure even to their closest relationship partners.

Lack of interpersonal coordination is also evident in insecure people's behavior during conflicts. As reviewed in the previous section, insecurely attached people are less likely to understand their partners' positions, integrate their own and their partners' perspectives, and negotiate a satisfactory resolution of the conflict. Here we add that insecure people's difficulties with interpersonal coordination are also evident in less conflictual exchanges. For example, Whiters and Vernon (2006) collected self-reports of embarrassment and found that attachment-anxious people were more likely to experience embarrassing situations in which they failed to perform an expected social role or to follow a coherent strategy or script in social interactions.

New findings from our laboratories also reveal that insecurely attached people have interpersonal coordination problems while attempting to promote closeness and cooperation. Study participants (40 Israeli undergraduates who had previously completed the ECR) were invited to engage in a problem-solving interaction (desert survival task) with another undergraduate whom they had not previously met. Participants were explicitly instructed to promote closeness and cooperation during the interaction, but their partners were unaware of this instruction. The interaction was videotaped, and five judges (undergraduate psychology students) who were blind to participants' attachment scores and the instructions they had received, rated participants' and partners' behaviors. Specifically, they received a brief list of eight interpersonal goals (including the goal of promoting closeness and cooperation) and were asked to mark the goals that participants seemed to pursue during the interaction. In addition, they rated the extent to which participants' behaviors were effective in attaining the desired goal, and the extent to which participants attended and adequately responded to their partners' comments, felt relaxed and calm during the interaction, and promoted closeness and cooperation. They also rated the extent to which partners were responsive to participants' bids and seemed to feel comfortable during the interaction. All ratings were made on 5-point scales.

The judges marked the goal of promoting closeness and cooperation in the vast majority of videotaped interactions (93%), implying that participants complied with the experimental instructions regardless of attachment style. In addition, interjudge reliabilities for all of the ratings were high, ranging from .82 to .91, implying that interpersonal coordination is an observable phenomenon. More important, there were significant associations between participants' attachment scores and judges' ratings (averaged across the five judges). As can be seen in Table 9.4, attachment-anxious and avoidant participants were rated by judges as displaying less effective goal-oriented behaviors, seeming to feel less relaxed and calm during the interaction, reacting in less appropriate ways to their partners' responses, and promoting less closeness and cooperation. Furthermore, partners of more attachment-anxious or avoidant participants were rated by judges as seeming less calm and relaxed during the interaction, and these associations remained significant even after partners' attachment scores on the ECR were statistically controlled. These findings highlight insecure people's difficulties in attaining interpersonal goals, but they represent only an initial step in systematically assessing attachment style differences in interpersonal coordination. Further research should examine the pursuit of other kinds of interpersonal goals in different kinds of laboratory and naturalistic settings.

PATTERNS OF INTERPERSONAL EXPERIENCE

Attachment style differences in interpersonal regulation are likely to be evident in people's experiences of interpersonal exchanges. Secure individuals are likely to appraise social interactions as good opportunities for closeness, mutual enjoyment, and personal growth; enter interactions with optimism, enthusiasm, and joy; emphasize the positive, appetitive aspects of social relations; and behave in ways that promote productive interdependence. Avoidant people's subjective experiences likely reflect their lack of nurturance and deficits in interpersonal skills. They are unlikely to enjoy most interactions or to behave in ways that promote closeness, intimacy, and interdependence. Anxious people's interpersonal experience is likely to be negatively biased by their hypersensitivity to rejection. Interpersonal exchanges involving emotional closeness and affection may cause them to experience positive emotions, arouse feelings of optimism and hope, and encourage approach behavior, because such interactions provide opportunities for merger, protection, approval, and support. But anxious people are unlikely to sustain positive emotions over time, because even minimal signs of partner unavailability, lack of interest, betrayal, or rejection will reactivate attachment-related worries, fears, and hyperactivating defenses. As a result, anxiously attached people's experiences are likely to be marked by disappointment, injury, anger, and conflict-related distress.

In the following sections we review three lines of research concerning attachment style differences in interpersonal experience. (In Chapter 10, we review studies examining these patterns of responding specifically in the context of couple relationships.)

Diary Studies

In one line of research, diary techniques are used to study how people react to daily interactions with different kinds of relationship partners (parents, acquaintances, friends,

TABLE 9.4. Pearson Correlations and Standardized Regression Coefficients (β) Showing Associations between Attachment Dimensions and Judges' Ratings of Interpersonal Coordination

Judges' ratings	ECR anxiety		ECR avoidance	
	r	β	r	β
Behavioral effectiveness	−.41**	−.43**	−.35*	−.37*
Attention to partner's responses	−.21	−.20	−.05	−.06
Responsiveness to partner's signals	−.45**	−.46**	−.41**	−.42**
Feelings of calmness	−.32*	−.34*	−.35*	−.37*
Closeness promotion	−.33*	−.34*	−.40*	−.41**
Cooperation promotion	−.35*	−.36*	−.32*	−.34*
Partner's responsiveness	−.22	−.23	−.17	−.18
Partner's comfort and enjoyment	−.36*	−.37*	−.33*	−.34*

Note. N = 40.
*$p < .05$; **$p < .01$.

romantic partners). In an early diary study, J. A. Feeney, Noller, and Patty (1993, Study 2) asked participants to record all interactions lasting 10 minutes or longer over a 6-week period and to describe the kinds of activities engaged in (e.g., chatting, kissing) and the kind of partner involved in each interaction. Compared with secure individuals, avoidant ones engaged in fewer interactions during the 6-week period, had fewer "chats," and interacted with a smaller number of friends. Anxious people engaged in fewer interactions with strangers, suggesting that such interactions would not have provided whatever it was that anxious people were looking for (presumably affection, closeness, and approval).

Six subsequent studies used the Rochester Interaction Record (RIR; H. T. Reis & Wheeler, 1991) to examine daily interactions over the course of 1–2 weeks (Kafetsios & Nezlek, 2002; Kerns & Stevens, 1996; Pierce & Lydon, 2001; Pietromonaco & Barrett, 1997; Sibley et al., 2005; Tidwell, Reis, & Shaver, 1996). Participants in these studies completed a fixed-format record for every interaction that lasted 10 minutes or longer and rated the interaction on various attachment-related dimensions (e.g., intimacy, support, responsiveness) and the extent to which the exchange elicited particular positive and negative emotions.

Despite methodological differences in the assessment of attachment (Hazan & Shaver's [1987] ratings, the RQ, the AAS; see Chapter 4, this volume), avoidant people displayed consistent patterns of responses across the five studies and across interactions with different kinds of partners. Compared with secure people, avoidant ones reported lower levels of satisfaction, intimacy, self-disclosure, supportive behavior, and positive emotions during daily interactions, as well as higher levels of negative emotions (e.g., boredom, tension). In addition, Tidwell et al. (1996) found that more avoidant people interacted less often and for shorter times with opposite-sex partners, and Kafetsios and Nezlek (2002) reported that avoidant people believed that their partners had experienced more negative emotions during the recorded interactions. Thus, avoidant people seemed to steer clear of intimate exchanges and feel uninvolved, tense, and bored during daily interactions.

Anxious people were similar to secure ones in their reports of intimacy, closeness-promoting behavior, and satisfaction, but different in reports of higher levels of negative emotions and feelings of rejection, especially when interacting with opposite-sex partners (Kafetsios & Nezlek, 2002; Tidwell et al., 1996). Tidwell et al. also found that attachment anxiety was associated with more variability or lability in emotional responses and closeness-promoting behavior; that is, more anxious people experienced and displayed more ups and downs across interactions, including interactions with the same partner. This finding fits well with other evidence concerning anxious people's ambivalence and the dramatic influence of perceived availability or unavailability of attachment figures on their emotions and emotion regulation (Chapter 7, this volume). This influence was also documented by Pierce and Lydon (2001), who found that although attachment-anxious people habitually reported low-quality daily interpersonal interactions, they tended to report more intimate and better quality interactions with partners with whom they felt more secure.

Pietromonaco and Barrett (1997) noted another interesting feature of anxious people's diary entries. During discordant interactions, they reported higher levels of satisfaction and self-disclosure, as well as stronger positive emotions than did secure people. In fact, they reported more positive perceptions of interactions as the level of conflict *increased*. According to Pietromonaco and Barrett, this fits with anxious people's goal of gaining their partners' attention and increasing partners' involvement in the relationship. Since conflict involves disclosure of private thoughts and feelings, anxious people may perceive their partners' self-disclosures and expressed emotions as signs of interest and engagement. However, this kind of reaction may be limited to conflicts that do not generate clear-cut signs of rejection or disapproval. In Chapter 10 we review numerous studies indicating that anxious individuals have very negative reactions to conflicts occurring within their couple relationships.

Using a different methodology, Ducharme, Doyle, and Markiewicz (2002) asked adolescents to rate their attachment orientations to parents and to complete a diary record every evening for a week. Each evening, participants wrote an open-ended description (telling what happened and how they felt) of one interaction with parents and one interaction with peers that occurred during that day. The narratives were content-analyzed and coded for levels of expressivity, positive and negative emotions, and conflict-management strategies. Unexpectedly, the findings failed to reveal attachment style differences in daily expressivity, but they did reveal theoretically interpretable differences in negative emotions and conflict-management strategies. Adolescents who were anxiously or avoidantly attached to their mothers reported more negative emotions while interacting with parents than did securely attached adolescents, and avoidant adolescents reported withdrawing more and negotiating less in conflictual interactions with parents and peers. In addition, the combination of insecure attachment to both the mother and the father resulted in the lowest level of expressivity and the highest level of negative emotions.

Interestingly, Gallo and Matthews (2006) recently showed that insecurely attached people's negative experiences of daily interpersonal interactions tend to be manifested in cardiovascular responses. High school students completed a self-report measure of anxious and avoidant attachment, and underwent 36 hours of ambulatory blood pressure and heart rate monitoring, while they concomitantly reported on their current or most recent interpersonal interactions. Replicating previous findings, avoidant attachment was associated with fewer interactions with friends, and attachment anxiety was associated with less pleasant and more conflictual interpersonal exchanges both during and outside school hours. More important, attachment anxiety was associated with heightened ambulatory diastolic and systolic blood pressure during interactions with friends. Similarly, avoidance was associated with heightened ambulatory diastolic blood pressure during conflictual interpersonal interactions. These findings suggest that attachment insecurities amplify stress-related physiological reactions to daily interpersonal interactions, which may increase the risk of physical health problems (Chapter 8, this volume).

Reactions to Specific Kinds of Social Interactions

Another line of research addresses attachment style differences in responses to certain kinds of social interactions. Here we focus on four broad categories of interpersonal relations: those in which a target participant's partner behaves negatively or positively toward the participant, and those in which the participant behaves negatively or positively toward the partner. (See Table 9.5 for prototypical attachment-related patterns of reactions to these interpersonal events.)

Episodes in Which a Partner Behaves Badly

Conflicts, offenses, and transgressions are unavoidable in interpersonal relations, because no two people's interests, attitudes, and behaviors are in perfect synch all the time. Eventually, everyone is bound to feel frustrated, offended, let down, betrayed, or wronged by a relationship partner (e.g., Gottman, 1994). The most common responses to such events are seeking distance from the partner, seeking to harm the partner in acts of revenge, or regulating anger constructively and forgiving the offending partner (e.g., Fincham, 2000). Distancing and revenge can erode interpersonal bonds, but forgiveness often results in the restoration of relational harmony (e.g., Fincham, 2000). In Chapter 7, we reviewed evidence linking attachment security with functional, constructive expressions of anger (nonhostile protests), and linking attachment insecurity with less functional forms of anger (animosity, hostility, vengeful criticism, or vicious retaliation). Here, we focus instead on attachment style differences in forgiving an offending relationship partner.

Forgiveness requires difficult regulatory maneuvers—inhibiting the impulse to retaliate and inflict pain, while choosing a more constructive, collaborative response (McCullough, 2000). This often requires understanding a transgressor's needs and motives, and making generous attributions and appraisals concerning the transgressor's traits and hurtful actions (e.g., Fincham, 2000; McCullough, 2000; McCullough, Worthington, & Rachal, 1997). People who are inclined to forgive a transgressor feel a degree of empathy for him or her, view the transgressor as inherently human and likable, and lay some of the blame for the behavior on extenuating circumstances. From an attachment perspective, these regulatory efforts are likely to be facilitated by a secure person's emotional stability and positive working models of others. Secure people are likely to offer relatively benign explanations of their partners' hurtful actions (see Chapter 6, this volume) and be inclined to forgive the partner.

In a recent study, we examined attachment-related differences in the experience of forgiveness and the tendency to forgive a transgressor (Mikulincer, Shaver, & Slav, 2006). The disposition to forgive was assessed with the Forgiving Scale (McCullough et al., 1997) and the Transgression-Related Interpersonal Motivations Inventory (TRIM; McCullough et al., 1998). The experience of forgiveness was assessed by a new self-report scale tapping thoughts and feelings associated with forgiving a transgressor (e.g., feelings of vulnerability or humiliation, being cleansed, and understanding the offending partner's action). (This scale was based on people's open-ended descriptions of particular examples of forgiveness.) More avoidant people were less inclined to forgive and more likely to withdraw or seek revenge. They also reported more intense feelings of vulnerability or humiliation, a stronger sense of relationship deterioration, and less empathy and

TABLE 9.5. An Integrative Summary of Attachment-Related Reactions to Four Kinds of Interpersonal Situations

Interpersonal situations	Attachment security	Avoidant attachment	Attachment anxiety
Interaction partner behaves badly	Functional anger, forgiveness	Suppressed anger, resentment, hostility, revenge, withdrawal, lack of forgiveness	Resentment, hostility, dysfunctional anger, despair, sadness, ambivalence
Interaction partner behaves positively	Happiness, joy, love, gratitude	Indifference, detachment, lack of gratitude	Ambivalent feelings of happiness, love, fear, anxiety
Self behaves badly toward interaction partner	Guilt, reparation	Resentment, hostility	Shame, despair
Self behaves positively toward interaction partner	Happiness, joy, love, pride	*Hubris*	Ambivalent feelings of happiness, anxiety, fear of success

understanding associated with forgiving the offending partner. In other words, avoidance was associated with a more negative experience of forgiveness, which fits with avoidant people's negative working models of others and their unwillingness to risk vulnerability and expend energy to repair damaged relationships.

Attachment anxiety was not significantly associated with dispositions to forgive, withdraw, or seek revenge, but anxiously attached people reported stronger feelings of vulnerability and humiliation associated with "forgiving" a wayward partner. We place forgiving in quotation marks because the genuineness and depth of forgiveness was in doubt; that is, attachment anxiety was associated with experiencing forgiveness in conjunction with lowered self-worth. We suspect that an anxious individual's reactions to a partner's hurtful behavior are influenced by two conflicting forces. On the one hand, the inclination to intensify negative emotions and ruminate on threats (Chapter 7, this volume) interferes with forgiveness. On the other hand, the desperate need for a partner's love and the willingness to sacrifice some self-respect in order not to provoke a breakup may cause the attachment anxious individual to suppress resentment and use "forgiveness" as a negotiation strategy.

Episodes in Which a Partner Behaves Positively

Another common kind of interpersonal exchange occurs when positive behavior on the part of one's partner satisfies one's needs, improves one's welfare, or advances the quality of the relationship. Scholars with different theoretical perspectives agree that the most common response to a partner's positive behavior is a blend of joy (being pleased about obtaining a desirable outcome), love, and respect and admiration (viewing the partner's actions as praiseworthy), which may fuse with feelings of gratitude (e.g., Frei & Shaver, 2002; Heider, 1958). In fact, research indicates that when people are asked to recall a favorable experience attributed to another person's behavior, their most frequent responses are happiness and gratitude (e.g., van Overwalle, Mervielde, & De Schuyter, 1995; Walker & Pitts, 1998; Weiner, 1985).

Although, at first sight, the link between a partner's positive behavior and one's own feelings of gratitude seems intuitively natural, it depends on a person's interpersonal goals and perceptions. One precondition for experiencing gratitude following a partner's supportive behavior is appraisal of the behavior as truly positive (Heider, 1958); that is, one reacts to a partner's behavior with gratitude mainly when one perceives it as authentically congruent with one's own goals. Another prerequisite for experiencing gratitude is recognizing a partner's good intentions (Weiner, 1985). From an attachment perspective, feelings of gratitude during positive interactions should go hand in hand with feeling protected, accepted, and valued, and forming positive models of a partner as available, supportive, and loving. Therefore, attachment security should be associated with the disposition to feel grateful.

In a recent study (Mikulincer, Shaver, & Slar, 2006) we explored the links between attachment and gratitude. Compared to less avoidant people, those scoring high on avoidance were less disposed to feel gratitude (assessed by the six-item Gratitude Questionnaire–6; McCullough, Emmons, & Tsang, 2002). Moreover, when asked to recall a time when they felt grateful to a relationship partner, avoidant people tended to remember more negative experiences, involving more narcissistic threats (e.g., "I felt I was risking my personal freedom," "I thought I was giving up my dignity") and distrust, and less happiness and love. These negative responses reflect avoidant people's unwillingness to depend on or be supported by others, or to express emotions, such as gratitude, that can be interpreted as indicating relational closeness or interdependence.

Attachment anxiety was not significantly associated with dispositional gratitude, but it was associated with a more ambivalent experience of gratitude-arousing interactions. More anxious people recalled security-related feelings (e.g., "I felt there was someone who cares for me"), happiness, and love, together with higher levels of narcissistic threats and inferiority feelings (e.g., "I felt weak and needy," "I felt vulnerable"). They often felt that they did not really deserve other people's kindness (Chapter 6, this volume) and worried that they would not be able to reciprocate fully or meet a partner's needs and expectations, which pollutes gratitude with discomfort and anxiety. In addition, for attachment-anxious individuals, positive interpersonal experiences may be reminiscent of previous experiences that began well but ended painfully, which can arouse negative memories and feelings, and hence interfering with gratitude (similar to Mikulincer & Sheffi's [2000] findings in their studies of positive affect induction; see Chapter 8, this volume).

Episodes in Which One Behaves Badly toward a Relationship Partner

Interpersonal exchanges in which one behaves badly toward a partner, fails to meet the partner's needs and expectations, or actually damages a partner's well-being or the quality of a relationship can evoke a wide array of emotional responses, ranging from self-conscious emotions such as guilt and shame, through fear of punishment or retaliation, to anger and hostile attitudes toward the damaged partner (e.g., Lazarus, 1991; Tangney, 1992). These different responses are likely to be associated with attachment-related processes.

Consider the case of the "self-conscious emotions," guilt and shame. Occurrence of these emotions implies that threatening or harming a partner's welfare is appraised as an undesirable failure to live up to one's own ideals or identity (Tangney, 1992). People who experience and express guilt or shame are likely to view protection of a partner's welfare and maintenance of harmonious interactions as important goals. In fact, these emotions are less evident when people take little responsibility for a partner's welfare or the fate of the relationship (M. S. Clark, Fitness, & Brisette, 2001). This seems characteristic of avoidant individuals, who try to minimize personal involvement and interdependence. For them, a partner's distress or injury does not necessarily arouse guilt or shame.

Attachment issues are also important for distinguishing between shame and guilt. Shame involves attentional focus on one's own objectionable personal qualities (which Janoff-Bulman [1979] called "characterological self-blame"), and attribution of one's negative behavior to global and stable aspects of the self. Moreover, shame is related to feelings of inferiority and a tendency to withdraw and hide from interactions with an offended partner. In contrast, guilt involves an attentional focus on the negative behavior itself (a reaction Janoff-Bulman called "behavioral self-blame"), and attribution of the negative behavior to unstable and controllable aspects of oneself. In addition, guilt is related to feelings of potency and mastery, and to the tendency to engage in reparative behavior to restore a partner's welfare and a harmonious relationship (e.g., Lazarus, 1991; Tangney, 1992).

It is therefore reasonable to suggest that although both secure and anxious people are motivated to maintain strong attachment bonds and react with self-conscious emotions when their actions hurt a partner, they differ in their senses of self-worth and mastery (Chapter 6, this volume); hence, they may experience and express different self-conscious emotions. Whereas secure people, who enjoy a stable sense of self-worth, may react to their own disagreeable behavior with guilt and a corresponding wish to repair the damage, anxious people, who often feel worthless and helpless, may attribute their hurtful behavior to personal deficiencies, which arouses shame.

Although few adult attachment studies have tested these hypotheses, Lopez, Gover, et al. (1997) discovered that ratings of attachment security were associated with higher scores on a guilt-proneness scale. Moreover, a blend of high anxiety and high avoidance (fearful avoidance) was associated with higher scores on a shame-proneness scale, and a combination of high avoidance and low anxiety (dismissing avoidance) was associated with lower shame scores. C. A. Gross and Hansen (2000) and Wei, Shaffer, Young, and Zakalik (2005) also found that people who scored high on attachment anxiety and avoidance were more shame-prone, and Magai et al. (2000) found attachment anxiety to be positively related to facial expressions of shame. In a recent study (Mikulincer & Shaver, 2005b) we asked participants to recall an episode in which they hurt a close relationship partner or failed to meet the partner's needs. After writing a brief description of the episode, participants rated the extent to which it caused them to feel guilty, ashamed, or hostile toward the partner. Whereas more attachment-anxious people reported more shame and less guilt, more avoidant people reported more hostility, less guilt, and less shame. In addition, as theoretically expected (because guilt tends to go with higher self-efficacy and efforts to rectify regrettable behavior), relatively secure people (those with low scores on both anxiety and avoidance) tended to experience more guilt.

Episodes in Which One Behaves Positively toward a Relationship Partner

The most common response to interactions in which one's own supportive behavior results in a partner's happiness is presumably an increase in one's own happiness, love, and pride (Weiner, 1985). As in the previous examples we considered, however, this straightforward linkage may depend on a person's attachment style. For avoidant people, who do not view promotion of a partner's welfare and maintenance of a comfortably interdependent relationship as major personal goals, a partner's happiness may not affect their own happiness and love. For anxiously attached people, who harbor serious doubts about their own value and efficacy (Chapter 6, this volume), engendering a partner's happiness may not result in a feeling of pride, because they cannot take credit for the partner's happiness and may attribute it to the partner's own good qualities. In fact, it seems possible that only securely attached people experience the full measure of joy, love, and pride.

Avoidant individuals may experience the kind of pride the ancient Greeks called *hubris*, described by Lewis (2000) as exaggerated pride resulting not from success in enhancing a partner's welfare but from confirming one's own brilliance, superiority, and grandiosity. This emotion is a manifestation of narcissism, which fits well with avoidant proclivities. In contrast, anxious individuals may react to a partner's happiness with "fear of success" feelings—distress caused by doubts about their worthiness to claim credit for a partner's welfare. They may worry that their success in meeting a partner's needs will increase his or her expectations, creating pressure on future performances.

Unfortunately, adult attachment researchers have not examined the role of attachment style in emotional reactions to a partner's happiness. In one of our studies (Mikulincer & Shaver, 2005b), however, we attempted to fill part of this empirical gap by asking people to recall a time when they made a partner happy, then rate the extent to which this evoked pride, other positive emotions, or negative emotions. More attachment-anxious people expressed greater distress in response to a partner's happiness; more avoidant people were less likely to express personal happiness in reaction to a happy partner; more secure people were happier when they made their partner happy. These are only preliminary findings, however. More systematic research is needed to determine how people with different attachment styles react to a partner's happiness.

The Cognitive Processing of Interpersonal Interactions

Attachment style is also likely to be associated with the cognitive processing of interpersonal interactions, which should facilitate the encoding and retrieval of aspects of the experience that coincide with a person's most accessible working models. For example, Belsky, Spritz, and Crnic (1996) assessed 3-year-olds' memory for positive and negative interpersonal events in a puppet show and found that secure children were more likely to remember and recognize positive than negative events. In contrast, insecure children recognized more negative than positive events. Similarly, Beinstein Miller and Noirot (1999) assessed young adults' recall of a story in which the main character experienced positive and negative interpersonal events, and found that more secure participants recalled more positive events. Fearfully avoidant participants displayed better recall of negative events. In a related study, Beinstein Miller (1999) found that more secure people exhibited better recall of story events that involved joint activities on the part of friends, whereas fearfully avoidant people better recalled the friends' separate activities.

B. Feeney and Cassidy (2003) expanded this line of research to adolescents' perceptions and memories of actual interactions with parents. Adolescents reported on their attachment security to parents, engaged in laboratory problem-solving discussions with each of their parents, then described their perceptions of the interactions both immediately after each one and again 6 weeks later. Secure adolescents' immediate perceptions of the discussions were more positive than those of insecure adolescents. Moreover, whereas secure adolescents later recalled having had more positive exchanges than they reported immediately following the discussions, insecure adolescents recalled having more negative exchanges than originally occurred. In other words, over time attachment orientations biased reconstruction of interpersonal memories in ways that confirmed dominant working models.

This memory bias was also observed in a diary study by Gentzler and Kerns (2006). College students completed questionnaires three times a day for 4 consecutive days and rated their immediate emotional reactions to events within each time period. Ten days later, participants were given descriptions of (1) the event that elicited the most negative affect during the 4-days study period and (2) the event that elicited the most positive affect. They were then asked to estimate how they initially felt when these events occurred. Insecure participants, whether anxious or avoidant, recalled having experienced less positive emotion than they reported immediately after their most positive interpersonal event. This kind of memory bias, occurring repeatedly in normal, everyday life, probably reduces the impact of positive interpersonal events and helps sustain insecure working models.

Interestingly, attachment-schematic processes also influence the amount of attention people pay to interpersonal exchanges and the consequent recall of this information. For example, Beinstein Miller (2001) asked young adults to act as participants or observers in short or long conversations with scripted confederates, then assessed the accuracy of their recall of the confederates' remarks. More avoidant individuals recalled confederates' remarks less accurately, and the association was stronger for long than for short conversations. Thus, avoidant people seem to remain detached and disinterested during interpersonal exchanges, especially during long conversations that demand more attention, and this interferes with subsequent memory for an interaction partner's remarks. (See Chapter 7, this volume, for a discussion of compatible results from a study by Fraley, Garner, & Shaver, 2000.)

Summary

A large literature indicates that secure people engage in positive, intimacy-promoting, and tension-reducing interpersonal behavior, and have a positive memory bias for interpersonal exchanges. In contrast, avoidant people are relatively disengaged during social interactions, easily become bored or tense, and are likely to forget their partners' feelings and remarks. They try not to become either positively or negatively emotional but when they do, they tend to be angry, hostile, or disparaging, and rarely experience unadulterated gratitude or forgiveness. Attachment-anxious people exhibit ambivalent blends of positive and negative reactions that reflect their characteristic conflict between desires for closeness and love on the one hand, and fears of rejection, disapproval, and abandonment on the other. They are capable of gratitude and forgiveness, but these emotions are often mixed with negative self-referential feelings rarely experienced by more secure people.

INTERPERSONAL PROBLEMS AND THE SENSE OF LONELINESS

In Chapter 10, we review the large literature on attachment-related problems in couple relationships. Here, we focus on insecure people's specific problems in interpersonal relations, their experience of loneliness, and their troubled friendships.

Profiles of Interpersonal Difficulties

Drawing from the general circumplex model (which applies to both secure and insecure people), L. M. Horowitz, Rosenberg, Baer, Ureno, and Villasenor (1988) identified interpersonal problems that characterize each octant of the circumplex. They then constructed a self-report scale—the Inventory of Interpersonal Problems (IIP)—to create a profile of each person's interpersonal difficulties. The major maladaptive patterns were labeled *overly autocratic* (e.g., "I try to control other people too much"), *overly competitive* (e.g., "I fight with other people too much"), *overly cold* (e.g., "I keep other people at a distance too much"), *overly introverted* (e.g., "I feel embarrassed in front of other people too much"), *overly subassertive* (e.g., "It is hard for me to be assertive with another person"), *overly exploitable* (e.g., "I let other people take advantage of me too much"), *overly nurturant* (e.g., "I put other people's needs before my own too much"), and *overly expressive/demanding* (e.g., "I want to be noticed too much"). Using the IIP, researchers create a profile of interpersonal problems for each individual based on his or her relative peaks and dips across the eight circumplex domains.

Bartholomew and Horowitz (1991) were the first to explore attachment-related interpersonal problems assessed with the IIP. Participants in their study completed the Peer Attachment Interview (see Chapter 4, this volume) and the IIP, and their friends also rated participants' problematic behavior using the IIP. Across both self- and friend-reports, attachment anxiety was associated with a higher overall level of interpersonal problems. There were also attachment-related differences in profiles of interpersonal problems. Whereas securely attached people did not show notable elevations in any parts of the circumplex of problems, avoidant people generally had problems with nurturance (being overly cold, introverted, or competitive), and anxious people had problems related to their insistent demands for love and support (being overly expressive). Interestingly, fearfully avoidant participants (those who scored high on both the anxious and avoidant attachment dimensions) had problems associated with lack of dominance (i.e., being overly subassertive and exploitable).

Bartholomew and Horowitz's (1991) findings have been conceptually replicated in diverse samples of college undergraduates (Bookwala & Zdaniuk, 1998; E. C. Chen & Mallinckrodt, 2002; Gillath, Mikulincer, et al., 2005), patients seeking services at a medical clinic (Noyes et al., 2003), and depressed women (Cyranowski et al., 2002). Moreover, some studies (Bookwala & Zdaniuk, 1998; Chen & Mallinckrodt, 2002; Gillath, Shaver, Mikulincer, et al., 2005; Noyes et al., 2003) have found that more anxiously attached people show a greater likelihood of being both overly expressive and overly subassertive. These findings highlight anxious people's ambivalence: They want and need a great deal, and sometimes express themselves intensely, but they lack confidence in their ability to get what they want, so they sometimes defer too readily to a partner's wishes or attempt to control their otherwise strong emotional reactions.

Loneliness

These interpersonal problems can easily cause feelings of dissatisfaction and loneliness (L. M. Horowitz et al., 1988). Loneliness arises when a person's social interactions and relationships are deficient in quality, quantity, or both (Peplau & Perlman, 1982), and it is a known risk factor for social withdrawal, mental health problems, and physical symptoms (e.g., Ernst & Cacioppo, 1999; Segrin, 1998). Its chronic, dispositional form is thought to result from a history of relationships with cool, rejecting, inconsistent, or unavailable attachment figures (e.g., Rubenstein & Shaver, 1982; Weiss, 1973).

Working explicitly from an attachment perspective, Weiss (1973) defined "loneliness" as an emotion that signals unsatisfied needs for proximity, love, and security due to the unavailability of attachment figures. In other words, loneliness is a form of separation distress that results from failure to have one's basic attachment needs fulfilled. As such, loneliness should be mitigated or precluded by a sense of attachment security. In contrast, attachment insecurities should render a person chronically vulnerable to loneliness (Berlin, Cassidy, & Belsky, 1995; Hazan & Shaver, 1987).

Attachment researchers have also hypothesized that anxious attachment, more than avoidant attachment, is conducive to loneliness (e.g., Berlin et al., 1995). Attachment-anxious people exaggerate their unsatisfied needs for love and security, which intensifies the psychological pain associated with insufficient or missing attachment relationships. Avoidant people try to deny or inhibit attachment needs; they may therefore feel less directly pained or frustrated by poor or absent relationships. As we have already shown in this chapter, avoidant individuals do experience a lack of engagement in social interactions, which leads them to feel bored, distant, tense, or irritated, but they can acknowledge those feelings without admitting a need for affection or connectedness. In fact, construing the problem as one of boredom or irritation puts the blame on something outside the avoidant person him- or herself. One can be bored and critical or dismissing of others without admitting personal needs, insufficiencies, or dependence on others. According to Hazan and Shaver (1987), this stance often allows avoidant people to admit that they are distant from others, without labeling themselves as lonely.

Table 9.6 summarizes published studies linking attachment style measures with loneliness in adolescence and adulthood. All studies in which attachment security in relationships with parents or peers was correlated with loneliness have produced inverse correlations. In addition, the vast majority of studies that included measures of attachment anxiety or compared anxious with secure people have found that anxious attachment is associated with loneliness. Moreover, most of the studies that have assessed avoidance or compared avoidant and secure individuals have found that avoidant attachment is also associated with loneliness. Findings are less consistent with respect to comparisons between anxious and avoidant attachment orientations: Some studies found no significant difference between the two insecure groups (when attachment was assessed categorically), but other studies have found greater self-reported loneliness among anxious than among avoidant people (see Table 9.6). Few studies have explored mediators of the associations between attachment insecurity and loneliness, but DiTommaso et al. (2003) found that the effects were mediated by deficits in interpersonal skills, and Larose and Bernier (2001) found that they were mediated by pessimistic appraisals of interpersonal relations and difficulties in obtaining social and emotional support.

The finding that avoidance, like attachment anxiety, is related to loneliness implies that avoidant people may not deactivate their attachment systems to the point of not caring at all about the absence of supportive relationships. This conclusion is consistent with findings we reviewed in Chapters 6, 7, and 13, which indicate that deactivating strategies are not sufficiently strong or complete to inhibit every inkling of the wish for greater security.

However, even if both anxious and avoidant people tend to feel lonely, only avoidant people seem to choose to withdraw socially and remain isolated. For example, Shaver and Hazan (1987) reported that whereas attachment-anxious people were less likely to expect to be lonely forever and described themselves as hopeful and active in their search for relationship partners, avoidant people were more likely to believe they would always be lonely. Interestingly, and sadly, longitudinal and cross-sectional studies of adults have indicated that these expectations tend to be fulfilled across the lifespan. In a nationally representative survey study of American adults, Mickelson et al. (1997) found that scores on anxious attachment declined with age, whereas scores on avoidant attachment remained about the same over the years. Klohnen and Bera

TABLE 9.6. A Summary of Findings Linking Attachment Orientations with Loneliness

Study	Attachment measure	Loneliness measure	Main findings
Studies assessing secure attachment to parents or peers			
Larose & Boivin (1997)	IPPA	UCLA scale	Security (–)
Larose & Boivin (1998)*	IPPA	UCLA scale	Security (–)
Long & Martin (2000)	HS ratings	UCLA scale	Security (–)
Larose et al. (2002)*	IPPA	UCLA scale	Security (–)
Moller et al. (2002)	ASQ	UCLA scale	Security (–)
Studies assessing attachment types			
Hazan & Shaver (1987)	HS types	UCLA scale	Anxious > Secure
Kobak & Sceery (1988)	AAI	UCLA scale	Avoidant > Secure
Hudson & Ward (1997)	RQ	UCLA scale	Anxious, Fearful > Secure
Goosens et al. (1998)	Projective test	LLCA	Fearful, Anxious, Avoidant > Secure
Man & Hamid (1998)	40-item scale	UCLA scale	Fearful > Anxious > Avoidant > Secure
Marsa et al. (2004)	ECR	UCLA scale	Fearful > Anxious > Avoidant > Secure
Studies based on attachment-style ratings			
DiTommaso et al. (2003)	RSQ	SELSA	Secure (–), Avoidant (+), Anxious (+), Fear (+)
Ireland & Power (2004)	HS ratings	UCLA scale	Secure (–), Avoidant (+), Anxious (ns)
Deniz et al. (2005)	RSQ	UCLA scale	Secure (–), Avoidant (+), Anxious (+), Fear (+)
Wiseman et al. (2005)	HS ratings	UCLA scale	Secure (–), Avoidant (+), Anxious (+)
Studies assessing attachment dimensions			
Kerns & Stevens (1996)	AAS	UCLA scale	Avoidance (+) Anxiety (+)
Sanford (1997)	AAS	UCLA scale	Avoidance (+) Anxiety (+)
Larose & Bernier (2001)	AAI	UCLA scale	Avoidance (ns) Anxiety (+)
		Withdrawal scale	Avoidance (+) Anxiety (ns)
Moller et al. (2003)	ASQ	UCLA scale	Avoidance (+) Anxiety (+)
Gillath, Shaver, Mikulincer, et al. (2005)	ECR	UCLA scale	Avoidance (+) Anxiety (+)
Wei, Russell, & Zakalik. (2005)	ECR	UCLA scale	Avoidance (+) Anxiety (+)
Wei, Shaffer, et al. (2005)	ECR	UCLA scale	Avoidance (+) Anxiety (+)
J. A. Feeney (2006)	ASQ	UCLA scale	Avoidance (+) Anxiety (+) for W
			Avoidance (ns) Anxiety (+) for M

Note. *, longitudinal design; M, men; W, women; (+), significant positive associations; (–), significant negative associations; (ns), nonsignificant effects; HS, Hazan and Shaver; LLCA, Louvain Loneliness Scale for Children and Adolescents; SELSA, Social and Emotional Loneliness Scale for Adults; UCLA, UCLA Loneliness Scale.

(1998) studied a group of women across a 30-year expanse of adulthood and obtained similar results.

Avoidant people are more likely than their secure and anxious agemates to say that during the preceding few years they have not felt in tune with other people, have not been part of a group of friends, and have not felt close to anyone (Shaver & Hazan, 1987). Similarly, Larose and Bernier (2001) found that avoidance, but not anxiety, was associated with social withdrawal, and Bookwala (2003), Davila, Steinberg, Kachadourian, Cobb, and Fincham (2004), and Kirkpatrick and Hazan (1994) found that avoidance increased the odds of being single or not being involved in serious dating.

Attachment Style and Friendship

Insecure people's lack of social adjustment has also been noted in studies assessing the quality of peer relationships and friendships. Several studies indicate that attachment insecurity in infancy (assessed in the Strange Situation) predicts less positive relations with peers and friends in childhood and preadolescence (e.g., Elicker, Englund, & Sroufe, 1992; K. Grossmann & Grossmann, 1991; Sroufe, 1983). Similarly, K. A. Park and Waters (1989) and Kerns (1994) found that insecure attachment to one's mother in the preschool years was associated with more controlling, less harmonious, and less happy interactions with friends later on. Schneider, Atkinson, and Tardif (2001) conducted a meta-analysis of such studies and found a moderate mean effect size ($r = .24$) linking attachment orientations with aspects of friendship from preschool to preadolescence.

Studies linking attachment security and friendship quality during adolescence and adulthood have yielded similar results. Attachment security is associated with friendships characterized by trust, self-disclosure, closeness, mutuality, and the use of more relationship-promoting conflict resolution strategies; attachment insecurity is associated with less satisfying friendships (e.g., Bippus & Rollin, 2003; Furman et al., 2002; Grabill & Kerns, 2000; Markiewicz, Doyle, & Brendgen, 2001; Mayseless, 1993; McCarthy, 1999; Weimer, Kerns, & Oldenburg, 2004; Zimmermann, 2004). Scharf et al. (2004) and Mayseless and Scharf (in press) found that self-rated secure attachment or a secure state of mind with respect to attachment (in the AAI) during late adolescence predicted greater intimacy and closeness in friendships 3 years later. Researchers who have assessed the quality of actual interactions between friends in the laboratory found that dyads with two secure members are more likely to interact in synchronous, intimate, and warm ways than dyads including at least one insecure person (K. A. Black & McCartney, 1997; Weimer et al., 2004). However, some studies have failed to find a link between attachment style and reports of friendship quality (Bartholomew & Horowitz, 1991; Kerns & Stevens, 1996). Despite the discrepant findings, there is sufficient evidence to suggest that attachment insecurity puts people at risk for troubled friendships.

CONCLUDING REMARKS

Researchers have been creative and productive in exploring connections between attachment theory and other approaches to the study of close relationships. Having found ways to probe mental processes associated with attachment security and insecurity, they have gone on to explore how these individual differences in attachment style play out in social interactions and interpersonal relations. Attachments styles are systematically related to some of the "Big Five" personality traits that provide an organizing framework for personality research, and they are related to the circumplex model of interpersonal traits, which is organized around two dimensions, running from cold to warm and from dominant to submissive.

Anxious and avoidant attachment are related to people's goals and wishes in interpersonal encounters, whether expressed in narrative accounts or in dream reports, and they influence patterns of communication, including expressiveness, sensitivity, and conflict management. Many of the individual differences reviewed in this chapter influence not only people's interpretations of their own and relationship partners' constructive and destructive relational behaviors but also emotions embedded in interpersonal relationships, such as guilt, shame, gratitude, forgiveness, and loneliness.

All forms of interpersonal regulation discussed in this chapter seem to fit well with the concepts of hyperactivation and deactivation (Chapter 2, this volume), and with the associated idea that people differ systematically in their characteristic degree of security versus insecurity and in their use of anxious or avoidant strategies. Attachment theory is based on the assumption that these relatively stable individual differences arise in the context of attachment relationships and are based more on experience than on genetic influences (Chapter 5, this volume). However, given that attachment style is associated with other dispositions known to be substantially affected by genes, such as the "Big Five" personality traits, it is important to learn more about the determinants of attachment style, using longitudinal designs, and to conduct adult twin studies and studies of particular genetic profiles to see whether and to what extent social experiences interact with genes to influence attachment style. (The few relevant studies are discussed briefly in Chapter 5, this volume.) Finally, now that there is an extensive network of associations between attachment style dimensions and other personality and relationship constructs, more research needs to be undertaken to reveal the mediating processes.

CHAPTER 10

Attachment Processes
and Couple Functioning

In this chapter we examine romantic relationships and marriages, sites of some of the most important emotional bonds in adulthood. We seek to understand whether and how the attachment style differences in interpersonal regulation reviewed in Chapter 9, this volume, influence couple relationships. Bowlby (1979) was the first to discuss individual differences in attachment-system functioning in the context of romantic and marital relationships, and Shaver et al. (1988) proposed that romantic attachment bonds in adulthood are similar to the ones infants form with their primary caregivers (see Chapter 1, this volume). Following their lead, and based on a great deal more evidence than Shaver et al. had available in 1988, we review and integrate what is now known about the influence of couple members' attachment styles on the success or failure of their romantic and marital relationships. We highlight (1) attachment-related processes affecting the formation, consolidation, and maintenance of long-term romantic relationships, and (2) the effects of these processes on relationship quality, satisfaction, and stability.

ATTACHMENT-RELATED PROCESSES THAT INFLUENCE INITIATION, CONSOLIDATION, AND MAINTENANCE OF COUPLE RELATIONSHIPS

In this section we consider three stages in the development of a couple relationship—flirtation/dating, consolidation, and maintenance—and examine the effects of attachment style on each stage. We do not discuss the termination phase of relationships in detail, because we already explained in Chapter 7 how attachment style affects coping with and adjustment to a relationship breakup or loss.

The Initial Stages: Flirting and Dating

Attachment strategies are evident even at the beginning of a romantic relationship. They influence flirting and dating, thereby affecting a person's likelihood of forming a long-lasting emotional bond with a new romantic partner. Flirtatious interactions and first dates, especially when aimed at something more than short-term sexual gratification, are likely to activate the attachment system. They are emotionally charged and can arouse hopes of care and support, as well as fears of disapproval and rejection. Hence, partners' thoughts, feelings, and behaviors when flirting and dating are shaped by attachment working models and associated patterns of interpersonal regulation. In this early stage of relationship development, one can sometimes detect the purest effects of chronic working models on relational behavior, because unacquainted interaction partners have minimal information about each other and have yet to establish a unique couple interaction pattern. Their fear and expectations are therefore likely to be influenced heavily by needs and projections.

These theoretical claims were explored in a recent study of attachment style and transference by Brumbaugh and Fraley (2006). In an initial session of the study, participants completed the Experiences in Close Relationships—Revised Scale (ECR-R) and provided a list of traits that described the partner in their most important previous romantic relationship. In the second session, they learned about two potential dating partners differing in the extent to which their traits resembled those of their former romantic partner (low, high) and used the ECR-R to indicate the level of attachment anxiety and avoidance they would feel if involved in a dating relationship with each of these potential partners. The findings nicely demonstrated that people transfer their attachment orientations to new potential dating partners even when there is little overlap between the new person's traits and those of a significant former partner. More attachment-anxious people anticipate feeling anxious with their new dating partner, and more avoidant people anticipate being more avoidant. This makes it likely that existing attachment working models and interpersonal dispositions will influence flirtatious interactions and first dates, and affect both the quality of these interactions and their ultimate fate.

Emotional Tone

As we discussed in Chapter 7, secure individuals typically manage tension and uncertainty constructively, transforming potential threats into challenges. They are likely to remain upbeat and fairly relaxed while flirting and getting to know someone, which can help their potential relationship partner relax and enjoy the interchange. In contrast, anxious and avoidant tendencies are likely to interfere with smooth and comfortable initial interactions. An attachment-anxious person is likely to be haunted by premonitions of rejection, rumination on possible signs of partner disapproval or rejection, and self-focused attention on needs and worries. Avoidant tendencies are likely to manifest themselves in egotism, detachment, inhibited self-expression, lax attention, and overemphasis on sexuality (see Chapter 12, this volume). These signs of avoidance are intended (perhaps unconsciously) to protect a person from threats to self-worth and pressures to self-disclose and become intimate or dependent. Although adult attachment researchers have yet to provide a systematic account of attachment style differences in flirting and dating behavior, there is some evidence that secure people score higher on self-report measures of joy, happiness, and interest in social interactions than do insecure individuals and are more likely to enjoy daily interactions with members of the opposite sex (see Chapter 9, this volume).

Self-Presentation and Self-Disclosure

We know that attachment insecurity can interfere with two interpersonal processes that play an important role in the initial stages of a romantic relationship—self-presentation and self-disclosure. "Self-presentation" refers to the way a person presents him- or herself to others, which can obviously influence an interaction partner's decision to continue or end a budding relationship (Schlenker, 1980). Self-presentation requires tactical choices about which aspects of the self to reveal, and these choices can be biased by insecurity. Anxious people's wish to achieve closeness, support, and love can cause them to present themselves as helpless, needy, or overeager. Avoidant people's desire for independence and self-containment can cause them to communicate to a dating partner that they do not really need a partner, although they may be interested in short-term sex.

A second interpersonal process of great importance early in a relationship is "self-disclosure." According to Altman and Taylor (1973), self-disclosure is systematically regulated at each stage of a developing relationship. Early on, disclosure is typically limited to relatively superficial public information, and rapid disclosure of very intimate information, concerns, and feelings is perceived as a sign of excessive neediness or some other form of maladjustment. As a relationship progresses, partners begin to exchange more personal information, including likes and dislikes, needs and fears, past relationships, personal secrets, and memories of painful experiences. At this stage, inhibition or evasion of self-disclosure is experienced as lack of trust or trustworthiness, or lack of interest in or commitment to the relationship, which can obviously disrupt its development. A history of security helps in this situation, because it allows a person to keep a partner's interests and disclosures in mind while disclosing him- or herself in synchrony with the partner's revelations. Also, to the extent that security fosters empathy and compassion (see Chapter 11, this volume, this volume), a secure person can encourage a partner's self-disclosure without causing him or her to feel vulnerable to misunderstanding or rejection.

Attachment research has established that avoidant tendencies are associated with low self-disclosure (see Chapter 9, this volume), whereas both security and attachment anxiety are associated with willingness to self-disclose. Despite the similarity between secure and anxious individuals in this respect, anxious ones tend to disclose indiscriminately, before their interaction partner is prepared for intense intimacy. They also tend to be relatively unresponsive to a partner's disclosures, perhaps because of nervousness, awkwardness, or intense self-focus (Grabill & Kerns, 2000; Mikulincer & Nachshon, 1991). It seems likely, therefore, that anxious self-disclosure is "too much, too soon"—reflecting a strong wish to merge with another person to quell anxiety, to perceive deep interpersonal similarity where no such similarity has been explored or established, to enlist other people's sympathy and support prematurely, and to focus on reducing fear of rejection rather than enhancing reciprocal intimacy. This is a natural but unfortunate consequence of focusing on one's own desperate needs rather than allowing oneself to appreciate a new interaction partner's qualities and comments.

Secure individuals' self-disclosures are guided by the goals of mutual enjoyment and intimacy. Mikulincer and Nachshon (1991), Keelan, Dion, and Dion (1998), and Grabill and Kerns (2000) found that the secure participants in their studies disclosed more personal information to a high- than to a low-disclosing partner (indicating their sensitivity to the partner's behavior). They were able to elicit more disclosures from the partner, were attentive to thoughts and feelings expressed by the partner, and expanded on them in their own replies. This combination of reciprocal self-disclosure and responsiveness to a partner's experiences and comments is likely to be the best strategy for forming the kinds of warm, trusting, and intimate bonds that secure individuals wish to create.

Self-disclosure was examined by S. A. Bradford, Feeney, and Campbell (2002) in an innovative study of dating interactions. Participants were asked to rate each conversation they had with a dating partner over a 7-day period, focusing on the amount and emotional tone of self-disclosure and their satisfaction with the disclosure process. More avoidant people reported fewer and less intimate disclosures in their everyday conversations with dating partners and felt less satisfied with the disclosure process. Attachment-anxious individuals made more negative disclosures, and their partners rated these disclosures as relatively unsatisfying and negative in tone.

Attachment Security as a Mate Selection Standard

Another source of insecure people's disadvantages in flirtatious and dating interactions is their lower psychological attractiveness compared with that of secure individuals. Beyond the usual features that attract one person to another (similarity to one's actual or ideal self, complementarity to one's needs and traits, physical appearance, and social status; e.g., Buss, 1998; Byrne, 1971), attachment security is a valued resource that people, regardless of their own attachment style, look for in potential romantic partners (e.g., Chappel & Davis, 1998; Klohnen & Luo, 2003). Most people are more attracted to secure than to insecure partners from the start, because secure partners offer the best opportunity for forming and maintaining mutually satisfying and stable couple relationships. In fact, because almost everyone wishes to achieve happiness, safety, and stability in close relationships, most people are interested in finding a partner who can help produce these desired outcomes.

Nine published studies have examined associations between attachment styles and attractiveness (Table 10.1 summarizes the methods and findings). In all of these studies, single undergraduates described their own attachment style and read descriptions of attachment style qualities of hypothetical or potential romantic partners. The findings were quite consistent across studies and provide strong support for the hypothesized use of attachment security as a mate-selection criterion. Participants in all nine studies, regardless of their own attachment style, were more attracted to secure than to insecure partners, reported more positive emotions and fewer negative emotions when imagining a relationship with secure rather than with insecure partners, and preferred to date secure rather than insecure people.

All of the studies but one (Frazier, Byer, Fischer, Wright, & DeBord, 1996, Study 2) also found that avoidant people were the most disadvantaged on initial dates. Although anxious and avoidant potential partners were both rated as less attractive than secure ones, study participants were more attracted to anxious than to avoidant people and felt better when imagining a date with an anxious person than when imagining a date with an avoidant person. According to Klohnen and Luo (2003), "This finding makes sense because individuals' preference with regard to emotional and physical closeness, as captured by the avoidance dimension, should play a more central role in initial attraction than how individuals think and feel about themselves vis-à-vis their relationships, as captured by the anxiety dimension" (p. 719).

Mating Preferences

Beyond their disadvantageous position when flirting and dating, insecure people are hindered by problematic mate preferences, which further jeopardize their chances of estab-

TABLE 10.1. A Summary of Findings Concerning Partner's Attachment Orientation and Consequent Attractiveness

Study	Attachment measure	Manipulation of partner's traits	Type of partner	Dependent variable	Main finding for partner's attachment style
Pietromonaco & Carnelley (1994)	HS ratings	Behavioral vignettes of three styles	Imaginary	Positive emotions	Secure > Anxious = Avoidant
				Negative emotions	Avoidant > Anxious > Secure
Baldwin et al. (1996, Study 3)	HS ratings	Questionnaire responses for each of three styles	Potential	Attractiveness	Secure > Anxious > Avoidant
Latty-Mann & Davis (1996)	RQ	Prototypical description of four styles	Ideal	Attractiveness	Secure > Anxious > Avoidant = Fear
Frazier et al. (1996, Study 2)	HS ratings	Questionnaire responses for each of three styles	Potential	Attractiveness	Secure > Anxious = Avoidant
Frazier et al. (1996, Study 3)	AAS	Questionnaire responses for each of three styles	Potential	Attractiveness	Secure > Anxious > Avoidant
Chappell & Davis (1998)	RQ	Behavioral vignettes matching four styles	Imaginary	Positive emotions	Secure > Anxious > Avoidant = Fear
				Negative emotions	Fear = Avoidant = Anxious > Secure
				Preference for date	Secure > Anxious = Avoidant = Fearful
Klohnen & Luo (2003, Study 1)	RQ, ECR	Behavioral vignettes; four styles	Imaginary	Attractiveness	Secure > Anxious > Avoidant = Fear
Klohnen & Luo (2003, Study 2)	RQ, ECR	Behavioral vignettes; four styles	Imaginary	Attractiveness	Secure > Anxious > Avoidant = Fear
Klohnen & Luo (2003, Study 3)	RQ, ECR	Questionnaire responses; three styles	Potential	Attractiveness	Secure > Anxious > Avoidant = Fear

Note. HS, Hazan and Shaver.

lishing a good relationship. In seven of the nine studies summarized in Table 10.1 (Baldwin et al., 1996; Frazier et al., 1996, Studies 1 and 2; Klohnen & Luo, 2003, Studies 1–3; Latty-Mann & Davis, 1996) insecure people were more attracted than secure ones to insecure potential partners (i.e., even though secure potential partners were favored overall, insecure people were more favorable than secure people toward insecure potential partners). In line with the well-documented connection between similarity and attraction (Byrne, 1971), anxious individuals were more attracted to anxious and fearful partners (with whom they would share anxiety), and avoidant people were more attracted to avoidant and fearful partners (with whom they would share avoidance). In addition, Pietromonaco and Carnelley (1994) found some support for a complementary pattern of mating preferences, in which avoidant individuals preferred anxiously attached partners who could confirm their working models of self (as stronger and more self-reliant than other people) and of others (viewing them as relatively weak, needy, and dependent). These patterns of attraction, while understandable and fully in line with hundreds of studies of either similarity or complementarity and attraction (e.g., Buss, 1998; Byrne, 1971), are likely to undermine insecure people's relationships, because relationships between two insecure people tend to fare less well, on average, than ones that include at least one secure person (as we show later in this chapter).

There is also evidence, beyond studies of hypothetical partner preferences, that insecure people really do tend to date less secure partners. In a sample of adult women who had been abused during childhood, McCarthy (1999) found that those with an anxious or avoidant attachment style were more likely than secure women to cohabit with a socially deviant (e.g., delinquent, drug-abusing) partner. Moreover, Collins et al. (2002) reported that avoidant attachment (assessed during adolescence) was predictive of involvement 6 years later in dating relationships with partners characterized by less healthy personality profiles: high negative affectivity, low autonomy, and high attachment anxiety. All of these qualities seem likely to interfere with achieving favorable relationship outcomes.

Interestingly, although the studies summarized in the previous paragraph indicated that avoidant people found other avoidant people relatively attractive, studies of actual dating relationships suggest that many avoidant people end up with anxious partners (e.g., Kirkpatrick & Davis, 1994; Kirkpatrick & Hazan, 1994). This suggests that the anxious member of the couple either takes the initiative with the avoidant one or is so desperate to be in a relationship that he or she is willing to get involved with a less generally desirable mate. Alternatively, it is possible that the avoidant member of the couple is willing to defer to the preferences and initiating role of the anxious one because of poor initiation skills.

The Consolidation Stage of a Long-Term Romantic Relationship

In the course of a romantic relationship, couples usually make a transition from falling or being in love to loving each other (Berscheid & Regan, 2004). Flirtation and dating give way to more extended joint activities, and the sharing of intimate information and discussion of personal histories and concerns are supplemented or replaced by discussions of long-term goals the couple might pursue together. In most cases, the importance of mutual support, nurturance, and intimacy as determinants of relationship quality increases as early infatuation and sexual passion recede in relative importance. The partners typically begin to make changes in their activities and living conditions that reflect their increasing commitment to each other (e.g., Brehm, 1992). These changes usually indicate that partners are setting the foundation for what they expect to be a lasting, committed, and mutually satisfying relationship.

During the transition, attachment styles can facilitate or hinder the consolidation of a long-lasting relationship (Morgan & Shaver, 1999). Secure individuals' positive beliefs about their partner's supportiveness and trustworthiness (see Chapter 6, this volume) favor optimistic expectations about the prospects of a lasting relationship. Moreover, these beliefs, together with the desire for a mutually satisfactory, intimate relationship, encourage secure people to commit themselves to a long-lasting relationship, to treat their partner as an attachment figure (a reliable source of comfort and support), and to serve the partner as an attachment figure (a sensitive and responsive caregiver). In contrast, the interpersonal goals of insecure people (either a self-focused quest for security and support or a self-protective effort to maintain autonomy and avoid intimacy), their preferred regulatory strategies (rumination about relationship threats and worries; emotional detachment and excessive self-reliance), and their negative working models (anxious and avoidant, respectively) are likely to distort beliefs and expectations about the relationship and interfere with the formation of a long-lasting, mutually intimate, supportive, and committed relationship.

Relational Beliefs and Attitudes

Attachment researchers have investigated the relational beliefs that contribute to consolidation of a romantic relationship. In Chapter 6, we reviewed evidence of insecure people's negative perceptions of relationship partners' intentions, trustworthiness, and supportiveness. In this section, we focus on how attachment insecurity biases beliefs and attitudes about romantic love and couple relationships.

In their original studies of adult attachment, Hazan and Shaver (1987) found that secure people held more optimistic beliefs about romantic love than their anxious or avoidant counterparts. Secure people were more likely to believe in the existence of romantic love, the possibility of maintaining intense love over a long period, and the possibility of finding a partner with whom one could really fall in love. Hazan and Shaver also found some interesting differences between anxious and avoidant individuals. Whereas anxious people were more likely than their avoidant counterparts to believe that it is easy to fall in love, avoidant people were more likely to believe that love either does not exist or is likely to disappear once a relationship is formed. That is, the too-easily activated attachment systems of anxious individuals seem to favor falling in love easily and indiscriminately, in hopes of merging with another person and increasing felt security. Avoidant people find it harder to fall in love and many even doubt that such a state is possible outside of movies and romantic stories. Even within a long-term relationship, anxious people are more likely to sustain their "passion," whereas an avoidant attachment style is associated with experiencing less passion over time (D. Davis et al., 2004).

Subsequent studies have replicated and extended Hazan and Shaver's (1987) initial findings about avoidant people's disbelief in the existence of romantic love (e.g., Jones & Cunningham, 1996). They have also revealed that anxious individuals are less confident than secure ones of being able to establish a successful relationship (Carnelley & Janoff-Bulman, 1992; Pietromonaco & Carnelley, 1994; Whitaker, Beach, Etherton, Wakefield, & Anderson, 1999) and more likely to emphasize potential losses when thinking about romantic relationships (Boon & Griffin, 1996). Moreover, anxious people tend to hold more dysfunctional relationship beliefs than secure people. They are more likely to believe, for example, that their behavior in relationships can be destructive (J. A. Feeney & Noller, 1992; Stackert & Bursik, 2003; Whisman & Allan, 1996). They are also more likely to perceive their relationships as inequitable, because their partners are not contributing as much as they should (Grau & Doll, 2003). Moreover, experimental priming of anxiety-related mental representations intensifies pessimistic expectations and perceptions of inequity (Grau & Doll, 2003; Whitaker et al., 1999), suggesting that attachment anxiety heightens the accessibility of negative beliefs about relationships.

Research has also revealed associations between attachment styles and "love styles" (i.e., attitudes about romantic love and couple relationships). One of the most influential theories in this topic area was developed by J. A. Lee (1977), who identified six love styles: *eros* (romantic, passionate love), *ludus* (game-playing, noncommitted love), *storge* (friendship, companionate love), *mania* (possessive, dependent, anxious love), *pragma* (logical, "shopping list," socially convenient love), and *agape* (selfless, altruistic, all-giving love). Research suggests that eros and agape contribute positively to the formation of a stable and mutually satisfying romantic relationship, whereas ludus and mania contribute negatively (e.g., Hendrick & Hendrick, 1989).

Six studies have examined associations between attachment style and Hendrick and Hendrick's (1986) Love Attitudes Scale (Collins & Read, 1990; J. A. Feeney & Noller, 1990; Fricker & Moore, 2002; Heaven, Da Silva, Carey, & Holen, 2004; Hendrick & Hendrick, 1989; Levy & Davis, 1988). Three findings recur across the six studies. First, secure attachment is associated with eros and agape—the love styles that facilitate the consolidation of lasting romantic bonds. Second, avoidance is associated with lower eros and higher ludus (game playing). Third, attachment anxiety is associated with mania. In addition, some of the studies suggest that avoidance is associated with lower agape scores

(Collins & Read, 1990; J. A. Feeney & Noller, 1900; Hendrick & Hendrick, 1989; M. B. Levy & Davis, 1988) and higher pragma scores (Collins & Read, 1990; Heaven et al., 2004).

Overall, then, attachment insecurity is associated with less constructive attitudes toward romantic love. Avoidant deactivating strategies seem to inhibit romantic and altruistic forms of love and favor game playing or practicality rather than romance. Consistent with this conclusion, R. W. Doherty, Hatfield, Thompson, and Choo (1994) found that more avoidant people scored lower on scales assessing passionate (erotic) and companionate (agapic) forms of love. Anxious people's desire for closeness and worries about rejection and unlovability seem to favor more intense, possessive, and dependent kinds of love (e.g., mania). J. A. Feeney and Noller (1990) and Sperling and Berman (1991) provided further support for this view: Attachment anxiety was associated with higher scores on scales tapping love addiction, "limerence" (Tennov, 1979), and desperate love. This desperate need for love may explain A. Aron, Aron, and Allen's (1998) finding of more frequent unreciprocated love among people with an anxious attachment style.

Intimacy

Attachment orientation is likely to affect the progression of intimacy during the consolidation phase of romantic relationships. Based on a theoretical analysis of secure people's working models, Pistole (1994) reasoned that secure people would be unlikely to experience much conflict related to closeness and distance. Their well-developed interpersonal sensitivity and conflict-management skills (see Chapter 9, this volume) should allow them to gauge accurately the amount of closeness sought by their partner, and be able to tolerate and communicate effectively about any momentary violations, in either direction, of desired personal boundaries.

Pistole (1994) also predicted that insecurely attached people would be less able to negotiate issues related to closeness and distance. Avoidant people's preference for interpersonal distance was expected to interfere with both their own intimacy-promoting behavior and their responsiveness to a partner's bids for proximity and intimacy. Anxious people's unmet needs for closeness were expected to cause them to seek closeness to such an extent that it would make their partners uncomfortable. Moreover, fear of rejection was expected to cause them to misinterpret a partner's desire for privacy or autonomy as a sign of rejection, which could tempt them to escalate demands for intimacy to such an extent that, paradoxically, it might cause their partner to withdraw or flee. Pistole noted that this kind of intrusion would be most unwelcome to avoidant partners, who view even normal intimacy and proximity as intrusive. This relational pattern, which in the marital research literature is called "demand–withdrawal" (Christensen, 1988) or "pursuit–withdrawal" (Bartholomew & Allison, 2006), is one of the major predictors of relationship violence and distress.

Associations between attachment style and relationship dynamics of this kind were found in two studies that involved asking dating partners to talk freely about their relationship (J. A. Feeney, 1999b; J. A. Feeney & Noller, 1991). A content analysis of their remarks revealed that secure people emphasized the importance of establishing a balance between closeness and independence; avoidant people emphasized the need to place limits on closeness and intimacy, and anxious people emphasized the importance of closeness and intimacy but not the importance of independence. In addition, these studies revealed that problems in regulating closeness and distance were most evident among anxious women and avoidant men. This is one of many indications in the relationship research literature that attachment style interacts with either biological sex or gender roles to influence relationship quality, a phenomenon that we discuss at greater length later in this chapter.

Additional evidence comes from self-report studies of couple intimacy (see Table 10.2 for a summary). Across numerous studies, secure people report greater intimacy in their relationships than do either anxious or avoidant people. This pattern appeared whether intimacy was assessed concurrently or as much as 6 years later (Collins et al., 2002). In addition, two studies suggest that the specific attachment style reported with reference to a particular relationship is more predictive of intimacy in that relationship than the more global attachment orientations assessed with general self-report scales or the AAI (Cozzarelli et al., 2000; Treboux et al., 2004). These findings highlight the importance of within-relationship attachment patterns established during the consolidation phase of a relationship (e.g., Pierce & Lydon, 2001).

In their study of the structure of romantic love, Mikulincer and Erev (1991) also found that avoidant people underestimated their partner's sense of intimacy, which might have served a defensive function. If avoidant people can deny or downplay a partner's sense of intimacy, they can more easily maintain their own independence and distance. (For similar findings in the sexual domain, see Chapter 11, this volume.) In addition, whereas avoidant people reported similarly low levels of both actual and desired intimacy in their relationships, anxiously attached people wanted more intimacy than they were experiencing (Mikulincer & Erev, 1991). It was not clear whether anxious people were simply unable to elicit the extreme level of intimacy they desired from their partners, or whether their needy, "hungry" style of relating caused their partners to establish greater self-protective distance.

Attachment-anxious people's difficulties in regulating closeness and distance within romantic relationships were documented in Lavy's (2006) studies of intrusiveness (i.e., attempting to increase intimacy, without concern for a partner's needs and desires). In one study, more attachment-anxious people reported engaging in more intrusive behavior in their couple relationships (e.g., asking their partners very personal questions and interfering with their plans to engage in some activities alone). In another study, Lavy measured the accessibility of intrusion-related thoughts and the potential effects of contextual activation of security representations (subliminal priming with the names of participants' attachment figures) on these thoughts. Study participants read three kinds of sentences (implying intrusiveness, nonintrusiveness in a relational context, or nonintrusiveness in a nonrelational context), half of which were grammatically correct, and half of which contained grammatical errors. Participants were asked to decide whether each sentence was grammatically correct. Short reaction times for sentences implying intrusiveness were taken as a sign of the accessibility of intrusion-related thoughts. Lavy found that more attachment-anxious people reacted faster to the intrusion-related sentences, and the experimental priming of attachment security reduced this accessibility. It therefore seems possible that increasing an anxious person's sense of security can reduce fears of rejection and make anxious intrusiveness less necessary.

In a third study, Lavy (2006) asked members of seriously dating couples to complete daily measures (over a 14-day period) of relationship satisfaction and intrusive behavior. More anxious participants typically acted more intrusively, but this association was moderated by relationship satisfaction on the previous day; that is, anxious people reported relatively high levels of intrusive behavior, mainly when they had been dissatisfied with their relationship the previous day. Both the priming results and this diary study imply that anxious intrusiveness is part of anxious people's efforts to create or restore the

TABLE 10.2. A Summary of Findings on Attachment Orientations and Intimacy in Couple Relationships

Study	Attachment measure	Intimacy measure	Main findings
Studies assessing attachment types			
Hazan & Shaver (1987, Study 1)	HS types	4 items	Secure > Avoidant, Anxious
Hazan & Shaver (1987, Study 2)	HS types	4 items	Secure > Avoidant, Anxious
J. A. Feeney & Noller (1991)	HS types	Open Accounts	Secure > Avoidant, Anxious
Mikulincer & Erev (1991)	HS types	TLS	Secure > Avoidant, Anxious
Senchak & Leonard (1992)^	HS types	MSI scale	Two partners secure > One or two partners insecure
Kirkpatrick & Davis (1994)	HS types	RRF Women	Secure > Anxious
		RRF Men	Secure > Avoidant
Crowell, Treboux, Gao, et al. (2002, Study 2)^	AAI	TLS	No significant differences
Paley et al. (2002)^	AAI	Interview	Secure > Insecure
Scharf et al. (2004)*	AAI	Interview	Secure > Insecure
Treboux et al. (2004, Study 1)	AAI	TLS	Ns differences
	CRI	TLS	Secure > Insecure
Treboux et al. (2004, Study 2)	AAI	TLS	Ns differences
	CRI	TLS	Secure > Insecure
Studies based on attachment style ratings			
M. B. Levy & Davis (1988)	HS ratings	TLS, RRF	Secure (+) Avoidant (−) Anxious (−)
Hendrick & Hendrick (1989)	HS ratings	TLS, RRF	Secure (+) Avoidant (−) Anxious (−)
Shaver & Brennan (1992)*	HS ratings	RRF	Secure (+) Avoidant (−) Anxious (−)
Fraley & Davis (1997)	RQ	FIR	Secure (+) Avoidant (ns) Anxious (−) Fearful (−)
You & Malley-Morrison (2000)	RQ	MSI scale	Secure (+) Avoidant (−) Anxious (ns) Fearful (ns)
Collins et al. (2002)*	HS ratings	TLS	Secure (ns) Avoidant (−) Anxious (ns)
Mayseless and Scharf (in press)*	HS ratings	Interview	Secure (+) Avoidant (−) Anxious (ns)
Studies assessing attachment dimensions			
Mayseless et al. (1997)^	ACS	SIS	Avoidance (−) Anxiety (ns)
Cozzarelli et al. (2000)	General RQ	IOS	Avoidance (ns) Anxiety (ns)
	Specific RQ	IOS	Avoidance (−) Anxiety (−)
Knobloch et al. (2001)	ASQ	Love Scale	Avoidance (−) Anxiety (−)
Treboux et al. (2004, Study 2)^	ECR	TLS	Avoidance (−) Anxiety (−)
Whiffen et al. (2005)^	RQ	MSI scale	Avoidance (−) Anxiety (ns)

Note. ^, married couples; *, longitudinal design; (−), significant inverse correlation; (+), significant positive correlation; (ns), nonsignificant effects; ACS, Attachment Concerns Scale; FIR, Factors in Intimate Relationship; HS, Hazan and Shaver; IOS, Inclusion–Other–Self; MSI, Miller Social Intimacy; RRF, Relationship Rating Form; SIS, Sharabany Intimacy Scale; TLS, Triangular Love Scale.

desired level of closeness. Like other anxious behaviors, these closeness-regulation efforts are likely to backfire if they cause a partner to feel intruded upon or suffocated.

Commitment

Attachment insecurities can also interfere with commitment. The avoidant preference for independence and anxious approach–avoidance ambivalence, combined with doubts about a partner's trustworthiness, can interfere with committing oneself to a lasting relationship. Moreover, avoidant distancing and anxious intrusiveness can deter partners from committing themselves to what they fear might be a troubled, unsatisfying relationship.

A large body of evidence supports the hypothesis that attachment insecurity is associated with lower commitment (see Table 10.3 for a summary). The same pattern of findings is obtained whether attachment style is assessed by self-reports or the Current Relationship Interview (CRI), but not when the AAI is used to assess state of mind with respect to attachment to parents. (This pattern of results suggests that there are important differences between the romantic and child–parent relationship contexts.) In a longitudinal study, Keelan, Dion, and Dion (1994) found that insecure people in dating relationships decreased their commitment over a 4-month period. In contrast, secure people maintained high levels of commitment over time. In addition, several studies found that partners of insecure people reported lower levels of commitment than partners of secure people (Kirkpatrick & Davis, 1994; Mikulincer & Erev, 1991; Paley, Cox, Burchinal, & Payne, 1999; Simpson, 1990).

Although attachment insecurities are associated with low levels of commitment to relationships, attachment-anxious and avoidant people differ substantially in their orientations to committed relationships. For example, Mikulincer and Erev (1991) found that anxious people were more likely than avoidant ones to *want* a highly committed relationship. In addition, Senchak and Leonard (1992) found that anxious men acquired marriage licenses much sooner (after 19 months of courtship) than secure men (49 months) or avoidant men (46 months). This raises the question of why anxious people seem relatively uncommitted to their relationships even though they apparently value commitment. According to Morgan and Shaver (1999), their tendency to commit too early, often before they know their partner very well, leaves anxious people more vulnerable to entanglement with a hurtful, uncommitted partner who frustrates their wishes for security and stability. Indeed, Hazan and Shaver (1987) found that anxious people tended to agree with the statement, "Few people are as willing and able as I am to commit themselves to a long-term relationship."

Differences in relationship commitment between anxious and avoidant people have also been examined within the framework of Rusbult's (1983) investment–cost model. Pistole, Clark, and Tubbs (1995) found that although both anxious and avoidant people reported relatively low levels of commitment to their couple relationships, anxious ones reported the highest relationship costs, whereas the avoidant ones reported the lowest investments. This implies that anxious people's lack of commitment stems from disappointment, pain, and frustration, whereas avoidant people's lack of commitment stems from unwillingness to invest in a long-term relationship.

Himovitch (2003) examined memory for commitment-related interpersonal exchanges and found that secure people exhibited faster recall than insecure people of episodes in which they or their partner strengthened their commitment to the relationship. In contrast, insecure people were more likely to emphasize the threats involved in commitment; they displayed faster recall of episodes that led to a decrease in commitment. However, whereas avoidant individuals more rapidly accessed memories of episodes in which they decreased their commitment to their partner, which we interpret as a case of attachment-system deactivation, anxious individuals more rapidly accessed memories of episodes in which a partner decreased commitment to them, which we interpret as another example of hypervigilance to signs of rejection, betrayal, and abandonment.

Construing a Couple Relationship as a Secure Base

In the consolidation phase of a developing relationship, part of what partners are consolidating is a relationship-specific sense of safety and security (based on appraisals of a part-

TABLE 10.3. A Summary of Findings on Attachment Orientations and Commitment in Couple Relationships

Study	Attachment measure	Commitment measure	Main findings
Studies assessing attachment types			
Mikulincer & Erev (1991)	HS types	TLS	Secure > Anxious
Kirkpatrick & Davis (1994)	HS types	RRF Women	Secure > Anxious
		RRF Men	Secure > Avoidant
Keelan et al. (1994)*	HS types	Investment scale	Secure > Insecure
Pistole et al. (1995)	HS types	Lund Scale	Secure > Avoidant, Anxious
Pistole & Vocaturo (1999)	RQ types	CI	Secure > Avoidant, Fearful
Paley et al. (1999)^	AAI	SIR	Ns difference
Crowell, Treboux, Gao, et al. (2002, Study 2)^	AAI	TLS, CI	Ns difference
Treboux et al. (2004, Study 1)^	AAI	TLS	Ns difference
	CRI	TLS	Secure > Insecure
Treboux et al. (2004, Study 2)^	AAI	TLS	Ns difference
	CRI	TLS	Secure > Insecure
Studies based on attachment style ratings			
M. B. Levy & Davis (1988)	HS ratings	TLS	Secure (+) Avoidant (−) Anxious (−)
Hendrick & Hendrick (1989)	HS ratings	TLS	Secure (+) Avoidant (−) Anxious (−)
Simpson (1990)	AAQ	Lund Scale	Secure (+) Avoidant (−) Anxious (−)
Shaver & Brennan (1992)*	HS ratings	RRF	Secure (ns) Avoidant (−) Anxious (ns)
Collins et al. (2002)*	HS ratings	TLS	Secure (ns) Avoidant (−) Anxious (ns)
Studies assessing attachment dimensions			
Tucker & Anders (1999)	AAQ	Lund Scale	Avoidance (ns) Anxiety (−) for W
			Avoidance (−) Anxiety (−) for M
Schmitt (2002)	RQ	TLS	Avoidance (ns) Anxiety (−) for W
			Avoidance (ns) Anxiety (ns) for M
Steiner-Pappalardo & Gurung (2002)	RQ	Lund Scale	Avoidance (ns) Anxiety (−)
Impett & Peplau (2002)	AAS	7-item measure	Avoidance (−) Anxiety (ns)
Himovitch (2003)	ECR	DCS—Partner subscale	Avoidance (−) Anxiety (−)
Treboux et al. (2004, Study 2)^	ECR	TLS	Avoidance (−) Anxiety (−)

Note. ^, married couples; *, longitudinal design; M, men; W, women; (−), significant inverse correlation; (+), significant positive correlation; (ns), nonsignificant effects; CI, Commitment Inventory; DCS, Dimensions of Commitment Scale; HS, Hazan and Shaver; RRF, Relationship Rating Form; SIR= Scale of Intimate Relations; TLS, Triangular Love Scale.

ner's availability and support) and of the relationship as a secure base from which they can engage in autonomous activities (L. J. Roberts & Greenberg, 2002; Zeifman & Hazan, 1997). However, construal of one's relationship as a secure base can be damaged by chronic attachment insecurity. First, as we reviewed in Chapter 6, insecurely attached people tend to question other people's supportiveness and expect even their romantic partners to be unavailable in times of need. Moreover, they tend to have problems seeking and acknowledging support (Chapter 7, this volume). Avoidant individuals are reluctant to seek proximity to, and obtain comfort from, their partners, and anxious individuals are sometimes reticent to express their need for support, especially when they worry that an open display of need will result in rejection. As a result, insecure people have difficulty experiencing their relationships as secure bases.

Attachment studies focusing on the transfer of safe haven and secure-base attachment functions from parents to romantic partners during adolescence provide interesting evidence for attachment style differences in construing a romantic relationship as a secure base. As we explained in Chapter 3, this transfer is expected to occur during late adolescence and young adulthood, when it enables the formation of an attachment bond to a romantic partner (Hazan & Zeifman, 1999). However, given that secure adolescents feel more at ease than insecure adolescents with intimacy-promoting behavior at the outset of a relationship, and are more confident that their parents will still love them even if they seek love, care, and comfort from another partner, they should show an earlier and stronger transfer of attachment functions from parents to romantic partners (Allen & Land, 1999). Indeed, five studies have found that greater attachment anxiety or avoidance during late adolescence is associated with a weaker tendency to use a romantic partner as a safe haven and secure base (J. A. Feeney, 2004a; J. A. Feeney & Hohaus, 2001; Fraley & Davis, 1997; Mayseless, 2004; Trinke & Bartholomew, 1997).

Anxiously attached people's inability to perceive their relationship as a secure base is also evident in their tendency to engage in excessive reassurance seeking from a romantic partner. In Chapter 9, we reviewed studies yielding strong correlations between attachment anxiety and excessive reassurance seeking. The correlations were corroborated in a recent study that assessed daily variations in reassurance seeking across a 2-week period in dating couples (Shaver et al., 2005). Participants who scored higher on attachment anxiety were more likely to seek daily reassurance from their dating partner. In addition, anxious men sought more reassurance following days on which they experienced relationship conflicts than following days on which little or no conflict was reported. Thus, it seems that anxious people seek reassurance as a way of quelling worries that interfere with relationship-specific security.

Maintenance of a Long-Term Relationship

The challenging and demanding task of maintaining a satisfying and stable relationship beyond the initial stages of ardent passion and deep self-disclosure depends largely on partners' interpersonal skills, the quality of their daily interactions, and their ability to manage disagreements and conflicts (see Noller & Feeney, 2002, for a review). Thus, it is reasonable to expect that attachment style differences in interpersonal skills and patterns of interpersonal experiences (see Chapter 9, this volume) will be reflected in the ways people do or do not successfully maintain their relationships. In the following sections, we review evidence linking attachment style with relationship maintenance processes.

Dyadic Communication

Verbal and nonverbal interchanges in which both partners feel free to express their thoughts and feelings in an affectionate and loving way seem to be critical for maintaining high-functioning, long-term relationships (e.g., Noller & Feeney, 2002). According to attachment theory, comfortable and open dyadic communication depends on partners' attachment security and is undermined or distorted by attachment insecurity. Avoidant people are less interested than nonavoidant ones in promoting warm and affectionate interactions, and may have difficulty expressing their concerns and feelings, and responding sensitively to a partner's needs and comments. Anxious people may have difficulty attending accurately and persistently to a partner's thoughts and feelings because of their self-focus and worries about being criticized or rejected.

Studies based on self-reports of couple communication indicate that secure people generally do communicate effectively and get involved less often than insecure people in demand–withdrawal interactions (Fitzpatrick, Fey, Segrin, & Schiff, 1993). Avoidant people report relatively high levels of emotional control (bottling up emotions and hiding feelings from romantic partners; J. A. Feeney, 1995a, 1999a) and less frequent use of affectionate "sweet talk" or baby talk to express affection in conversations with romantic partners (Bombar & Littig, 1996). J. A. Feeney (1999a) also found that attachment anxiety was associated with greater self-perceived suppression or control of negative emotions, perhaps reflecting reluctance to express neediness after having been criticized for doing so too often, or too intrusively, in the past.

Insecure people's problems with dyadic communication have also been documented in a diary study of newlywed couples (J. A. Feeney, Noller, & Callan, 1994). Partners recorded all conversations lasting 10 minutes or more over the course of a week. Couples in which the husband was avoidant reported lower levels of conversational involvement and satisfaction, and couples in which the wife was anxious reported higher levels of conflict and coercion during the conversation. These findings indicate again that the combination of attachment insecurity and traditional gender roles can undermine couple relationships.

This result is not limited to self-report measures. The association between avoidant attachment and a cool, distant, and disinterested communication style has been observed in studies of actual conversations between dating partners. For example, Guerrero (1996), who videotaped couples while they discussed important personal problems, found that avoidance was associated with lower levels of facial gaze, facial pleasantness, vocal pleasantness, general interest in the conversation, and attentiveness to the partner's comments. In another study, Tucker and Anders (1998) videotaped dating couples while they discussed positive aspects of their relationship and found that more avoidant people laughed less, touched their partners less, looked less at their partners, and smiled less during the interaction. In a related study, but one involving couple-level analyses, Le Poire, Shepard, and Duggan (1999) found that couples in which partners scored higher on avoidance tended to display less expressive nonverbal behavior during a conversation.

These observational studies also provide important information about the tense climate that anxiously attached people establish during conversations with their relationship partners. Guerrero (1996) found that attachment anxiety was associated with more vocal and physical signs of distress during taped conversations, and Tucker and Anders (1998) rated more anxious people as displaying less enjoyment during their conversations. Given anxious individuals' strong desire for intimacy, it may seem surprising that they do not seek greater proximity by gazing at and touching their partners during conversations. According to Tucker and Anders, "Preoccupied individuals are inclined to engage in intimate behaviors, but learn that relationship maintenance demands, in part, a suppression of their overt attempts to engage their partners, as 'clingy' behaviors might cause their partners to withdraw" (p. 121).

Attachment insecurities also tend to be associated with misperception of a relationship partner's signals. For example, Noller and Feeney (1994) and J. A. Feeney et al. (1994) asked both members of newlywed couples to send a set of nonverbal messages expressing particular emotional states and intentions to their spouse (e.g., sadness, anger, support seeking), and to decode the feelings and intentions expressed by the spouse. The more anxious husbands and more avoidant wives were less accurate in decoding their partners' nonverbal messages. The statistical association held up over time, too; it appeared even when accuracy was assessed 9 months later.

In a study of empathic accuracy (the ability to infer a partner's feelings correctly), Simpson, Ickes, and Blackstone (1995) found that people who described their dating relationship as less secure were less accurate when trying to infer their partners' feelings from a videotaped discussion of pictures of opposite-sex people with whom the partner might later interact. Using a similar procedure, Simpson, Ickes, and Grich (1999) unexpectedly discovered that more anxious individuals scored higher on empathic accuracy. However, among anxious participants, greater accuracy was associated with subsequent negative changes in relationship quality. These findings imply that for anxious individuals empathic accuracy may sometimes have negative relational consequences. According to Simpson et al., these negative consequences may be due to anxious people's correct detection of a partner's feelings that pose a threat to the relationship.

Guerrero and Burgoon (1996) also examined anxious people's wishes for closeness and merger during couple conversations. Dating and married couples participated in two conversations, and after the first, a randomly chosen member of the couple was asked to increase or decrease involvement in the second conversation. Anxious people became more involved in the conversations following a scripted increase or decrease in partner involvement; that is, anxious people tended to reciprocate a partner's increases in affection and to compensate with increased involvement when the partner showed signs of disinterest. This tendency to persist in an unpleasant interaction with a disinterested partner, which might seem laudable or beneficial, can take a destructive turn (as discussed later in this chapter) when anxious people prove unable or unwilling to leave a dysfunctional relationship.

Responding to a Relationship Partner's Actual or Potential Transgressions

In Chapters 7 and 9 we reviewed studies showing that insecure people are likely to react to an interaction partner's unfavorable behavior with more hostility and dysfunctional anger, and less forgiveness than secure people. Here we ask whether these destructive reactions are also evident in couple relationships, where they are likely to contribute to relationship dissatisfaction and instability.

Five studies designed to test interdependence theory (Rusbult et al., 1991) provide evidence of insecure people's maladaptive reactions to a romantic partner's transgressions (Gaines & Henderson, 2002; Gaines, Work, Johnson, Youn, & Lai, 2000; Gaines et al., 1997, 1999; Scharfe & Bartholomew, 1995). In general, attachment insecurities are associated with less "voice" (active attempts to solve a problem) and "loyalty" (understanding the temporary nature of a partner's behavior and waiting for improvement)—the two most accommodative, constructive responses to a partner's transgressions (Rusbult et al., 1991). Attachment insecurities also tend to be associated with more "exit" responses (attempts to harm the partner or leave the relationship) and "neglect" responses (ignoring the partner and refusing to discuss the problem)—the two most relationship-destructive responses. (Findings from these studies generalize to interethnic and same-sex couples [see Gaines & Henderson, 2002; Gaines et al., 1999]).

Conceptually similar findings were obtained in two studies of reactions to a relationship partner's betrayal of trust (Jang, Smith, & Levine, 2002; Mikulincer, 1998c). Compared with secure people, insecure ones were less likely to talk openly with their partner about his or her deception. In addition, more anxious people were more likely to ruminate about their partners' betrayal, talk around and avoid discussing partners' deception, and react with strong negative emotions—the usual hallmarks of attachment-system hyperactivation. Avoidant people, in contrast, increased their distance from the transgressing partner and denied the importance of the threatening episode, which exemplifies their general attempt to keep their attachment systems deactivated. However,

Mikulincer (1998b) measured lexical decision times to the word "worry" and found that avoidant people implicitly activated the word "worry" when primed with a trust-violation story. This discrepancy between self-reports of not being bothered by betrayal and implicit signs of worry may hint at the fragile nature of avoidant people's defenses. In fact, when responses to trust violations were assessed without the involvement of deliberate, controlled processing, avoidant people exhibited a more anxious pattern of reaction, a finding that recurs throughout this book (see Chapters 7, 9, and 13, this volume).

In a study of hurt feelings in couple relationships, J. A. Feeney (2004b) asked participants, who had previously completed the ECR, to recall and describe an event in which a close relationship partner said or did something that hurt their feelings. Then, participants answered questions tapping their emotional reactions to the recalled event, self-perceptions immediately following the event, perceptions of their partner's remorse, behavioral reactions (constructive, destructive) to the partner's negative behavior, and the long-term effects of the hurtful event on self-esteem and the relationship. Attachment-anxious participants were more likely to report that the hurtful event had negative long-term effects on their self-esteem, and this association was mediated by the report of more distress and more negative self-perceptions ("I'm stupid") following the event; that is, attachment-anxious individuals tended to react to hurtful events in close relationships with relatively strong distress and negative self-views, which in turn seemed to exacerbate their self-related doubts and worries.

The study also revealed that avoidant attachment was associated with more negative perceived effects of the hurtful event on the relationship, and this association was mediated by lower perceptions of partner remorse and more destructive behavioral reactions to the hurtful event; that is, more avoidant individuals were less likely to accept a partner's remorse and more likely to act destructively, which in turn seemed to aggravate relational tensions and conflicts. Overall, J. A. Feeney's (2004b) findings imply that hurtful events in close relationships have somewhat different meanings and effects for attachment-anxious and avoidant people, tending to exacerbate both anxious people's negative self-views and avoidant people's negative views of others and relationships.

A recent paper and a book chapter on the link between attachment style and forgiveness within couple relationships add to the evidence concerning insecure people's troubled reactions to a partner's transgressions (Kachadourian, Fincham, & Davila, 2004; Mikulincer, Shaver, & Slav, 2006). In two correlational studies of dating and married couples, Kachadourian et al. (2004) found that more attachment-anxious or avoidant people were less likely to forgive their romantic partners. In a diary study of daily fluctuations in the tendency to forgive a partner, Mikulincer, Shaver, & Slav (2006) found that both attachment anxiety and avoidance predicted lower levels of daily forgiveness across 21 consecutive days. Moreover, whereas secure people were more inclined to forgive their spouse on days when they perceived more positive spousal behavior, more insecure people (either anxious or avoidant) reported little forgiveness even on days when they perceived their spouse to be available, attentive, and supportive. In other words, attachment insecurities interfered with not only daily forgiveness but also the ability of a partner's positive behavior to restore understanding and empathy.

Attachment style is also implicated in jealousy-related thoughts, feelings, and behaviors in response to real or imagined partner transgressions. Secure people generally report low levels of jealousy, fairly mild or restrained emotional reactions to a partner's occasional interest in other people, and constructive strategies for coping with transgressions, such as openly discussing them with one's partner (Buunk, 1997; Collins & Read, 1990; Guerrero, 1998; Hazan & Shaver, 1987; Leak, Gardner, & Parsons, 1998; Radecki-Bush,

Farrell, & Bush, 1993; Sharpsteen & Kirkpatrick, 1997). It seems, therefore, that secure individuals usually interpret their own jealousy as a reason for taking constructive action to restore mutual understanding and continued relationship harmony.

In these same studies, attachment-anxious people tended to react dysfunctionally to partner transgressions or to a partner's interest in other attractive people: They reported relatively high levels of jealousy, suspicion, worries about relationship exclusivity, and experienced high levels of fear, guilt, shame, sadness, inferiority, and anger, and coped by expressing strong disapproval and engaging in intense surveillance (Buunk, 1997; Collins & Read, 1990; Dutton et al., 1994; Guerrero, 1998; Hazan & Shaver, 1987; Knobloch, Solomon, & Cruz, 2001; Radecki-Bush et al., 1993; Sharpsteen & Kirkpatrick, 1997). These reactions generally intensified distress and disharmony rather than relieving it. Dismissingly avoidant individuals, like their secure counterparts, reported low levels of chronic jealousy and did not react to jealousy-eliciting partner behavior with strong negative emotions. However, fearfully avoidant individuals were less likely than secure ones to engage in coping efforts aimed at restoring relationship quality (Guerrero, 1998). Instead, they preferred to avoid discussing the problem (Guerrero, 1998), another sign of deactivating strategies.

These studies show that people apply their characteristic attachment strategies when dealing with romantic partners' transgressions. As Gaines et al. (1997) mentioned, a partner's inconsiderate behavior threatens felt security; hence, it can cause insecure individuals to reprise long-standing attachment-related worries and cope by using well-practiced but ineffective strategies that aggravate rather than resolve relationship difficulties.

Conflict Management within Couple Relationships

In Chapter 9, we reviewed studies showing that insecure people *generally* have difficulty managing interpersonal conflict. Many studies also indicate that this deficiency occurs specifically in dating and marital relationships (see Table 10.4 for a summary). Insecure men and women tend less often than secure ones to express affection and empathy during conflicts, less frequently compromise, more frequently use coercive and destructive demand–withdrawal strategies, engage more often in attacks of various kinds, and end up experiencing more postconflict distress. At the couple level, Senchak and Leonard (1992) found that couples in which one or both partners were insecurely attached reported more withdrawal and verbal aggression during conflictual interactions than couples in which both partners were secure.

Researchers who have assessed partners' behavior during actual conflicts have also noticed insecure people's conflict-management difficulties (see Table 10.4). In the first of these studies, Kobak and Hazan (1991) used a Q-sort measure of marital attachment, and found that husbands and wives who were less secure in their marriage were more likely to display facial expressions of rejection while discussing a relational disagreement. In addition, insecure husbands were less likely to provide support during the discussion. Using more conventional self-report attachment scales (AAQ, ASQ), Simpson et al. (1996), J. A. Feeney (1998), and Campbell et al. (2005) found that insecurely attached men and women exhibit greater distress and less skillful communication tactics while discussing a major disagreement with their dating partner. J. A. Feeney (1998) also found that attachment insecurities are associated with fewer displays of warmth and affection during conflict discussions. However, Bouthillier et al. (2002) used the AAQ and failed to replicate these findings, perhaps due to differences between the samples in marital status, age, and culture, as well as the use of different behavioral coding schemes.

TABLE 10.4. A Summary of Findings on Attachment Orientations and Conflict Management in Couple Relationships

Study	Attachment measures	Conflict measures	Dependent variables	Main findings
Studies using self-report measures of conflict-management behaviors				
Senchak & Leonard (1992)^	HS ratings	MCI	Withdrawal	Both partners insecure > One or two partners secure
			Verbal aggression	Both partners insecure > One or two partners secure
J. A. Feeney (1994)^	ASQ	CPQ	Mutuality	Anxious (−) Avoidant (−) for W and M
			Destructive patterns, coercion	Anxious (+) Avoidant (+) for W and M
			Postconflict distress	Anxious (+) Avoidant (+) for W and M
J. A. Feeney et al. (1994)*^	ASQ	CPQ	Mutuality	Anxious (−) Avoidant (−) for W and M
			Destructive patterns, coercion	Anxious (+) Avoidant (ns) for W and M
			Postconflict distress	Anxious (ns) Avoidant (ns) for W; Anxious (+) Avoidant (ns) for M
N. Roberts & Noller (1998)^	RSQ	CPQ	Mutuality	Anxious (−) Avoidant (−) for W and M
			Destructive patterns	Anxious (+) Avoidant (ns) for W; Anxious (+) Avoidant (−) for M
			Postconflict distress	Anxious (+) Avoidant (ns) for W; Anxious (+) Avoidant (−) for M
Shi (2003)	Multi-item measure	ROCI	Compromising/integrating	Anxious (ns) Avoidant (−) for W and M
			Dominating strategies	Anxious (+) Avoidant (+) for W and M
			Obliging strategies	Anxious (−) Avoidant (−) for W and M
			Avoiding strategies	Anxious (ns) Avoidant (+) for W and M
Marchand (2004)^	AAS	CRBQ	Attacking	Anxious (+) Avoidant (+) for W and M
			Compromising	Anxious (−) Avoidant (−) for W; Anxious (ns) Avoidant (ns) for M
Marchand et al. (2004)^	AAS	CRBQ	Attacking	Anxious (+) Avoidant (+) for W and M
			Compromising	Anxious (−) Avoidant (−) for W; Anxious (ns) Avoidant (ns) for M
Heene et al. (2005)	AAS	CPQ	Constructive patterns	Anxious (ns) Avoidant (ns) for W; Anxious (ns) Avoidant (−) for M
			Demand–withdrawal	Anxious (+) Avoidant (+) for W; Anxious (+) Avoidant (ns) for M
			Avoidance	Anxious (+) Avoidant (+) for W; Anxious (+) Avoidant (ns) for M
Studies using observational measures of behaviors and feelings during conflict-resolution discussions				
Kobak & Hazan (1991)^	Q-sort	IDCS	Rejection behaviors	Security (−) for W and M
			Support validation	Security (ns) for W; Security (+) for M
Cohn, Silver, et al. (1992)^	AAI	Specific coding	Positive-conflict behaviors	Security (ns) for W; Security (+) for M
			Conflict escalation	Security (ns) for W; Security (−) for M
Simpson et al. (1996)	AAQ	Specific coding	Observer-coded distress	Anxious (+) Avoidant (ns) for W and M
			Observer-coded warmth	Anxious (ns) Avoidant (ns) for W; Anxious (ns) Avoidant (−) for M
			Quality of discussion	Anxious (−) Avoidant (ns) for W; Anxious (−) Avoidant (−) for M
J. A. Feeney (1998)	ASQ	Specific coding	Observer-coded distress	Anxious (ns) Avoidant (+) for W
			Observer-coded approach	Anxious (−) Avoidant (ns) for W; Anxious (ns) Avoidant (−) for M
			Quality of discussion	Anxious (ns) Avoidant (−) for W; Anxious (ns) Avoidant (−) for M

302

Study	Measure(s)	Coding	Behavior	Finding
Paley et al. (1999)^	AAI	IDCS	Positive affect	Secure > Anxious for W; Ns differences for M
			Withdrawal behavior	Secure < Avoidant for W; Ns differences for M
Babcock et al. (2000)^	AAI (only husbands)	SPAFF	Domineering, defensiveness	Secure < Avoidant, Anxious
			Stonewalling, contempt	Secure < Avoidant
Roisman et al. (2001)	AAI	Specific coding	Positive-conflict behaviors	Security (+) for W and M
			Negative-conflict behaviors	Security (−) for W and M
Bouthillier et al. (2002)^	AAI, AAQ	IDCS	Support validation	Secure > Avoidant, Anxious for W and M
			Positive communication	Ns differences for W; Secure > Avoidant, Anxious for M
			Withdrawal	Ns differences for W; Secure < Avoidant, Anxious for M
			Negative-conflict behaviors	Ns differences for W and M
Creasey (2002a)	AAI	SPAFF	Positive-conflict behaviors	Secure > Anxious, Avoidant for W; Ns differences for M
			Negative-conflict behaviors	Secure < Anxious, Avoidant for W and M
Crowell, Treboux, Gao, et al. (2002)^	AAI	RMICS	Positive-conflict behaviors	Security (+) for W; Security (ns) for M
			Negative-conflict behaviors	Security (−) for W; Security (ns) for M
Roisman et al. (2002)	AAI	Specific coding	Positive-conflict behaviors	Security (+) for W and M
Wampler et al. (2003)^	AAI	Georgia Marriage Q-sort	Negative affect	Security (−) for W and M
			Respect, negotiation	Security (+) for W and M
			Avoidance	Security (−) for W; Security (ns) for M
			Open communication	Security (+) for W and M
Creasey & Ladd (2004)	AAI	SPAFF	Negative-conflict behaviors	Secure < Avoidant (controlling for gender)
Alexandrov et al. (2005)^	Couple Attachment Interview	CPSSRS	Conflict escalation	Security (−) for W and M
			Positive emotion	Security (ns) for W and M
			Negative emotion	Security (−) for W and M
Campbell et al. (2005)	AAQ	Specific coding	Observer-coded distress	Anxious (+) Avoidant (ns) for W and M
			Conflict escalation behavior	Anxious (+) Avoidant (ns) for W and M
Creasey & Ladd (2005)	AAI	SPAFF	Negative-conflict behaviors	Secure < Avoidant, Anxious for W and M
			Domineering, defensiveness	Secure < Avoidant, Anxious for W and M
			Contempt	Ns differences for W and M
Roisman et al. (2005)	AAI, CRI	Specific coding	Positive-conflict behaviors	Security in the AAI, CRI (+)

Note. ^, married couples; *, longitudinal design; M, men; W, women; (−), significant inverse correlation; (+), significant positive correlation; (ns), nonsignificant effects; CPQ, Communication Patterns Questionnaire; CPSSRS, Couple Problem-Solving Style Rating System; CRBQ, Conflict Resolution Behavior Questionnaire; HS, Hazan and Shaver; IDCS, International Dimensions Coding System; MCI, Margolin Conflict Inventory; RMICS, Revised Marital Interaction Coding System; ROCI, Rahim Organizational Conflict Inventory; SPAFF, Specific Affect Coding System.

Interestingly, Bouthillier et al. (2002) also used the AAI and found the expected relationship between insecurity and destructive behavior during conflictual interactions with a romantic partner (see Table 10.4). This pattern of findings has been conceptually replicated in 10 other studies that have used the AAI to assess adult attachment. Individuals categorized as insecure based on the AAI have been coded as displaying less positive affect than their secure counterparts during conflict discussions, less open communication, less attentiveness to their partner's statements, and more relationship-destructive behavior, such as expressing contempt, withdrawal, and stonewalling (see Table 10.4). Overall, although there are some discrepancies in the specific measures that revealed secure versus insecure differences in the different studies (see Table 10.4), as a group, the studies provide strong converging evidence that an insecure state of mind with respect to attachment to the mother (or to both parents) is associated with more negative behavior during conflicts in both dating and married couples.

Differences between people classified by the AAI as dismissing and those classified as preoccupied are less marked and seem to be overshadowed by the secure–insecure contrast. However, Paley et al. (1999) found that whereas anxious women expressed less positive affect during discussions of conflicts, avoidant women were more likely to withdraw from the discussion. Babcock, Jacobson, Gottman, and Yerington (2000) found that avoidant husbands displayed more stonewalling and contempt during conflictual interactions than anxious husbands, and Creasey and Ladd (2005) reported that the specific effects of anxious and avoidant attachment (assessed by the RQ) were observed mainly among people classified by the AAI as insecure/unresolved. Among these people, anxiety was associated with more expressions of contempt for the partner, and avoidance was associated with more domineering behavior.

The ability of the AAI to predict behavior in conflictual interactions may be related to the fact, discussed in Chapter 4, this volume, that the AAI itself is based on a behavioral interaction (with an interviewer)—an interaction in which emotional issues are discussed face-to-face. That is, the AAI is a more behavioral measure of state of mind with respect to attachment than are the various self-report measures, so it makes sense that the AAI is often a better predictor of communicative behavior during a dyadic interaction. More research is needed on the different kinds of communication variables that correlate with each of the different kinds of adult attachment measures.

Turning back for a moment to studies based on self-report measures, there is also evidence linking attachment insecurities and heightened physiological reactivity to an actual relationship conflict (S. I. Powers, Pietromonaco, Gunlicks, & Sayer, 2006). In the S. I. Powers et al. study, young heterosexual couples were asked to spend 15 minutes discussing an unresolved conflict and attempt to resolve the problem. Salivary cortisol levels (an index of physiological reactivity of the HPA axis) were assessed seven times before, during, and after the conflict negotiation task. Growth modeling of cortisol data showed that attachment insecurities are associated with greater physiological reactivity to the conflict-resolution task, and that gender moderates the effects of the specific kind of attachment insecurity (anxiety or avoidance). Whereas avoidance was associated with women's cortisol reactivity before and during the task, attachment anxiety predicted the curvature of men's cortisol trajectory (more anxious men showed a more rapid increase of cortisol before the task; these high levels remained high throughout the task and began to decline at a slower pace after the task). These findings are important, because they begin to show that attachment-style differences are not confined only to behaviors and cognitions, but also have strong physiological underpinnings.

S. I. Powers et al. (2006) attempted to explain the observed gender differences in terms of gender-related expectations and norms concerning conflictual interactions. Previous studies have indicated that women are expected to take an active, leading role during such interactions (e.g., articulate relationship concerns and guide a discussion of areas of disagreement); men are generally assigned a less active role (e.g., Christensen & Heavey, 1990). As a result, the conflict negotiation task may be particularly stressful for avoidant women, who prefer to distance themselves rather than confront relationship problems, and for anxious men, who tend to express distress and take a controlling position in the discussion. This mismatch between gender role expectations and the habitual strategies of avoidant and anxious people in conflictual interactions may heighten physiological reactivity, thereby affecting the subjective experience of stress and distress.

Studies using self-report attachment measures have also found that attachment anxiety is associated with intensification of the negative consequences of conflict discussions. For example, Simpson et al. (1996) found that anxiously attached people reported a stronger decline than secure people in love and commitment after discussing a major relationship problem with a dating partner. Gallo and Smith (2001) also found that anxious wives, compared with secure wives, reacted to a discussion about a relationship disagreement with more negative appraisals of their husbands. These findings were conceptually replicated and extended in Campbell et al.'s (2005) diary study of dating couples' daily conflicts. More anxious participants reported more conflictual interactions across 14 consecutive days. They also reacted to days of intense conflict with a sharper decline in relationship satisfaction and a more pessimistic view of the relationship's future. Interestingly, although their partners did not report a corresponding heightening of relational worries, anxious people thought that their partners were less satisfied and less optimistic about the future of the relationship on days of intense rather than mild conflict.

In a correlational study, Fishtein, Pietromonaco, and Feldman Barrett (1999) found that more attachment-anxious people construed their romantic relationships in more complex terms as the level of conflict increased. According to Fishtein et al., this finding implies that anxiously attached individuals are attuned to the positive sides of relational conflicts, because conflictual interactions provide an opportunity to elicit a partner's attention and responsiveness. This finding might also be explained as resulting from anxious people's tendency to ruminate about conflicts, which creates more associative links between different mental representations of the relationship and increases the cognitive complexity of the overall relationship schema. This is an interesting and important issue, and more research is needed concerning the ways in which anxiously attached people organize information about their couple conflicts.

Expressions of Positive Regard for a Romantic Partner

Maintenance of a long-term relationship depends on the extent to which partners experience and express respect, admiration, and gratitude to each other and the extent to which they are able to create a climate of appreciation and friendship instead of criticism and contempt (Gottman, 1994). According to Markman, Stanley, and Blumberg (1994), expressing positive regard for a romantic partner is one of four crucial relationship values; the other three are commitment, intimacy, and forgiveness. These expressions increase a partner's sense of love and lovability, deepen mutual trust, and promote what Wieselquist, Rusbult, Foster, and Agnew (1999) called "mutual growth cycles" in relationships. In these cycles, one partner's trust increases his or her dependence on the relationship, commitment to the relationship, and pro-relationship behaviors, which in turn increase the other partner's trust, dependence, commitment, and prorelationship behaviors, thereby heightening both partners' involvement and satisfaction.

There is accumulating evidence that insecure people's negative working models of others inhibit or interfere with expressions of respect, admiration, and gratitude toward a romantic partner. As shown in Chapter 6, this volume, insecure people make more negative appraisals of their romantic partners than do secure people and also express less respect for their partners (Frei & Shaver, 2002). In Chapter 9, we showed that avoidance inhibits or interferes with gratitude, and attachment anxiety encourages ambivalent experiences of gratitude. In a recent diary study, Mikulincer et al. (2006) explored these issues in the context of marital relationships and found that avoidance predicted lower levels of daily gratitude toward a spouse across 21 consecutive days. Moreover, whereas less avoidant husbands reported more gratitude on days when they perceived more positive behavior on the part of their wives, more avoidant husbands reported relatively low levels of gratitude even on days when they noticed their wives' positive behavior.

There is also evidence that more avoidant people report having less positive feelings toward a romantic partner after outperforming the partner, or being outperformed by him or her, on cognitive tasks (Scinta & Gable, 2005). That is, avoidant people tend to bask in the glow of a superior performance even if this basking damages a romantic partner's self-worth. Moreover, they tend to deny their partners the benefits of a successful performance. Overall, it seems that avoidant individuals' narcissistic tendencies, lack of nurturance, and deficits in interpersonal sensitivity inhibit or distort expressions of positive regard for a romantic partner, expressions that, when not distorted, contribute strength and longevity to a relationship.

Family Dynamics

With the transition to parenthood, a couple usually becomes transformed into a family system (e.g., Minuchin, 1985), in which family members participate in different kinds of relationships (marital and parent–child relationships, but possibly also deepened relationships with extended family members and new relationships with child care providers). Many tasks and interactions have to be planned, coordinated, and integrated to facilitate the smooth functioning of the family and its subsystems. Poor functioning of some of the subsystems can generate problems that spread to other subsystems and eventually cause major problems for the family as a whole.

Although adult attachment research has focused primarily on dyadic relationships (couple relationships, parent–child relationships), some studies have examined attachment-related variations in family dynamics. The rationale for these studies is simple: If attachment insecurities reduce the quality of couple relationships, the damage and difficulties can spread to other family subsystems and interfere with the functioning of the family as a whole. Using the AAI, Dickstein et al. (2001; Dickstein, Seifer, Albus, & Magee, 2004) found that spouses classified as insecure scored lower than secure spouses on self-report measures and clinical ratings of family functioning, and Paley et al. (2005) found that the quality of family interaction (when mother, father, and a 2-year-old child were videotaped during a 15-minute play task) was dramatically impaired by fathers' attachment insecurities, particularly when there were high levels of marital discord.

Using self-report attachment scales, Diehl, Elnick, Bourbeau, and Lavouvie-Vief (1998) found that insecure spouses reported a less positive family climate than did secure spouses, and three other studies (Finzi-Dottan, Cohen, Iwaniec, Sapir, & Weizman, 2003; Mikulincer & Florian, 1999b; Pfaller, Kiselica, & Gerstein, 1998) found that less secure spouses scored lower on two dimensions of family dynamics: *family cohesion* (the extent of emotional bonding between family members) and *family adaptability* (the extent to which a family is able to adjust its rules in response to changes). Avoidant individuals' lack of nurturance and anxious people's deficits in interpersonal skills can interfere with family cohesion. In addition, insecure people's defensive attempts to avoid either distance or closeness can interfere with the adjustment of family bonds to specific demands and changes.

Leon and Jacobvitz (2003) assessed attachment style influences on another contributor to family cohesion—the quality of family rituals (e.g., family dinners, birthday celebrations). The authors hypothesized that because family rituals symbolize investment in family relationships, foster closeness and cohesion, and require expressivity, sensitivity, and conflict management, secure people would engage in more satisfying and meaningful rituals than would insecure people. Indeed, mothers' attachment security (assessed with the AAI prior to the first child's birth) was associated with reports of more flexible family rituals when the child was 7 years old. Moreover, couples in which at least one spouse was secure reported more flexible family rituals than couples in which both spouses were insecure. Finally, couples in which both spouses were secure attributed more meaning and importance to family rituals.

Summary

Our literature review confirms that attachment security facilitates the formation, consolidation, and maintenance of lasting and satisfying couple relationships. In contrast, attachment insecurities interfere with favorable interpersonal processes. For example, defenses inherent to avoidant attachment interfere with comfortable flirtation and progression of a relationship toward intimacy, commitment, and generally productive conflict resolution. Anxious attachment engenders tension and ambivalence, suspicion and intrusiveness, and conflict escalation rather than resolution. In addition to these specifically interpersonal processes, insecure individuals experience general difficulties when coping with stress (Chapter 7, this volume) that are bound to influence relationships given the inevitability of a certain amount of conflict and stress. Moreover, as we show in subsequent chapters, attachment insecurity impairs one's ability to provide support and comfort to a partner undergoing stress (Chapter 11), interferes with a satisfying sex life (Chapter 12), and puts people at risk for emotional problems and psychological disorders (Chapter 13)—all of which can obviously damage and derail a couple relationship over the long haul.

ATTACHMENT ORIENTATION AND RELATIONSHIP ADJUSTMENT

One implication of our discussion of attachment-related influences on the initiation, consolidation, and maintenance of a couple relationship is that attachment insecurity places a relationship at risk for maladjustment and dissolution. In the remainder of this chapter we focus on three major relationship outcomes: dissatisfaction and unhappiness, instability and breakups, and violence.

Relationship Satisfaction

"Satisfaction" refers to having needs met, and within long-term couple relationships, the needs have to do with wishes for love, intimacy, affection, acceptance, understanding, support, and security, as well as more individualistic wishes for autonomy, growth, and competence. In terms of attachment theory, relationship satisfaction depends on the extent to which partners effectively meet their needs for proximity, a safe haven, and a secure base. That is, relationship satisfaction can be expected to increase as partners become available and reliable sources of closeness and intimacy, effective providers of support and security (safe havens), and secure bases from which they can engage in autonomous growth-oriented activities (J. A. Feeney, 1999c; Mikulincer, Florian, Cowan, & Cowan, 2002).

Attachment theory also suggests that relationship dissatisfaction arises from attachment-related worries and insecurities (Kobak, Ruckdeschel, & Hazan, 1994). For example, attachment injuries (experiencing a partner's unavailability, infidelity, abuse, or rejection) can cause especially strong relationship distress whenever they activate defensive patterns of attachment-system hyperactivation or deactivation that foster either angry, clingy demands for a partner's attention, or cold detachment from a disappointing or frustrating partner. Moreover, these injuries can also interfere with the restoration of relational harmony, if they are incorporated into insecure working models that generate pessimistic expectations about the partner and the relationship (e.g., S. M. Johnson, 2003). Because every relationship is likely to include partner transgressions, misunderstandings, and at least minor attachment injuries from time to time, attachment insecurities put couples at risk for more lasting relationship distress and dissatisfaction.

Relationship satisfaction has been examined in studies of dating couples (see Table 10.5 for a summary). Supporting an attachment-theoretical analysis, less secure people—whether anxious, avoidant, or both—generally report lower satisfaction with their dating relationships. This link between attachment insecurities and relationship dissatisfaction has been found in both homosexual and heterosexual couples (Elizur & Mintzer, 2001; Mohr, 1999; Ridge & Feeney, 1998). Some studies considered potentially confounded variables and found that insecurely attached people's relationship dissatisfaction cannot be explained by other personality factors, such as the "Big Five" traits, depression, self-esteem, or sex role orientation (e.g., Carnelley, Pietromonaco, & Jaffe, 1994; Jones & Cunningham, 1996; Noftle & Shaver, 2006; Shaver & Brennan, 1992; Whisman & Allan, 1996), increasing our confidence in the uniqueness of the contribution of attachment-related variables to relationship satisfaction.

Studies of married couples have also examined links between attachment insecurities and marital dissatisfaction (see Table 10.6). However, the results and conclusions seem to depend on the way attachment is assessed. The vast majority of studies based on self-report assessments of attachment style have found that insecure spouses have lower marital satisfaction than do secure ones. In contrast, five of the seven studies based on the AAI failed to find a significant link between attachment insecurity and marital dissatisfaction. Although method variance (self-report vs. interview) might account for some of the discrepancies, Alexandrov et al. (2005), Dickstein et al. (2001), Treboux et al. (2004), and Shields, Travis, and Rousseau (2000) used interview methods (e.g., the CRI) to assess attachment orientations in marriage (see Chapter 4, this volume, for a description of measures) and found higher marital satisfaction among secure than among insecure spouses. This implies that current attachment insecurities related specifically to adult close relationships (whether assessed by self-report scales or interviews) are better

TABLE 10.5. A Summary of Findings on Attachment Orientations and Satisfaction in Dating Relationships

Study	Attachment measure	Satisfaction measure	Main findings
Studies assessing attachment types			
Pistole (1989)	HS types	DAS	Secure > Avoidant, Anxious
Mikulincer & Erev (1991)	HS types	MAT	Secure > Anxious
J. A. Feeney et al. (1993)	HS types	1 item	Secure > Avoidant, Anxious
Keelan et al. (1994)*	HS types	1 item	Secure > Insecure
Kirkpatrick & Davis (1994)	HS types	RRF	Secure > Anxious for W; Secure > Avoidant for M
Pistole et al. (1995)	HS types	RRF	Secure > Anxious, Avoidant
Keelan et al. (1998)	RQ	9 items	Secure > Avoidant, Fearful
McCarthy (1999)	HS types	APFA	Secure > Avoidant
Stein et al. (2002)	AAS, RQ	DAS	Secure > Insecure
Fricker & Moore (2002)	HS types	GMREL	Secure > Avoidant, Anxious
Stackert & Bursik (2003)	HS types	RAS	Secure > Avoidant, Anxious
Studies based on attachment style ratings			
M. B. Levy & Davis (1988)	HS ratings	RRF	Secure (+) Anxious (−) Avoidant (−)
Hendrick & Hendrick (1989)	HS ratings	RRF	Secure (+) Anxious (−) Avoidant (−)
Simpson (1990)	AAQ	11 items	Secure (+) Anxious (ns) Avoidant (−) for W; Secure (+) Anxious (−) Avoidant (−) for M
Hammond & Fletcher (1991)*	HS ratings	PRQC	Secure (+) Anxious (−) Avoidant (−)
Carnelley & Janoff-Bulman (1992)	HS ratings	1 item	Secure (ns) Anxious (−) Avoidant (ns)
Shaver & Brennan (1992)*	HS ratings	RRF	Secure (+) Anxious (−) Avoidant (−)
Brennan & Shaver (1995)	HS ratings	RRF	Secure (+) Anxious (−) Avoidant (−)
Bookwala & Zdaniuk (1998)	RQ	11 items	Secure (+) Anxious (−) Avoidant (ns) Fearful (−)
Elizur & Mintzer (2003)	HS secure	3 items	Secure (+) (sample of homosexual men)
Neyer & Voigt (2004)	HS secure	RAS	Secure (+)
Roisman et al. (2005)	SS, AAI, CRI	Battery of scales	Security in SS and CRI (+) Security in AAI (ns)
Studies assessing attachment dimensions			
Collins & Read (1990)	AAS	DAS	Anxious (−) Avoidant (ns) for W; Anxious (ns) Avoidant (−) for M
Carnelley et al. (1994, Study 1)	RQ	1 item	Anxious (−) Avoidant (−) (sample of women)
Carnelley et al. (1996, Study 1)	48 items	1 item	Anxious (−) Avoidant (−) for W and M
Collins (1996, Study 2)	AAS	15 items	Anxious (−) Avoidant (−) for W and M
Frazier et al. (1996)	AAS	5 items	Anxious (ns) Avoidant (−) for W; Anxious (−) Avoidant (−) for M
Jones & Cunningham (1996)	ASQ	6 items	Anxious (−) Avoidant (−) for W and M
Whisman & Allan (1996)	AAS	DAS	Anxious (ns) Avoidant (−) for W and M
Morrison, Urquiza, et al. (1997)	AAS	MSI	Anxious (−) Avoidant (−)
J. A. Feeney (1999a)	HS ratings	QMI	Anxious (ns) Avoidant (−) for W and M
Tucker & Anders (1999)	AAQ	11 items	Anxious (−) Avoidant (ns) for W; Anxious (−) Avoidant (−) for M
Cozzarelli et al. (2000)	RQ	RAS	Anxious (−) Avoidant (ns)
Frei & Shaver (2002)	ECR	RAS	Anxious (−) Avoidant (−)
Schmitt (2002)	RQ	5 items	Anxious (ns) Avoidant (−) for W; Anxious (ns) Avoidant (ns) for W
Steiner-Pappalardo & Gurung (2002)	RQ	DAS	Anxious (−) Avoidant (−)
Shi (2003)	New scale	RAS	Anxious (−) Avoidant (−) for W and M
Kachadourian et al. (2004)	RQ	PRQC	Anxious (−) Avoidant (−)
N. Sumer & Cozzarelli (2004)	RQ, RSQ	DAS, QMI	Anxious (−) Avoidant (−)
Williams & Riskind (2004)	ECR	RAS, DAS	Anxious (−) Avoidant (−)
Shaver et al. (2005, Study 1)	ECR	PRQC	Anxious (ns) Avoidant (−) for W and M
Shaver et al. (2005, Study 2)	ECR	PRQC	Anxious (ns) Avoidant (−) for W and M

Note. *, longitudinal design; M, men; W, women; (−), significant inverse correlation; (+), significant positive correlation; (ns), nonsignificant effects; APFA, Adult Personality Functioning Assessment; DAS, Dyadic Adjustment Scale; GMREL, General Model of Relationships; HS, Hazan and Shaver; MAT, Marital Adjustment Test; MSI, Marital Satisfaction Inventory; PRQC, Perceived Relationship Quality Components Inventory; QMI, Quality of Marriage Index; RAS, Relationship Assessment Scale; RRF, Relationship Rating Form; SS, Strange Situation.

TABLE 10.6. A Summary of Findings on Attachment Orientations and Satisfaction in Marital Relationships

Study	Attachment measure	Satisfaction measure	Main findings
Studies assessing attachment types			
Kobak & Hazan (1991)	Q Sort	DAS	Secure > Insecure for W and M
Senchak & Leonard (1992)	HS types	FAM	Both partners secure > One or two partners insecure
Cohn, Silver, et al. (1992)	AAI	MAT	No significant differences for W and M
Berman et al. (1994)	HS types	DAS	Both partners secure > One or two partners insecure
Fuller & Fincham (1995)*	HS types	MAT	No significant differences for W / Secure > Avoidant, Anxious for M
Medway et al. (1995, Study 1)	RQ	RAS	No significant differences (sample of women)
Medway et al. (1995, Study 2)	RQ	RAS	Secure > Insecure (sample of women)
Gerlsma et al. (1996)	HS types	RISS	No significant differences for W / Secure > Avoidant, Anxious for M
DeKlyen (1996)	AAI	LWS	No significant differences (sample of women)
Klohnen & Bera (1998)*	HS types	3 items	Secure > Insecure (sample of women)
Mikulincer, Horesh, et al. (1998)	HS types	DAS	Secure > Avoidant, Anxious for W and M
Pfaller et al. (1998)	HS types	FSS	Secure > Avoidant, Anxious for W and M
Volling et al. (1998)	HS types	1 item	No significant differences for couple types
Shields et al. (2000)	Interview	DAS	Secure > Insecure for W and M
Dickstein et al. (2001)	AAI, MAI	DAS	Secure > Insecure for W; Ns differences for M
Crowell, Treboux, & Waters (2002, Study 2)*	AAI	FBS	No significant differences for W and M
Wampler et al. (2003)	AAI	DAS	No significant differences for W and M
Dickstein et al. (2004)	AAI, MAI	DAS	No significant differences for W and M
Treboux et al. (2004, Study 1)	AAI, CRI	DAS	Secure > Insecure
Treboux et al. (2004, Study 2)	AAI	DAS	Ns differences
	CRI		Secure > Insecure
Ben Ari & Lavee (2005)	ECR	ENRICH	Both partners secure > Both partners insecure
Studies based on attachment style ratings			
Lussier et al. (1997)	HS ratings	DAS	Secure (ns) Anxious (–) Avoidant (–) for W and M
Diehl et al. (1998)	RQ	Family APGAR	Secure (+) Anxious (ns) Avoidant (ns) Fearful (–) for W and M
Amir et al. (1999)	HS ratings	DAS	Secure (+) Anxious (–) Avoidant (–) (sample of women)
H. Cobb et al. (2001)*	RQ-secure	MAT	Secure (+) for W and M
Sumer & Knight (2001)	RQ	QMI	Secure (+) Anxious (–) Avoidant (–) Fearful (–) for W and M
Meyers & Landsberger (2002)	HS ratings	DAS	Secure (+) Anxious (–) Avoidant (–) (sample of women)
R. L. Scott & Cordova (2002)	HS ratings	DAS	Secure (+) Anxious (–) Avoidant (–) for W / Secure (+) Anxious (ns) Avoidant (–) for M
Meredith & Noller (2003)	RQ	QMI	Secure (ns) Anxious (–) Avoidant (ns) (sample of women)
Banse (2004)	RQ	RAS	Secure (+) Anxious (–) Avoidant (–) Fearful (–) for W and M
Alexandrov et al. (2005)	Interview	MAT	Secure (ns) Anxious (ns) Avoidant (–) for W and M
Heene et al. (2005)	AAS	DAS	Secure (+) Anxious (–) Avoidant (–) for W / Secure (ns) Anxious (–) Avoidant (–) for M
Hollist & Miller (2005)	MAQ	DAS	Secure (ns) Anxious (–) Avoidant (–) for W and M
Studies assessing attachment dimensions			
Carnelley et al. (1994, Study 2)	RQ	DAS	Anxious (–) Avoidant (–) (sample of depressed women)
J. A. Feeney (1994, 1–10 years)	ASQ	QMI	Anxious (–) Avoidant (–) for W and M
J. A. Feeney (1994, 11–20 years)	ASQ	QMI	Anxious (–) Avoidant (–) for W and M

(cont.)

TABLE 10.6. *(cont.)*

Study	Attachment measure	Satisfaction measure	Main findings
Studies assessing attachment dimensions (cont.)			
J. A. Feeney (1994, over 20 years)	ASQ	QMI	Anxious (–) Avoidant (–) for W and M
J. A. Feeney et al. (1994)*	ASQ	QMI, DAS	Anxious (–) Avoidant (ns) for W; Anxious (–) Avoidant (–) for M
Rholes et al. (1995, Study 1)	AAQ	DAS	Anxious (–) Avoidant (ns) (sample of women)
Carnelley et al. (1996, Study 2)	48 items	DAS	Anxious (–) Avoidant (–) for W and M
J. A. Feeney (1996)	ASQ	QMI	Anxious (–) Avoidant (–) for W and M
Davila et al. (1998, Study 1)	AAS	MAT	Anxious (–) Avoidant (–) for W and M
Davila et al. (1998, Study 2)	AAS	MAT	Anxious (–) Avoidant (–) for W and M
Roberts & Noller (1998)	RSQ	DAS	Anxious (–) Avoidant (–) for W and M
Davila et al. (1999)*	AAS	MAT	Anxious (–) Avoidant (–) for W and M
J. A. Feeney (1999b)	ASQ	QMI	Anxious (–) Avoidant (–) for W and M
Davila & Bradbury (2001)*	AAS	MAT	Anxious (–) Avoidant (–) for W and M
Gallo & Smith (2001)	AAS	QRI	Anxious (–) Avoidant (ns) for W and M
DiFilippo & Overholser (2002)	ECR	DAS	Anxious (–) Avoidant (–) for W and M
J. A. Feeney (2002)	ASQ	QMI	Anxious (–) Avoidant (ns) for W and M
Kurdek (2002)	RSQ	3 items	Anxious (–) Avoidant (–) (sample of heterosexual, gay, and lesbian couples)
Berant et al. (2003)*	HS ratings	ENRICH	Anxious (–) Avoidant (–) (sample of women)
Feeney et al. (2003)	ASQ	MSI	Anxious (–) Avoidant (–) for W and M
Kachadourian et al. (2004)	RQ	MAT	Anxious (–) Avoidant (–) for W and M
Marchand (2004)	AAS	MCLI	Anxious (–) Avoidant (ns) for W; Anxious (–) Avoidant (–) for M
Treboux et al. (2004, Study 2)	ECR	DAS	Anxious (–) Avoidant (–) for W and M
Rholes et al. (2006)	AAQ	DAS	Anxious (–) Avoidant (–)
Birnbaum (2007)	ECR	RAS	Anxious (–) Avoidant (ns) (sample of women)

Note. *, longitudinal design; M, men; W, women; (–), significant inverse correlation; (+), significant positive correlation; (ns), nonsignificant effects; DAS, Dyadic Adjustment Scale; FAM, Family Assessment Measure; FBS, Family Behavior Survey; FSS, Family Satisfaction Scale; HS, Hazan and Shaver; LWS, Love Withdrawal Scale; MAQ, Multidimensional Attachment Questionnaire; MAT, Marital Adjustment Test; MCLI, Marital Comparison Level Inventory; MSI, Marital Satisfaction Inventory; QMI, Quality of Marriage Index; QRI, Quality of Relationship Index; RAS, Relationship Assessment Scale; RISS, Relational Interaction Satisfaction Scale.

predictors of marital dissatisfaction than "state of mind with respect to attachment" to parents and other childhood caregivers. This conclusion converges with previously reviewed findings on the link between attachment orientations and romantic intimacy (e.g., Treboux et al., 2004).

Tables 10.5 and 10.6 provide answers to two important questions frequently asked in the attachment literature. The first concerns gender differences in the attachment–satisfaction link and the possibility that women's relationship satisfaction is more influenced by attachment insecurities than men's (because of women's greater investment in relationships and their interdependent self-construals). However, as can be seen in Tables 10.5 and 10.6 there is no consistent gender difference along these lines. In fact, the vast majority of studies have yielded significant associations between attachment insecurities and relationship dissatisfaction in both women and men.

The second question concerns differences between anxious and avoidant individuals (or between correlations involving anxious and avoidant attachment dimensions). Although most studies suggest that both kinds of insecurity are associated with relationship dissatisfaction (see Tables 10.5 and 10.6), detailed examination of the results within genders reveals differential effects of anxiety and avoidance. Whereas anxiety and avoidance are equally predictive of women's dissatisfaction, avoidance rather than anxiety appears to be more consistently associated with relationship dissatisfaction in men. That is, avoidant men seem to be at greater risk than anxious men for relationship dissatisfaction. It is possible that the male role's emphasis on independence and emotional control exacerbates, or is exacerbated by, attachment avoidance. Or perhaps women are especially unhappy with avoidant men, which translates into complaints and conflicts that undermine avoidant men's satisfaction.

Most of the reviewed studies are based on cross-sectional designs, making it impossible to discount the possibility that the observed associations between attachment insecurities and relationship dissatisfaction reflect influences of dissatisfaction on insecurity rather than the reverse, or mutual effects on these variables of some unmeasured third variable (see Chapter 5, this volume, for a review of effects of relational events on attachment security). However, even studies with prospective longitudinal designs consistently find that attachment insecurities predict subsequent reductions in relationship satisfaction (see Tables 10.5 and 10.6). For example, Davila et al. (1999) reported that higher anxiety and avoidance scores within the first 6 months of marriage predicted larger decreases in marital satisfaction over the next 3 years (assessed every 6 months). Making the story more complex, however, Davila et al. also found that attachment insecurities and marital dissatisfaction affected each other over time, suggesting a cycle of insecurity and dissatisfaction that worsens over time.

Three diary studies examined the attachment–satisfaction link in daily rather than global reports of relationship satisfaction (Campbell et al., 2005; J. A. Feeney, 2002a; Shaver et al., 2005). In all three studies, dispositional measures of attachment insecurities were associated with lower daily reports of relationship satisfaction across study periods ranging from 1 to 3 weeks. Two of these studies (the Shaver et al. study being the exception) also found that participants' insecurities, mainly along the anxiety dimension, caused them to be more reactive to daily fluctuations in their partners' positive and negative behaviors. That is, compared to secure spouses, anxious ones reacted with greater daily ups and downs in satisfaction, depending on the extent to which their partners were available and supportive. This result may mean that anxious partners' doubts about their lovability and their partners' love cause them to assign greater significance to daily events that signal approval or rejection. According to Campbell et al. (2005), this "myopic," here-and-now focus on daily relationship events helps to explain anxious individuals' dissatisfaction, because evaluating a relationship based on daily fluctuations exacerbates doubts and insecurities (today's available partner can be tomorrow's rejecting partner) and intensifies a maladaptive cycle of clinging behavior and relationship distress.

Some investigators have examined possible mediators of the link between attachment insecurities and relationship dissatisfaction (see Table 10.7). Findings indicate that maladaptive ways of coping, negative beliefs about relationship partners, and problems in conflict management underlie the heightened relationship dissatisfaction of anxious and avoidant people. Moreover, whereas negative affectivity also contributes to anxious people's relationship dissatisfaction, lack of nurturance and deficits in interpersonal expressivity and sensitivity are additional mediators of avoidant people's dissatisfaction. The issue of mediation is complex, and research is not likely to identify just one or two isolated mediators. Nevertheless, exploring the mechanisms by which attachment insecurities are played out in couple relationships is important for both theoretical and clinical reasons.

Up to this point, we have focused mainly on the detrimental effects of attachment insecurities on relationship satisfaction. However, there is also evidence that attachment security can protect relationship quality during life transitions and stressful periods. Satis-

TABLE 10.7. A Summary of Findings Concerning Mediators of the Attachment–Satisfaction Link

Study	Main findings
Mediators of the link between attachment anxiety and dissatisfaction	
J. A. Feeney (1994)	Problems in negotiation and conflict resolution
Lussier et al. (1997)	Lack of reliance in problem solving strategies
Davila et al. (1999)	Negative affectivity
Gallo & Smith (2001)	Negative explanations of their own and partner's behaviors
Frei & Shaver (2002)	Lack of respect for partner
Marchand (2004)	Problems in negotiation and conflict resolution
Sumer & Cozzarelli (2004)	Negative explanations of their own and partner's behaviors
Mediators of the link between avoidance and dissatisfaction	
J. A. Feeney (1994)	Problems in negotiation and conflict resolution
J. A. Feeney (1996)	Sensitivity to a relationship partner's needs
Lussier et al. (1997)	Maladaptive patterns of coping
Morrison, Urquiza, et al. (1997)	Lack of nurturance
J. A. Feeney (1999b)	Deficits in emotional expressivity (emotional control)
Berant et al. (2003)	Negative appraisals of relationship tasks
	Maladaptive patterns of coping
Cobb et al. (2001)	Negative perceptions of partner's support
Meyers & Landsberger (2002)	Negative perceptions of partner's support
Marchand (2004)	Problems in negotiation and conflict resolution

faction is endangered by a broad array of extrarelational stressors (e.g., illness or injury, financial difficulties, problems at work); changes in a partner's roles, identity, preferences, and values; and normative transitions that demand personal and dyadic readjustment (e.g., parenthood, aging). During trying times, securely attached people's optimistic and constructive ways of regulating emotions and coping with stress (Chapter 7, this volume) facilitate restoration of emotional equanimity; maintenance of a calm, confident, and affectionate climate within a relationship; and flexible readjustment of couple dynamics to fit new reality constraints. Moreover, attachment security not only allows relationship readjustments but also sometimes even increases camaraderie and relationship satisfaction during stressful periods.

In a study of married women dealing with infertility problems, Amir et al. (1999) found that attachment security buffered the detrimental effects of prolonged infertility on marital satisfaction. Women suffering from sustained infertility problems reported lower marital satisfaction than women who became aware of such problems not long before the study. However, this effect was observed mainly among attachment-anxious women. Secure women were more able to maintain marital satisfaction despite the chronic distress and recurrent frustration associated with prolonged infertility.

Interesting buffering effects of attachment security have also been noted during the transition to parenthood. For example, Rholes et al. (2001) and Simpson and Rholes (2002a) reported that wives' negative prenatal perceptions of spousal support (assessed 6 weeks before the birth of a first child) predicted decreases in marital satisfaction 6 months later, but this detrimental effect of insufficient spousal support occurred mainly among anxious women. Paley, Cox, Harter, and Margand (2002) found that couples who exhibited escalation of negative emotions (one spouse's negative emotion being followed by an increase in the other spouse's negative emotion) while discussing a marital problem prior to the birth of their first child also showed decreases in affection and intimacy 3 and 12 months after the birth. But, again, the decrease occurred mainly among insecure husbands and their wives. Secure husbands and their wives showed little or no decrease in affection or intimacy, even if they had displayed negative emotion escalation during the high-stress transition to parenthood.

Overall, the findings imply that attachment security is a psychological resource that facilitates relationship satisfaction despite stressful experiences and relationship changes. Insecure individuals, in contrast, are at risk for relationship deterioration during stressful periods and may need interventions that bolster relational stability during demanding times.

Relationship Stability

Even if attachment insecurity is conducive to relationship dissatisfaction, does it also contribute over time to breakups and divorces? The answer to this question appears to be "yes." In the very first study of romantic attachment, Hazan and Shaver (1987) found that people who described themselves as having an avoidant or anxious attachment style had shorter relationships (4.9 and 6 years, respectively) than secure people (10 years) and were more likely to report having been divorced (10% of anxious and 12% of avoidant participants vs. 6% of secure participants). Subsequent studies have also found that insecure people have briefer relationships and are more likely to divorce (e.g., Birnbaum et al., 1997; R. W. Doherty et al., 1994; J. A. Feeney & Noller, 1990, 1992; E. M. Hill, Young, & Nord, 1994). In a study of individuals who entered another marriage following a divorce, the avoidant ones were more likely to divorce again (Ceglian & Gardner, 1999).

Beyond these cross-sectional studies, several prospective longitudinal studies (with the exception of Whisman & Allan, 1996) have indicated that attachment insecurity predicts subsequent breakups of dating relationships (Crowell & Treboux, 2001; Duemmler & Kobak, 2001; Kirkpatrick & Davis, 1994; Kirkpatrick & Hazan, 1994; Shaver & Brennan, 1992). In a 3-year longitudinal study, Kirkpatrick and Davis (1994) found interesting gender differences in this respect: Couples that included an avoidant woman and/or an anxious man were highly predisposed to break up within the 3-year study period. In contrast, the pairing of an anxious woman with an avoidant man, even though both partners reported relatively high levels of relationship distress, was resistant to dissolution. Unfortunately, this intriguing pattern of gender effects has not been replicated in other studies. For example, Duemmler and Kobak (2001) found that avoidance was predictive of relationship dissolution 2 years later among both men and women.

In a 4-year follow-up of Hazan and Shaver's (1987) original newspaper survey study, Kirkpatrick and Hazan (1994) found theoretically sensible differences between anxious and avoidant people's patterns of relationship stability or instability. Findings for anxious respondents seemed to reflect both their frustrating search for love and their reluctance to leave an unhappy relationship. People with an anxious attachment style at the time of the initial survey were most likely to have broken up at least once since completing the initial questionnaire, but they were also just as likely as secure people to be involved with the same romantic partner 4 years later. According to Kirkpatrick and Hazan, this pattern of results implies that anxious people tend to break up, then get back together with the same person, perhaps multiple times. D. Davis et al. (2003) found something similar in a study of reactions to breakups: Their more anxious respondents were more likely to feel sexually attracted to their former partners, and were more likely to become reinvolved with the person through sexual activities.

Attachment-anxious people's reluctance to leave unhappy relationships was further documented by Davila and Bradbury (2001), who followed newlywed couples for 4 years and examined whether attachment insecurities within the first 6 months of marriage predicted staying in unsatisfactory marriages. Although both avoidance and anxiety predicted marital dissatisfaction over time, only attachment anxiety put spouses at risk for staying in unhappy marriages. Attachment anxiety was higher among individuals who were married but chronically dissatisfied, compared to those who were happily married and those who divorced, even after controlling for divorce attitudes, neuroticism, and self-esteem. Thus, it seems that anxious adults' overdependence on relationship partners, fears of abandonment and separation, and doubts about their ability to handle life challenges alone lead them to maintain relationships at all costs, even if it implies staying in an unhappy marriage. (Later, in the section dealing with relationship violence, we discuss similar findings concerning anxious adults' difficulties in leaving a violent relationship). According to Davila and Bradbury, spouses' attachment anxiety "may make them unhappy in their marriage and at the same time keep them in their marriage. Hence, the stability of such marriages may be grounded in insecurity rather than satisfaction" (p. 388).

Kirkpatrick and Hazan's (1994) findings for avoidant individuals suggested, in contrast, they these people were ready to exit a close relationship as soon as they experienced relationship distress. They were the most likely of the three attachment "types" (assessed in that study with a categorical self-report measure) to report no longer being involved with a partner 4 years later. Moreover, they were most likely to say they were not currently seeing anyone and not looking for a partner or going out with more than one partner (see Chapter 9, this volume, for related findings on loneliness and social withdrawal).

Conceptually similar findings were reported by Klohnen and Bera (1998) among women who participated in their 31-year longitudinal study (see details in Chapter 5, this volume). Women who described themselves as securely attached at age 52 were more likely than avoidant women to be married at age 52. In addition, secure midlife women had reported higher commitment than avoidant women to getting married and starting a family at age 21, and this early difference in commitment seemed to have been borne out in behavior 6 years later, at age 27, when secure women were more likely to be married and to report fewer marital tensions. Although we have to keep in mind that variations in relationship trajectory might have affected women's self-reported attachment style at age 52 (see Chapter 5, this volume), Klohnen and Bera conducted several analyses of other kinds of self-report and observational measures showing that the avoidant women at age 52 would probably have classified themselves as avoidant earlier in adulthood as well.

Overall, the studies of attachment style and relationship stability and satisfaction indicate that attachment security contributes to these two aspects of romantic and marital relationships, and that the two major forms of insecurity diminish satisfaction and contribute to relationship dissolution. Avoidant individuals are especially likely to be dissatisfied with their relationships (when they are in them) and to address their dissatisfaction by leaving. Anxious individuals are also vulnerable to dissatisfaction, but they seem more likely to deal with it by staying in an unfulfilling relationship, unless their partners leave them. Perhaps to them, being alone seems even less likely to be fulfilling than sticking with a struggling relationship. As we will see, this reluctance to leave makes anxious adults vulnerable to psychological and physical abuse. Secure individuals can stay with a committed long-term relationship when problems can be resolved, but they also have the self-confidence and perhaps supportive social network to help them successfully leave a dangerous or persistently dissatisfying relationship.

Relationship Violence

Attachment insecurity contributes to abuse and violence within couple relationships—the most painful and dangerous kind of relationship maladjustment. Insecure partners' deficient conflict-management skills incline them to try coercive tactics, insults, and threats (see Table 10.4) that can escalate conflict and set the stage for aggression and reciprocal violence. Anxious individuals' controlling behavior can escalate to coercion and aggression when a partner is not responsive to bids for proximity and loyalty, or can incite a partner to behave aggressively to free him- or herself from overly insistent, intrusive demands. Avoidant individuals' coolness, detachment, and lack of nurturance can induce a partner, particularly if he or she is overly dependent and demanding (i.e., anxiously attached), to behave aggressively to gain attention, respect, or love.

Viewed from an attachment perspective, couple violence is an exaggerated form of protest against perceived partner unavailability and lack of responsiveness (e.g., Bartholomew & Allison, 2006; Mayseless, 1991). According to this perspective, aggression is precipitated by a partner's undesirable behavior (e.g., rejection, inattentiveness), or by insecurities about the future of a relationship, and is aimed at discouraging a partner's withdrawal or departure (Pistole & Tarrant, 1993). This reasoning is consistent with findings that indicate physical and psychological abuse typically occur during couple conflicts about real or imaginary threats of rejection, infidelity, or abandonment (e.g., M. Crawford & Gartner, 1992; Dutton & Browning, 1988). In light of this theoretical analysis, it is easy to understand why anxious adults, who are chronically afraid of rejection and separation, and are often pessimistic about the future of their relationships, are inclined to perpetrate acts of violence against a romantic partner. These destructive acts of protest can be further intensified by anxious individuals' difficulties in managing anger (Chapter 7, this volume) and their ineffective communication of strong needs for love and attention. As a result, they are more likely than secure individuals to strike out aggressively as a means of gaining or regaining proximity to their partner during couple disagreements and conflicts. This kind of behavior is evident even in infancy, and it led Bowlby (1969/1982) to emphasize "protest" following infants' separation from an attachment figure, and Ainsworth et al. (1978) to code angry "resistance" during infants' reunions with an attachment figure in the Strange Situation.

Some attachment researchers have suggested that avoidant individuals are also more likely than their secure counterparts to engage in acts of violence during couple conflicts because of their hostility, narcissism, and dysfunctional approach to conflict management (e.g., Bookwala & Zdaniuk, 1998; Mayseless, 1991). However, Bartholomew and Allison (2006) reasoned that avoidant people's tendency to withdraw from interpersonal conflicts and suppress overt expressions of anger and hostility (Chapter 7, this volume) might actually discourage outright aggression toward a relationship partner. Even Bartholomew and Allison mention, however, that avoidant people can become violent when involved in negative reciprocity and a demand–withdrawal behavioral dynamic with a partner (who is likely to be anxiously attached). They give a harrowing example from one of their studies in which a man refused to keep arguing with his wife after they had been up most of the night fighting (he was trying to relax with a newspaper before leaving for work). His anxious partner stabbed him in the back with a kitchen knife, which definitely got his attention and caused him to become enraged in return. Bartholomew and Allison point out that the correlation between one partner being violent and the other partner also being violent is above .60 in most studies of couple violence, which suggests that people with violent tendencies either choose one another as mates, or that one partner's violence provokes the other partner's violence in turn. Probably both causal pathways exist; that is, if there is reciprocity of negative affect in a couple and/or a demand–withdrawal pattern in their interactions, the partners may mutually goad each other to become more abusive.

We also suspect that avoidant individuals display aggression indirectly, even if they are not prone to violence. They are likely to engage in "passive aggression," which includes expressions of indifference, disrespect, and contempt, and to use violence as a means of distancing themselves from a partner who will not leave them alone (Bartholomew & Allison, 2006; N. Roberts & Noller, 1998). These reactions, which fit comfortably with attachment-system deactivation, can easily be perceived by a partner as psychologically abusive, which might cause the partner to react aggressively. Thus, even if not directly aggressive themselves, avoidant partners may be involved in mutually violent and abusive acts within a couple.

Consistent with expectations, there is evidence linking attachment insecurities with perpetration of violence within couples, although the findings are stronger and more consistent for anxiety than for avoidance (see Table 10.8). Although the attachment perspective on couple violence is not gender-specific, most of the studies have focused on men's violence toward women. But some studies have obtained similar findings when assessing women's violence toward men.

Anxiously attached people's proneness to couple violence has been documented in three kinds of studies. First, compared with nonviolent samples, men and women who engage in acts of violence within couple relationships score higher on attachment anxiety (either anxiety scores per se or anxiety as an aspect of fearful avoidance). Second, battering men who score higher in attachment anxiety tend to report more severe and frequent acts of abuse toward romantic partners, and more coercive behavior during couple conflicts. Third, most researchers who have examined the association between attachment style and couple violence in unrestricted samples of adolescents and young adults have consistently found that young men and women who score higher on attachment anxiety (often assessed in the form of preoccupied or fearful self-ratings) are more likely to engage in couple violence. These associations cannot be explained by relationship length or interpersonal problems (Bookwala & Zdaniuk, 1998) and seem to be mediated by ineffective conflict management (N. Roberts & Noller, 1998) and attempts to control a partner's behavior (Follingstad, Bradley, Helff, & Laughlin, 2002).

With regard to avoidant attachment, most of the studies summarized in Table 10.8 did not turn up significant associations with relationship violence. However, Holtzworth-Munroe et al. (1997, Study 1) found that avoidance was significantly higher among battering men than among nondistressed men, and Rankin, Saunders, and Williams (2000) found that higher avoidance in a sample of African American men who had been arrested for partner abuse was associated with perpetration of more frequent and severe acts of abuse toward romantic partners. In addition, more than one-third of the studies that assessed the link between attachment style and violence in unrestricted samples of adolescents and young adults found that men and women who scored higher on avoidance reported higher levels of violence against romantic partners. This kind of association has been found even prospectively, when avoidance was assessed during adolescence and perpetration of violence was assessed 6 years later (Collins et al., 2002). From Table 10.8, we conclude that when fearful and dismissing forms of avoidance were distinguished, only fearful avoidance was related to violence. Thus, the few associations with avoidance might actually be due to fearful avoidance, which is a combination of anxiety and avoidance. If this is correct, it suggests that anxiety is the major culprit in facilitating violence.

TABLE 10.8. A Summary of Findings on Attachment Orientations and Couple Violence

Study	Attachment measure	Violence measure	Main findings
Studies that compared attachment scores of violent and nonviolent samples			
Dutton et al. (1994)^	RSQ (M)	PMWI	Secure: V < NV Anxious, Fearful: V > NV; Avoidant: V = NV
Holtzworth-Munroe et al. (1997, Study 1)^	AAS (M)	CTS	Anxious: V > NV; Avoidant: V > NV
Holtzworth-Munroe et al. (1997, Study 2)^	RQ (M)	CTS	Secure: V < NV; Anxious, Fearful: V > NV; Avoidant: V = NV
Bookwala & Zdaniuk (1998)^	RQ (M, W)	CTS	Secure: V = NV; Anxious, Fearful: V > NV; Avoidant: V = NV
Tweed & Dutton (1998)^	RQ (M)	PMWI	Secure: V = NV; Anxious, Fearful: V > NV; Avoidant: V = NV
Babcock et al. (2000)^	AAI (M)	CTS	Secure: V < NV
Studies of associations between attachment and couple violence			
Henderson et al. (1997)	RQ (M)	PMWI	Anxious (+) Avoidant (ns) Secure (ns) Fearful (+)
Landolt & Dutton (1997)	RSQ	PMWI	Anxious (+) Avoidant (ns) Secure (−) Fearful (+) (gay sample)
O'Hearn & Davis (1997)	RQ (W)	AC	Anxious (+) Avoidant (ns) Secure (ns) Fearful (+)
Kesner & McKenry (1998)^	RQ (M)	CTS	Anxious (ns) Avoidant (ns) Secure (−) Fearful (+)
N. Roberts & Noller (1998)^	RSQ (W, M)	CTS	Anxious (+) Avoidant (ns) for W and M
Wekerle & Wolfe (1998)	HS ratings (W, M)	CIRQ	Anxious (+) Avoidant (+) Secure (ns) for W and M
Rankin et al. (2000)^	RSQ (V-M)	MWA	Anxious (+) Avoidant (+)
Mauricio & Gormley (2001)^	RQ (V-M)	CTS	Secure (−)
Bookwala (2003)	RQ (W, M)	CTS	Anxious (ns) Avoidant (ns) Secure (ns) Fearful (+) for W and M
Collins et al. (2002)*	HS ratings (M)	CTS	Anxious (ns) Avoidant (+) Secure (ns)
Crowell, Treboux & Waters (2002)^*	AAI (W, M)	FBS	Secure (−) for W and M (verbal aggression)
Crowell, Treboux, et al. (2002)^*	AAI (W, M)	FBS	Secure (ns) for W and M
Follingstad et al. (2002)	HS ratings (W, M)	CTS	Anxious (+) Avoidant (ns) Secure (ns) for W and M
Treboux et al. (2004, Study 1)	AAI, CRI (W, M)	FBS	Secure (−) for W and M
Treboux et al. (2004, Study 2)^	AAI, CRI ECR (W, M)	FBS	Secure (ns) for W and M Anxious (+) Avoidant (+) for W and M
Henderson et al. (2005)	Interview	CTS	Anxious (+) Avoidant (ns) for W and M
W. S. Rogers et al. (2005)	AAQ	CTS	Anxious (+) Avoidant (+) for W and M

Note. ^, married couples; *, longitudinal design; NV, non-violent samples; V, violent samples; M, men; W, women; (−) significant inverse correlation; (+) significant positive correlation; (ns) nonsignificant effects; AC, Abuse Checklist; CIRQ, Conflict in Relationship Questionnaire; CTS, Conflict Tactics Scale; FBS, Family Behavior Survey; HS, Hazan and Shaver; MWA, Measure of Wife Abuse; PMWI, Psychological Maltreatment of Women Inventory.

Interestingly, *victims* of partner abuse have also been found to suffer from attachment insecurities, with some studies finding elevations in attachment anxiety (Bond & Bond, 2004; Henderson, Bartholomew, Trinke, & Kwong, 2005; O'Hearn & Davis, 1997; N. Roberts & Noller, 1998; Wekerle & Wolfe, 1998) and others finding elevations in avoidance (Bond & Bond, 2004; Kesner & McKenry, 1998; Wekerle & Wolfe, 1998). Of course, because of the cross-sectional nature of the studies, the findings might indicate either that attachment insecurity puts people at risk for becoming victims of partner abuse or that abuse can increase attachment insecurity, or both (see Chapter 5, this volume, for a review of the effects of abusive relationships on attachment style). Also, given the previously mentioned mutuality of violence, most of the victims are also perpetrators. Therefore, logically, the same variables have to predict both perpetration and victimization.

Longitudinal studies indicate that abused women who previously scored higher on attachment anxiety had more problems in resolving their feelings of separation 6 months after leaving their romantic partner. For example, they engaged in more frequent sexual contact and emotional involvement with their old partner after separation (Henderson, Bartholomew, & Dutton, 1997; see also D. Davis et al., 2003). This finding fits with Davila and Bradbury's (2001) conclusion that anxious people are unable or unwilling to leave unhappy relationships. More important, it suggests that such people may form a "traumatic bond" with an abusive partner that puts them at risk for further abuse.

A Systemic Perspective on Attachment Style and Relationship Adjustment

Before concluding this section, we should note that although most of the reviewed studies focused mainly on the contribution of one person's attachment style to his or her relationship adjustment, some studies moved beyond the individual as the unit of analysis and considered three kinds of dyadic effects: (1) "partner effects"—the extent to which each partner's attachment style affects the other partner's relationship adjustment; (2) "couple-type effects"—the extent to which particular pairings of secure and insecure styles affect relationship adjustment; and (3) "interactive" effects—the extent to which the effects of each partner's attachment style on relationship adjustment are altered by the other partner's attachment style. These studies reveal the complex ways in which both partners' attachment systems influence the quality of a couple relationship.

Partner Effects

Living with a cool, distant, emotionally detached partner or with a clingy, controlling, chronically distressed partner can easily erode a person's relationship satisfaction and raise doubts about the wisdom of maintaining the relationship. It is therefore reasonable to expect significant effects of one partner's attachment insecurities on the other partner's relationship dissatisfaction. More than 30 published studies have examined these partner effects (see Table 10.9), and most have found that partners of insecurely attached people (either anxious or avoidant) report lower relationship satisfaction than do partners of secure people. However, since most of the studies relied on cross-sectional designs, the findings might just as well imply that relational dissatisfaction on the part of one couple member arouses attachment insecurities in the other. Fortunately, there are five prospective longitudinal studies, four of which provide support for the path going from one partner's attachment insecurity to subsequent decreases in the other partner's level of relationship satisfaction (see Table 10.9).

In a 3-year follow-up study of newlywed couples, Davila et al. (1999) noted recursive dyadic links between one partner's attachment insecurity and the other partner's dissatisfaction. Specifically, husbands' attachment anxiety and avoidance and wives' avoidance within the first 6 months of marriage predicted subsequent decreases in the other partner's reports of marital satisfaction over the 3-year study period. Moreover, decreases in husbands' satisfaction predicted subsequent increases in wives' attachment anxiety. Variation in wives' satisfaction did not have a significant effect on husbands' attachment scores, so the findings reveal only one kind of recursive dyadic link, by which husbands' insecurities heightened wives' dissatisfaction, and husbands' dissatisfaction heightened wives' insecurities. However, more prospective studies are needed before we can confidently accept and interpret such effects.

TABLE 10.9. A Summary of Findings Concerning Effects of Partner's Attachment Style on Relationship Satisfaction

Study	Women's satisfaction	Men's satisfaction
Studies based on ratings of attachment security		
Kobak & Hazan (1991)^	Men's security (+)	Women's security (+)
Shields et al. (2000)^	Men's security (+)	Women's security (+)
Cobb et al. (2001)*^	Ns effects of men's attachment	Women's security (+)
Alexandrov et al. (2005)^	Men's security (+)	Women's security (+)
Studies based on ratings of attachment anxiety and avoidance		
Collins & Read (1990)	Men's anxiety (ns) avoidance (−)	Women's anxiety (−) avoidance (ns)
Simpson (1990)	Men's anxiety (ns) avoidance (−)	Women's anxiety (−) avoidance (ns)
J. A. Feeney (1994, 1–10 years)^	Men's anxiety (−) avoidance (ns)	Women's anxiety (−) avoidance (−)
J. A. Feeney (1994, 11–20 years)^	Men's anxiety (ns) avoidance (−)	Women's anxiety (−) avoidance (−)
J. A. Feeney (1994, over 20 years)^	Men's anxiety (−) avoidance (ns)	Women's anxiety (−) avoidance (−)
J. A. Feeney et al. (1994)*^	Men's anxiety (ns) avoidance (ns)	Women's anxiety (ns) avoidance (ns)
Kirkpatrick & Davis (1994)	Men's anxiety (ns) avoidance (ns)	Women's anxiety (−) avoidance (ns)
Brennan & Shaver (1995)	Men's anxiety (−) avoidance (−)	Women's anxiety (−) avoidance (−)
Carnelley et al. (1996, Study 1)	Men's anxiety (ns) avoidance (ns)	Women's anxiety (−) avoidance (ns)
Carnelley et al. (1996, Study 2)^	Men's anxiety (−) avoidance (−)	Women's anxiety (−) avoidance (−)
J. A. Feeney (1996)^	Men's anxiety (−) avoidance (ns)	Women's anxiety (ns) avoidance (ns)
Frazier et al. (1996)	Men's anxiety (−) avoidance (ns)	Women's anxiety (ns) avoidance (ns)
Jones & Cunningham (1996)	Men's anxiety (−) avoidance (−)	Women's anxiety (−) avoidance (ns)
Whisman & Allan (1996)	Men's anxiety (ns) avoidance (ns)	Women's anxiety (ns) avoidance (−)
Lussier et al. (1997)^	Men's anxiety (−) avoidance (−)	Women's anxiety (−) avoidance (ns)
Davila et al. (1998, Study 1)^	Men's anxiety (−) avoidance (ns)	Women's anxiety (−) avoidance (−)
Davila et al. (1998, Study 2)^	Men's anxiety (−) avoidance (−)	Women's anxiety (−) avoidance (−)
Mikulincer, Horesh, et al. (1998)^	Men's anxiety (−) avoidance (−)	Women's anxiety (−) avoidance (−)
N. Roberts & Noller (1998)^	Men's anxiety (−) avoidance (−)	Women's anxiety (−) avoidance (−)
Davila et al. (1999)*^	Men's anxiety (−) avoidance (−)	Women's anxiety (ns) avoidance (−)
J. A. Feeney (1999b)^	Men's anxiety (−) avoidance (ns)	Women's anxiety (−) avoidance (ns)
Gallo & Smith (2001)	Men's anxiety (−) avoidance (ns)	Women's anxiety (ns) avoidance (ns)
J. A. Feeney (2002a)^	Men's anxiety (−) avoidance (ns)	Women's anxiety (−) avoidance (ns)
Schmitt (2002)	Men's anxiety (ns) avoidance (ns)	Women's anxiety (ns) avoidance (ns)
Kachadourian et al. (2004)^	Men's anxiety (ns) avoidance (ns)	Women's anxiety (−) avoidance (−)
J. A. Feeney et al. (2003)^	Men's anxiety (ns) avoidance (ns)	Women's anxiety (ns) avoidance (ns)
Banse (2004)^	Men's anxiety (−) avoidance (ns)	Women's anxiety (−) avoidance (−)
Shaver et al. (2005, Study 1)	Men's anxiety (−) avoidance (−)	Women's anxiety (ns) avoidance (−)
Shaver et al. (2005, Study 2)	Men's anxiety (−) avoidance (−)	Women's anxiety (−) avoidance (−)

Note. ^, married couples; *, longitudinal design; (−), significant inverse correlation; (+), significant positive correlation; (ns), nonsignificant correlation.

A detailed analysis of Table 10.9 also provides information about a frequently discussed gender difference in partner attachment effects. Two of the early attachment studies (Collins & Read, 1990; Simpson, 1990) found that men's satisfaction was more adversely affected by women's anxiety than by women's avoidance, and that women's satisfaction was more detrimentally affected by men's avoidance than by their anxiety. The most common explanation of these findings was based on gender differences in needs for closeness and autonomy (e.g., Koski & Shaver, 1997). Men's relationship satisfaction might depend on their satisfying a need for autonomy, which can be more easily frustrated by overly anxious, clinging female partners than by avoidant women. In contrast, women's relationship satisfaction might be heavily dependent on their desire for closeness, which can be more easily frustrated by avoidant than by anxious men.

However, as can be seen in Table 10.9, these gender differences have not been replicated in subsequent studies. In the case of women's satisfaction, the findings suggest that men's anxiety is the most consistent predictor of dissatisfaction. In the case of men's satisfaction, there is some evidence that women's anxiety is also a more consistent predictor than women's avoidance, but several studies also find significant effects of women's avoidance. Overall, then, the best single conclusion we can reach from the reviewed findings is that although both major kinds of attachment insecurity are associated with partner dissatisfaction, one partner's anxious attachment style seems especially likely to erode the other partner's satisfaction, regardless of gender. Longitudinal studies (e.g., Robins, Caspi, & Moffitt, 2002) suggested that neuroticism (which is partly determined by genes) has a similar negative effect on relationship satisfaction. Further research is needed to examine the unique contributions of anxious attachment and neuroticism to the erosion of partners' satisfaction over time.

Couple-Type Effects

Findings from the few studies that have examined couple-type effects on relationship satisfaction are not consistent. Three studies (Berman, Marcus, & Berman, 1994; Dickstein et al., 2001; Senchak & Leonard, 1992) found that secure couples (i.e., couples in which both partners were securely attached) reported greater satisfaction than mixed couples (in which only one partner was secure) and doubly insecure couples. No difference was found between mixed and insecure couples, implying that attachment insecurity in one partner has negative effects on couple satisfaction. This negative effect of one partner's attachment insecurity has also been noted in studies assessing regulation of closeness (J. A. Feeney, 1999b), dyadic communication (Tucker & Anders, 1998), responses to a partner's transgressions (Gaines et al., 1999), and conflict-management strategies (Bouthillier et al., 2002).

However, Cohn, Silver, Cowan, Cowan, and Pearson (1992), Mikulincer and Florian (1999c), and Wampler, Shi, Nelson, and Kimball (2003) found no significant difference between couple types. Moreover, other researchers have concluded that a secure partner can sometimes buffer the negative effects of an insecure partner on relationship outcomes. Specifically, compared with couples in which both partners are insecure, mixed couples in which one partner is secure report higher marital quality and more intimacy-promoting behavior (Ben-Ari & Lavee, 2005; Volling et al., 1998), higher emotional expressivity (J. A. Feeney, 1995a), and calmer emotions and prorelationship behaviors during a conflict discussion (Cohn et al., 1992; Paley et al., 1999). In addition, S. I. Powers et al. (2006) found that men interacting with a secure partner during a conflict-resolution task exhibited less physiological reactivity (assessed with salivary cortisol), although women's cortisol levels did not depend on their partner's security. Overall, it is difficult to reach a definitive conclusion because of the small number of studies and the failure of some studies to include both dimensions of insecurity. As J. A. Feeney (2003) noted, an avoidant person creates very different relational problems for anxious and avoidant partners.

Interaction Effects

In the research literature on couple relationships, there is extensive evidence that interactional processes resulting from both partners' behavior predict relationship adjustment (for a review, see Bradbury, Fincham, & Beach, 2000). In the attachment domain, although some studies have failed to find interactive effects of partners' attachment orientations on relationship satisfaction (e.g., Jones & Cunningham, 1996; Kirkpatrick & Davis, 1994) and on other relational cognitions and behaviors (e.g., Creasey, 2002a; Paley et al., 1999; Mikulincer & Florian, 1999c), there is now substantial evidence that two combinations of insecure attachment styles interfere with relationship adjustment: (1) the pairing of an anxious person with an avoidant one, and (2) the pairing of two anxious people (e.g., Allison, Bartholomew, Mayseless, & Dutton, 2005; J. A. Feeney, 1994; N. Roberts & Noller; 1998).

Couples in which an anxious person is paired with an avoidant one tend to produce destructive pursuit–distancing or demand–withdrawal patterns of relating. In such couples, the anxious partner's needs and demands frustrate the avoidant partner's preference for distance, and the avoidant partner's tendency to create distance frustrates the anxious partner's intense desire for closeness. As a result, both partners are dissatisfied and can become abusive or violent when attempting to influence their partner's undesirable behavior.

In a study of the early years of marriage, J. A. Feeney (1994) found that a wife's attachment anxiety, coupled with a husband's avoidance, reduced both partners' marital satisfaction. N. Roberts and Noller (1998) and Allison et al. (2005) extended these findings to relationship violence and noted that the combination of an avoidant individual (either male or female) with an anxious one intensified the effects of each partner's attachment style on the perpetration of violence against the other partner. In addition, Babcock et al. (2000) found that anxiously attached men engaged in couple violence mainly when their partners attempted to remain distant during conflicts.

Attachment studies also reveal the destructive effect of pairing two anxious partners: One partner's anxiety exacerbates the other partner's anxiety, and the combination erodes marital satisfaction (J. A. Feeney, 1994; Gallo & Smith, 2001), amplifies negative responses to a partner's distancing (J. A. Feeney, 2003), and increases couple violence (Allison et al., 2005). J. A. Feeney (2003) described these anxious–anxious couples as engaging in "mutual attack and retreat," and Bartholomew and Allison (2006) labeled them "pursuing–pursuing." In such couples, both partners feel misunderstood and rejected, both are excessively focused on their own insecurities, and both try to control the other's behavior. Bartholomew and Allison say about these pursuit–pursuit couples: "When both partners showed preoccupied tendencies, they tended to compete for support and attention from each other. Moreover, neither partner was able to recognize or meet their partner's needs, leading to mutual frustration and, at times, aggression" (p. 116).

Overall, the evidence strongly indicates that attachment insecurities put couples at risk for relationship maladjustment. At the individual level, attachment insecurities are associated with relationship dissatisfaction and troubled relational behavior, sometimes including violence. At the dyadic level, there is increasing evidence that partners of insecure individuals also suffer from relationship distress and dissatisfaction. Moreover, whereas specific combinations of anxious and avoidant partners within a couple (anxious–avoidant, anxious–anxious) tend to exacerbate relationship dissatisfaction and violence, the presence of a relatively secure partner within a relationship sometimes buffers the detrimental effects of the other partner's insecurity.

CONCLUDING REMARKS

From flirting and dating through relationship consolidation, maintenance, adjustment to stresses and changes, and in some cases to relationship dissolution, attachment issues are ubiquitous in couple relationships, including marriages. Moreover, individual differences in attachment style are systematically related to relationship behaviors and outcomes. Although many of the studies we reviewed in this chapter are based on cross-sectional and correlational designs, there are enough longitudinal studies and a few suggestive experiments and diary studies to indicate that individual differences in attachment style truly play a causal role in relationship development and outcomes. Of course, given that attachment styles themselves are caused, in whole or in part, by relationship experiences, the causality runs both ways, and it runs from one partner's behaviors through the other partner's perceptions, feelings, and behaviors, and back to the original partner's perceptions, feelings, and further behaviors. From both theoretical and clinical standpoints, what matters most is that relational oddities and dysfunctions ranging from inhibited self-disclosure during the early phases of a relationship to mutual violence in dating relationships and marriages, can be systematically understood in terms of attachment theory, and that the research to date both supports the theory and suggests potentially fruitful interventions, which we discuss at length in Chapter 14.

In general, the associations between attachment style and relationship functioning are consistently observed in both men and women; that is, there are no consistent, meaningful gender differences in the link between attachment insecurities, and the various relational problems and dysfunctions reviewed in this chapter. Moreover, the link between attachment insecurities, and relational problems has been found in both homosexual and heterosexual couples. There are some indications, however, that gender moderates partner interaction effects. For example, as we mentioned earlier, the findings suggest that when attachment styles correspond with gender roles (anxious women being coupled with avoidant men), relational outcomes are worse, which is ironic, because most people probably believe that masculine men and feminine women are natural and successful matches. More research is needed to illuminate further the potential roles of gender, psychological masculinity and femininity, and culturally determined gender roles and identities in moderating the relational effects of attachment orientations at both individual and dyadic levels.

It is also important to note that although attachment insecurities are related to relational problems, insecure attachment does not inevitably lead to dysfunctional or unsatisfactory relationships. The associations between attachment style and the various aspects of relationship functioning, satisfaction, and stability are generally moderate in size and, in some cases, are not consistent across studies. This means that there is some overlap in the couple dynamics of secure and insecure individuals and relationships. Part of this overlap is likely due to the couple-type and interactional effects resulting from both partners' attachment orientations. But even the few studies that have considered such effects find that attachment style makes only a moderate-size contribution to couple functioning. There are, therefore, many other important factors involved, and these also deserve researchers' attention.

CHAPTER 11

∎ ∎ ∎

Relations between the Attachment and Caregiving Systems

In many of the beautiful and moving pictures of the Madonna and Child created over the centuries, we see two sides of an attachment relationship: the secure, trusting, happy infant and the warm, loving, security-providing parent. Attachment researchers focused first on the child's side of this relationship, because Bowlby's (1944, 1969/1982) original questions had to do with the effects of a child's early secure or insecure attachment on later personality development and psychopathology. But the answers to his questions lay mostly on the parent's side of the relationship, because the child's outcomes were viewed as largely determined by primary caregivers' mental states and observable behaviors. To provide answers to his questions in terms of his era's ethology and evolutionary psychology, Bowlby had to imagine that there was not only an "attachment behavioral system" in the infant but also a "caregiving behavioral system" in the parent.

One of the major contributions of subsequent attachment research has been to complete the causal circle by showing that the parameters of the caregiving system, as these can be inferred from observing and interviewing adults, are shaped by the caregiver's prior attachment experiences (e.g., Main et al., 1985; E. Waters et al., 2000). In other words, an adult's caregiving behavioral system is influenced, in large part, by his or her experiences with caregivers earlier in development.

Caregiving has been designated not only as a primary ingredient of parental behavior, but also as a major component of romantic and marital relationships, and in fact as a key constituent of all forms of prosocial behavior. For young children, parents are usually the primary providers of protection, support, and security, and differences in the ways they fulfill or mishandle this role have dramatic consequences for children's socioemotional development in general, and for their attainment of felt security in particular (see Chapter 5, this volume). Similarly, romantic partners are frequently called upon to provide comfort, support, and security to one another in times of need, and the quality of the support they are willing and able to provide is one of the major determinants of relationship quality and stability (Collins & Feeney, 2000; Chapter 10, this volume).

Anyone who works at a university, as we both do, has seen many romantic parallels to the Madonna's soothing affection for the infant Jesus in the behavior of one loving romantic partner toward another. Young lovers often sit on campus benches or lean against stately trees and speak softly and affectionately to each other, gently rearranging each other's wayward hair or twisted collar, and providing reassuring hugs and caresses. They often look at each other with the same loving regard one sees when parents unself-consciously admire and appreciate their children. Anyone who is married, as both of us are, has repeatedly occupied both the caregiving and care-receiving roles in a mutually supportive relationship. Moreover, anyone who is familiar with world religions and cultural history realizes that the human need for sympathy and care, and the importance of mature adults who are able to provide it, are central themes in all major religions. When viewed as products of an innate caregiving behavioral system, all forms of sensitive, responsive, compassionate care, indeed of "love" in the broadest sense, can be seen to bear family resemblances to one another, and the reasons for these similarities need to be better understood by psychologists.

In this chapter, we begin by considering theoretical ideas about the interplay of the attachment and caregiving behavioral systems, then review empirical studies of the relations between attachment styles and compassionate, caring behavior in parent–child relationships, adult romantic couples, and broader interpersonal contexts.

THE CAREGIVING SYSTEM AND ITS RELATION TO THE ATTACHMENT SYSTEM

Defining the Caregiving Behavioral System

According to attachment theory (Bowlby, 1969/1982), human beings are born with a capacity to develop *caregiving behaviors* aimed at providing protection and support to others who are either chronically dependent or temporarily in need. Bowlby claimed that these caring behaviors, as they emerge in development, are organized around a psycho-evolutionary adaptation (the *caregiving behavioral system*) that emerged over the long course of evolution because it increased the inclusive fitness of humans by increasing the likelihood that children, siblings, and tribe members with whom a person shared genes would survive to reproductive age and succeed in producing and rearing offspring (W. D. Hamilton, 1964). According to this inclusive fitness logic, the proliferation of a particular person's genes depends on not only his or her own reproductive success (based on transmitting genes through sexual reproduction) but also the extent to which people who share copies of one's genes are able to survive and reproduce. Therefore, behaviors aimed at helping others can have a beneficial effect on gene proliferation and may have been critical for our ancestors, whose reproductive success was challenged by illness, predation, injuries, natural disasters, and scarce resources.

Although the caregiving system presumably evolved primarily to increase the viability of an individual's own offspring and close relatives (George & Solomon, 1999), it may also have been more generally adapted to respond to the needs of other tribe members. Today, through educational elaboration, it can be extended to include genuine concern for anyone in need. (This involves socializing children to view all human beings as "members of a single family," as "brothers and sisters," etc.) Although most of us probably care more, and more easily, for people to whom we are closely related, either psychologically or genetically, our caregiving systems can be made more widely available to all suffering human beings and even to members of other species. Just as attachment-related motives, once they became universally present in the human psychological repertoire, can affect a wide variety of social processes, caregiving motives can be applied more broadly than to one's immediate genetic relatives. If the development of a person's caregiving system occurs under favorable social circumstances, compassion, loving-kindness, and generosity can become common ways of feeling and behaving. Of course, if the caregiving system does not develop under favorable circumstances, due to lack of parental modeling, training, and support, or to separations, losses, or negative interactions with parents and other adults that create insecurities and defenses, the developing child is likely to be less generous and less willing to focus compassionately on other people's (or creatures') needs and suffering.

Normative Parameters of the Caregiving System

The first logical step in conceptualizing the caregiving system is to specify the goal state for which the system seems to have been "designed" (by evolution). According to attachment theory, the set-goal of the caregiving system is to reduce other people's suffering, protect them from harm, and foster their growth and development (e.g., Collins, Guichard, et al., 2006; George & Solomon, 1999; Gillath, Shaver, & Mikulincer, 2005; Kunce & Shaver, 1994). In other words, the caregiving system is designed to accomplish the two major functions of a security-providing attachment figure: to meet another person's needs for protection and support in times of danger or distress (Bowlby [1969/ 1982] called this "providing a safe haven"), and to support others' exploration, autonomy, and growth when exploration is safe and viewed by the explorer as desirable (Bowlby and Ainsworth called this "providing a secure base for exploration"). Theoretically speaking, activation of the caregiving system transforms an individual, for the time being, into a "stronger and wiser" attachment figure and motivates him or her to meet another person's needs for proximity, safety, and security. In other words, the goals of the caregiver and the needy other become, for the moment, fully congruent, and both have the goal of making sure the dependent person's needs for safety and security are met.

According to Collins, Guichard, et al. (2006), caregiving needs and behaviors are likely to be activated in one or both of two kinds of situations: (1) when another person has to cope with danger, stress, or discomfort, and is either seeking help or would clearly benefit from it; and (2) when another person has an opportunity for exploration, learning, or mastery, and either needs help in taking advantage of the opportunity or seems eager to talk about, celebrate, or be validated for certain aspirations or accomplishments. In either case, a person becomes motivated to provide care and support based on his or her *appraisal* of the other's need for assistance or encouragement, not directly from the other person's need in itself. That is, a person would not adopt the role of caregiver if he or she failed to notice a needy person's expressions of distress or bids for support and encouragement, and to view the person's needs as legitimate. Moreover, a prospective caregiver can sometimes intrusively offer support and encouragement even in the absence of another person's explicit expressions of need, and this sometimes causes annoyance and resistance rather than gratitude. There are many opportunities for missed signals, incorrectly inferred needs, neglect of others' autonomy, and meddling in other people's lives when no help is needed or requested, which means there are many points at which individual differences in appraisals and reactions can have effects.

Once a person's caregiving system is activated (whether appropriately or not), he or she calls upon a repertoire of behaviors aimed at restoring the other person's welfare and felt security. Caregiving behaviors include attempts to relieve a needy person's distress and to support his or her coping efforts, for example, by showing interest in the person's problems, affirming his or her ability to deal with the situation, expressing love and affection, and providing instrumental aid as needed (Collins, Guichard, et al., 2006; B. C. Feeney, 2004, B. C. Feeney & Collins, 2004). A caregiver's behavior can also provide a secure base for another person's exploration, growth, and development, by supporting the person's desire to take on new challenges and acquire new skills, showing genuine interest in the person's goals and plans, affirming his or her ability to deal with challenges, providing advice and resources, not interfering with the person's exploratory activities, and admiring and applauding successes (Collins, Guichard, et al., 2006; B. C. Feeney, 2004, B. C. Feeney & Collins, 2004).

A key part of the caregiving system's primary strategy is the adoption of what Batson (1991) called an empathic stance toward another person's needs (e.g., by taking the other's perspective in order to help him or her effectively reduce suffering and distress or pursue growth and development. According to Collins, Guichard, et al. (2006), an empathic stance includes sensitivity and responsiveness, the two aspects of parental caregiving emphasized by Bowlby and Ainsworth. Sensitivity includes attunement to, and accurate interpretation of, another person's signals of distress, worry, or need, and responding in synchrony with the person's proximity- and support-seeking behavior. It also includes noticing both the needy person's implicit or explicit signals and the relevant contextual constraints, which determine what kind of support might be most beneficial in a particular situation (George & Solomon, 1999). Responsiveness includes generous intentions; validating the troubled person's needs and feelings; respecting his or her beliefs, attitudes, and values; and helping him or her feel loved, cared for, and understood (H. T. Reis & Shaver, 1988).

Both sensitivity and responsiveness are necessary, in general, for achieving the caregiving system's set-goal (meeting the other person's actual needs). Insensitive caregivers are likely to dismiss or misinterpret a needy person's signals and either evade the caregiving role or insert themselves awkwardly or intrusively into the needy person's affairs (e.g., insisting on solving the problem when the person, although frustrated, wishes to solve it independently). Lack of sensitivity and responsiveness can cause a careseeker to feel misunderstood, disrespected, or burdensome, which exacerbates distress rather than providing a secure base (Collins, Guichard, et al., 2006).

Dealing with another person's suffering can evoke two different kinds of emotional reactions in a potential caregiver (Batson, 1991): empathic compassion and personal distress. The two are often commingled, making it difficult for some people to tell whether the optimal response is to help the other person or to turn away to avoid one's own negative feelings. Although both compassion and personal distress are signs that one person's distress has triggered potentially caring reactions in another, the two states are quite different in attentional focus and motivational implications. The main focus of compassion is the other person's needs or suffering, and the natural implication is that the distress should be alleviated for the sufferer's benefit. In contrast, the main focus of personal distress is the self's own discomfort, which might be alleviated either by helping or by ignoring, or fleeing, the situation. Moreover, whereas compassion sustains caregiving without any direct payoff to the caregiver (*unconditional caregiving*), personal distress is likely to be translated into helping only if helping is the best way to reduce the caregiver's own discomfort (Batson, 1991). Under conditions of "easy escape," when potential caregivers can reduce their distress by means other than helping, personal distress does not motivate empathic care (Batson, 1991).

When caregiving works properly, it benefits the person being cared for—by solving a problem, increasing the person's sense of safety and security, or bolstering the person's own coping ability (Collins, Guichard, et al., 2006). Appropriate care also benefits the support provider, even though its primary goal is to benefit the other. It promotes an inner sense of what Erikson (1950/1993) called "generativity"—the sense that one is more than an isolated self and is able to contribute significantly to others' welfare. The sense of generativity includes very positive feelings about oneself as having good moral qualities and being able to perform good deeds; strong feelings of self-efficacy; confidence in one's interpersonal skills; and heightened feelings of love, communion, and connectedness (Shaver & Mikulincer, 2006). In addition, the benefits bestowed on both the care provider and the care recipient often strengthen their relationship and make it more satisfying (e.g., Collins & Feeney, 2000; B. C. Feeney, 2004).

Individual Differences in Caregiving

Although we assume that everyone is born with the potential to become an effective care provider, smooth and effective operation of the caregiving system depends on both intra- and interpersonal factors. Caregiving can be impaired by feelings, beliefs, and concerns that dampen or conflict with sensitivity and responsiveness. It can also be impaired by a careseeker's failure to express needs appropriately, by his or her rebuff of a caregiver's help, or by external obstacles to support provision. As Collins, Gichard, et al. (2006) noted, "It is clear that effective caregiving is a difficult process that is likely to be easier for some people than for others, and in some relationships compared to others" (p. 160).

Effective care provision requires both intra- and interpersonal regulation of the kinds we discussed in previous chapters. First, it involves emotion regulation processes (see Chapter 7, this volume) that help caregivers deal effectively with the discomfort caused by witnessing another person's distress. Deficient emotion regulation can cause a caregiver to feel overwhelmed by anxiety (Batson's "personal distress"), to slip into the role of another needy person rather than serving as a care provider, or to distance oneself physically, emotionally, or cognitively from the needy person to soothe one's own feelings, even if it means abdicating the caregiving role. Caregivers also need to encourage and bolster appropriate emotion regulation strategies on the part of the needy other. If this is not handled thoughtfully and sensitively, attempts to help may turn into additional causes of strain and dysfunction (Rook, 1998).

Second, effective caregiving requires self-regulation of goals and motives (see Chapter 8, this volume). Addressing another person's problems often requires suspension of one's own goals and plans. The other person's needs take precedence over one's own agenda. One has to diagnose the other person's problem, develop a plan for assisting the person sensitively and effectively, and suppress interfering motives or behavioral tendencies that increase distance from the needy person or interfere intrusively with the person's own coping efforts. Poor self-regulation can derail the caregiving process and exacerbate rather than alleviate the other person's suffering.

Third, effective caregiving requires interpersonal regulation (see Chapter 9, this volume), which includes synchronizing and coordinating the caregiver's and careseeker's behavior to solve the problem at hand. This kind of coordination can be achieved most readily, and in some cases only, if the caregiver can flexibly chart a course between distance and closeness and between dominance and submissiveness. Excessive distance limits a caregiver's ability to attend to the other's needs and remain accessible and responsive to signals or calls for help. Excessive closeness leads to overidentification with the suffering person's emotional state, which can overwhelm a caregiver. Excessive closeness blurs the boundary between caregiver and careseeker, resulting in misinterpretations of the seeker's signals. Often, such blurring is based on assumed similarity and the projection of the caregiver's own feelings and thoughts onto the needy person. Batson (1991) pointed out that effective care depends on the ability to distinguish between another person's welfare and one's own.

In Chapter 9 we discussed the dominance–submission dimension of dyadic interactions. In a caregiving context, excessive dominance leads to overly controlling behavior, interferes with cooperation with the careseeker, causes disrespect for the careseeker's beliefs and preferences, and reduces sensitive responsiveness. Excessive submissiveness may cause caregivers to sacrifice themselves rather than act judiciously, which undermines the role of "stronger and wiser" attachment figure—a role that is occupied most effectively if the caregiver truly is stronger and more knowledgeable or resourceful in a particular situation.

Collins, Guichard, et al. (2006) discussed four factors that hamper the intrapersonal and interpersonal regulation necessary for optimal caregiving: (1) social skills deficits, (2) depletion of psychological resources, (3) lack of motivation to help, and (4) acting on egoistic motives when "helping." Social skills deficits interfere with accurate decoding of a needy person's signals and communications. Without sufficient psychological resources, it is difficult to attend empathically to a needy person's distress while also developing effective plans to intervene. Lack of willingness to take responsibility for another person's welfare disrupts caregiving from the start.

Attachment Styles and Patterns of Care

Bowlby (1969/1982) noticed that different behavioral systems, such as attachment and exploration, sometimes interfere with each other. Because of the urgency and priority of threats to oneself (especially during early childhood), Bowlby thought activation of the attachment system was likely to inhibit activation of other behavioral systems, thus interfering with nonattachment activities (see Chapter 8, this volume, for a discussion of the "attachment–exploration balance"). This kind of interference can also occur in caregiving situations (Kunce & Shaver, 1994), because a potential caregiver may feel so threatened that obtaining care for him- or herself seems more urgent than providing care to others. At such times even adults are likely to be so focused on their own vulnerability that they lack the mental resources necessary to attend compassionately to others' needs for help and care.

Only when a degree of safety is attained and a sense of security is restored can most people perceive others to be not only sources of security and support but also human beings who need and deserve comfort and support themselves. This inner sense of security helps to explain why in emergency situations many healthy parents focus first on their children's safety even if it means putting themselves in harm's way. This is presumably why flight attendants need to remind parents before takeoff that, in case of emergency, they must affix their own oxygen mask before trying to put a mask on their child. Not realizing their own immediate vulnerability, secure parents might turn attention first to their children's welfare.

In general, a sense of security allows a person to attend less to his or her own needs and shift attention to the domains of other behavioral systems, such as caregiving. According to our current understanding of this process, attachment security does not activate caregiving efforts directly, but instead provides a psychological foundation for accurate empathy and altruistic helping. Security protects a caregiver from being overwhelmed by others' suffering or threatened by the interdependence involved in providing care. In addition, secure adults are ones who have generally witnessed good care provided by their attachment figures, and this gives them positive models for their own behavior (Collins & Feeney, 2000).

Securely attached people's positive working models (Chapter 6, this volume) sustain effective caregiving. Secure adults are likely to view themselves as efficacious (i.e., have positive models of self) and others as deserving of respect and support (positive models of others). Their comfort with intimacy and interdependence allows them to approach others in need, which is important, because it is often necessary to acknowledge other people's needs for sympathy and support if one is to help them through a crisis (Lehman, Ellard, & Wortman, 1986). Secure people's emotion regulation skills (Chapter 7, this volume) help them maintain emotional balance while addressing others' needs, a task that otherwise arouses self-doubt and personal distress (Batson, 1991). As a result, securely attached people can focus fully on others' needs and supply a safe haven and secure base even when being helpful and encouraging yields no obvious benefit to them other than a feeling of being an effective, helpful human being.

Insecure people, in contrast, are likely to have difficulties providing effective care (Collins, Guichard, et al., 2006; George & Solomon, 1999; Shaver & Hazan, 1988). Although anxiously attached people may have some of the skills and qualities needed for effective caring (e.g., comfort with intimacy and closeness), their deficits in intra- and interpersonal regulatory skills (Chapters 6, 7, and 9, this volume) make them vulnerable to personal distress, which interferes with sensitive and responsive care. Their tendency to intensify distressing thoughts and emotions (Chapter 7, this volume) can interfere with focusing clearly and accurately on other people's pain and suffering, drawing attention inward rather than outward, toward what others need. If personal distress is prolonged during an extended crisis, it can produce emotional overload, "burnout," or emotional exhaustion. Anxiously attached people easily become sidetracked by self-focused worries and concerns, misplaced projections, and blurred interpersonal boundaries (Chapter 6, this volume), making it difficult to help others in appropriate ways. Moreover, their need for closeness and approval (Chapter 9, this volume) can cause them to become overly involved and enmeshed, and their lack of self-confidence (Chapter 6, this volume) can make it difficult for them to adopt the role of a "stronger and wiser" pillar of support.

Although attachment-anxious individuals are often motivated to care for others, they may do so in ways intended to satisfy their own unmet needs for closeness, acceptance, and inclusion. According to Collins, Guichard, et al. (2006), these self-centered impulses result in intrusive caregiving that is insensitive to a needy partner's signals. Anxious people may try to get too close or too involved when a partner does not want help, which can generate resentment, anger, and conflict that in turn leave the anxious caregiver feeling unappreciated or falsely accused (Collins, Guichard, et al., 2006). To make matters worse, attachment-anxious people sometimes hesitate to provide a secure base for their partner's exploration and growth, because a freely exploring partner might move away from the relationship (Collins, Guichard, et al., 2006).

Avoidant people, who often maintain what they perceive to be a safe distance from their partners, are likely to react coolly or unresponsively to suffering partners and try to avoid being taken advantage of or "sucked in." Avoidant people do not generally approve of expressions of need and vulnerability, whether their own or those of their partners, and they have no desire to get entangled with someone whose weaknesses and needs are all too visible. For them, besides being a potential drain on their own resources, a suffering person threatens to mirror their own suppressed weaknesses and vulnerabilities. Studies we reviewed in Chapter 6 show that avoidant people project their own negative qualities onto others, then distance themselves from both the qualities and the people thought to possess them.

When obliged by social norms or interpersonal commitments to help others, avoidant people are likely to express disapproval, to lack sympathy and compassion, and to behave insensitively. At times, their reactions to others' suffering may take the form of pity rather than sympathy or compassion. Pity portrays the sufferer as inferior to oneself and causes a person either to withdraw rather than help or to help while showing disgust or disdain (Ben-Zeev, 1999). In some cases, avoidant people's negative models of others and associated hostile attitudes toward them (Chapter 6, this volume) may even transform pity into gloating (i.e., actually enjoying another person's suffering; "The idiot is being stewed in his own juices"; "He made his bed, now let him lie in it"). This is the motive behind hostile, dismissive humor—avoidant people's most characteristic form of humor (Kazarian & Martin, 2004; Saroglou & Scariot, 2002).

ATTACHMENT STYLES AND PARENTAL CAREGIVING

Attachment and caregiving have been examined most often in the context of parent–child relationships. Bowlby (1969/1982) noted that "what a mother brings to the [caregiving] situation is . . . complex; it derives not only from her naive endowment but from a long history of interpersonal relations within her family of origin" (p. 342); that is, Bowlby conceptualized parents as having developed their caregiving systems in tandem with their attachment systems and the associated working models (George & Solomon, 1999). Many researchers have assessed parents' attachment orientations and determined whether and how they affect mental representations of parenting and sensitivity, and responsiveness to children's needs, difficulties, and development. Most such studies have focused on mothers' (rather than fathers') working models and behavior, and have relied mainly on the AAI rather than self-report measures to assess adult attachment patterns. Nevertheless, the major findings have been replicated in the few studies that have focused on fathers or used self-report scales rather than interviews to assess adult attachment.

Mental Representations of Parental Caregiving

According to recent extensions of attachment theory (George & Solomon, 1999; Slade & Cohen, 1996), just as children develop mental representations of their parents, adults preparing for parenthood, and those who have already become parents, develop mental representations of themselves as caregivers, their child as a developing care recipient, and the parent–child relationship. These mental representations, like other working models of self and others, guide caregiving behaviors during parent–child interactions and influence parents' expectations, feelings, and actions (George & Solomon, 1999). If attachment insecurities influence working models of parenting and actual care provision, they should show up when adults' feelings and self-doubts about parenting and views of children and parent–child relationships are assessed.

People who score high on avoidance or anxiety are in fact less positive than their secure peers when it comes to judging their ability to relate to children and imagining relationships with their own future children (Rholes, Simpson, Blakely, Lanigan, & Allen, 1997; Rholes et al., 1995). Moreover, avoidant college students are less interested in having children and anticipate less satisfaction from caring for infants (Rholes et al., 1995, 1997). Attachment-anxious students have more exaggerated, unrealistic, and perfectionist conceptions of their imagined performance as parents (Snell, Overbey, & Brewer, 2005). These views may stem from a combination of wishing to be loved and wishing to overcome doubts about their parenting skills. Because participants in these college student studies had no children at the time they were questioned, the findings reflect internal working models of self-as-parent rather than actual experiences with offspring.

Conceptually similar results were obtained in studies of adults who were already parents. Using either the AAI or self-report attachment scales, these studies revealed that insecure parents experience less joy and pleasure than secure ones in relationships with their children (Rholes, Simpson, & Friedman, 2006; Scher & Dror, 2003; Slade, Belsky, Aber, & Phelps, 1999). The insecure parents also described themselves as less competent as parents (Volling et al., 1998), had more worries about separation from their children (Lutz & Hock, 1995; Mayseless & Scher, 2000; Scher & Mayseless, 1994), and reported less competence in handling their children's distress (DeOliveira et al., 2005). In addition, Rholes et al. (1995) found that parents' avoidance scores were associated with feeling less close to their children (but see Meredith & Noller [2003] for nonsignificant findings), and Mayseless and Scher (2000) reported that more attachment-anxious mothers attributed less importance to the development of their children's social skills and independence. Whereas anxious parents' hunger for closeness and recognition interfered with providing a secure base for exploration and discouraged their children's growth and autonomy, avoidant parents' distance interfered with fostering and enjoying intimacy with their children. Interestingly, more avoidant mothers also reported less satisfaction with parenting at the time of divorce (O. Cohen & Finzi-Dotan, 2005) and felt less competent when caring for stepchildren (Ceglian & Gardner, 2000). All of these findings indicate that individual differences in attachment style and associated differences in working models of relationships, assessed in young adults before marriage and childbirth, continue to exist and influence behavior and outcomes when adults actually become parents or stepparents.

Insecure parents also seem to have somewhat negative mental representations of children. In a sample of nonparents, Rholes et al. (1997) found that self-reports of avoidance were associated with imagining prospective children as less secure and less affectionate, and this association was not explained by participants' scores on the "Big Five" personality factors. Moreover, insecure mothers compared to secure mothers (according to self-report scales) viewed their infants as more prone to distress and less sociable (Pesonen, Raikkonen, Keltikangas-Jarvinen, Strandberg, & Jarvenpaa, 2003; Pesonen, Raikkonen, Strandberg, Keltikangas-Jarvinen, & Jarvenpaa, 2004; Priel & Besser, 2000; but see Meredith & Noller, 2003, for nonsignificant findings). Interestingly, Pesonen et al. (2003, 2004) replicated these findings in a sample of fathers.

Using the AAI, Zeanah et al. (1993) discovered that avoidant mothers (compared with secure mothers) interpreted infants with ambiguous emotional expressions in photographs as experiencing more negative emotions, and they attributed more negative characteristics to an infant who was videotaped during a separation from his mother. In an extension of these findings to adolescence, Kobak, Ferenz-Gillies, Everhart, and Seabrook (1994) found that insecure mothers (assessed with the AAI), compared with secure ones, perceived their adolescent daughters as less able to regulate impulses and distress.

Parental Caregiving Behavior

In one of the first studies of attachment-related predictors of maternal sensitivity, Haft and Slade (1989) administered the AAI to mothers of 9- to 23-month-old infants and videotaped interactions between them and their children, later coding the tapes for a mother's notice of and attunement to her child's emotions and needs. As expected, secure mothers were more attuned to their babies than were insecure mothers. Moreover, secure mothers attuned to both positive and negative emotions, and were consistent in reacting to their babies' needs. Anxious mothers attuned inconsistently to both positive and negative emotions, whereas avoidant mothers did not attune to negative emotions and seemed to ignore them. Avoidant mothers' dismissal of their infants' negative affect was also documented by Milligan, Atkinson, Trehub, Benoit, and Poulton (2003) in their study of mothers' emotional expressivity while singing to their infants. Unlike secure mothers, who sang less playfully to distressed than to nondistressed infants, the emotional tone of avoidant mothers did not vary as a function of their infants' levels of distress. They seemed not to acknowledge their infants' negative emotions and displayed high levels of playfulness that seemed more designed to keep their own spirits up than to respond appropriately to their infants' distress.

Attachment-related sensitivity and responsiveness of mothers to their infants have also been examined during videotaped free-play sessions and unstructured observations of everyday mothering behavior at home (K. Grossmann, Fremmer-Bombik, Rudolph, & Grossmann, 1988; Pederson, Gleason, Moran, & Bento, 1998; Raval et al., 2001; Slade et al., 1999; Tarabulsy et al., 2005; M. J. Ward & Carlson, 1995). Several teams of investigators, using the AAI, found that insecure mothers (whose behavior was coded by judges who were blind to the mothers' attachment classifications) were less attentive and responsive than secure mothers to their infants' needs, and more distressed and intrusive when interacting with their infants (but see Volling et al. [1998] for a failure to replicate this association using a self-report measure of adult attachment). It is noteworthy that M. J. Ward and Carlson (1995) and Raval et al. (2001) found attachment-related differences in parental behavior even when the AAI was administered before the children's birth, thus precluding an alternative explanation in terms of effects of children's temperament on mothers' attachment orientations.

Several studies have examined whether mothers with different adult attachment patterns differ in the quality of support they provide to their preschool children when the children attempt to solve increasingly difficult puzzles or problems (E. K. Adam, Gunnar, & Tanaka, 2004; Bosquet & Egeland, 2001; Crowell & Feldman, 1989; Eiden, Teti, & Corns, 1995; Rholes et al., 1995). With the exception of Rholes et al., who assessed mothers' attachment styles using self-report scales, the researchers administered the AAI months before or at the same time as the assessment of maternal caregiving. Despite differences in assessment methods, all of the studies found that compared to insecure mothers, secure mothers were rated by independent judges as warmer, more supportive, and more helpful toward their children. In addition, whereas avoidant mothers were cool, controlling, and task-focused when assisting their children (Crowell & Feldman, 1989), anxious mothers gave confusing instructions (Crowell & Feldman, 1989), seemed distressed during problem solving (Eiden et al., 1995), and were intrusive when trying to help their children (E. K. Adam et al., 2004; Bosquet & Egeland, 2001). Thus, as expected, anxious mothers were willing to help their children with problem solving, but they were confused, distressed, and intrusive, which impaired the quality of support they could provide.

Additional AAI studies included videotaping mothers' behavior during joint activities with their preschool children—activities such as playing, drawing, writing a story, and reading a book (Biringen et al., 2000; Bus & van IJzendoorn, 1992; Cohn, Cowan, Cowan, & Pearson, 1992; Crandell, Fitzgerald, & Whipple, 1997; Crowell, O'Connor, Wollmers, Sprafkin, & Rao, 1991; Oyen, Landy, & Hilburn-Cobb, 2000; Pearson, Cohn, Cowan, & Cowan, 1994; van IJzendoorn et al., 1991). As expected, secure mothers displayed more warmth, responsiveness, and supportiveness toward their children than did insecure mothers. They also tended to engage in more synchronous give-and-take interactions with their children, provided better task organization and structure, and had fewer difficult interactions with their children. (In general, differences between anxious and avoidant mothers were given less attention in these studies than differences between secure and insecure mothers.)

Van IJzendoorn et al. (1991) and Cohn, Cowan, et al. (1992) included fathers in their studies and were among the few researchers to examine effects on caregiving behavior of the father's state of mind with respect to attachment (based on the AAI). Although van IJzendoorn et al. (1991) found no significant attachment effects on fathers' sensitivity, Cohn, Cowan, et al. (1992) reported that secure fathers were warmer and more supportive, and provided better task organization and structure when interacting with their children. They also observed that insecure mothers married to secure husbands were more supportive and helpful toward their children than were insecure mothers married to insecure husbands, suggesting that the mother's parenting behavior was influenced by both her own attachment dynamics and the secure or insecure context provided by her husband. As we explain below, the same kind of dual influence—from both dispositions and contexts—is evident when adults are called upon to provide care to other adults.

In one of the studies just reviewed, Pearson et al. (1994) found that parents' "earned security" (a coherent state of mind regarding attachment, seen in the AAI, despite difficult early relationships with parents) was associated, like "continuous security," with warm and supportive interactions with children. In another study, Phelps, Belsky, and Crnic (1998) examined effects of earned and continuous security on daily maternal sensitivity and responsiveness on both high-stress and low-stress days (assessed by mothers' reports of daily hassles). The results indicated that the experience of daily hassles impaired the quality of caregiving among insecure mothers but not among those who were coded as evincing earned or continuous security on the AAI. That is, earned or continuous security seemed to buffer the detrimental effects of stress on caregiving and allowed mothers to remain sensitive to their children's needs despite their own momentary distress.

It is important to note that even though the vast majority of studies provide strong evidence for a link between adult attachment orientation and parental caregiving, they have generally assessed parental caregiving in nonthreatening situations, when children's attachment systems were unlikely to have been activated. One exception is a study by Crowell and Feldman (1991). They videotaped mothers' behavior when their children were exposed to an attachment-related threat: separation from mother in the lab. The secure mothers were more affectionate with their children and prepared them better for the separation. They left the room with little anxiety and quickly established closeness upon reunion. The anxious and avoidant mothers differed in their emotional reactions to leaving their children alone: Whereas avoidant mothers showed little distress, anxious mothers were agitated and found it difficult to leave the room. This kind of personal distress might have interfered with anxious mothers' effective caregiving when they returned to the room and needed to help their children recover from the separation.

Two subsequent studies yielded conceptually similar findings based on assessing mothers' behavior during children's exposure to attachment-unrelated threats (Edelstein et al., 2004; Goodman, Quas, Batterman-Faunce, Riddlesberger, & Kuhn, 1997). Goodman et al. (1997) asked parents to describe their interactions with their children after the children underwent a threatening and painful medical procedure (voiding cysto-urethrogram fluoroscopy). The authors found that secure parents (assessed with self-report scales) were more likely than insecure parents to discuss the procedure with their children and physically comfort them afterward. Edelstein et al. (2004) videotaped children's and parents' behavior when each of the children received an inoculation at an immunization clinic, and found that more avoidant parents (assessed with a self-report scale) were less responsive to their children, particularly if the children became highly distressed; that is, when the children were most upset and most in need of parental support, avoidant parents failed to provide effective care.

In an extension of this kind of research to parents of adolescents, Kobak, Ferenz-Gillies, et al. (1994) videotaped mother–adolescent conversations about the adolescents' leaving home for work or college. As expected, anxiously attached mothers (based on the AAI) had the greatest difficulty maintaining a calm state of mind during the conversation and providing a secure base for their children's exploration. These mothers displayed more verbal and nonverbal signs of anxiety (than secure mothers) with respect to their adolescents' imminent departure, and more verbal intrusions in response to the adolescents' attempts at autonomy, which in turn hindered adolescents' ability to discuss future goals and plans. Similar findings were reported by D. Diamond and Doane (1994) in a study of conversations between parents and severely disturbed adolescents receiving long-term inpatient treatment.

Beyond interfering with sensitive and responsive caregiving, attachment insecurities are sometimes involved in more abusive, life-threatening parental behavior. For example, in a study of mothers who had mistreated their children—a study that also included each mother's husband or lover—Crittenden, Partridge, and Claussen (1991) found that more than 90% of the adults (both women and men) were classified (based on the AAI) as having an insecure state of mind with respect to attachment. In a nonabusing control group, matched for socioeconomic status (SES), the proportion of insecure parents was dramatically lower, 60%, suggesting that parents' attachment insecurity is a major correlate of mistreating or abusing their children. Similarly, Adshead and Bluglass (2005) noted the overrepresentation of disorganized states of mind (88%) in a sample of mothers demonstrating Munchausen syndrome by proxy, an unusual form of child maltreatment in which a mother induces medical symptoms in her child, so that the child has to be taken to a hospital for treatment. In another example study, Moncher (1996) found that attachment insecurities (assessed with self-report scales) put mothers at higher risk for child abuse, as determined by their responses on measures that distinguish between abusive and nonabusive mothers.

There is also evidence that mothers with severe disturbances in attachment security (the AAI insecure/unresolved loss group, described in Chapter 4, this volume) are more likely to display what Main and Hesse (1990) called "frightening/frightened" behavior during interactions with their infants (Goldberg et al., 2003; Lyons-Ruth et al,, 2005; Schuengel, van IJzendoorn, Bakermans-Kranenburg, & Blom, 1998; Schuengel et al., 1999). These atypical maternal behaviors are a blend of threatening behavior toward the infant (e.g., suddenly looming too close), expressions of fear of the infant or the infant's actions (e.g., exaggerated startle when the infant falls down), and dissociated states of mind (e.g., inexplicable changes in voice quality), which tend to be experienced as frightening by infants (Main & Hesse, 1990). According to Schuengel et al. (1999), "Fear of their attachment figure presents infants with a paradox: Instead of a safe haven, their parents become a source of alarm. Infants may become disorganized because they are unable to reconcile their fear with their attachment to the same person" (p. 54).

ADULT CHILDREN'S PROVISION OF CARE TO PARENTS

The studies reviewed so far offer converging evidence that attachment insecurities contribute to insensitive caregiving, which fails to provide a safe haven and secure base for a child's healthy development. Interestingly, a few researchers have extended this line of research to the other end of the adult age spectrum, seeking to learn what happens when adult children are called upon to care for their aging parents. Cicirelli (1993) hypothesized that secure adult children would be more empathic toward their parents' needs and would reciprocate their parents' earlier warmth, affection, and concern. In contrast, attachment insecurities were expected to cause adult children to be more self-focused, and more likely to react with emotional detachment or overwhelming distress when their early sources of safety became weak, needy, and vulnerable. Indeed, Eberly and Montemayor (1998, 1999) found that adolescents who reported more secure attachment to parents showed more supportive and affectionate behavior toward their mother and father in both cross-sectional and 2-year longitudinal studies. Along the same lines, Cicirelli (1993) and Townsend and Franks (1995) found that adult children who maintained stronger attachment bonds with their dependent parents reported greater amounts of care and lower caregiver burden regardless of their parents' level of functional dependence.

Additional studies reveal that anxious or avoidant adult children whose parents are institutionalized have more difficulty than their secure counterparts as caregivers (Crispi, Schiaffino, & Berman, 1997), and avoidant adult children whose parents suffer from progressive dementia are more likely to choose to institutionalize the parent rather than to provide care at home (Markiewicz, Reis, & Gold, 1997). Moreover, adult daughters who scored higher on attachment anxiety or avoidance reported providing less emotional support to their community-dwelling mothers regardless of the mothers' actual need for care (B. D. Carpenter, 2001). In this sample of daughters, avoidant attachment was also associated with experiencing caregiving as a burden. Sörensen, Webster, and Roggman (2002) asked middle-age adults about their preparation for future care of older parents, and found that attachment anxiety and avoidance were associated with less preparedness for care provision, suggesting that insecure adult children have problems with the idea of caregiving even before care is explicitly needed.

In an innovative study, Steele et al. (2004) examined associations between adult daughters' AAI classifications and the behavior of their mentally impaired mothers with various degrees of dementia, during a reunion episode following a 45- to 60-minute separation. As the authors explain, this procedure is somewhat like Ainsworth's Strange Situation (see Chapter 4, this volume), which is used to assess the attachment patterns of 12- to 18-month-old infants. Steele et al. found that adult daughters' attachment security was positively associated with joyful and "secure" behavior on the part of the older adult mothers, including proximity seeking, contact maintaining, and overall responsiveness, even after controlling for severity of the mothers' dementia. These findings fit well with Crowell and Feldman's (1989) study on reactions of secure mothers and their infants to separation and reunion, and they clearly suggest that secure adult daughters, like secure mothers, tend to provide sensitive and responsive care that allows the careseeker (the older adult mother in Steele et al.'s study) to remain calm and confident during separation and react with joy upon reunion.

CAREGIVING IN ROMANTIC RELATIONSHIPS

Attachment-related differences in caregiving can be examined in adult close relationships, just as they have been investigated in parent–child relationships. In the past 20 years, researchers who study romantic and marital relationships have acknowledged that a person's ability and willingness to respond sensitively and responsively to a relationship partner are major determinants of relationship quality, stability, and satisfaction (e.g., Collins & Feeney, 2000; Julien & Markman, 1991). Moreover, adult romantic love involves not only the attachment system, which helps maintain proximity to a relationship partner, but also the caregiving system, which causes one partner to attend and respond to the other's signals and needs (Shaver & Hazan, 1988). As a result, romantic and marital relationships provide good opportunities to discover how attachment styles shape caregiving orientations.

Self-Report Studies

The first study to examine the link between attachment and caregiving within romantic relationships was conducted by Kunce and Shaver (1994). Based on an extensive review of the literature describing parental care for children, these researchers developed an adult Caregiving Questionnaire (included here in Appendix G) that assesses responsive, controlling, and compulsive patterns of caregiving in couple relationships. Two correlated dimensions tap responsive caregiving: *proximity maintenance* to a needy partner (e.g., "When my partner is troubled or upset, I move closer to provide support or comfort") and *sensitivity* to a partner's signals and needs (e.g., "I am very attentive to my partner's nonverbal signals for help and support"). *Controlling* caregiving is assessed by items measuring the extent to which the caregiver adopts a domineering, uncooperative stance during the caregiving process and fails to respect a partner's ability to solve the problem at hand (e.g., "When I help my partner with something, I tend to do things my way"). *Compulsive* caregiving items assess overinvolvement with the partner's distress and a tendency to merge with the needy partner (e.g., "I frequently get too 'wrapped up' in my partner's problems and needs"). Kunce and Shaver found that scores on these dimensions were stable over a 1-month period in a sample of young couples, and that a person's self-description of caregiving behavior was validated by his or her partner's independent reports.

Using Kunce and Shaver's (1994) scale, four studies found that secure individuals exhibited the most favorable pattern of care within dating and married couples: Compared with an insecure individual, a secure individual was more likely to provide support to the needy partner and be sensitive to his or her needs, and less likely to adopt a controlling stance or be overinvolved in caregiving (B. C. Feeney & Collins, 2001; J. A. Feeney, 1996; J. A. Feeney & Hohaus, 2001; Kunce & Shaver, 1994). As expected, avoidant individuals exhibited a neglectful, nonresponsive style of caregiving: They scored relatively low on proximity maintenance and sensitivity, reflecting their tendency to maintain distance from a needy partner (restricting accessibility, physical contact, and sensitivity), and tended to adopt a controlling, uncooperative stance resembling their domineering behavior in other kinds of social interactions (Chapter 9, this volume). Anxious individuals tended to score relatively high on the compulsive caregiving scale, probably because of their personal distress and overinvolvement with their partners' problems.

Using another self-report scale tapping quality of care for a romantic partner (active engagement in support provision, respect of a partner's needs, reciprocal care), Carnelley, Pietromonaco, and Jaffe (1996) found that both dating and married people who scored higher on avoidance reported poorer caregiving. Among married (but not dating) couples, individuals scoring higher on attachment anxiety also reported less favorable care provision. B. C. Feeney (2005) found that attachment insecurities also interfered with providing a secure base for a dating partner's explorations. Specifically, more avoidant people reported being less available and responsive when a dating partner engaged in exploratory activities or pursued important personal goals. Anxious people's desire for closeness was expressed in their report of more intrusive behavior that interfered with a partner's exploratory activities.

Insecure people's deficits in caregiving were also evident in their narrative accounts of actual examples of the care they provided to their spouses (J. A. Feeney & Hohaus, 2001). Avoidant people's narratives were characterized by lack of support for a needy spouse and dissatisfaction with the caregiving experience. Anxious people's narratives were characterized by poor handling of the caregiving task (e.g., less reliance on problem-focused strategies) and a negative attitude toward their spouses' needs. In the same study, J. A. Feeney and Hohaus found that both attachment anxiety and avoidance were associated with less willingness to care for a dependent spouse, and this association was mediated by lack of sensitivity to the spouse's needs (as measured by Kunce & Shaver's [1994] scales). The same pattern was evident among both husbands and wives.

Beyond identifying insecure adults' caregiving deficits within romantic and marital relationships, researchers have begun to identify the cognitive and motivational processes that explain these deficits. For example, B. C. Feeney and Collins (2001) found that avoidant people's lack of sensitivity and responsiveness to their partners' needs was mediated by lack of knowledge about how to provide support, lack of a prosocial orientation, and lack of relationship commitment and intimacy. Anxious people's overinvolvement during caregiving was mediated by their high sense of interdependence combined with lack of relationship trust and heightened egoistic, self-focused attention (B. C. Feeney & Collins, 2001). These findings fit well with our contention earlier in this chapter that avoidant people's caregiving deficits stem from a lack of empathic concern for others' needs, whereas anxious people's deficits are a result of self-focused worries.

Pursuing this line of research, B. C. Feeney and Collins (2003) and B. C. Feeney (2005) assessed motives for providing (or not providing) care to a romantic partner and found that secure adults tended to endorse more altruistic reasons for helping (e.g., helping out of concern for one's partner or to reduce a partner's suffering). In contrast, avoidant people reported more egoistic reasons (e.g., to avoid a partner's negative reactions or to get something explicit in return), and their reasons for not helping reflected their deactivating strategies. For example, they disliked coping with a partner's distress, lacked a sense of responsibility for the partner, and perceived the partner as too dependent. Although anxiously attached adults endorsed some altruistic reasons for helping (helping out of concern for the partner or because they enjoyed helping), they also reported egoistic reasons reflecting unmet desires for closeness and security: helping in order to gain a partner's approval and increase the partner's relationship commitment. When asked why they sometimes chose not to provide a secure base for the partner's exploration, anxious people attributed their reluctance to worries that the partner's independent pursuits might damage the relationship. These findings led Collins, Guichard, et al. (2006) to conclude that "although anxious caregivers may be heavily engaged in caregiving behavior, their caregiving efforts are often in the service of their own attachment needs" (p. 176).

Interestingly, B. C. Feeney and Collins (2003) found that these motives for helping explained why anxious and avoidant people differed in the care they provided to their romantic partners. Avoidant individuals' lack of responsiveness and sensitivity was associated with more egoistic reasons for helping, such as feeling obligated to help or expecting to get something in return. Anxious people's compulsive, intrusive pattern of support was associated with using care provision as a means of satisfying unmet attachment needs.

Overall, the findings support the view that effective caregiving is marked by not only responsiveness, sensitivity, and respect for a partner's needs but also altruistic motives focused on the partner's welfare and development. This kind of care is more common among secure adults. Research also indicates that attachment insecurities can interfere with or overload the caregiving system with attachment-related worries, concerns, and defenses, which results in less responsive, less sensitive, more intrusive caregiving.

Observational Studies of Caregiving Behavior in Romantic and Marital Relationships

Insecure people's deficits in providing care to their partners have also been documented in laboratory studies of actual caregiving behavior. In the first such study, Simpson et al. (1992) unobtrusively videotaped dating couples while the female partner waited to endure a stressful task (see Chapter 7, this volume, for a fuller description of this study), and judges then rated the female partners' expressions of distress and the male partners' caregiving behavior. The results supported the hypothesis that avoidant men would react to a partner's distress with neglect. Specifically, whereas secure men recognized partners' worries and provided greater support (more emotional support and more supportive verbal comments) as their partners showed higher levels of distress, men who scored high on avoidance provided less support as their partners' distress increased (the same pattern observed by Edelstein et al. [2004] in their study of parents whose children were receiving painful inoculations at a medical clinic). Using a similar experimental paradigm, Simpson et al. (2002) exposed male members of couples to a stressful procedure and found that more avoidant female partners provided less support regardless of their partners' expressions of distress.

Using Simpson et al.'s (1992) sample, Rholes et al. (1999) coded male partners' expressions of anger toward the female partner while she was waiting to perform the stressful task and during a poststress recovery period (after couples were told that the female partner would not really have to endure the stressful procedure). During the stressful waiting period, avoidant men expressed more anger toward their partners, especially if the partners expressed high levels of distress. During the recovery period, these men showed greater anger and interacted less positively with their partners, and this was especially so if the partners had sought support during the stressful period. Taken together, this series of studies provided excellent behavioral evidence that avoidant individuals react to their romantic partners' expressions of distress and requests for help with decreased support and heightened displeasure, possibly reflecting their reluctance to deal with distress and their preference for emotional distance and detachment. As mentioned, the findings are remarkably similar to those obtained in studies of avoidant parents reacting to distressed children.

Simpson's and Rholes's observational studies have provided a revealing portrait of avoidant individuals' lack of sensitivity and responsiveness, but unlike self-report studies, they have revealed few deficiencies in anxious people's caregiving behavior. It's possible that Simpson et al.'s (1992) measures failed to capture the overinvolvement and intrusiveness characteristic of anxious caregivers, because the caregivers were evaluated along a single dimension—the extent to which they offered emotional support. No attempt was made to assess their own distress or their intrusiveness. Another possible explanation for the null findings regarding anxious caregiving is that overinvolvement in caregiving may be evident mainly in highly stressful or protracted situations (compared with the vague threats created in laboratory settings).

The deficiencies in anxious adults' approach to caregiving in couple relationships have been easier to see in experiments conducted by Collins and her colleagues. In the first such study, Collins and Feeney (2000) videotaped dating couples while one partner disclosed a personal problem to the other (the "caregiver"). Caregivers scoring higher on attachment anxiety were coded (by independent judges) as less supportive during the interaction, especially when a partner's needs were not very clear (i.e., when the partner engaged in less obvious support seeking). In contrast, secure "caregivers" tended to provide relatively high levels of support regardless of whether a partner's needs were clearly expressed. Interestingly, attachment insecurities were also found to bias people's appraisals of the support they provided: Anxious and avoidant individuals evaluated their support as even less helpful than it actually was (as coded by independent judges).

In two subsequent laboratory experiments, B. C. Feeney and Collins (2001) and Collins et al. (2005) provided a finer-grained analysis of the unique caregiving deficits of avoidant and anxious persons. In these studies, dating couples were brought to the lab, and one member of the couple (the "careseeker") was informed that he or she would perform a stressful task—preparing and delivering a speech that would be videotaped. The other member of the couple (the "caregiver") was led to believe that his or her partner was either extremely nervous (high-need condition) or not at all nervous (low-need condition) about the speech task, and was given the opportunity to write a private note to the partner. In both studies, the note served as a behavioral measure of caregiving and was rated for the degree of support it conveyed. In addition, the caregiver's attentiveness to the partner's needs was assessed by counting the number of times the caregiver checked a computer monitor for messages from the partner while the caregiver was working on a series of puzzles (in a separate room). To assess the caregiver's state of mind, Collins et al. (2005) added measures of empathic feelings toward the partner, rumination about the partner's feelings, willingness to switch tasks with the partner, partner-focused attention (the extent to which the caregiver was distracted by thoughts of the partner while working on puzzles), and causal attributions regarding the partner's feelings.

The studies provided strong evidence of avoidant individuals' hypothesized nonresponsive caregiving. More avoidant people wrote less emotionally supportive notes in both high- and low-need conditions, and provided less instrumental support in the high- than in the low-need condition, precisely when the partner most needed support. Moreover, avoidant participants reported less empathic feelings toward their partners, were less willing to switch tasks with partners, and were less distracted by thoughts about partners while doing puzzles.

The findings also provided clear-cut evidence of the anxious caregiver's overinvolvement during the experiment and lack of sensitivity to the partner's needs. Specifically, anxiously attached participants were easily distracted by thoughts about their partners, reported relatively high levels of empathy and rumination, but failed to write more supportive notes as partners' needs increased. In addition, they perceived their partners more negatively in the high-need condition (they perceived their partners as weaker and more vulnerable), due perhaps to projection of their own feelings or to the frustration they felt when realizing that their own source of security was not as strong as they had hoped (Collins et al., 2005).

Overall, these studies show that attachment insecurities interfere with caregiving in adult couple relationships, just as they do in parenting. As in parent–child relationships, avoidant romantic/marital partners' defenses interfere with the sensitive and responsive caregiving needed by troubled romantic partners. Anxious people have difficulties providing care to partners. Their anxious self-focus, combined with confusion, disorganization, and a wish that their partners would occupy the role of "stronger and wiser" caregiver, can cause their caregiving intentions to go astray. They remind us, sadly, of the joke about the self-preoccupied conversationalist: "Well, that's enough about me. So, what do *you* think about me?"

CAREGIVING IN THE WIDER SOCIAL WORLD: EMPATHY, COMPASSION, AND ALTRUISM

The discovery of connections between attachment style and caregiving in both the parent–child and romantic/marital domains led researchers to explore the possibility that attachment insecurity interferes with compassion toward suffering strangers, members of minority groups, and members of the community with special needs (e.g., the housebound elderly). If all forms of loving-kindness draw from the same caregiving well, then contamination of that well by attachment-related worries and defenses is likely. And in fact, even before we became interested in the broader implications of attachment and caregiving, studies of preschoolers had shown that the attachment insecurities evident in the Strange Situation at age 1 were associated with less empathic concern for an adult stranger's or other children's distress years later, as indicated by teachers' ratings and researchers' observations of children's behavior (e.g., Kestenbaum, Farber, & Sroufe, 1989; van der Mark, van IJzendoorn, & Bakermans-Kranenburg, 2002). Moreover, secure attachment to parents during adolescence had been found to contribute positively to compassionate, empathic responses to needy people (Laible, Carlo, & Raffaelli, 2000; Markiewicz et al., 2001; but for nonsignificant findings, see Saroglou et al., 2005).

In studies of adult attachment, there is now converging evidence that avoidant people score lower on measures of sensitive, responsive reactions to other people's needs. Specifically, more avoidant people report less empathic concern (e.g., B. C. Feeney & Collins, 2001; Joireman, Needham, & Cummings, 2002; Lopez, 2001; Wayment, 2006), less inclination to take the perspective of a distressed person (Corcoran, & Mallinckrodt, 2000; Joireman et al., 2002), less ability to share another person's feelings (Trusty, Ng, & Watts, 2005), less sense of communion with others, and less willingness to take responsibility for others' welfare (Collins & Read, 1990; Shaver, Papalia, et al., 1996; Zuroff, Moskowitz, & Cote, 1999). Avoidant people are less likely to be cooperative and other-oriented (Van Lange, de Bruin, Otten, & Joireman, 1997), to write comforting messages to a distressed person (Weger & Polcar, 2002), or to offer effective help in relation to hypothetical scenarios (Drach-Zahavy, 2004). Moreover, Priel et al. (1998) found that avoidant adolescents were perceived by peers as less supportive than their secure classmates, indicating that their selfishness was not just a matter of self-perception.

With regard to attachment anxiety, research once again suggests a pattern of overinvolvement and intrusiveness during encounters with people in distress. In particular, although Lopez (2001) found a positive association between attachment anxiety and a measure of emotional empathy, people who score relatively high on measures of attachment anxiety also report higher levels of personal distress while witnessing others' distress (Britton & Fuendeling, 2005; Joireman et al., 2002), offer less effective help to physically ill people in hypothetical scenarios (Drach-Zahavy, 2004) and, compared to less anxious people, rate intrusive and neglectful caregiving responses to elderly people's needs as less abusive and more typical (Malley-Morrison, You, & Mills, 2000). Moreover, anxious individuals score higher on a measure of unmitigated communion, which taps a compulsive need to help others even when they are not asking for assistance, and even when the help comes at the expense of one's own health and legitimate needs (Fritz & Helgeson, 1998; Shaver, Papalia, et al., 1996).

In an observational laboratory study, Westmaas and Silver (2001) videotaped people while they interacted with the experimenter's confederate, who they thought had recently been diagnosed with cancer. The authors found that both kinds of attachment insecurity created specific impediments to effective caregiving. As expected, avoidant participants were rated by observers as less verbally and nonverbally supportive, and as making less eye contact during the interaction. Moreover, they rated their own interactions as less warm and supportive. Attachment anxiety was not associated with supportiveness, but more anxious participants reported greater discomfort while interacting with the confederate and were more likely to report self-critical thoughts after the interaction (as measured in free-thought listings). These are clear signs of emotional overinvolvement and self-related worries, which we know can sometimes interfere with caregiving.

In an attempt to examine the link between attachment and altruistic behavior more directly, McKinney (2002) found that insecure attachment of adolescents to their parents was associated with less involvement in voluntary altruistic activities, such as caring for the elderly or donating blood. Gillath, Shaver, Mikulincer, et al. (2005) extended this line of research by assessing young adults' attachment orientations and their motives for volunteering in their communities in three countries (Israel, the Netherlands, and the United States). The results were similar in all three countries. Avoidant attachment was associated with engaging in fewer volunteer activities and being involved for less altruistic reasons. Attachment anxiety was not directly related to engaging in volunteer activities but was associated with more egoistic reasons for volunteering (e.g., hoping for social acceptance and approval), another indication of anxious people's self-focus. The association between attachment and volunteering could not be explained by other factors, such as self-esteem and interpersonal trust.

Insecure people's relative lack of a prosocial orientation is also manifested in career choice. For example, Horppu and Ikonen-Varila (2004) focused on students at a college for kindergarten teachers and assessed students' state of mind with respect to attachment (using the AAI) and their motives for studying to be kindergarten teachers. Insecurely attached students, either anxious or avoidant, endorsed less altruistic, less prosocial motives for being teachers. Similarly, Roney et al. (2004) found that less secure occupational therapy students (identified with self-report scales) were less likely to say they chose a therapeutic career because they wanted to help people. In a sample of medical students, Ciechanowski, Russo, Katon, and Walker (2004b) found that less secure students (according to self-report scales) were more likely to choose non-primary-care specialties, because primary care demands intense and long-term patient–physician relationships that can cause patients to become attached to their physician.

Recently, a number of investigators, ourselves included, have adopted well-validated priming techniques (see Chapter 3, this volume, for a description of these techniques) for examining the effects of both dispositional attachment orientations and contextually activated representations of attachment security or insecurity on feelings and attitudes toward needy people (Bartz & Lydon, 2004; Mikulincer, Gillath, et al., 2001, 2003; Mikulincer, Shaver, et al., 2005). For example, Bartz and Lydon (2004) primed attachment-related representations by asking people to think about a close relationship in which they felt either secure, anxious, or avoidant, and then assessed the implicit and explicit activation of communion-related thoughts (thoughts about devoting themselves to others and maintaining supportive and warm interactions with them). Implicit activation was assessed in a word fragment completion task (which identified the number of word fragments completed with a communion-related word); explicit activation was assessed with the Communion scale of the Extended Personality Attributes Questionnaire. Contextual priming of representations of avoidant attachment led to lower levels of implicit or explicit communion-related thoughts than contextual priming of secure attachment. These findings suggest a causal relation between avoidance and inhibition or interference with a communal orientation.

Along the same lines, Mikulincer, Gillath, et al. (2001, Study 1) performed an experiment assessing compassionate responses to others' suffering. Dispositional attachment anxiety and avoidance were assessed with the ECR scales, and the sense of attachment security was activated by having participants read a story about support provided by a loving attachment figure. This condition was compared with the activation of neutral or positive affect. Following the priming procedure, all participants rated their current mood, read a brief story about a student whose parents had been killed in an automobile accident, and rated how much they experienced compassion (e.g., compassion, sympathy, tenderness) and personal distress (e.g., tension, worry, distress) when thinking about the distressed student.

As expected, dispositional attachment anxiety and avoidance were inversely related to compassion, and attachment anxiety (but not avoidance) was positively associated with personal distress. The findings paralleled earlier studies of parental and romantic caregiving: Whereas avoidance seemed to reduce responsiveness to others' needs, anxiety appeared to increase self-preoccupation and a form of distress that, while possibly aroused through empathy, failed to motivate people to take care of a needy other. In addition, enhancement of attachment security, but not simple enhancement of positive affect, strengthened compassion and inhibited personal distress in reaction to others' distress. These findings were replicated in four additional studies (Mikulincer, Gillath, et al., 2001, Studies 2–5).

In another set of three experiments, Mikulincer, Gillath et al. (2003) found theoretically predictable attachment-related variations in value orientations. Avoidant attachment, assessed with the ECR, was inversely associated with endorsement of two self-transcendent values, benevolence (concern for close others) and universalism (concern for all humanity), supporting our notion that avoidant strategies interfere with concern for others' needs. In addition, experimental priming of mental representations of attachment figure availability, compared with enhancing positive affect or exposing participants to a neutral priming condition, strengthened endorsement of these two prosocial values. These findings fit well with van IJzendoorn and Zwart-Woudstra's (1995) discovery that secure attachment (assessed with the AAI) is associated with more mature, humanistic moral reasoning.

In a recent series of studies, Mikulincer et al. (2005) examined the actual decision to help or not to help a person in distress. In the first two experiments, participants watched a confederate perform a series of increasingly aversive tasks. As the study progressed, the confederate became increasingly distraught about the aversive tasks, and the actual participant was given an opportunity to take the distressed person's place, in effect sacrificing self for the welfare of another. Shortly before the scenario just described, participants were primed with either representations of attachment figure availability (the name of a participant's security provider) or attachment-unrelated representations (the name of a close person who did not function as an attachment figure, the name of a mere acquaintance). This priming procedure was conducted at either a subliminal level (rapid presentation of the name of a specific person) or supraliminal level (asking people to recall an interaction with a particular person). At the point of making a decision about replacing the distressed person, participants completed brief measures of compassion and personal distress.

In both studies, dispositional avoidance was related to lower compassion and lower willingness to help the distressed person. Dispositional attachment anxiety was related to personal distress, but not to either compassion or willingness to help. In addition, as we described in Chapter 3, subliminal or supraliminal priming of representations of a security-providing figure decreased personal distress and increased participants' compassion and willingness to take the place of a distressed other.

In two additional studies, Mikulincer et al. (2005, Studies 3–4) examined whether the contextual heightening of attachment security overrides egoistic motives for helping, such as mood-enhancement (Schaller & Cialdini, 1988) and empathic joy (K. D. Smith, Keating, & Stotland, 1989), and results in genuinely altruistic helping. Specifically, participants were divided into two priming conditions (security priming, neutral priming), read a true newspaper article about a woman in dire personal and financial distress, and rated their emotional reactions to the article (compassion, personal distress). In one study, half of the participants anticipated mood enhancement by means other than helping (e.g., expecting to watch a comedy film). In the other study, half of the participants were told that the needy woman was chronically depressed and her mood might be beyond their ability to repair (*no empathic joy* condition). Schaller and Cialdini (1988) and K. D. Smith et al. (1989) had found that these two conditions, expecting to improve mood by other means or anticipating no sharing of joy with the needy person, reduced egoistic motives for helping, because a person gains no mood-related benefit from helping the needy person. However, these conditions failed to inhibit altruistic motives for helping, which persisted even when egoistic motives were absent (Batson, 1991).

Our studies also showed that expecting to improve one's mood by means other than helping or expecting not to be able to share a needy person's joy when helped reduced compassion and willingness to help in the neutral priming condition but failed to affect these emotional and behavioral reactions in the security priming condition. That is, the contextual priming of attachment security led to heightened compassion and willingness to help even when there was no egoistic reason for helping. These findings fit well with our theoretical view that the sense of attachment security reduces selfishness (defensive self-protection) and allows a person to activate his or her caregiving behavioral system, direct attention to others' distress, take the perspective of a distressed other, and engage in altruistic behavior with the primary goal of benefiting the other person. For secure people, helping others does not serve personal protection goals, because they already feel safe and secure. Rather, their sense of attachment security frees energy and attention to be used by the caregiving system, allowing them to adopt an empathic attitude toward others' distress.

Interestingly, our findings also indicated that expecting to improve one's mood by watching a comedy film or anticipating no sharing of joy with the needy person reduced compassion and willingness to help only among people who scored high on avoidant attachment. For these insecure people, helping others provides one possible route to feeling better about themselves; hence, they were more willing to help when an egoistic payoff was likely. Such egoistic concerns held less sway over people who were either dispositionally less avoidant (i.e., more secure in one sense) or under the influence of a security-enhancing prime. It seems, therefore, that attachment security counteracts some of the egoistic motives underlying avoidant people's reluctance to help.

Overall, across several correlational and experimental studies, attachment security was associated with greater compassion, greater willingness to help, and greater participation in altruistic activities. Avoidant attachment predicted lower levels of compassion and altruistic helping. Attachment anxiety was linked with heightened personal distress that did not translate into greater willingness to help. All of these results support the hypothesis that altruistic motives for caregiving and the ability to provide sensitive, responsive care are conditional upon a certain degree of attachment security.

CONCLUDING REMARKS

All of the findings reviewed in this chapter are compatible with the theoretical claim that the attachment system affects the operation of the caregiving system. Thus, attachment theory provides a well-validated conceptual framework for further examination of the developmental and social-relational roots of compassion and altruism, as well as the processes and mechanisms that underlie compassionate behavior.

It's interesting that ideas stemming at first from close scrutiny of the parent–child relationship have proven to apply not only to other close relationships but also to all kinds of social relationships in which concern for others' welfare arises. It seems that all forms of sensitive, responsive, and compassionate care across the lifespan (e.g., caregiving in parent–child relationships, in adult romantic relationships, in relationships between middle-aged adults and their infirm elderly parents) and in different contexts (e.g., in close relationships and in the wider social world, where thousands of strangers need help and support) have a common basis and resemble each other. This implies that the research literatures on parenting, romantic caregiving, social support, helping, empathy, counseling and psychotherapy, and leadership and management (see Chapters 14 and 15, this volume, for discussions of attachment and caregiving in the contexts of client–therapist and follower–leader relationships) are fundamentally related, and that further theoretical and empirical efforts should be made to create an overarching perspective on them.

More work is also needed to create better measures of compassion and to determine how attachment security and the different forms of insecurity relate to other prosocial emotions, personality traits, and moral qualities. Researchers should also examine whether participation in compassionate, loving activities in one's role as a parent, lover, and member of civil society can "feed back on" attachment security, by bolstering a person's sense of being loved and needed, and by helping to create prosocial working models of self. It is important to explore further how various experiences and techniques, including psychotherapy, family therapy, meditation and other religious practices, and participation in religious or charitable organizations can enhance a person's sense of security and thereby foster compassion and altruism (see Chapter 16, this volume).

As we stated at the outset of this chapter, there may be a circular, reciprocal connection between attachment security and compassionate, generous caregiving. It is important to study the extent to which interventions can break into the circle at any point—or at more than one point simultaneously—and have beneficial effects on individuals, relationships, and humanity in general.

CHAPTER 12

■ ■ ■

Attachment and Sex

In the same way that Bowlby (1969/1982) viewed attachment and caregiving as two distinct behavioral systems, he viewed sexual motivation and behavior as having their own biological functions and being governed by a separate behavioral system. However, he and Ainsworth (1991; Ainsworth & Bowlby, 1991) said little in their writings about sexual motives and behavior, partly because their work focused on children and dealt with adults mainly in their role as parents. This sidestepping of sexuality represented a dramatic shift in emphasis compared with Freud, whose theory gave a central role to sexual "libido"—a theoretical emphasis that was probably always present in the back of Bowlby's (e.g., 1969/1982, p. xxvii) mind. In part, the shift away from sexuality and toward attachment was necessary if Bowlby (and other object relations theorists of his generation, e.g., Winnicott, 1965) was going to understand children's relationship-seeking behavior in its own terms, and not as an immature form of sexual desire.

Once we turn our attention to later stages of the lifespan, however, especially adolescence and young adulthood, on which many recent attachment studies have focused, it is impossible to ignore sexuality. In fact, in theorizing about "romantic love conceptualized as an attachment process," Hazan and Shaver (1987; Shaver et al., 1988) specifically proposed that what we think of as romantic love in everyday terms involves at least three behavioral systems: attachment, caregiving, and sex. Evolutionary psychologists who study mate selection, romantic love, and jealousy (e.g., Buss, 1998) also place heavy emphasis on sex, because mating strategies and sexual reproduction are crucial for human evolution, and jealousy is often aroused by sexual rivals.

In this chapter we conceptualize the "sexual behavioral system" in ways parallel to our analyses of the attachment and caregiving systems in previous chapters. We consider how the sexual system is activated in adolescents and adults, how it operates, what affects its operation, and whether it can take hyperactivated and deactivated forms. We also consider how individual differences in sexual system functioning are related to attachment style. In particular, we review published evidence, present new findings from our laboratories, and propose new ideas about ways in which attachment style contributes to sexual motives, feelings, and attitudes. We also examine the role of attachment-related processes in moderating the links between sexuality and relationship quality, and the effect of insecure attachment on failure to resolve the Oedipus complex. The latter topic brings us full circle, back to Freud.

THE SEXUAL SYSTEM AND ITS INTERPLAY WITH THE ATTACHMENT SYSTEM

The Sexual Behavioral System

According to attachment theory, sexual behavior is governed by an inborn sexual behavioral system, and both sexual behavior in general and individual differences in sexual attitudes and activities reflect, in part, the activation and functioning of this system (Shaver & Hazan, 1988; Shaver & Mikulincer, in 2006). From an evolutionary perspective, the major function of the sexual system is obviously to pass genes from one generation to the next, and its innate aim (what Bowlby, 1969/1982, called its "set-goal") is for a person to have sexual intercourse with an opposite-sex partner and either become pregnant oneself (in the case of women) or impregnate one or more partners (in the case of men) (Buss & Kenrick, 1998). As evolutionary psychologists have explained, however, the proximal motivation for an act (i.e., wishing to have sex with an attractive person or wishing to become sexually aroused and achieve orgasm) need not be the same as the distal (i.e., evolutionary) reason for the existence of the motives and feelings involved (i.e., the importance of sexual reproduction). People can obviously seek sexual pleasure without hoping that pregnancy will result, and modern methods of birth control (as well as homosexuality) make it possible to separate the two goals, but many aspects of sexual motivation and attraction (e.g., being attracted to people whose qualities indirectly suggest health, fertility, and "good genes"; Gangestad, Simpson, Cousins, Garver-Apgar, & Christensen, 2004) are still governed by neural and hormonal systems that evolved for reproductive purposes.

In this chapter we forgo a detailed discussion of homosexuality, which has been thoughtfully analyzed from an attachment perspective by Mohr (1999) and L. M. Diamond (2003, 2006). Most of the relational dynamics we discuss when considering relations between the attachment and sexual systems apply to both homosexual and heterosexual couples (see Mohr, 1999, for references). We mention some of the parallel heterosexual and homosexual research findings as we conduct our literature review, but we do not tackle the issue of heterosexual or homosexual "object choice" per se.

Sexual intercourse is an effortful, and in some respects risky, activity that, at least when voluntary, requires a considerable degree of coordination between partners. Thus, we speculate that over the course of human evolution, selection pressures have produced subordinate functional behavioral and psychological processes (goals and brain mechanisms) that solve particular adaptive problems associated with mate acquisition, intercourse, and reproductive success (Birnbaum & Gillath, 2006; Buss & Kenrick, 1998). These goals, mental processes, and behaviors are the primary features of the sexual behavioral system.

In conceptualizing this system, it is important to differentiate between its aims and underpinnings, and those of romantic attraction (L. M. Diamond, 2003; Fisher, 1998). According to Fisher, the sexual system drives a person to want to have sex with *any* appropriate member of the species, whereas romantic attraction involves the choice of a specific partner with whom one already has, or may be able to form, an affectional bond that goes beyond merely having sex; that is, the sexual system is involved in romantic attraction (the desire to be near and to have sex with a particular person), but it does not fully explain romantic attraction. In fact, there are countless cases in which sexual relations occur without affectional bonds, such as one-night stands; sex with casual, even anonymous, partners; and rape. Moreover, romantic attraction involves specific psychological mechanisms that may have nothing to do with sex per se, such as craving emotional closeness and union with the beloved, signs of emotional dependency on the relationship and the partner (e.g., separation anxiety), and willingness to sacrifice for the beloved (Fisher, 1998; Fisher, Aron, Mashek, Li, & Brown, 2002). These are signs of attachment and caregiving, the two behavioral systems that complement the sexual system when a person experiences romantic attraction. Because, as we mentioned earlier, romantic love involves a combination of attachment, caregiving, and sex, sexual attraction is only one element of romantic attraction.

L. M. Diamond (2003) went a step further and argued that the sexual system does not have to be involved at all in romantic attraction; that is, humans can form romantic bonds without experiencing sexual desire for the beloved, such as when a child develops a crush on a favorite teacher, or when an adult maintains high levels of proximity and physical contact with a particular person over an extended period and comes to love the person, but not necessarily in a sexual way (Hazan & Zeifman, 1994). Still, the formation of a romantic relationship is frequently initiated by a combination of sexual attraction (Berscheid, 1984) and romantic infatuation (Hazan & Zeifman, 1994). L. M. Diamond (2003) reviewed extensive and wide-ranging evidence that romantic love sometimes develops asexually but then arouses sexual desire for the beloved, even if this desire runs counter to a person's usual sexual orientation (heterosexual or homosexual). In other words, even though sex and the other behavioral system components of romantic love, such as attachment and caregiving, are functionally independent, they still influence each other, provide opportunities for each other, spill over into each other, and contribute jointly to relationship formation, development, and quality.

Normative Patterns and Individual Differences in Sexual Functioning

The sexual system is automatically activated by noticing and *subjectively appraising* an attractive, sexually interested (possibly flirtatious), and presumably fertile partner (Fisher, 1998). The primary strategy for achieving the sexual system's set-goal is to approach a potential partner, entice or persuade the person to have sex, then engage in genital intercourse (Fisher, 1998). The most direct way to move toward sexual relations is to assert one's sexual interest in a potential partner. Of course, it is possible to achieve this goal by less assertive, more subtle, or craftily manipulative methods, but indirect methods are more likely to be misinterpreted or dismissed, and they can produce conflict or resistance rather than mutual sexual attraction. Assertiveness does not necessarily require a domineering, controlling stance, coercion, or aggression. A sexually interested person can be appropriately assertive, while still being sensitive to a partner's signals, desires, and concerns. Of course, sexual gratification *can* be sought through various forms of coercion, including rape (D. Davis, 2006; Thornhill & Palmer, 2000), but the personal, interpersonal, and social costs of such actions are too high to make them feasible or attractive to most people, and as we show throughout this and other chapters, relatively secure people tend to be considerate of others' needs, so they probably would not engage in coercive sex even if they could get away with it.

Like the activation of other behavioral systems, sexual system activation has a well-defined emotional signature. Encountering an attractive, sexually interested, potentially fertile partner triggers intense interest, an increase in autonomic arousal, and intense excitement. This excitement is followed by great pleasure, physiological relief, and joy, if it carries partners through to sexual intercourse and orgasm (Kaplan, 1974). This well-known cycle is often accompanied by pleasurable dissociative states, in which a person freely abandons self-control, abandons him- or herself to erotic sensations, and temporarily lets go of other worries and concerns (Kaplan, 1974). Orgasm not only feels good as a form of sensory gratification but it can also produce deep relaxation, gratitude, and affection—psychological states that are likely to foster physical health and psychological well-being.

In spite of all these pleasurable feelings and benefits, however, sexual arousal, sexual activities, and reaching orgasm can be accompanied by negative feelings, ambivalence, worries about one's lovability and sexual performance, religious guilt, memories of previous disappointments or instances of sexual abuse, and worries about the meaning of the sexual episode, the future of the relationship, and so on (Barlow, 1986; Kaplan, 1974). Moreover, because sex is often wrapped up with romantic love, which theoretically involves the attachment and caregiving systems, sexual attraction and the attainment of sexual pleasure can be accompanied by warm and affectionate feelings toward a sexual partner who is viewed as an attachment figure, a target of caregiving, or both. To the extent that a person's socialization and personal history incline him or her to feel insecure with respect to any of the three behavioral systems involved in romantic love—attachment, caregiving, and sex—it is unlikely that the sexual system will function optimally.

What are the causes of poor sexual system functioning? Beyond a partner's sexual inhibitions and worries, and other external obstacles that block the way to sexual intercourse, orgasm, and impregnation, we suspect that problems in both intra- and interpersonal regulation are important. Lack of regulation of the intense excitement associated with sexual arousal can create a powerful sense of urgency for sexual gratification, which fuels impulsive actions aimed at gaining immediate satisfaction without taking a partner's concerns or circumstances into account (D. Davis, 2006). In addition, sexual relations can be disrupted by poor regulation of sex-related worries and anxieties, which may include fear of disapproval or rejection and discomfort with closeness and intimacy. This is where attachment anxiety and avoidance are likely to influence the sexual behavioral system.

Problems in coordinating one's own and a partner's sexual interests can easily cause difficulties. Ignoring or misperceiving a partner's wishes makes insensitive behavior likely, and ignoring or suppressing one's own wishes encourages or allows a partner's insensitive behavior. Sexual relations require a flexible balance between distance and closeness, self-concern and concern for a partner, dominance (taking the lead) and submissiveness (allowing a partner to take the lead). Communication skills and accurate empathy are valuable under those circumstances, but they are often lacking. (Most people have much less direct training and practice in the sexual domain than in interpersonal relations more generally.) Viewed in terms of the issues we discussed in Chapter 9, sensitivity and flexible role switching require movement within the interpersonal circumplex. Deficits in interpersonal competencies (expressiveness, sensitivity, and conflict management) and depletion of psychological resources due to fatigue, illness, or attending to worries, easily interfere with comfortable, mutually enjoyable sex.

Of course, lack of sexual motivation or desire (said by couple therapists to be a common problem in modern societies) can discourage sexual activity from the start. But even an ardent desire for sex, if motivated by insecurity, may interfere with mutual satisfaction. For example, having sex for self-reassuring or self-enhancing reasons (countering doubts about one's attractiveness, attempting to gain social prestige) likely makes one overly self-focused, anxious, and inconsiderate of one's partner. Having sex to gain attention, to bolster flagging self-esteem, or to hang on to a wayward partner encourages a needy, self-preoccupied, dependent approach to sex that may cause a partner to feel "used" as a caregiver rather than treated as an attractive, deserving, coequal sex partner. Repeated or extreme forms of urging someone to have sex to assuage one's feelings of insecurity or self-doubt are also likely to breed relationship difficulties and dissatisfactions. Like every form of neurotic behavior, these approaches to sexuality create more problems than they solve and lead a person further away from the desired state of security.

The Interplay of Attachment and Sex

In their initial writings on "romantic love conceptualized as an attachment process," Hazan and Shaver (1987; Shaver & Hazan, 1988; Shaver et al., 1988) put forward several hypotheses concerning how individual differences in attachment-system functioning, which appear early in childhood (during the first year of life), might influence sexual system parameters, which generally become manifest later in development, when hormonal changes bring about the capacity for genital sexuality. Shaver and Hazan's (1988) analysis was based on Bowlby's (1969/1982) claim that activation of the attachment system inhibits or distorts the operation of other behavioral systems, such as the exploration system, and interferes with activities associated with those systems. The same kind of inhibition or distortion can occur when a distressed and vulnerable person encounters an attractive, sexually available, prospective relationship partner. For such people, the partner is likely to be appraised as a possible protector or ego-booster rather than simply as a sexual partner, because needy people are preoccupied with attaining protection, approval, and support rather than with sexual involvement (or, sometimes, with support provided in the context of sexual involvement).

This reasoning led Shaver and Hazan (1988) to hypothesize that securely attached people would be attentive to actual signals of sexual arousal and attraction, be able to perceive a partner's interests accurately, and therefore be able to engage in mutually satisfying genital sex, if it was mutually desirable. A secure person's comfort with closeness, self-disclosure, and interdependence (see Chapter 9, this volume) creates a positive foundation for sexual engagement, which is one of the most intimate of all human activities. In addition, a secure person's positive models of others (see Chapter 6, this volume) may make it easier to view sexual partners as caring and well-intentioned (lacking inclinations to engage in sexual coercion, violence, or exploitation), which allows a secure person to enjoy intimate sex. Moreover, a secure person's positive models of self (Chapter 6, this volume) support feelings of being desired and esteemed during sexual activities, and help to maintain a sense of confidence in the ability to gratify one's own and a partner's sexual needs. These positive mental representations allow secure adults to relax their defenses and be less preoccupied with sexual performance, which, when combined with enjoyment of closeness, is conducive to "letting go" sexually and experiencing maximal sexual pleasure (Shaver & Mikulincer, in 2006).

The crucial role that attachment security plays in the regulation of emotions, goal-oriented behavior, and interpersonal exchanges (see Chapters 7 through 9, this volume) can have further desirable effects on sexual functioning. Secure people's effective emotion regulation techniques allow them to maintain a comfortable, relaxed state of mind during sexual activities and be free of worries that interfere with enjoyable sexual intercourse. The sense of attachment security also favors cognitive openness and relaxed exploration of novel possibilities (see Chapter 8, this volume), which allow for shared sexual exploration. In addition, secure people's willingness and ability to balance their own and others' concerns (see Chapter 9, this volume) allow them to move flexibly from one position to another in the interpersonal circumplex during sex.

Beyond supporting sexual intimacy, openness, and satisfaction, "felt security" probably inclines a person to establish a long-term couple relationship rather than pursuing short-term sex with numerous relatively anonymous partners. In previous relationships with supportive attachment figures, secure individuals have learned that intimacy, mutual understanding, and mutual care are highly rewarding and mutually beneficial for relationship partners. Secure people are more likely than insecure ones to have grown up in a considerate home, with security-providing attachment figures. As we have mentioned in other chapters, they are less likely to have lived through parental divorce or witnessed spousal violence. They are also less likely to be divorced themselves, and are on average better able to alter their hierarchy of attachment figures, so that a stable romantic or marital partner replaces a parent as the primary figure. Thus, secure people are more likely than insecure ones to search for and find a romantic/sexual partner with whom they can satisfy their sexual desires within a long-term couple relationship (Gillath & Schachner, 2006).

This does not mean that secure individuals never enjoy sex without commitment or that they necessarily equate sex with romantic love. Because they generally possess a stable and authentic sense of self-worth, they do not have to use sex as a means of feeling loved, admired, or accepted. If they wish, they can have sex simply for the pleasures involved, which may sometimes carry them beyond the bounds of a committed relationship. In so doing, they would be expected to retain an accurate understanding of their own motives, and the consequences for their relationship partners and for themselves. We are suggesting not a tight link between security and monogamy, although for various reasons there may be such a link empirically, but rather the ability of secure individuals to have sex with or without affectional bonds and with or without defensive distortions due to attachment insecurities. We expect them to be able to channel their sexual desires and activities in whatever directions they choose—including, but not being limited to, the creation of a mutually fulfilling, long-term romantic relationship or marriage.

Insecure adults are likely to have more sexual problems and to be less able to enjoy conflict-free sex. Avoidant people's discomfort with closeness and negative models of others may interfere with psychological intimacy and interpersonal sensitivity in sexual situations. In addition, avoidant people may be willing to engage in sex without any consideration of establishing a long-term relationship, or even with the conviction that they do not want to be burdened by a long-term relationship. In other words, avoidance may be associated with measurable erotophobia (i.e., fearing or backing away from sex), sexual abstinence, or preference for impersonal, uncommitted sex. Moreover, avoidant individuals' frequent reliance on distancing as a strategy of emotion regulation (see Chapter 7, this volume) and their problems with exploration and cognitive openness (see Chapter 8, this volume) make them especially likely to dismiss sexual needs or to inhibit sexual desire rather than explore what a sexual partner wants or needs and talk openly about interpersonal problems that arise during sexual relations. In addition, because avoidant strategies are associated with extreme self-reliance, personal control, and defensive self-image inflation (see Chapter 6, this volume), avoidant people may use sex to maximize control over a partner, to gain social prestige, or to enhance self-esteem, all without much regard for a partner's feelings.

In fact, avoidant people's sexual behavior may be focused selfishly on their own needs in combination with dismissal of or blindness to a partner's sexual wishes. Avoidance also, paradoxically, may promote sexual promiscuity powered by insecurity, narcissism, or a wish to elevate one's self-image or standing in the estimation of one's peers. This kind of self-promotion through sexual conquest can occur in the absence of intense sexual interest and without much enjoyment of sex per se (Schachner & Shaver, 2004). Another way to have sex without interpersonal entanglements is to masturbate, a solitary activity that eliminates concerns about intimacy, vulnerability, and cooperation or coordination with another person.

Attachment anxiety is likely to be associated with a complex, ambivalent approach to sexuality. Because sex is an obvious route to closeness and intimacy, attachment-anxious people can hold a positive attitude toward sex and use it as a means of fulfilling unmet needs for security and love. However, while focusing on their own wishes for protection and security, they may have trouble attending accurately to a partner's sexual wishes and preferences. Moreover, attachment-anxious people's negative models of self, worries about rejection and disapproval, and regulatory difficulties (e.g., distress amplification) may make it difficult for them to relax and "let go" sexually, thereby making sexual pleasure less intense and more tinged with ambivalence. For them, sexual arousal may be accompanied by worries and doubts about their sexual attractiveness, the extent to which they are loved and valued, their ability to gratify a partner, and a partner's lack of sensitive responsiveness to their sexual needs. Thus, although anxious people are likely to place a high value on sex, often for reasons beyond sex itself, they may still have personal sexual problems and interpersonal difficulties with sexual partners.

Perhaps the most dangerous kinds of sexual difficulties for anxious individuals can be traced to their general methods of regulating interpersonal relations. Their intense desire for closeness can result in intrusive sexual behavior and cause them to engage in unsafe sex while pursuing maximal intimacy (e.g., without a condom), which can be deadly for themselves and their partners. In addition, their worried, dependent position in a relationship can create problems in communication about sex, difficulties with sexual assertiveness, and an increased vulnerability to sexual coercion. They may agree to arrangements and activities they do not like simply as a means of avoiding a partner's disapproval.

Anxious and avoidant people's different combinations of motives may also affect their construal of the links between sex and romantic love. Avoidant people's preference for interpersonal distance and emotional detachment favors viewing sex and love as quite distinct; indeed, in the first studies of avoidance within the adult close-relationship domain, Hazan and Shaver (1987) found that avoidant people tended to view romantic love as a Hollywood fiction that does not exist in real life. In contrast, anxious individuals' unmet attachment needs and their compulsive need for love and security might cause them to equate sex with romantic love, hence using sexual interest and sexual activities as a "barometer" of romantic relationship quality (D. Davis et al., 2003, in press); that is, they may interpret good or frequent sex as an indication of their partner's love and a partner's lack of sexual desire or refusal to engage in sexual activities as indicating an absence of love.

In a recent discussion of attachment-oriented psychotherapy, Laschinger, Purnell, Schwartz, White, and Wingfield (2004) extended Bowlby's (1973) distinction between "the anger of hope" and "the anger of despair" to the sexual realm. They proposed that attachment security is conducive to a "sexuality of hope," in which sexual desire provides a bridge between one's subjective world and a partner's subjectivity, and fosters genuine intimacy and a mutually satisfying relationship. In contrast, attachment insecurities can lead either to a sexuality of despair—"the sexuality of one whose subjectivity has been denied by past or present attachment failure, a sadomasochistic sexuality that denies the other [his or her] subjectivity" (Laschinger et al., 2004, p. 154)—or to melancholic sexuality, "an arctic wasteland, cold and devoid of relationships" (p. 156). Theoretically, attachment-anxious individuals are vulnerable to a sexuality of despair, and avoidant individuals are vulnerable to melancholic sexuality.

EMPIRICAL ASSOCIATIONS BETWEEN THE ATTACHMENT AND SEXUAL SYSTEMS

When Shaver and Hazan (1988) first offered hypotheses concerning the interplay of the attachment and sexual behavioral systems, there was no empirical evidence to show how attachment insecurities might affect sex. With the progress of research on adult attachment, however, this empirical gap is being filled. In the following sections, we present a brief summary of the evidence. We review studies that have examined associations between attachment style and (1) engagement in sexual activities; (2) attitudes toward casual, uncommitted sex; (3) the subjective experience of sexual activities; (4) sexual motives; (5) sexual self-confidence; communication, and exploration; (6) sexual risk taking; and (7) and sexual coercion.

Engagement in Sexual Activities

Several researchers have looked for an association between attachment style and engagement in sexual activities, providing strong support for the hypothesized inhibitory relation between avoidant attachment and sexual system activation. In a sample of American adolescents, Tracy, Shaver, Albino, and Cooper (2003) found that avoidant adolescents were less likely ever to have had sex, had engaged in fewer noncoital sexual behaviors (e.g., making out, petting) before trying intercourse; and after they did begin having intercourse, had it less frequently than their less avoidant agemates. A negative association between avoidant attachment and frequency of sexual intercourse has also been noted in studies of young adults (Bogaert & Sadava, 2002; Gentzler & Kerns, 2004; Hazan, Zeifman, & Middleton, 1994) and in a diary study in which participants were asked to report all interactions with members of the opposite sex that lasted 10 minutes or longer over a 6-week period (J. A. Feeney et al., 1993). Interestingly, Bogaert and Sadava (2002) found that although avoidant individuals reported engaging less frequently in sexual activities with a relationship partner, they masturbated more frequently—a solitary activity that fits with Bowlby's conception of avoidant self-reliance.

In a study of married couples and cohabiting but unmarried couples, Brassard, Shaver, and Lussier (2007) found that more avoidant men and women reported having sex less often and were more likely to report trying to avoid sex with their partner (a pattern of motives and behavior that their partners confirmed). The study also revealed several interesting dyadic interaction patterns. First, more avoidant men reported having less frequent sex if their female partner was attachment-anxious. It seemed likely that attachment-anxious women wanted a great deal of physical proximity and intimacy, causing avoidant men to back away. Second, and similarly, avoidant women were more sex-avoidant if their male partners were attachment-anxious. There was also a significant interaction between women's and men's avoidant attachment, such that a woman perceived her partner as more sex avoidant if both she and he scored high on avoidant attachment. All of these findings indicate that avoidant attachment contributes to sex avoidance even within the context of a committed, long-term relationship.

Studies have also revealed consistent gender differences in the link between attachment anxiety and sexual activities. Among young men, attachment anxiety, like avoidant attachment, is associated with less frequent sexual activity over a 6-week period (J. A. Feeney et al., 1993) and with older age at first intercourse (Gentzler & Kerns, 2004). However, among young women, attachment anxiety is associated with greater likelihood of ever having had sex during adolescence (Cooper, Shaver, & Collins, 1998) and with younger age at first intercourse (Bogaert & Sadava, 2002; Gentzler & Kerns, 2004). In other words, whereas attachment anxiety seems to inhibit either sexual system activation or its expression in actual sexual activities among young men, it increases the likelihood of sexual activity in young women (conceptually similar findings were reported by D. Davis, Follette, & Vernon, 2001).

According to D. Davis et al. (2006), these findings may be explained by anxiously attached people's deference to partners' needs, coupled with traditional sex roles that assign the task of initiating sexual relations to men more than to women. D. Davis et al. found that both men and women who scored high on attachment anxiety were more likely to sacrifice their own sexual needs and defer to a partner's sexual preferences, probably because of their intense desire for acceptance, love, and approval. As a result, when anxious women defer to male partners, they are likely to reach the higher rate of sexual intercourse that men prefer, whereas when anxious men defer to female partners, they are more likely to inhibit sexuality in line with the traditional female gender role. This matter deserves further study, because it contributes to relationship dissatisfaction at times and probably plays a role in anxious women's greater rates of unwanted pregnancy and sexually transmitted disease (Cooper et al., 2006).

Attitudes toward Casual, Uncommitted Sex

Beyond abstaining from sex, avoidant individuals seem to construe sexual activities in ways that make intimacy and interdependence unlikely. Several studies that have assessed attitudes toward casual sex (e.g., acceptance of casual sex without love, acceptance of uncommitted sex) found that avoidant attachment is associated with more positive attitudes toward casual sex (E. S. Allen & Baucom, 2004; Brennan & Shaver, 1995; J. A. Feeney et al., 1993; Gentzler & Kerns, 2004; Simpson & Gangestad, 1991). In a study of sexual attitudes in 47 nations, Schmitt (2005) found a significant positive correlation in most countries between self-reported avoidance and willingness to have uncommitted, casual sex.

A similar association between avoidance and sexual permissiveness was found in a sample of gay men and lesbians (Ridge & Feeney, 1998). However, Scharfe and Eldredge (2001) found that a positive attitude toward casual sex was associated with fearful, but not dismissing, avoidance in a sample of undergraduates involved in committed heterosexual relationships. There is also evidence that adolescents and young adults who scored higher on avoidance were more interested in emotionless sex, were less likely to be involved in sexually exclusive relationships, and were more likely to have sex with a stranger and engage in "one-night stands" (Bogaert & Sadava, 2002; Cooper et al., 1998;

J. A. Feeney, Peterson, Gallois, & Terry, 2000; Gangestad & Thornhill, 1997; Hazan et al., 1994; Paul, McManus, & Hayes, 2000; Stephan & Bachman, 1999). Interestingly, a similar positive attitude toward uncommitted sex has been noted in attachment-anxious women (E. S. Allen & Baucom, 2004; Bogaert & Sadava, 2002, J. A. Feeney et al., 2000; Gangestad & Thornhill, 1997), perhaps due to their deference to male sexual partners' preferences.

Consistent with the notion that avoidant individuals detach sex from intimacy and commitment, Schachner and Shaver (2002) found that "mate poaching" (i.e., appropriating someone else's mate) and being available for "poaching"—in the context of short- but not long-term relationships—were associated with avoidance. Interestingly, these associations between avoidance and sexual promiscuity were not explained by differences in sexual drive (Schachner & Shaver, 2002), which was no higher in avoidant than in nonavoidant individuals. Thus, the associations must have been due to some other ingredient of avoidance that attracts a person to short-term sexual relations. Avoidant individuals' tendency to dissociate sex from romantic love was also evident in K. N. Levy, Kelly, and Jack's (2006) finding that individuals with avoidant attachment reported greater jealousy in response to possible sexual infidelity than in response to possible emotional infidelity, whereas nonavoidant individuals were more bothered by emotional than by sexual infidelity. According to K. N. Levy et al., avoidant individuals are more concerned with their partners' sexual investment than with their emotional investment in a relationship, and they project their own interests in extradyadic, short-term sex onto their partners.

In a recent series of three laboratory experiments, Gillath and Schachner (2006) constructed a 12-item scale to assess interest in long-term sexual mating (e.g., "I'm looking for a potential spouse and hope to get married before too long") and short-term sexual relations (e.g., "I have no objection to 'casual' sex, as long as I like the person I'm having sex with"). Across the three studies, Gillath and Schachner found that more avoidant people showed a stronger preference for short-term sexual mating and a weaker preference for long-term mating, compared with less avoidant people. In their third study, they manipulated the accessibility of avoidance-related representations (asking people to think about a relationship in which they felt avoidant) and found that contextual priming of avoidance increased interest in short-term sex and weakened interest in a long-term sexual relationship. In all three studies, Gillath and Schachner also manipulated the accessibility of security-related representations (asking participants to think about people to whom they turn for support or about a past relationship in which they felt secure). Contextual priming of attachment security increased interest in a long-term sexual relationship and reduced avoidant people's preference for short-term sex.

These findings fit well with Belsky, Steinberg, and Draper's (1991) hypothesis that children who experience harsh and insensitive parenting not only develop an insecure attachment style but also develop a preference for short-term mating strategies, which place emphasis on casual sex and reproduction rather than relational commitment and parenting. The results also fit with a study by E. M. Hill et al. (1994), which showed that less secure individuals, especially the avoidant ones, had experienced relatively low parental investment when they were growing up (i.e., their parents were relatively unavailable or insensitive); they grew up to have similarly dismissive attitudes toward parenting and to prefer short-term sex. More specifically, E. M. Hill et al. found that poor childhood relationships with parents predicted attachment insecurity in adulthood, which in turn predicted a low-investment, short-term mating strategy. Rholes et al. (1995, 1997, 2006) also showed that more avoidant young adults were less likely to want children or to think they would be good parents.

Interestingly, Gillath and Schachner (2006) found that attachment anxiety was related to preference for a long-term mating strategy, presumably because of a desire for reliable love, acceptance, and protection. Indeed, as reviewed in Chapter 10, this volume, anxious people sometimes have relationships as enduring as those of secure people, although they are also more likely than people with other attachment styles to be rejected as a result of pressuring their partners for more love and for greater intimacy and commitment. Their experiences with difficulties and rejections in previous relationships may explain Gillath and Schachner's finding that security priming failed to increase preference for a long-term relationship in the case of anxious individuals, even though it did increase interest in such a relationship among avoidant and even secure people. It seems possible that when anxious individuals were asked to think about a relationship, or a time in a relationship, when they felt secure and well cared for, they were reminded of relationships or times within a relationship that seemed good in some respects but not good enough, or that led from peaks of satisfaction to subsequent disappointment or devastation. This fits with evidence we summarized in Chapter 7, that attachment-anxious people have heightened mental access to negative attachment-related memories and tend to ruminate on negative experiences and emotions. They also react to a positive mood induction with cognitive constriction and lowered creativity—just the opposite of the effect of positive mood inductions on secure individuals.

The Subjective Experience of Sexual Activities

There is extensive evidence concerning the adverse effects of attachment insecurities on the subjective experience of sexual activities. Both attachment anxiety and avoidance are associated with fewer positive and more negative feelings during sex (Birnbaum, 2007; Birnbaum, Reis, Mikulincer, Gillath, & Orpaz, 2006; Brassard et al., 2007; Gentzler & Kerns, 2004; Tracy et al., 2003); higher levels of sexual anxiety (D. Davis et al., 2006); lower levels of sexual arousal, intimacy, and pleasure (Birnbaum, 2007; Hazan et al., 1994); and less positive appraisals of one's own sexual qualities (Cyranowski & Andersen, 1998). However, whereas avoidant people tend to dismiss the importance of sex and fail to express feelings of love and affection for their partners during sex (Birnbaum, 2007; Birnbaum et al., 2006; Brennan, Wu, & Loev, 1998; Hazan et al., 1994; Tracy et al., 2003), anxious individuals express a strong desire for their partner's emotional involvement during sex (Birnbaum et al., 2006) and have an erotophilic orientation to sex (Bogaert & Sadava, 2002). In line with our theoretical reasoning, avoidance seems to be associated with a negative conception of sex, whereas attachment anxiety is associated with an ambivalent approach to sex, in which aversive feelings coexist with sexual excitement and strong wishes for sex and love.

Attachment insecurities are also associated with less frequent orgasmic experiences in women (Birnbaum, 2007; D. L. Cohen & Belsky, 2006), lower sexual satisfaction (Birnbaum, 2007; D. Davis et al., 2006; Fricker & Moore, 2002; Morrison, Urquiza, et al., 1997), and more dissatisfaction with control over sexual activities (D. Davis et al., 2006). However, D. Davis et al. also found that anxious and avoidant people differed in the specific aspects of sex that elicited dissatisfaction. Anxious people scored higher on measures tapping emotional dissatisfaction during sex (e.g., "I would like to have my partners be more romantic"), possibly reflecting their tendency to equate sex and love, and their difficulties in meeting unrealistic wishes for extreme approval and affection. Supporting this interpretation, D. Davis et al. found that anxious individuals were more likely to use sex as a barometer of relationship status (e.g., "When my partner doesn't want to have sex, it makes me worry about whether he still loves me"), which in turn explained their lack of satisfaction during sex. In contrast, avoidant individuals scored higher on measures of dissatisfaction with the physical aspects of sex ("I'm dissatisfied with the physical enjoyment I get out of sex"), perhaps reflecting not only distancing from emotional aspects of sex but also perhaps suggesting that sex without full interest and engagement (and accompanied by distaste for mutual intimacy and affection) is unsatisfying. The latter interpretation fits with Hazan et al.'s (1994) discovery that avoidant people reported less enjoyment of touching, cuddling, and kissing (see also Brennan et al., 1998). Interestingly, Hazan et al. (1994) also reported that, for both sexes, anxious attachment was associated with enjoyment of holding and caressing, but not of behaviors that were more clearly sexual.

Sexual Motives

Several studies have examined the association between attachment style and sexual motives, providing strong support for the hypothesis that attachment orientation affects a person's reasons for having sex. In their study of adolescent sexuality, Tracy et al. (2003) found that more attachment-anxious adolescents were more likely to say they had sex to avoid a partner's rejection, and avoidant adolescents were less likely than nonavoidant ones to say they had sex to express love and affection for their partner. In addition, avoidant adolescents were more likely to say their first intercourse was motivated by a desire to lose their virginity, which might have been aimed at increasing self-esteem or peer acceptance rather than getting psychologically closer to their partner. In an Internet survey assessing 10 motives for sex, D. Davis et al. (2004) extended Tracy at al.'s (2003) findings to a diverse sample of sexually active adults. Anxiously attached people were more likely to report having sex to foster closeness, gain a partner's reassurance, reduce stress, and manipulate a partner. In contrast, avoidant people were less likely to report having sex as a means of fostering closeness and gaining partners' reassurance. Although these findings revealed which motives were *not* endorsed by avoidant adults, they failed to identify what positively motivated these people to have sex.

In an attempt to learn more about avoidant people's motives for sex, Schachner and Shaver (2004) asked a sample of young adults to complete two standard measures of sexual motivation, the Sex Motives scale and the Affective and Motivational Orientation Related to Erotic Arousal (AMORE) scale, as well as some new items devised especially for their study. They found that more avoidant people endorsed more self-enhancement and self-affirmation reasons for engaging in sex. Specifically, they were more likely to have sex to fit in with their social group, to comply with peer pressure, and to be able to brag about it. In addition, replicating D. Davis et al.'s (2004) findings, Schachner and Shaver (2004) found that avoidant people were less likely to have sex to increase intimacy or to express affection for a partner, and attachment-anxious people were more likely to have sex to feel loved, to avoid a partner's rejection, and to induce a partner to love them more.

Conceptually similar findings were obtained in a study of gay males and lesbians (Ridge & Feeney, 1998) and in a study of motives for extradyadic involvement (E. S. Allen & Baucom, 2004). Ridge and Feeney (1998) found that more avoidant gay and lesbian individuals were more likely to hold an instrumental view of sex as a means for gaining social prestige and status, whereas attachment-anxious homosexuals were more likely to construe sex as a route to intimacy and communion. In addition, E. S. Allen and Baucom (2004) found that attachment anxiety was associated with intimacy-related motives for having sex outside a marital or primary dating relationship (e.g., "I was lonely and I needed to feel cared about," "I was feeling neglected in my primary relationship"). Conversely, more avoidant people reported more autonomy-related motives for extradyadic involvement (e.g., "I wanted a little freedom," "I wanted some space from my primary partner"). In line with our theoretical analysis of anxious attachment, E. S. Allen and Baucom also found that more anxiously attached adults were more likely to report obsessive extradyadic affairs ("I was obsessed with the other person").

Most of these findings were replicated in a recent longitudinal study (Cooper et al., 2006) that assessed attachment orientations during adolescence and examined sexual motives 7 years later (during young adulthood). The authors found that avoidant people's sexual motives mediated their tendency to engage in casual sex. Specifically, women who scored higher on avoidance during adolescence were more likely in young adulthood to use sex to bolster their self-esteem, and this motivation was associated with having more casual sex partners. Similarly, men who scored higher on avoidance during adolescence were more likely to have sex for a variety of nonsocial reasons (e.g., self-affirmation, coping with distress), and these sexual motives appeared to predispose them to have more casual sex as young adults; that is, avoidant people's desire for prestige and self-affirmation attained through sexual activities, free from any desire for intimacy, seemed to encourage promiscuous, uncommitted sex.

Cooper et al. (2006) also found some interesting gender differences in the longitudinal effects of attachment anxiety on sexual motives and behaviors. On one hand, women who scored higher on attachment anxiety during adolescence were more likely to have sex to bolster their self-esteem and to please or appease their partners during young adulthood; ironically, they were also more likely to cheat on their sexual partners. On the other hand, highly anxious adolescent men were less likely to use sex to cope with negative emotions or to bolster their self-esteem, and less likely to cheat on their sexual partners during young adulthood. These findings suggest that the sexual motives of anxiously attached adolescents and adults are moderated by gender-specific norms for sexual behavior. Whereas an anxious woman's intense desire for love, affection, and approval may cause her to acquiesce to male sexual partners' demands, including ones that are not ideal from her standpoint, anxious men's equally intense desire for love, affection, and approval may cause them to be more compliant with their female partners' wishes. Also, to the extent that men's attachment anxiety is incompatible with a male gender role stressing assertiveness, confidence, and dominance, anxious men may behave fairly differently from nonanxious men because the anxious men are less self-confident (Cooper et al., 2006). However, since attachment theory does not specifically predict gender differences in the expression of attachment-related needs, more research is needed to delineate the specific paths by which gender-specific norms affect the interplay of the attachment and sexual systems.

Overall, research conducted so far suggests that the sexual motives of anxious and avoidant people are affected by attachment-related goals and tendencies. For avoidant people, minimizing intimacy and gaining social status and power seem to be important motives that govern sexual relations; for anxiously attached people, holding on to a partner, assessing the partner's attraction and affection, and complying with the partner's wishes seem to interfere with comfortable, freely chosen, and mutually regulated sexual relations.

Sexual Self-Confidence, Communication, and Exploration

Attachment insecurities are likely to erode a person's confidence in his or her sexual attractiveness and prowess. Higher scores on attachment anxiety and avoidance are associated with lower appraisals of ability to gratify one's sexual needs (Tracy et al., 2003), lower sexual self-esteem (Shafer, 2001), and lower self-perceptions of physical attractiveness and sensuality (Bogaert & Sadava, 2002; Shafer, 2001). (These findings recur despite the fact that actual physical attractiveness does not seem to be reliably associated with attachment security or insecurity [Tidwell et al., 1996].) In addition, J. A. Feeney et al. (2000) found that people who scored relatively high on either attachment anxiety or avoidance endorsed a more external, sex-related locus of control and felt that sexual relations are controlled by the partner or situational factors. Attachment anxiety has also been associated with lower self-appraisals of ability to negotiate sexual encounters (J. A. Feeney et al., 2000), stronger concerns about sexual performance (Birnbaum et al., 2007; Hazan et al., 1994), and more worries about losing sexual partners (Schachner & Shaver, 2002). Perhaps these worries explain D. Davis and Vernon's (2002) finding that anxiously attached women are more likely than less anxious women to have cosmetic surgery to increase their physical attractiveness.

Research also indicates that attachment insecurities are associated with the inhibition of open sexual exploration and communication. Specifically, individuals scoring higher on attachment anxiety or avoidance tend to report less willingness to experiment sexually within a romantic relationship (Hazan et al., 1994) and to openly express their sexual needs and preferences (D. Davis et al., 2006). In addition, J. A. Feeney et al. (1999) found that attachment anxiety, but not avoidance, was associated with reluctance to speak with sexual partners about AIDS-related issues, and that both forms of attachment insecurity were associated with less openness in discussing safe sex, contraception, and other sexual matters with a partner J. A. Feeney et al. (2000). However, they also found that anxiety and avoidance related differently to willingness to discuss specific topics related to sexual risks. In reports of men's actual discussions with their sexual partners, avoidance was positively associated with discussions about transmission of sexual diseases, whereas anxiety was negatively related to discussions about the use of contraceptives.

These findings were conceptually replicated by J. Feeney et al. (2001), who found that attachment orientation, measured at an initial time point, was predictive of satisfaction with sexual communication 9 months later in a sample of married couples making the transition to parenthood, and also in a sample of married couples without children. Specifically, husbands from the two samples who scored higher on either attachment anxiety or avoidance were less likely to be satisfied with sexual communication. In addition, wives' avoidant attachment was associated with less satisfaction with sexual communication, but this association was significant only in the sample of married couples without children. According to J. A. Feeney et al., new mothers' sexual behavior may be more affected by variables related to the birth of the first child and the demands of infant care than by their attachment insecurities.

J. A. Feeney et al. (2001) also reported some interesting partner effects: Husbands' attachment anxiety and avoidance predicted wives' reports of lower satisfaction with sexual communication 9 months later. However, wives' attachment insecurities did not significantly affect husbands' satisfaction with sexual communication. It seems possible that husbands' insecurities block open communication about sex, which in turn frustrates wives' sexual needs and desire to have open and relaxed discussions about sexual relations. Insecure women's inhibition of sexual communication may be less relevant for men's sexual satisfaction, both because men may feel that anything resulting in sexual gratification is acceptable and because the male gender role does not encourage intimate discussions of sexual concerns.

Although both attachment anxiety and avoidance are associated with problems in sexual communication, D. Davis et al. (2006) found different pathways by which the two forms of attachment insecurity contribute to inhibited expression of sexual needs. Sexual anxiety and deference to a partner's needs (designed to please the partner and avoid offense or conflict) were found to explain the link between attachment anxiety and inhibited expression of sexual needs. Specifically, D. Davis et al. found that participants scoring high on attachment anxiety were also more sexually anxious and more likely to defer to a partner's sexual preferences. These mediators, in turn, were associated with inhibited sexual communication. In a quite different pattern, negative feelings about relationship partners and lack of love for them explained avoidant people's deficits in sexual communication.

Practicing or Failing to Practice Safe Sex

Several studies indicate that attachment anxiety interferes with safe sex. Specifically, more anxious adults have more negative beliefs about condom use (e.g., condoms are boring; they reduce intimacy); are less likely to use condoms; are more likely to engage in deviant, painful sexual activities (e.g., bondage); report lower perceived risk of contracting AIDS; and are less willing to change their risky sexual practices (Bogaert & Sadava, 2002; J. A. Feeney et al., 1999, 2000; Hazan et al., 1994). In addition, attachment anxiety is associated with the use of alcohol and drugs before sex (J. A. Feeney et al., 2000), higher rates of unplanned pregnancy among adolescent girls (Cooper et al., 1998), and higher rates of unprotected sex among people who are HIV-positive (Ciesla, Roberts, & Hewitt, 2004). It therefore seems likely that anxiously attached people's desire to get close to their sexual partners, while hoping not to "turn them off," leads them to put their own and their partners' health at risk.

Interestingly, people who scored high on avoidance reported more positive attitudes toward condoms and were more likely to use them (J. A. Feeney et al., 2000)—one case in which selfishness and willingness to forgo intimacy may be health-promoting. However, avoidant people's openness to having casual sex with relative strangers, without talking about their and their own partners' sexuality and sexual histories can sometimes result in unsafe sex. This possibility is reinforced by avoidant men's tendency to use alcohol and drugs in sexual situations, probably to reduce anxious awkwardness or sex-related tension (J. A. Feeney et al., 2000; Tracy et al., 2003). Tracy et al. found that this link between avoidance and heightened use of alcohol and drugs in connection with sex cannot be explained by individual differences in general substance abuse; instead, it is mediated by avoidant individuals' doubts about their sexual performance.

In summary, the attachment-related psychological dynamics of both anxious and avoidant individuals tend to favor unsafe sexual practices, and although it may happen for different reasons, unsafe sex and contraction of sexually transmitted diseases are more common among insecure than among secure people. This conclusion fits with A. L. Miller et al.'s (2002) finding that adolescents who reported insecure working models of attachment at least once during a two-wave study (with assessments 1 year apart) were more likely to use alcohol and drugs during sex than adolescents who reported attachment security at both points in time.

Sexual Coercion

Attachment insecurities have been implicated in both perpetrators' use of coercive sexual tactics and victims' responses to sexual coercion. Tracy et al. (2003) and Gentzler and Kerns (2004) found that higher attachment anxiety and avoidance were associated with higher rates of physical coercion on the part of sexual partners and more involvement in unwanted but consensual sex. Impett and Peplau (2002) also found that women scoring high on attachment anxiety were more accepting of unwanted sex portrayed in hypothetical scenarios. These authors also found that sexually active women's anxiety and avoidance, respectively, were related to different reasons for acquiescing to unwanted sexual advances. Whereas anxiously attached women more often accepted unwanted sex to reduce relational conflicts and to avoid rejection and abandonment, avoidant women more often had unwanted sex to avoid intimate and self-disclosing discussions about relationship problems or issues. For anxious women, acceptance of unwanted sex was a way to maintain a form of closeness and assuage fears of abandonment; for avoidant women, it was a way to avoid, conflict, intimacy, and emotional involvement.

There is also evidence that both attachment anxiety and avoidance in men are associated with using physical force and other coercive strategies in the context of sexual relations (K. E. Davis, Ace, & Andra, 2002; Smallbone & Dadds, 2000, 2001; Tracy et al., 2003). In Brassard et al.'s (2007) study of cohabiting and married couples, however, only men's attachment anxiety was associated with pressuring a female partner to have sex. For anxious men, who have difficulty articulating their strong desires for love, attention, and reassurance, coercive sexual behavior may be a means to gain or regain proximity to what they perceive to be an unreliable or insufficiently responsive partner. (See Chapter 10, this volume, for similar findings concerning couple violence.) For avoidant men, sexual coercion may be another means of gratifying a need for self-affirmation and dominance (D. Davis et al., 2004). Additionally, sexual coercion may be a way to avoid mutuality and psychological intimacy during sexual intercourse.

In a recent study of attachment and attitudes toward rape, D. Davis, Carlen, and Gallio (2006) found that more attachment-anxious and avoidant men were more likely to hold adversarial sexual beliefs and to score relatively high on a rape acceptance scale. Participants were also asked to think about three sexual coercion scenarios—an alleged stranger rape, a date rape, and the rape of an ongoing partner who refused to have sex—and to rate the validity of the victim's claim, the extent to which the rapist's actions were justified or he had a right to expect sex, and the psychological and social effects that the rape would have on the victim. Attachment-anxious men were less likely to accept the validity of the victim's claim in all three types of rape scenarios, and avoidant men were more likely to say the rapist was justified and had a right to expect sex in both the date rape and the ongoing relationship rape scenarios. Interestingly, women's avoidance scores were related to believing that all three kinds of rape would have negative effects on how the victim was perceived by others—a finding that fits with avoidant people's tendency to have sex to enhance their public or social identity (D. Davis et al., 2004).

D. Davis (2006) analyzed the various attachment-related pathways to sexual coercion and concluded that anxiously attached people may be most prone to coerce and to rape a partner within established couple relationships when a partner's behavior threatens relationship continuity or stability (e.g., when a partner threatens to leave the relationship). Under these conditions, anxious people may desperately want to engage in sex with the partner as a way to reestablish closeness and connectedness. D. Davis also concluded that avoidant men are most likely to coerce and to rape partners during pickups, first dates, or occasional dating situations as a means of gaining access to sexual intercourse (exhibiting what Lalumiere, Harris, Quinsey, & Rice [2005] called the "young male syndrome"), without having to cope with more intimate and involved communication. In D. Davis's (2006) terms, "The patterns of sexual coercion of avoidant men can be expected to resemble those of narcissists, whereby the view of women as sex objects and the possession of generally adversarial sexual attitudes promotes negative construals of women generally and of sexual negotiations specifically" (p. 324). This negative approach to sex fits with other evidence of avoidant individuals' negative working models of others (see Chapter 6, this volume).

Summary

Panning back from this diverse sampling of empirical evidence concerning attachment style and sexuality, we see that both attachment anxiety and avoidance are associated with theoretically predictable patterns of sexual motives, cognitions, and behaviors. Anxious individuals tend to sexualize their desire for acceptance, affection, and security, thereby assimilating sexual desire into their hunger for attachment security. Unfortunately, this subordination of sexuality to attachment goes hand in hand with lack of sexual self-confidence, unsafe sexual practices, and the use or acceptance of coercion. These tactics, ironically, undermine genuine intimacy and mutuality, and increase the likelihood of disappointing sexual encounters, which in turn lead to the breakup of what people hoped would be stable, mutually satisfying couple relationships.

Avoidant people's discomfort with closeness and negative models of others sometimes cause them to abstain from sexual intercourse; rely on masturbation; engage in casual, uncommitted sex; experience various forms of discomfort during sex; forgo mutual sexual exploration; and seek self-enhancement or peer admiration through sex. Relatively secure individuals are more likely to be genuinely interested in sex, able to sustain mutual sexual intimacy and enjoyment, and able to activate attachment, caregiving, and sexual systems simultaneously, if desired, without distortion or interference.

Overall, when we conceptualize attachment and sex as domains of distinct behavioral systems, we see that the parameters of the attachment system strongly affect the operation of the sexual system. There may also be reciprocal causal processes by which sexual experiences alter attachment security or patterns of insecurity, but no systematic studies have been designed to test this idea (see Chapter 16, this volume, for a review of preliminary findings).

ATTACHMENT, SEX, AND RELATIONSHIP QUALITY

Beyond biasing sexual system functioning, attachment insecurities distort the potential contribution of sexuality and sexual intercourse to relationship quality and satisfaction. There is growing evidence that sexual interactions in which both partners gratify their sexual needs contribute to relationship satisfaction and stability (for a review, see Sprecher & Cate, 2004) and heighten feelings of love and commitment (e.g., Sprecher & Regan, 1998; Waite & Joyner, 2001). In addition, both clinical observations and empirical studies indicate that sexual dysfunctions heighten relational tensions and increase conflict. Moreover, relational conflicts can interfere with sexual desire and satisfaction (for reviews, see Metz & Epstein, 2002; Sprecher & Cate, 2004). Nevertheless, the empirical findings have not always been consistent or compelling, and most of the studies suffer from methodological deficiencies (e.g., the use of cross-sectional designs from which it is impossible to draw causal conclusions; Sprecher & Cate, 2004).

Recently, Birnbaum et al. (2006) proposed that attachment style moderates the association between sexuality and relationship quality. They reasoned that because anxiously attached people have sex to meet their needs for security and affection (D. Davis et al., 2004; Schachner & Shaver, 2004; Tracy et al., 2003), they are likely to rely heavily on sexual experiences when assessing relationship quality; that is, anxiously attached people are likely to equate gratifying sexual experiences with a sense of being loved, valued, and protected, which temporarily quells their fears of rejection, unlovability, and abandonment. By the same token, they are likely to interpret frustrating and disappointing sexual experiences as signs or portents of a partner's disapproval and frustration, which can easily be interpreted as omens of abandonment.

Based on this theoretical analysis, Birnbaum et al. (2006) hypothesized that attachment anxiety would amplify the effects of sexual experiences on perceived relationship quality. In contrast, because avoidant people have sex for nonrelational reasons and tend to dismiss the relational and affectionate aspects of sexual experiences, they are likely to detach sex from love; that is, avoidant people are not likely to take seriously the possible relational implications of positive or negative sexual experiences, or to rely on these experiences for assessing relationship quality. Hence, Birnbaum et al. hypothesized that avoidance would dramatically weaken the effects of sexual experiences on perceived relationship quality.

To test these hypotheses, Birnbaum et al. (2006) measured the attachment styles of both members of heterosexual, cohabiting couples, then asked them to complete daily diary measures of interactions with their partner and the quality of their relationship for a period of 42 consecutive days. Each time they had sex during the 42-day period, study participants were asked to report their thoughts and feelings during and after the sexual episode. Thus, Birnbaum et al. were able to explore whether attachment style moderates the extent to which having sex on a given day and the quality of that sexual experience contribute to reports of relationship quality and behaviors (positive, negative) the next day (after controlling for relationship quality and behavior on the previous day).

The findings supported both the linkage between sex and relationship quality, and the moderating role of attachment style. Having sex or experiencing positive feelings during sexual intercourse on one day had a significant positive effect on the next day's interactions with the partner and on appraisals of relationship quality. However, these effects were amplified by attachment anxiety and dampened by avoidance. Specifically, the links between having sex or sex-related feelings and next-day relationship quality/behaviors were (1) *stronger* among highly anxious individuals than among less anxious individuals and (2) *weaker* among highly avoidant individuals than among less avoidant ones.

The study also revealed the power of gratifying sexual experiences to reduce anxiously attached people's relational worries. The usual negative effects of attachment anxiety on daily interactions and appraisals of relationship quality were notably weakened on days following sexual activities with the partner, and days on which sexual intercourse was experienced as especially positive. These findings fit well with other diary studies of relationship satisfaction (reviewed in Chapter 10, this volume) showing that attachment anxiety causes people to react with greater daily ups and downs in satisfaction depending on the extent to which relational events (e.g., partner's supportive behavior, having good sex) satisfy their unmet needs for love and security. Perhaps anxious individuals' doubts about their own lovability and their partners' love cause them to adopt a myopic, here-and-now focus on daily relationship events, hence assigning greater significance to events, including sexual intercourse, that signal approval or rejection.

Interestingly, although there was a strong association between daily sexual experiences and subsequent relationship quality for both anxious men and anxious women, there were also some notable gender differences. Whereas anxious women's appraisals of their interactions with their partners were mainly affected by the feelings they experienced while having sex the previous day, highly anxious men's relational appraisals were affected mainly by the mere fact of having engaged in sexual activities; that is, for anxious men, having sex per se had a salutary effect on their assessment of their relationship. For anxious women, having sex per se was not enough to assuage relational worries; instead, the quality of their sexual experiences determined their feelings about the relationship. In both cases, however, anxious people were using sex as a barometer of relationship quality (D. Davis et al., 2004, 2006).

Overall, Birnbaum et al.'s (2006) findings indicate that attachment anxiety creates a stronger link between sexual experiences and relationship quality. Attachment-anxious people, particularly women, seem to conflate sex and love, making it likely that feelings about sex will be translated into feelings about the relationship in general. Birnbaum et al.'s findings also imply that avoidant adults tend to dissociate sex from other aspects of romantic love, such as attachment and caregiving.

RESOLUTION OF THE OEDIPUS COMPLEX AND THE ATTAINMENT OF MATURE SEXUALITY

We turn now to a more controversial and surprising example of the interplay between attachment and sexuality, namely, the adverse effects of attachment insecurities on resolution of the Oedipus complex (which is thought by psychoanalysts to be part of the normal development of mature sexuality). Although many psychoanalytic theorists who preceded Bowlby failed to consider the role of primary caregivers as attachment figures, they did contend that gratifying and loving interactions with primary caregivers during the first few years of life, and the consequent consolidation of "good object" representations, facilitate resolution of the Oedipus complex (e.g., Klein, 1945/1989; Lupinacci, 1998; Tognoli, 1987). In contrast, early painful experiences with primary caregivers can generate hostility, anger, envy, and unrealistic desires for merger and exclusivity, while encouraging the use of archaic, schizoid–paranoid defenses (e.g., splitting, projection) that jeopardize effective handling of oedipal issues and give rise to conflicts in the sexual and romantic realms.

In a creative merger of attachment theory and other psychoanalytic ideas, Eagle (1997) proposed that early experiences with responsive and supportive attachment figures, and the consequent development of attachment security, are likely to promote adequate resolution of the Oedipus complex. In our view, as we explained in Chapter 8, attachment security is an inner resource that allows effective coping with many normative developmental transitions, including resolution of the Oedipus complex. Whereas secure children's positive working models of others allow them to appreciate their parents' goodwill and love, despite competition with the same-sex parent and loss of an imagined exclusive relationship with the opposite-sex parent, secure children's positive working models of self allow them to maintain a sense of self-worth and self-efficacy despite their "inferior" position in the oedipal triangle.

These mental representations, combined with a sense of competence and autonomy, openness to new and challenging experiences, ability to empathize with parents' feelings, and reliance on constructive ways of coping, facilitate a smooth transition through the oedipal period. In other words, secure children, adolescents, and adults can integrate pre-oedipal and oedipal parental representations without feeling hostile or resentful. Moreover, they can become deeply involved with romantic partners, without attempting to recreate the oedipal situation, and can direct both sexual desire and tender caregiving toward their adult romantic partners.

In contrast, negative attachment experiences in childhood and the consolidation of insecure patterns of attachment are likely to interfere with resolution of the oedipal conflict. For avoidant children, who possess negative models of primary caregivers, the oedipal triangle can further increase pre-oedipal hostility and anger, exacerbate their defensively detached stance in close relationships, and eventually extend this detachment into the sexual realm. For anxiously attached children, the oedipal triangle can be experienced as traumatic, because it frustrates their infantile wish to control and merge with a primary caregiver, and inflames their unmet needs for security and love. As a result, anxious children are likely to have difficulty abandoning their oedipal object and may continue to search for a similar person in their adult romantic relationships. This in turn perpetuates the oedipal drama and causes the anxious person to confuse sexual desire with yearning for love, acceptance, and merger. This lack of resolution of the oedipal conflict may exacerbate anxious adults' difficulties in establishing long-lasting couple relationships, their strong ambivalence toward sexuality and love, and their sexualization of the needs for security and affection.

We are currently testing some of these ideas empirically. In particular, we are exploring the extent to which unconscious activation of oedipal imagery has differential effects on secure and insecure adults' patterns of sexual and relational impulses. In a recent study, Barabi, Mikulincer, and Shaver (2006) examined the effects of subliminal exposure to an oedipal scene (an erotic picture of a nude child touching the genital area of a nude adult woman) on men's ratings of the sexual attractiveness of other women. If anxiously attached men continue to harbor oedipal remnants and express them in their sexual relationships, unconscious activation of oedipal representations should increase their sexual desire and heighten their perception of available women as attractive. This effect should be absent in less anxious men, who might even react to oedipal representations with disgust or distaste and, as a consequence, view possible sexual partners as less attractive.

Male undergraduates, who reported on their attachment orientations during a class period, were invited to participate in an experiment in which they were asked to rate the attractiveness and sexual allure of a series of women appearing in magazine advertisements. Before recording each rating, however, the men were exposed for 20 milliseconds (which is too brief a time to allow conscious perception) either to the oedipal picture or to one of four control pictures (a nude woman, a nude child, a dressed child with a dressed woman in a nonerotic posture, a geometrical figure). We found that men who scored high on attachment anxiety and were exposed subliminally to the oedipal picture rated the women as more attractive and more sexually arousing compared with ratings in the control conditions. In contrast, men who scored low on attachment anxiety and were exposed subliminally to the oedipal picture rated the women as less attractive and less sexually arousing compared with ratings in the control conditions. Interestingly, although the parallel results for avoidance were not statistically significant, more avoidant men reacted similarly to anxious men: They rated pictured women's attractiveness higher following subliminal exposure to the oedipal picture. These findings, though quite preliminary, are compatible with the hypothesis that attachment insecurity impedes resolution of the Oedipus complex and may interfere with mature sexuality.

Recent studies of pedophiles provide additional evidence for a link between attachment insecurity and failure to achieve mature sexuality. Seven studies have examined differences in self-reported attachment orientation between incarcerated pedophiles and control samples—incarcerated nonsexual offenders, some of whom had engaged in violence and some of whom had not, or healthy nonoffenders. Five of these studies (Bogaerts, Vanheule, & Declercq, 2005; Lyn & Burton, 2004; Marsa et al., 2004; Sawle & Kear-Colwell, 2001; T. Ward, Hudson, & Marshall, 1996) found that pedophiles scored higher than other incarcerated men on attachment anxiety and were more likely to exhibit a fearful attachment style (high anxiety combined with high avoidance). Hampering a clear conclusion on the matter, however, two other studies (Baker & Beech, 2004; Smallbone & Dadds, 1998) found no significant difference in attachment orientation between pedophiles and other criminals. Despite the conflicting results, the preponderance of supportive evidence suggests that future studies should focus on links between attachment insecurity and sexual pathology.

We do not mean to imply that insecure attachment is necessarily involved in any particular case of sexual offending. As Burk and Burkhart (2003) noted, there are contextually induced sexual offenses (e.g., a young adult with no previous history of sexual offense may molest a dating partner on a single occasion while intoxicated) that may be unrelated to the offender's attachment patterns. Moreover, we are not implying that insecure attachment is sufficient to produce sexual offenses, or that every insecure person is a potential sexual criminal. According to attachment theory, insecure attachment creates serious deficits in the regulation of emotions, goal-oriented behavior, and interpersonal exchanges, which in turn favor reliance on self-focused, controlling, coercive tactics that can lead to interpersonal conflicts, distress, and even violence (see Chapter 10, this volume). However, for sexual offenses to occur, these deficits usually have to be combined with other situational, sociocultural, and temperamental factors (e.g., lack of behavioral inhibition), as well as a particular history of sexual experiences that set the stage for violence and sexually deviant behavior (Burk & Burkhart, 2003).

CONCLUDING REMARKS

Although research on the interplay of the attachment and sexual systems is relatively new, we can already see that many predictable associations exist. Because individual differences in attachment are thought to arise developmentally, before anything like mature sexuality appears, and also because attachment measures for adolescents and adults were created and tested in numerous studies, before anyone began to connect them with an attachment-theoretical conception of the sexual behavioral system, most studies have been conceptualized in terms of the influence of attachment style on sexual motivation and behavior. Nevertheless, given that attachment style can change as a result of experiences in relationships, it seems likely that sexual experiences, beginning with sexual abuse in childhood (in cases where that occurred) and continuing through adolescence and adulthood, affect attachment security and forms of insecurity (see Chapter 5, this volume). Moreover, because sexual relations are often embedded in attachment and/or caregiving relationships, there are likely to be systematic associations and interactions between caregiving and sexuality. Certainly there are many examples in literature and film in which a person has sex with someone as a way of helping the person feel better—about life, about him- or herself, or about previous relational events. It is not difficult to imagine ways in which sexual interest and involvement can be partially motivated by compassion, empathy, and altruism. There are therefore many interesting and important issues waiting to be explored empirically, before we have a full theoretical understanding of the interplay among attachment, caregiving, and sex.

PART IV

CLINICAL AND ORGANIZATIONAL APPLICATIONS OF ATTACHMENT THEORY

CHAPTER 13

Attachment Bases of Psychopathology

Attachment theory (Bowlby, 1969/1982, 1973) was a theory of psychopathology from the start. Based on his informal preuniversity counseling experiences (see Chapter 1, this volume) and subsequent training in child psychiatry, Bowlby (1944) wondered about the etiology of juvenile delinquency in general and young "juvenile thieves" in particular, many of whom had suffered what he called "maternal deprivation" (e.g., loss of the mother, separation from the mother, inadequate mothering, poor or inconsistent care from foster parents or professionals in institutional settings). Like other psychoanalysts, including object relations theorists (e.g., Fairbairn, 1954; Klein, 1940), self psychologists (e.g., Kohut, 1977, 1984), and relational theorists (e.g., L. Aron, 1996; J. Benjamin, 1992; Blatt & Behrends, 1987), Bowlby assumed that the explanation of disordered behavior lay somewhere in childhood, especially in early relationships with primary caregivers. However, what was unique about attachment theory was its reliance on empirical evidence from a wide range of sciences and its articulation of empirically testable propositions explaining why and how early relationships contribute to mental health and psychopathology.

According to our elaboration of the theory, the broaden-and-build cycle of attachment security provides the foundation for mental health and is built from repeated experiences with loving, caring, and sensitive attachment figures. On the other side of the security coin, attachment insecurities, negative models of self and others, and both intra- and interpersonal regulatory deficits rooted in discouraging experiences with unavailable, rejecting, or neglectful attachment figures put a person at risk for psychological disorders.

In this chapter we focus on empirical associations between attachment insecurities and various forms of psychopathology. We review studies of both clinical and nonclinical samples aimed at determining whether and how attachment anxiety and avoidance in adulthood relate to proneness to distress (negative affectivity), affective disorders (depression and anxiety), posttraumatic stress disorder, suicidal tendencies, eating disorders, conduct disorders (substance abuse, criminal behavior), personality disorders, dissociative disorders, and schizophrenia. In this review, we do not attempt to follow the

DSM-IV (American Psychiatric Association, 1994) classification system or relate attachment insecurities to specific DSM-IV diagnoses. Rather, we organize the review in terms of different lines of research that have connected attachment insecurities to psychopathology. In this sense, our review is more theoretical than clinical, because we are interested in general processes rather than formal diagnoses, which tend to change over time in response to both advances in research and political battles within the mental health field.

We also discuss the salutary effects of attachment security and review evidence concerning the decrease in psychopathological symptoms produced by experimentally augmented attachment security. We extend our discussion of these therapeutic effects of secure attachment in Chapter 14, this volume, where we consider Bowlby's (1988) perspective on psychotherapy.

THEORETICAL BACKGROUND AND INITIAL QUESTIONS AND CONSIDERATIONS

According to attachment theory and research, insecurely attached people harbor serious doubts about their self-worth and self-efficacy. They lean toward hopeless and helpless patterns of causal explanation; are susceptible to rejection, criticism, and disapproval; and suffer from self-criticism and destructive perfectionism (Chapter 6, this volume). These destructive cognitive processes leave insecure people vulnerable to distress, supplying a pervasive psychological context that, according to proponents of cognitive models of psychopathology (e.g., Abramson et al., 1989; A. Beck, 1976), is conducive to demoralization and mental illness. For example, A. Beck posited that dysfunctional beliefs about self and world (e.g., "It is awful to be disapproved by others," "I am nothing if a person I love doesn't love me," or "I am nothing if I can't get A's in college") are major diatheses (vulnerabilities) for psychopathology. From an attachment perspective, these vulnerability factors emerge and are consolidated during repeatedly frustrating or emotionally damaging interactions with unsupportive and inconsistent attachment figures.

Moving from cognitions to emotions (two closely related mental states), we note that the attachment system plays an important role in emotion regulation (Chapter 7, this volume), which is necessary for mental health and deficient in most forms of psychopathology. Attachment theorists view the sense of attachment security as an inner resource for managing negative emotions and restoring emotional composure, and as a resilience factor that fosters constructive, adaptive strategies for coping with life's problems (e.g., Cassidy, 1994; Mikulincer & Shaver, 2005a; Sroufe & Waters, 1977b). As we explained in Chapter 7, these strategies reduce the impact of distressing events, allow a person to experience and acknowledge negative emotions without undue distortion or repression, and maximize the adaptive potential of emotion-related action tendencies. This ability to manage distress counters negative affectivity and sustains longer periods of positive affectivity, making it less likely that a person will succumb to maladaptive emotional states and psychopathology.

Attachment theory portrays insecure attachment as a risk factor for negative affectivity, prolonged distress, and psychopathology. Specifically, anxious attachment interferes with the down-regulation of negative emotions and encourages intense and persistent distress, which continues even after objective threats subside (Chapter 7, this volume). As a result, attachment-anxious people experience an unmanageable stream of negative thoughts and feelings that contribute to cognitive disorganization and, in some cases, culminate in psychopathology. In particular, anxious attachment fuels chronic attachment-related and attachment-unrelated worries, depressive reactions to actual or potential failures and losses, and intrusive symptoms following traumatic events (e.g., unwanted trauma-related thoughts). Moreover, problems in emotion regulation can provoke destructive outbursts of anger and impulsive behavior.

Avoidant attachment is also a source of emotional and adjustment problems (e.g., Cassidy, 1994; Shaver & Mikulincer, 2002a). Although avoidant people often maintain a defensive facade of security and composure, they do so by blocking normal emotions and leaving suppressed distress unresolved, which can impair their ability to deal with inevitable adversities (Chapter 7, this volume). This impairment is particularly likely during prolonged, demanding stressful experiences that require active confrontation of a problem and mobilization of external sources of support. In these cases, avoidant people may feel inadequate to cope and may undergo a marked decline in functioning, including what M. J. Horowitz (1982) called "avoidance-related" posttraumatic symptoms (e.g., psychic numbing, behavioral inhibition).

Insecure individuals' difficulties with behavioral self-regulation (Chapter 8, this volume) further exacerbate their vulnerability to psychopathology. Their relative inability to create effective plans, organize efforts to solve problems, inhibit interfering action tendencies, and disengage from unobtainable goals lead to repeated experiences of frustration, failure, and distress in close relationships, at school, and at work. These experiences cause insecure people to have doubts about their identity and low self-efficacy for dealing with demanding life tasks. They can become victims of a self-fulfilling and self-amplifying cycle in which problems in self-regulation reinforce negative models of self and exacerbate difficulties in emotion regulation, which in turn increase the likelihood of self-regulatory failures and difficulties in fulfilling important roles. This self-exacerbating cycle of insecurity, pessimism, frustration, and life dissatisfaction renders insecure individuals increasingly vulnerable to psychological disorders.

The destructive cycle is intensified by insecure people's problems in interpersonal regulation. As we discussed in Chapter 9, insecurely attached adults are more frequently involved in conflicts and tend to adopt maladaptive strategies of conflict resolution that aggravate rather than mitigate interpersonal distress. Moreover, their lack of interpersonal sensitivity and problems in maintaining a flexible balance between self-concern and concern for others tend to erode relationship quality and engender relationship instability and, in some cases, violence (Chapter 10, this volume). Insecure individuals' inability or unwillingness to care sensitively for a relationship partner in times of need (Chapter 11, this volume) and their sexual inhibitions and difficulties (Chapter 12, this volume) can alienate relationship partners; arouse feelings of rejection, anger, and isolation; and contribute to relationship failure. According to interpersonal theories of psychopathology (e.g., Hammen, 1991; Joiner & Coyne, 1999), these negative relationship experiences, which are attributable in part to the way insecure people relate to their partners and regulate social interactions, provide additional pathways to psychological disorders.

In other words, attachment insecurities, having, as they do, cognitive, emotional, and social–interactional aspects, predispose a person to psychological maladjustment for several reasons. Although each separate aspect of an insecure attachment style might be imagined to make specific contributions to psychopathology, they form such a densely interwoven web of cognitions, emotions, motives, behaviors, and patterns of relating to others that they may create a general vulnerability to breakdown rather than a specific dysfunctional outcome. Thus, searching for a single, or most important, mediating mechanism seems to be a fruitless task. The different difficulties seem to reinforce each other in self-expanding cycles of maladjustment, just as the broaden-and-build cycle of attachment security seems to foster overall adjustment rather than any single personal strength.

This way of thinking about the links between attachment style and mental health has important implications for psychotherapy and for evaluations of particular therapeutic interventions (see Chapter 14, this volume). Any intervention that successfully modifies one component of the web of mediators may in turn affect other components, and ultimately lead to a change in the entire network and, therefore, in the individual's mental health. This line of reasoning implies, for example, that either a cognitive intervention aimed at changing dysfunctional beliefs about the self or an interpersonal intervention aimed at changing maladaptive patterns of relatedness can produce similar therapeutic outcomes (a fact that has always bothered therapy researchers seeking to show that one method is superior to others). Just as changes in beliefs about the self can modify the regulation of emotions and interpersonal exchanges, improvements in patterns of relating to others can have beneficial effects on mental representations of self.

It is important to remember that to the extent dysfunctional beliefs and patterns of relatedness were established during interactions with inconsistent or rejecting attachment figures and were woven into a fairly consistent psychological network over many years, the pathogenic network of psychological elements will resist therapeutic change. Thus, every intervention, whether cognitive, interpersonal, or psychodynamic, should be accompanied by security-promoting interactions with the therapist and the concomitant construction of more secure working models of attachment. (In Chapter 14, we elaborate further on Bowlby's [1988] notion that a therapist should provide a safe haven and secure base for a client, like any other security-enhancing primary attachment figure.)

Beyond considering mediators of the association between attachment insecurities and psychopathology, we address three major questions concerning the pathogenic effects of attachment-system dysfunctions. First, are particular forms of attachment insecurity linked to particular forms of mental disorder? The answer to this question is likely to be "no." Interactions with inconsistent, unreliable, or insensitive attachment figures interfere with development of a solid, stable, and secure psychological foundation, interfere with all forms of healthy self-regulation, and cause a person to lack resilience in the face of stress. Such problems constitute a general vulnerability to psychological disorders, whose detailed realization in symptoms probably depends on organic and environmental factors. By the same token, the creation or restoration of a sense of attachment security during therapy should be a nonspecific source of strength that allows a broaden-and-build cycle of personal growth to occur and improves mental health almost regardless of the specific form of pathology.

We do not mean to suggest that there is no connection at all between kinds of attachment insecurity and particular forms of psychological distress or dysfunction. In fact, separation anxiety, complicated grief due to the loss of a close relationship partner, and posttraumatic reactions to physical, sexual, or psychological abuse from an attachment figure represent clear-cut cases of dysfunctions of the attachment system and can be directly linked to insecurities generated by the unavailability or insensitivity of an attachment figure. Moreover, specific attachment insecurities have been associated with specific personality disorders (as we explain later in this chapter). Whereas attachment anxiety is associated with dependent, histrionic, and borderline personality disorders, avoidant attachment is associated with more schizoid, avoidant forms of personality disorder. We are merely emphasizing the possibility that beyond these theoretically sensible connections between attachment history, particular forms of attachment insecurity, and specific mental disorders, attachment insecurities also contribute nonspecifically to many kinds of psychopathology because of their negative effects on central psychological resources; feelings such as optimism, hope, and self-worth; and intra- and interpersonal regulatory skills.

A second question is this: Can attachment insecurities by themselves produce psychopathology? Beyond specific attachment disorders in which attachment-related worries are the main cause and theme of the disorder, we doubt that attachment insecurities are sufficient causes of mental disorders. Many insecure people identified by our measures do not seem to suffer from a diagnosable mental disorder. Due to innate factors (e.g., intelligence, temperament), life history, or other environmental and socioeconomic factors, these insecure people can maintain their mental health despite relatively negative mental representations and deficits in regulatory skills. In our view, serious mental disorders result from multiple converging processes, and attachment insecurities act as catalysts of other pathogenic processes by reducing psychological and social resources, and weakening a person's resilience. For example, attachment insecurities can increase a person's likelihood of developing a psychological disorder following exposure to natural or man-made traumatic events, life transitions, or actual or anticipated loss of important material or psychological assets. Moreover, they can amplify the effects of other pathogenic factors, such as poverty, physical illnesses, and learning disabilities.

A third question: Is the link between attachment insecurity and psychopathology unidirectional? Our answer: Probably not. The causal pathway is likely to be bidirectional. Although attachment insecurities can contribute to psychological disorders, mental afflictions can also exacerbate attachment insecurity and lead to more severe attachment-system dysfunctions. In Chapter 5 we reviewed evidence that psychological vulnerabilities and disorders contribute to the intensification of attachment insecurities over time. In such cases, a disorder can be viewed as a source of stress and distress that automatically activates the attachment system and brings to mind attachment-related worries about being loved, cared for, accepted, and supported during a crisis. These worries can be amplified by the social stigma associated with psychological disorders, and the insults and ostracism that mentally ill people frequently experience, even from their closest relationship partners (e.g., Joiner & Coyne, 1999).

NEGATIVE AFFECTIVITY AND PRONENESS TO DISTRESS

Before examining attachment style connections with specific disorders, we review studies providing evidence of associations between attachment style and general proneness to distress in nonclinical populations. In these studies, the tendency to report negative moods and to complain about emotional problems and adjustment difficulties is usually called *neuroticism*—a superordinate trait in the five-factor model of personality related to experiencing unpleasant and disturbing emotions (McCrae & Costa, 1989)—or *negative affectivity*—"the extent to which a person is feeling upset or unpleasantly engaged rather than peaceful" (L. A. Clark & Watson, 1991, p. 321). Some investigators have also used self-report measures of the occurrence and severity of a broad array of psychiatric symptoms (e.g., the Symptom Checklist–90 [SCL-90] or the Mental Health Inventory) and have computed global distress scores rather than scores for particular disorders.

More than 30 studies that examined correlations between attachment measures and neuroticism scales (see Table 13.1 for a summary of methods and results) found that both major forms of attachment insecurity (anxiety and avoidance), but especially anxiety, are associated with neuroticism. Whereas all of the studies, without exception, yielded significant correlations between attachment anxiety and neuroticism, only two-thirds of them produced significant correlations with avoidance. Moreover, the correlations between attachment anxiety and neuroticism were generally higher (with a mean value around .40) than the correlations between avoidance and neuroticism (averaging around .20). These findings indicate that although anxious individuals' expression and intensification of distress, and avoidant individuals' attempts to suppress or evade distress might originally have seemed liked adaptive ways to relate to specific attachment figures, these strategies are associated later on with emotional disturbance. Additional evidence comes from three studies that found significant negative associations between security of attachment to parents and peers on the one hand, and neuroticism on the other (Beitel & Cecero; 2003; Neyer & Voigt, 2004; Wilkinson & Walford, 2001).

Conceptually similar findings were obtained in studies examining attachment-related variations in negative affectivity and psychiatric symptoms (see Table 13.2 for a summary of methods and findings). These studies focused on different age groups, ranging from adolescents to elderly adults, and sampled either undergraduates or members of the broader adult community, some of whom were experiencing stressful events (e.g., a heart attack, an abortion) or chronic stressful conditions (e.g., chronic pain, HIV-AIDS). Although most of the studies employed cross-sectional designs, some were prospective in nature and others assessed the long-term effects of attachment style on later indices of distress and negative affectivity over periods ranging from 6 months to 6 years.

The results are fairly consistent regarding the effects of attachment security. All of the studies using the Inventory of Peer and Parent Attachment (IPPA) or the Parental Attachment Questionnaire (PAQ) as measures of security found secure attachment to parents to be associated with lower levels of negative affectivity and less severe psychiatric symptomatology (see Table 13.2). Similar findings were obtained in studies examining states of mind with respect to attachment to parents (using the Adult Attachment Interview [AAI]) and self-reported attachment style in romantic relationships. In both cases, insecurely attached individuals scored higher than their more secure peers on measures of negative affectivity and general distress (Table 13.2). Torquati and Raffaelli (2004) asked undergraduates to report their emotions six or seven times a day for a week, and found that insecure people (according to the Adult Attachment Scale [AAS]) experienced more frequent and intense negative emotions than did secure people. Interestingly, this difference was strongest during everyday situations in which participants were not involved in social interaction. When alone, insecure undergraduates were more likely than their secure counterparts to feel lonely, irritable, and anxious.

Research also provides information about the emotional correlates of attachment anxiety and avoidance. Studies based on categorical measures of attachment style indicate that the anxious form of insecurity is more related to self-reported distress than is the avoidant form. With the exception of J. P. Allen, Hauser, and Borman-Spurrell's (1996) study, all of the studies summarized in Table 13.2 found that attachment-anxious people had higher negative affectivity scores and more severe psychiatric symptoms than did secure people. In contrast, the only two studies that found such a difference between avoidant and secure individuals relied on Hazan and Shaver's (1987) avoidance prototype, which seems to include elements of attachment anxiety and to tap the fearful rather

TABLE 13.1. A Summary of Findings on Attachment Orientations and the Big-Five Trait of Neuroticism

Study	Attachment measure	Personality measure	Anxiety	Avoidance
Shaver & Brennan (1992)	HS ratings	NEO-PI	+	+
J. A. Feeney et al. (1994)	ASQ	EPQ	+	ns
Griffin & Bartholomew (1994a)	RQ	NEO-PI	+	ns
Griffin & Bartholomew (1994a)	RSQ	NEO-PI	+	+
J. E. Roberts et al. (1996)	AAS	EPI	+	+
Shaver, Papalia, et al. (1996)	RQ	NEO-PI	+	ns
Buunk (1997)	HS ratings	DPQ	+	+
Becker et al. (1997)	New scale	BFM	+	+
Carver (1997, Study 3)	MAQ	NEO-FFI	+	ns
Carver (1997, Study 4)	MAQ	NEO-FFI	+	ns
Carver (1997, Study 4)	RQ	NEO-FFI	+	−
Markiewicz et al. (1997)	AAQ	NEO-PI	+	+
Mickelson et al. (1997)	HS ratings	BFM	+	+
Davila et al. (1998, Study 2)	AAS	EPQ	+	+
Davila et al. (1998, Study 2)	AAS	NEO-FFI	+	+
Moreira et al. (1998)	HS types	EPI	+	+
Mikulincer & Florian (2000, Study 5)	ECR	EPI	+	ns
Backstrom & Holmes (2001)	RSQ	NEO-PI	+	+
Davila & Bradbury (2001)	AAS	EPQ	+	+
Rholes et al. (2001)	AAQ	IPIP	+	ns
Shafer (2001)	ASQ	BBM	+	+
D. Davis & Vernon (2002)	ECR	NEO-PI	+	+
Gallo et al. (2003)	AAS	BFA	+	+
Noyes et al. (2003)	RSQ	NEO-FFI	+	ns
Bakker et al. (2004)	ASQ	FFPQ	+	−
D. Davis et al. (2004)	ECR	NEO-PI	+	+
Edelstein et al. (2004)	RSQ	NEO-PI	+	ns
Heaven et al. (2004)	AAS	IPIP	+	+
Gillath, Shaver, Mikulincer, Nitzberg, et al. (2005)	ECR	EPI	+	ns
Picardi, Toni, et al. (2005)	ECR	BFQ	+	+
Mikulincer et al. (2005, Study 3)	ECR	EPI	+	ns
Mikulincer et al. (2005, Study 4)	ECR	EPI	+	ns
Mikulincer et al. (2005, Study 5)	ECR	EPI	+	ns
Noftle & Shaver (2006, Study 1)	ECR	BFI	+	+
Noftle & Shaver (2006, Study 2)	ECR	NEO-PI	+	+

Note. (−), significant inverse correlation; (+), significant positive correlation; (ns), nonsignificant correlation; BBM, Brief Bipolar Markers; BFA, Big Five Adjectives; BFM, Big Five Markers; BFI, Big Five Inventory; BFQ, Big-Five Questionnaire; DPQ, Dutch Personality Questionnaire; EPI, Eysenck Personality Inventory; EPQ, Eysenck Personality Questionnaire; FFPQ, Five-Factor Personality Questionnaire; HS, Hazan and Shaver; IPIP, International Personality Item Pool; MAQ, Multidimensional Attachment Questionnaire; NEO-FFI, NEO Five-Factor Inventory; NEO-PI, NEO Personality Inventory.

than the dismissing form of avoidance (Brennan et al., 1991). Compatible findings were obtained in studies using continuous measures of attachment style. Whereas the vast majority of these studies turned up significant associations between attachment anxiety, negative affectivity, and psychiatric symptomatology, fewer than half found such associations with avoidant attachment (Table 13.2).

It is important to note that although attachment insecurities, mainly of the anxious variety, are related to neuroticism and negative affectivity, one should not simply collapse

TABLE 13.2. A Summary of Findings on Attachment Orientations and Measures of Negative Affectivity and Psychiatric Symptomatology (General Distress)

Study	Attachment scale	Affect/symptom scale	Main findings
Studies assessing secure attachment to parents or peers			
Armsden & Greenberg (1987)	IPPA	ASI	Security (−)
Kenny & Donaldson (1991)	PAQ	HSCL	Security (−) for W, Security (ns) for M
E. Bradford & Lyddon (1993)	IPPA	SCL-90	Security (−)
Cavell et al. (1993)	IPPA	SCL-90	Security (−)
Davila et al. (1997)*	HS ratings	SCID-Interview	Security (−)
Wilkinson & Walford (2001)	IPPA	PANAS	Security (−)
Moller et al. (2002)	ASQ	HSCL	Security (−)
Davila & Cobb (2003)*	RQ	SCID-Interview	Security (−)
Davila & Sargent (2003)*	AAS	PANAS	Security (−)
Zhang & Labouvie-Vief (2004)*	RQ	CPI	Security (−)
L. N. Johnson et al. (2003)	IPPA	OQ	Security (−)
Studies assessing attachment types			
Kobak & Sceery (1988)	AAI	SCL-90	Secure < Anxious
Dolan et al. (1993)	HS types	HSCL	Secure < Anxious, Avoidant
J. P. Allen et al. (1996)	AAI	SCL-90	Ns differences
Birnbaum et al. (1997)	HS types	MHI	Secure < Anxious
Pietromonaco & Barrett (1997)	RQ	WAI	Secure < Anxious, Fearful
Klohnen & Bera (1998)*	HS types	Q-sort	Secure < Avoidant
Meyers (1998)	HS types	Q-sort	Secure < Anxious, Avoidant
Mikulincer & Florian (1998)	HS types	MHI	Secure < Anxious, Avoidant
Mikulincer, Horesh, et al. (1998)	HS types	MHI	Secure < Avoidant < Anxious
Z. Solomon et al. (1998)	HS types	SCL-90	Secure < Avoidant < Anxious
Kemp & Neimeyer (1999)	RQ	BSI	Secure, Avoidant < Anxious, Fearful
Creasey (2002b)	AAI	BSI	Secure < Anxious
Roisman et al. (2002)	AAI	YASR	Secure < Insecure
Kerr et al. (2003)	HS types	PANAS	Secure < Anxious
E. K. Adam et al. (2004)	AAI	MPQ	Secure < Anxious
Roisman et al. (2006)	AAI	YASR	Secure < Insecure
Studies based on attachment style ratings			
J. A. Feeney & Ryan (1994)	HS ratings	MPQ	Secure (−), Anxious (+), Avoidant (ns)
Magai et al. (1995)	RQ	DES	Secure (ns), Anxious (+), Avoidant (+), Fearful (+)
Amir et al. (1999)	HS ratings	MHI	Secure (ns), Anxious (+), Avoidant (ns)
Beinstein Miller & Noirot (1999)	RQ	PANAS	Secure (−), Anxious (+), Avoidant (ns), Fearful (+)
Mikulincer & Florian (1999c)	HS ratings	MHI	Secure (−), Anxious (+), Avoidant (+)
Mikulincer et al. (1999)	HS ratings	SCL-90	Secure (−), Anxious (+), Avoidant (+)
Magai et al. (2000)	AAI (RQ)	Multiple scales	Secure (−), Anxious (+), Avoidant (−), Fearful (+)
Pielage et al. (2000)	RQ	SCL-90	Secure (−), Anxious (ns), Avoidant (ns), Fearful (+)
Leak & Cooney (2001)	RQ	Multiple scales	Secure (−), Anxious (+), Avoidant (+), Fearful (+)
Neria et al. (2001)	HS ratings	MHI, SCL-90	Secure (−), Anxious (+), Avoidant (+)
Meyers & Landsberger (2002)	HS ratings	BSI	Secure (−), Anxious (ns), Avoidant (+)
Bakker et al. (2004)	ASQ	RHS	Secure (−), Anxious (+), Avoidant (ns)
Magai et al. (2004)	RSQ	DES	Secure (ns), Anxious (+), Avoidant (ns)

(cont.)

TABLE 13.2. (*cont.*)

Study	Attachment scale	Affect/symptom scale	Main findings
Studies assessing attachment dimensions			
Griffin & Bartholomew (1994b)	RQ	3 items	Anxiety (+), Avoidance (ns)
Hardy & Barkham (1994)	RQ	SCL-90	Anxiety (+), Avoidance (+)
West et al. (1995)	RAQ	SCL-90	Anxiety (+)
Cozzarelli et al. (1998)	RQ	SCL-90	Anxiety (+), Avoidance (+)
Davila et al. (1998)	HS ratings	PANAS	Anxiety (+), Avoidance (+)
Lopez et al. (1998)	RQ	PPI	Anxiety (+), Avoidance (ns)
Berant et al. (2001a)	HS ratings	MHI	Anxiety (+), Avoidance (+)
Berant et al. (2001b)*	HS ratings	MHI	Anxiety (+), Avoidance (+)
Field & Sundin (2001)*	RAQ	SCL-90	Anxiety (+), Avoidance (ns)
McGowan (2002)	RQ	PANAS	Anxiety (+), Avoidance (ns)
Lopez et al. (2002)	ECR	HSCL, PPI	Anxiety (+), Avoidance (+)
Stein et al. (2002)	AAS, RQ	BSI	Anxiety (+), Avoidance (ns)
Moller et al. (2003)	ASQ	HSCL	Anxiety (+), Avoidance (+)
Moreira et al. (2003)	RSQ	BSI	Anxiety (+), Avoidance (ns)
Shorey et al. (2003)	ASQ	MHI	Anxiety (+), Avoidance (+)
Wearden et al. (2003)	AAS	PANAS	Anxiety (+), Avoidance (+)
Safford et al. (2004)	AAS	MASQ	Anxiety (+), Avoidance (+)
Mallinckrodt & Wei (2005)	ECR	OQ	Anxiety (+), Avoidance (+)
Vogel & Wei (2005)	ECR	HSCL	Anxiety (+), Avoidance (+)
Wearden et al. (2005)	RQ	PANAS	Anxiety (+), Avoidance (ns)
Wei, Vogel, et al. (2005)	ECR	DASS	Anxiety (+), Avoidance (+)

Note. *, longitudinal design; (–), significant inverse correlation; (+), significant positive correlation; (ns), nonsignificant effects; M, men; W, women; ASI, Affective Status Index; BSI, Brief Symptom Inventory; CPI, California Personality Inventory; DASS, Depression, Anxiety, and Stress Scales; DES, Differential Emotion Scale; HS, Hazan and Shaver; HSCL, Hopkins Symptom Checklist; MASQ, Mood and Anxiety Symptom Questionnaire; MHI, Mental Health Inventory; MPQ, Multidimensional Personality Questionnaire; OQ, Outcome Questionnaire; PANAS, Positive and Negative Affect Scale; PPI, Personal Problems Inventory; RHS, RAND Health Survey; SCL-90, Symptom Checklist-90; WAI, Weinberger Adjustment Inventory; YASR, Young Adult Self-Report.

these constructs into a single distress category. There is more to attachment insecurity than its overlap with negative affectivity (see Chapter 4, this volume). Moreover, as detailed in previous chapters, measures of attachment insecurity contribute statistically to variance in behavioral self-regulation, interpersonal regulation, relationship quality, and the functioning of other behavioral systems even after measures of neuroticism and negative affectivity have been statistically controlled. (The converse is rarely the case in the studies we reviewed; that is, neuroticism rarely explains variance in other variables, at least in studies related to the attachment domain, after measures of attachment insecurity have been considered.) Safford, Alloy, Crossfield, Morocco, and Wang (2004) reported that even the effects of attachment anxiety and avoidance on depression, a prime form of "negative affectivity," could not be fully accounted for by individual differences in general negative affectivity.

We therefore continue to view attachment insecurities as different from negative affectivity. The former are more likely to be relevant when social relationships and social aspects of personality are considered. Negative affectivity, in contrast, may be due to a combination of inherited temperament and personal experiences, including, but not limited to, negative relationships with attachment figures. In the latter case, attachment insecurities may be viewed as predisposing factors for negative affectivity that arises in response to threats and life stresses.

AFFECTIVE DISORDERS: DEPRESSION AND ANXIETY

The theoretical links between attachment insecurities and the development of depression and anxiety disorders were formulated by Bowlby (1973, 1980) in the second and third volumes of his attachment trilogy. With regard to depression, Bowlby (1980) suggested that the loss of attachment security during infancy, childhood, or adolescence contributes to the development of later depression. This loss, which can result from either the death of a primary attachment figure or repeated failure to form a secure relationship with a caregiver, encourages the formation of pessimistic, hopeless representations of self and world. Moreover, an "abandoned" child is likely to feel powerless and helpless in attempting to keep a dead or neglectful parent present or to gain support, love, approval, or admiration from an inconsistently responsive or rejecting parent. (A. Green [1986] referred to these childhood cognitions and feelings as "the dead mother complex," because although the mother is not literally, physically dead, she is emotionally absent or unavailable to the child.) Bowlby (1980), like the authors of cognitive models of depression (e.g., Abramson et al., 1989; A. Beck, 1976), believed that these childhood cognitions and feelings are conducive to depression, especially when an insecure individual encounters subsequent losses, traumatic events, or hardships.

According to Bowlby (1973), attachment figure unavailability and the resulting attachment insecurities can also be transformed into anxiety disorders, because the attachment system has failed to accomplish its basic protective function, and the unsupported child feels unsafe while navigating and exploring the world. For insecure individuals, the world is a dangerous place, full of unexpected threats and perils, and devoid of a safe haven or secure base. Moreover, insecure individuals (mainly those who are consciously anxious) who harbor serious doubts about their ability to cope alone with threats and dangers are burdened with remaining constantly vigilant with respect to potential threats (see Chapters 6 and 7, this volume). These core beliefs and feelings can heighten fearful reactions to threats and challenges, and the tendency to escape from or evade potential threats—the clinically familiar fear and avoidance components of most anxiety disorders (American Psychiatric Association, 1994).

Depression and Anxiety in Nonclinical Samples

Bowlby's ideas have received strong support from longitudinal studies of the long-term effects of negative attachment-related experiences in childhood on affective disorders in adulthood. For example, Harris, Brown, and Bifulco (1990) found that death of a parent or prolonged separations from a parent in early childhood heightened the risk of depression in adulthood. This association between early traumatic attachment experiences and later depression seems to be stronger among people who had insecure working models prior to the loss (Cummings & Cicchetti, 1990) and among those who experienced inadequate, insensitive care following the traumatic event (Harris, Brown, & Bifulco, 1986). There is also evidence that prolonged separations from parents, parental divorce, or extremely inadequate caregiving during childhood are associated with heightened risk for agoraphobia or panic disorder in adolescence and adulthood, as originally suggested by Bowlby (G. W. Brown & Harris, 1993; Faravelli, Webb, Ambronetti, Fonnesu, & Sesarego, 1985). In addition, several studies have found that adults with depression or anxiety disorders, compared with healthy controls, tend to describe their parents as more rejecting, unavailable, and unsupportive (e.g., Cassidy, 1995; Enns, Cox, & Clara, 2002; Gotlib, Mount, Cordy, & Whiffen, 1988).

More than 100 studies have examined associations between adult attachment and the severity of depression and anxiety symptoms, as assessed by self-report scales (e.g., Beck Depression Inventory [BDI], Spielberger's State–Trait Anxiety Inventory [STAI]) or interview (e.g., the Structured Clinical Interview for DSM-IV [SCID]) in nonclinical samples (see Tables 13.3 and 13.4 for a summary of methods and findings). As can be seen in Tables 13.3 and 13.4, security of attachment to parents or peers, secure states of mind with regard to attachment (assessed with the AAI), and endorsement of a secure attachment style in close relationships are consistently related to lower levels of depression and anxiety (however, notice that three studies summarized in Table 13.3 found no significant association between AAI classification and depression). Also, without exception, studies show that a preoccupied state of mind in the AAI, endorsement of an anxious (categorical) attachment style in close relationships, or higher ratings of attachment anxiety on self-report scales are associated with depression and anxiety. With regard to avoidant attachment, the picture is less consistent, but around half of the studies concluded that avoidant individuals suffer from depression and anxiety more than do secure individuals. Of importance, depression and anxiety are more consistently associated with fearful avoidance than with dismissing avoidance, suggesting that the anxious or fearful aspects of fearful avoidance are linked with vulnerability to depression and general anxiety.

It is worth noting that although attachment anxiety is more strongly associated with depression than is avoidant attachment, researchers who have assessed multiple facets of depression report that this difference is less evident when examining the contribution of each attachment dimension to particular depressive symptoms (Batgos & Leadbeater, 1994; Davila, 2001; Murphy & Bates, 1997; Zuroff & Fitzpatrick, 1995). In these studies, both attachment anxiety and avoidance were associated with depression, but the two dimensions differed with respect to which forms or facets of depression they predicted. Whereas attachment anxiety is related to interpersonal aspects of depression, such as overdependence, lack of autonomy, and neediness (the form of depression that Blatt [1974] called *anaclitic*), avoidance is related to achievement-related aspects of depression, such as perfectionism, self-punishment, and self-criticism (which Blatt called *introjective depression*). On the one hand, anxious individuals' hyperactivation of their attachment systems favors overdependence and lack of autonomy (see Chapter 9, this volume), which in turn contributes to interpersonal forms of depression. On the other hand, avoidant individuals' extreme and compulsive self-reliance favors unrealistic positive appraisals of self (see Chapter 6, this volume), which in turn contribute to self-criticism and depression when an individual receives external feedback that he or she is weak, mistaken, or imperfect.

Because most of the studies summarized in Tables 13.3 and 13.4 were based on cross-sectional designs, their findings may indicate either that attachment insecurities are conducive to depression and anxiety or that these disorders can erode attachment security. Although the second possibility is plausible (see Chapter 5, this volume), studies using prospective designs have found that attachment insecurities predict subsequent increases in depression over periods of time ranging from 1 month to 2 years (see Tables 13.3 and 13.4). In addition, Haaga et al. (2002) showed that whereas attachment insecurity predicts variations in depression over time, the experimental manipulation of either elated or depressed mood does not significantly affect subsequent reports of attachment insecurities. Similarly, Roisman, Fortuna, and Holland (2006) found that experimental inductions of elated or depressed mood did not affect subsequent states of mind with respect to attachment (secure–insecure classification based on the AAI). These mood inductions produced differences in the valence (degree of positivity or negativity) of par-

TABLE 13.3. A Summary of Findings on Attachment Orientations and Depression in Nonclinical Samples

Study	Attachment scale	Depression scale	Main findings
Studies assessing secure attachment to parents or peers			
Berman & Sperling (1991)	New scale	BDI	Security (−)
Papini et al. (1991)	IPPA	CDI	Security (−)
Cotterell (1992)	IPPA	BDI	Security (−)
de Jong (1992)	IPPA	BSI	Security (−)
Nada-Raja et al. (1992)	IPPA	DISC-C	Security (−)
Papini & Roggman (1992)	IPPA	CDI	Security (−)
Kenny et al. (1993)	PAQ	CDI	Security (−)
Papini & Roggman (1993)	IPPA	CES-D	Security (−)
Kenny & Perez (1996)	PAQ	HSCL	Security (−)
Styron & Janoff-Bulman (1997)	HS ratings	BDI	Security (−)
Gittleman et al. (1998)	RQ	CES-D	Security (−)
Kenny et al. (1998)*	PAQ	CDI	Security (−)
Noom et al. (1999)	IPPA	6 items	Security (−)
Laible et al. (2000)	IPPA	CDI	Security (−)
Vivona (2000, Study 1)	IPPA	BDI	Security (−)
Vivona (2000, Study 2)	IPPA	BDI	Security (−)
Engels-Rutger et al. (2001)	IPPA	DML	Security (−)
Muris et al. (2001)	IPPA	CDI	Security (−)
Lopez & Gormley (2002)*	RQ	CES-D	Security (−)
Wautier & Blume (2004)	ASQ	BDI	Security (−)
Zhang & Labouvie-Vief (2004)*	RQ	CES-D	Security (−)
Studies assessing attachment types			
Kobak et al. (1991)*	AAI	DPI	Secure < Insecure
Mikulincer et al. (1993)	HS types	SCL-90	Secure < Anxious
Pearson et al. (1993)	AAI	CES-D	Secure < Insecure
Radecki-Bush et al. (1993)	HS types	BDI	Secure < Anxious, Avoidant
Pearson et al. (1994)	AAI	CES-D	Secure < Insecure
Kobak & Ferenz-Gillies (1995)	AAI	DPI	Secure < Anxious
Priel & Shamai (1995)	HS types	BDI	Secure < Anxious, Avoidant
Cole-Detke & Kobak (1996)	AAI	CES-D	Secure < Anxious
Salzman (1996)	Interview	CES-D	Secure < Anxious
Cooper et al. (1998)	HS types	SCL-90	Secure < Avoidant < Anxious
Torquati & Vazsonyi (1999)	AAS	BDI	Secure < Insecure
Bosquet & Egeland (2001)	AAI	CES-D	Ns differences
Muris et al. (2001)	HS types	CDI	Secure < Anxious
Ciechanowski, Walker, et al. (2002)	RSQ	MHI	Secure < Anxious, Avoidant, Fearful
Riggs & Jacobvitz (2002)	AAI	CES-D	Secure > Avoidant for W but not M
E. K. Adam et al. (2004)	AAI	BDI	Ns differences
Dickstein et al. (2004)	AAI	BDI	Secure < Insecure
		SCID-Interview	Secure < Insecure
Treboux et al. (2004)	AAI, CRI	BDI	Secure < Insecure
DeOliveira et al. (2005)	AAI	CES-D	Secure < Avoidant, Unresolved
Tarabulsy et al. (2005)	AAI	CES-D	No significant differences
Studies based on attachment style ratings			
J. E. Roberts et al. (1996, Study 1)	HS ratings	IDD	Secure (−), Anxious (+), Avoidant (+)
Mickelson et al. (1997)	HS ratings	CDI	Secure (−), Anxious (+), Avoidant (+)
Murphy & Bates (1997)	RQ	BDI	Secure (−), Anxious (+), Avoidant (ns), Fearful (+)
Shapiro & Levendosky (1999)	AAS	CDI	Secure (−), Anxious (+), Avoidant (+)
Davila (2001, Study 2)*	Interview	SCID-Interview	Secure (−), Anxious (+), Fearful (+)
Onishi et al. (2001)	ECR	GBI	Secure (−), Anxious (+), Avoidant (ns), Fearful (+)
Haaga et al. (2002, Study 1)	RQ	BDI	Secure (−), Anxious (+), Avoidant (ns), Fearful (ns)
R. L. Scott & Cordova (2002)	HS ratings	BDI	Secure (−), Anxious (+), Avoidant (ns) for W
			Secure (−), Anxious (+), Avoidant (+) for M
Wayment & Vierthaler (2002)	ASQ	SCL-90	Secure (−), Anxious (+), Avoidant (+)
Davila et al. (2004, Study 1)	RQ	IDD	Secure (ns), Anxious (+), Avoidant (ns), Fearful (ns)
Davila et al. (2004, Study 2)*	Interview	SCID-Interview	Secure (−), Anxious (+), Avoidant (ns), Fearful (ns)
S. Reis & Grenyer (2004, Study 2)	RQ	BDI	Secure (−), Anxious (+), Avoidant (ns), Fearful (+)

(cont.)

TABLE 13.3. (*cont.*)

Study	Attachment scale	Depression scale	Main findings
Studies based on attachment style ratings (cont.)			
Heene et al. (2005)	AAS	SCL-90	Secure (−), Anxious (+), Avoidant (+)
Irons & Gilbert (2005)	HS ratings	CDI	Secure (−), Anxious (+), Avoidant (+)
Irons et al. (2006)	RQ	CES-D	Secure (−), Anxious (+), Avoidant (ns), Fearful (+)
Studies assessing attachment dimensions			
Carnelley et al. (1994, Study 1)	RQ	CES-D	Anxiety (+), Avoidance (+)
Hammen et al. (1995)*	AAS	SCID-Interview	Anxiety (+), Avoidance (+)
Whisman & McGarvey (1995)	INVAA	BDI	Anxiety (+), Avoidance (ns)
J. E. Roberts et al. (1996, Study 2)*	AAS	IDD	Anxiety (+), Avoidance (+)
J. E. Roberts et al. (1996, Study 3)*	AAS	IDD	Anxiety (+), Avoidance (+)
Burge et al. (1997)	AAS	SCID-Interview	Anxiety (+), Avoidance (ns)
West et al. (1998)	RAQ	CES-D	Anxiety (+)
Torquati & Vazsonyi (1999)	AAS	BDI	Anxiety (+), Avoidance (+)
Whiffen et al. (1999)	AAS	BDI	Anxiety (+), Avoidance (+)
Cozzarelli et al. (2000)	RQ	BDI	Anxiety (ns), Avoidance (ns)
Oliver & Whiffen (2003)	AAS	BDI	Anxiety (+), Avoidance (+)
Whiffen et al. (2000)	AAS	BDI	Anxiety (+), Avoidance (+)
Davila (2001, Study 1)	AAS, RQ	BDI	Anxiety (+), Avoidance (+)
R. DeFronzo et al. (2001)	RSQ-avoidance	BDI	Avoidance (+)
Lopez et al. (2001)	ECR	DACL	Anxiety (+), Avoidance (ns)
Reese-Weber & Marchand (2002)	AAS-anxiety	CES-D	Anxiety (+)
Williamson et al. (2002)	RQ	CES-D	Anxiety (+), Avoidance (+)
Besser & Priel (2003)	RQ	CES-D	Anxiety (+), Avoidance (ns)
Simpson et al. (2003)	AAQ	CES-D	Anxiety (+), Avoidance (+)
Strodl & Noller (2003)	ASQ	BDI	Anxiety (+), Avoidance (+)
Wei et al. (2003)	AAS	BDI	Anxiety (+), Avoidance (+)
Bifulco et al. (2004)	ASI	SCID-Interview	Anxiety (+), Avoidance (+)
Marchand (2004)	AAS	CES-D	Anxiety (+), Avoidance (ns) for W Anxiety (+), Avoidance (+) for M
Marchand et al. (2004)	AAS	CES-D	Anxiety (+), Avoidance (ns) for W Anxiety (+), Avoidance (+) for M
Pesonen et al. (2004)	AAS, RQ	CES-D	Anxiety (+), Avoidance (+)
Safford et al. (2004)	AAS	BDI	Anxiety (+), Avoidance (+)
Treboux et al. (2004)	ECR	BDI	Anxiety (+), Avoidance (+)
Wei, Russell, et al. (2004)	ECR	DASS	Anxiety (+), Avoidance (+)
Wei, Mallinckrodt, et al. (2004)	ECR	BDI	Anxiety (+), Avoidance (+)
Williams & Riskind (2004)	ECR	BDI	Anxiety (+), Avoidance (+)
Besser & Priel (2005)	RQ	CES-D	Anxiety (+), Avoidance (ns)
Carmichael & Reis (2005)	ECR	CES-D	Anxiety (+), Avoidance (+) for W Anxiety (+), Avoidance (ns) for M
Gamble & Roberts (2005)	AAS	IDD	Anxiety (+), Avoidance (+)
Hankin et al. (2005, Study 1)*	AAS	IDD	Anxiety (+), Avoidance (+)
Hankin et al. (2005, Study 2)*	AAS	IDD	Anxiety (+), Avoidance (+)
Hankin et al. (2005, Study 3)*	AAQ	BDI	Anxiety (+), Avoidance (+)
Maunder et al. (2005)*	ECR	CES-D	Anxiety (+), Avoidance (+)
Picardi, Mazzoti, et al. (2005)*	ECR	ZDS	Anxiety (ns), Avoidance (+)
Shaver et al. (2005, Study 1)	ECR	CES-D	Anxiety (+), Avoidance (ns)
Shaver et al. (2005, Study 2)	ECR	CES-D	Anxiety (+), Avoidance (ns)
Wei, Mallinckrodt, et al. (2005)	ECR	CES-D	Anxiety (+), Avoidance (+)
Wei, Russell, & Zakalik (2005)*	ECR	CES-D	Anxiety (+), Avoidance (ns)
Wei, Shaffer, et al. (2005)	ECR	ZDS, CES-D	Anxiety (+), Avoidance (+)
Whiffen (2005)*	ECR	CES-D	Anxiety (+), Avoidance (+)
Rholes et al. (2006)	AAQ	CES-D	Anxiety (+), Avoidance (+)
Wei, Heppner, et al. (2006)	ECR	CES-D	Anxiety (+), Avoidance (+)

Note. *, longitudinal design; (−), significant inverse correlation; (+), significant positive correlation; (ns), nonsignificant effects; M, men; W, women; BDI, Beck Depression Inventory; BSI, Brief Symptom Inventory; CDI, Children's Depression Inventory; CES-D, Center for Epidemiological Studies—Depression; DACL, Depression Adjectives Checklist; DASS, Depression, Anxiety, and Stress Scales; DISC-C, Diagnostic Interview Schedule for Children; DML, Depressive Mood List; DPI, Depression Personality Inventory; GBI, General Behavior Inventory; HS, Hazan and Shaver; HSCL, Hopkins Symptom Checklist; IDD, Inventory to Diagnose Depression; MHI, Mental Health Inventory; SCL-90, Symptom Checklist–90; ZDS, Zung Depression Scale

TABLE 13.4. Summary of Findings on Attachment Orientations and Measures of Different Kinds of Anxiety

Study	Attachment scale	Anxiety scale	Main findings
Studies assessing secure attachment to parents or peers			
Papini et al. (1991)	IPPA	CMAS	Security (–)
Nada-Raja et al. (1992)	IPPA	DISC-C	Security (–)
Papini & Roggman (1992)	IPPA	CMAS	Security (–)
Kenny & Perez (1996)	IPPA	HSCL	Security (–)
Gittleman et al. (1998)	RQ	STAI	Security (–)
Laible et al. (2000)	IPPA	CMAS	Security (–)
Vivona (2000, Studies 1–2)	IPPA	BAI	Security (–)
Muris et al. (2001)	IPPA	SCAS	Security (–)
Wautier & Blume (2004)	RQ	BAI	Security (–)
Studies assessing attachment types			
Mikulincer et al. (1993)	HS types	SCL-90	Secure < Anxious
Priel & Shamai (1995)	HS types	STAI	Secure < Avoidant < Anxious
Cooper et al. (1998)	HS types	SCL-90	Secure < Anxious, Avoidant
Torquati & Vazsonyi (1999)	AAS	STAI	Secure < Insecure
Muris et al. (2001)	HS types	SCAS	Secure < Anxious, Avoidant
Muris & Meesters (2002)	HS types	SCAS	Secure < Anxious, Avoidant
E. K. Adam et al. (2004)	AAI	IPAT	Secure < Anxious
Studies based on attachment style ratings or dimensions			
Doi & Thelen (1993)	AAS	STAI	Anxious (+), Avoidant (+)
Burge et al. (1997)*	AAS	SCID-Interview	Anxious (+) Avoidant (ns)
Mickelson et al. (1997)	HS ratings	SCID-Interview	Secure (–), Anxious (+), Avoidant (+)
Thelen et al. (1998)	AAS	STAI	Anxious (+), Avoidant (+)
R. DeFronzo et al. (2001)	RSQ-avoidance	STAI	Avoidant (ns)
Lopez et al. (2001)	ECR	STAI	Anxious (+) Avoidant (+)
Onishi et al. (2001)	ECR	KAS	Secure (–), Anxious (+), Avoidant (ns), Fearful (ns)
Sheehan & Noller (2002)	ASQ	STAI	Anxious (+) Avoidant (ns)
Weems et al. (2002)	ECR	SCL-90	Anxious (+) Avoidant (+)
Strodl & Noller (2003)	ASQ	MIA	Anxious (+) Avoidant (ns)
Wei et al. (2003)	AAS	STAI	Anxious (+) Avoidant (+)
Safford et al. (2004)	AAS	BAI	Anxious (+) Avoidant (+)
Sonnby-Borgstrom & Jonsson (2004)	RSQ	STAI	Anxious (+) Avoidant (ns)
Wei, Russell, et al. (2004)	ECR	DASS	Anxious (+) Avoidant (+)
Williams & Riskind (2004)	ECR	BAI	Anxious (+) Avoidant (+)
Costa & Weems (2005)	ECR	SCl-90	Anxious (+) Avoidant (ns)
Hankin et al. (2005, Study 1)*	AAS	STAI	Anxious (+) Avoidant (+)
Hankin et al. (2005, Study 2)*	AAS	STAI	Anxious (+) Avoidant (+)
Hankin et al. (2005, Study 3)*	AAQ	MASQ	Anxious (+) Avoidant (+)
Irons & Gilbert (2005)	HS ratings	SCAS	Secure (–), Anxious (+), Avoidant (+)
Picardi, Mazzoti, et al. (2005)*	ECR	STAI	Anxious (+) Avoidant (ns)
Watt et al. (2005)	ECR	ASI	Anxious (+) Avoidant (ns)

Note. *, longitudinal design; (–), significant inverse correlation; (+), significant positive correlation; (ns), nonsignificant effects; ASI, Affective Status Index; BAI, Beck Anxiety Inventory; CMAS, Children's Manifest Anxiety Scale; DASS, Depression, Anxiety, and Stress Scales; DISC-C, Diagnostic Interview Schedule for Children; HS, Hazan and Shaver; HSCL, Hopkins Symptom Checklist; IPAT, Institute for Personality and Ability Testing; KAS, Kaiser Anxiety Scale; MASQ, Mood and Anxiety Symptom Questionnaire; MIA, Mobility Inventory for Agoraphobia; SCAS, Spence Children's Anxiety Scale; SCL-90, Symptom Checklist–90; STAI, State–Trait Anxiety Inventory.

ticipants' memories of early interactions with their mothers (recalled during the AAI) but not in the coherence with which these memories were reported. (As we explained in Chapter 4, the AAI is scored primarily in terms of discourse coherence rather than semantic content.)

In a further attempt to overcome the limitations of cross-sectional designs, we recently conducted a study in which we experimentally manipulated attachment-related mental representations and examined their effects on anxiety symptoms. Specifically, we focused on spider phobia and examined whether the contextual activation of attachment-related mental representations affects a frequently observed phobic response—the tendency to avoid spider-related stimuli whenever possible (e.g., Thorpe & Salkovskis, 1995). The study comprised two sessions. In the first session, at the beginning of a semester, 160 Israeli undergraduates completed the Experiences in Close Relationships (ECR) Anxiety and Avoidance scales and the Spider Phobia Questionnaire (SPQ; Watts & Sharrock, 1984). According to their total SPQ scores, two groups of participants were selected to participate in the second session. One group—the phobic group ($N = 40$)—included participants who scored above the 75th percentile on spider phobia. The other group—the nonphobic group ($N = 40$)—included participants who scored below the 25th percentile. Two to 3 weeks later, the 80 participants were invited to an experimental session in which we contextually primed representations of attachment security (visualizing a supportive, caring relationship partner, $N = 28$), representations of attachment insecurity (visualizing a rejecting, nonsupportive relationship partner, $N = 24$), or neutral representations (visualizing a drugstore clerk, $N = 28$). All participants then viewed a series of 12 pictures on a computer monitor and were told that they would be asked questions about each picture at the end of the session. Participants advanced through the pictures at their own pace by pressing the space bar on the keyboard when they wanted to move to the next picture. The set of pictures included four pictures of spiders and eight neutral pictures (e.g., flowers, horses). Avoidance of spider pictures was calculated by averaging the viewing time for the spider pictures while covarying the time spent viewing neutral pictures (to control for variation in general viewing times).

The phobic participants had a shorter mean viewing time for spider pictures than the nonphobic participants, which is the typical phobic response, but the effect was qualified by a significant interaction with visualization condition. Compared to visualization of a neutral attachment figure, visualization of a security-enhancing figure led phobic participants to show less aversion to spider pictures (see Figure 13.1). No significant difference between experimental (attachment visualization) conditions was found among nonphobic participants. Thus, the activation of attachment security representations seemed to counter phobic symptoms.

Figure 13.1 reveals another important difference between visualization conditions: Visualization of a rejecting (insecurity-inducing) attachment figure led to stronger aversion responses (shorter viewing times for spider pictures) than visualization of a neutral figure among phobic participants. This effect was not significant among nonphobic participants; that is, the tendency of phobic participants to view spider pictures for a shorter time (relative to nonphobic participants) was intensified following the visualization of a rejecting figure. It seems that the contextual activation of attachment insecurities strengthens phobic avoidance symptoms.

There were also significant associations (1) between attachment anxiety and spider phobia (SPQ score) in the total sample [$r(158) = .39$, $p < .01$], and (2) between attachment anxiety and avoidance, and shorter viewing time of spider pictures among phobic participants [$r(38) = .43$, $p < .01$; $r(38) = .34$, $p < .05$]. Taken together, the experimental and correlational findings indicate that attachment insecurities are involved in the generation of phobic symptomatology and that the restoration of attachment security can have healing effects on phobic people (see Chapter 14, this volume for further discussion of the therapeutic implications).

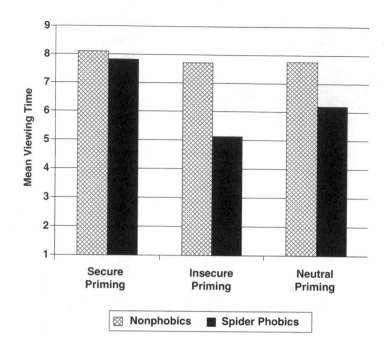

FIGURE 13.1. Mean viewing time for spider pictures (in seconds) as a function of priming conditions and intensity of spider phobia.

Depression and Anxiety in Special and Clinical Samples

The contribution of attachment insecurities to the development of affective disorders has also been documented in special populations whose low socioeconomic status (SES), stressful life history, poor physical health, or psychiatric status put them at risk for depression. Specifically, insecure states of mind with respect to attachment (according to the AAI) and higher scores on self-report measures of attachment anxiety or avoidance have been associated with more severe symptoms of depression in samples of high-risk women (Bifulco, Moran, Ball, & Bernazzani, 2002; Bifulco, Moran, Ball, & Lillie, 2002; McCarthy, 1999), patients with chronic pain (Ciechanowski, Sullivan, Jensen, Romano, & Summers, 2003), patients with diabetes (Ciechanowski et al., 2001; Ciechanowski, Katon, & Russo, 2005), HIV-positive patients (Ciesla et al., 2004), violent incarcerated men (Rankin et al., 2000), and outpatients with eating disorders, drug abuse, or social anxiety (Eng, Heimberg, Hart, Schneier, & Liebowitz, 2001; Miljkovitch et al., 2005). Some of these studies go beyond cross-sectional correlations to show that attachment insecurities prospectively predict an increase in severity of depression over a 1-year period (Bifulco, Moran, Ball, & Bernazzani, 2002; Ciechanowski et al., 2003, 2005).

Similar associations have been found in studies assessing postpartum depression (Besser, Priel, & Wiznitzer, 2002; Bifulco et al., 2004; J. A. Feeney, Alexander, Noller, & Hohaus, 2003; McMahon, Barnett, Kowalenko, & Tennant, 2005; Meredith & Noller, 2003; Simpson, Rholes, Campbell, Tran, & Wilson, 2003). In these studies, women's attachment anxiety (assessed during pregnancy or soon after delivery) prospectively predicted more severe postnatal depression over periods ranging from 6 to 9 months. Only one study (Besser et al., 2002) found a significant association between women's avoidant attachment and postpartum depression.

Using self-report attachment scales, studies with samples of clinically depressed patients shed further light on the link between attachment insecurities and depression. For example, a blend of attachment anxiety and avoidance (Bartholomew's [1990] fearful avoidant pattern) has been associated with more severe depressive symptomatology among people diagnosed with depression (Carnelley et al., 1994, Study 2; DiFilippo & Overholser, 2002; Reinecke & Rogers, 2001; S. Reis & Grenyer, 2004, Study 1). Attachment insecurities have also been prevalent in samples of women with recurrent depression (Cyranowski et al., 2002) and outpatients with dysthymia—a mild but chronic unipolar depression (West & George, 2002). Furthermore, as compared to control groups (nonpatients or patients with other psychiatric disorders), outpatients or inpatients diagnosed with a major depressive episode reported higher levels of attachment insecurities, and were less likely to endorse a secure style description and more likely to endorse a fearful avoidant style description (Armsden et al., 1990; Cawthorpe, West, & Wilkes, 2004; Haaga et al., 2002, Study 2; Myhr, Sookman, & Pinard, 2004; Pettem, West, Mahoney, & Keller, 1993; S. Reis & Grenyer, 2004, Study 3; Rosenfarb, Becker, & Khan, 1994; Whiffen, Kallos-Lilly, & MacDonald, 2001). Similarly, Eng et al. (2001) found that outpatients diagnosed with social anxiety reported higher levels of attachment anxiety and avoidance than age-matched nonclinical participants.

Using the AAI, five studies found a prevalence of insecure states of mind with respect to attachment in patients with clinically diagnosed depression (Cole-Detke & Kobak, 1996; Fonagy et al., 1996; Patrick et al., 1994; Rosenstein & Horowitz, 1996; Tyrrell & Dozier, 1997). Similarly, Manassis, Bradley, Goldberg, Hood, and Swinson (1994) found that women outpatients diagnosed with anxiety disorder were more likely than age-matched nonclinical women to be classified as insecure by the AAI. However, the findings are less consistent with respect to the type of insecurity that is more prevalent in depressed patients: Whereas some studies indicate that depression is associated with a preoccupied state of mind (Cole-Detke & Kobak, 1996; Fonagy et al., 1996; Rosenstein & Horowitz, 1996), other studies find depression to be more associated with a dismissing state of mind (Patrick, Hobson, Castle, Howard, & Maughan, 1994; Tyrrell & Dozier, 1997).

According to Dozier, Stovall, and Albus (1999), this discrepancy might be due to differences in defining the "depressed" group. For example, Rosenstein and Horowitz (1996) excluded depressed patients who were comorbid for antisocial disorders—a kind of disorder that is consistently associated with avoidant attachment (as discussed later in this chapter). This exclusion might explain why these researchers found a higher prevalence of attachment anxiety than avoidance in the "pure" depressed group. In contrast, Patrick et al. (1994) excluded patients who met any criterion for borderline personality disorder—a disorder associated with attachment anxiety (see the "Personality Disorders" section of this chapter)—and found a higher prevalence of avoidance than anxiety in the depressed group.

Beyond these methodological differences, it is important to note that Fonagy et al. (1996) and Tyrrell and Dozier (1997) found that different subtypes of depression were related to different states of mind with respect to attachment (assessed with the AAI). Whereas patients with bipolar or schizoaffective types of depression exhibited a relatively high rate of dismissing attachment, patients with a major depressive episode were more likely to exhibit a secure state of mind. According to Fonagy et al. (1996), an acute episode of depression can be a temporary reaction to a traumatic loss rather than the product of core attachment insecurities. These insecurities seem to be more conducive to chronic depressive disorders.

Mediating, Moderating, and Dyadic Factors

Attachment studies have also begun to reveal some of the mediators of the association between attachment style and affective disorders. Findings obtained to date implicate a network of interrelated cognitive, coping, and interpersonal processes by which attachment insecurities render a person vulnerable to depression or anxiety. Among the cognitive mechanisms, research has revealed a mediating role for low self-esteem (e.g., Hankin, Kassel, & Abela, 2005; J. E. Roberts, Gotlib, & Kassel, 1996), low self-efficacy expectancies (e.g., Mallinckrodt & Wei, 2005; Strodl & Noller, 2003), perceptions of lack of social support (e.g., Vogel & Wei, 2005; Simpson, Rholes, Campbell, Tran, et al., 2003), maladaptive perfectionism (e.g., Wei, Mallinckrodt, Russell, & Abraham, 2004), self-splitting (Lopez, Mitchell, & Gormley, 2002), and hopelessness (e.g., Hankin et al., 2005; Roberts et al., 1996).

There is also evidence for mediation by various emotion regulation processes. For example, attachment style and affective disorders are connected through pessimistic expectations about emotional control (e.g., Creasey, 2002b; Strodl & Noller, 2003; Williams & Riskind, 2004) and difficulties in problem solving (e.g., Lopez et al., 2001; Wei et al., 2003). Moreover, whereas the association between attachment anxiety and affective disorders is partially explained by heightened reliance on emotion-focused coping, the association between avoidance and these disorders is mediated by heightened reliance on distancing coping, high levels of emotional control, and reluctance to engage in support seeking (e.g., Berant et al., 2001a; Birnbaum et al., 1997; Cozzarelli et al., 1998; Kotler et al., 1994; Wei, Vogel, et al., 2005).

Research also indicates that interpersonal difficulties, such as lack of emotional expressiveness, problems in assertiveness, excessive reassurance seeking, inability to meet closeness and autonomy needs, and feelings of loneliness, act as additional mediating paths between attachment insecurities and affective disorders (e.g., Engels-Rutger, Finkenauer, Meeus, & Dekovic, 2001; Shaver et al., 2005; Wei, Russell, & Zakalik, 2005; Wei, Shaffer, et al., 2005). For example, Hankin et al. (2005, Study 3) reported that negative interpersonal events (e.g., relationship breakups, divorce) during a 2-year period mediated the prospective effects of attachment anxiety and avoidance on later depression. Specifically, more attachment-anxious and avoidant individuals reported more negative interpersonal events over the 2 years, which in turn increased the incidence of depression during that period.

Adult attachment studies have also begun to reveal personal and contextual factors that mitigate or exacerbate attachment style influences on affective disorders. For example, Wautier and Blume (2004) found that a stable sense of personal identity mitigated the differences between secure and insecure adolescents in depression and anxiety, and R. L. Scott and Cordova (2002) reported that marital satisfaction dramatically weakened the detrimental effects of spouses' attachment insecurities on severity of depression. In addition, there is solid evidence that supportive husbands can reduce the likelihood of postpartum depression among anxiously attached wives (J. A. Feeney et al., 2003; Simpson, Rholes, Campbell, Tran, et al., 2003). Specifically, anxiously attached women (compared with more secure women) did not show heightened postpartum depression when they perceived more support and less anger from their husbands (Simpson, Rholes, Campbell, Tran, et al., 2003), or when husbands themselves reported more effective support of their wives during pregnancy (J. A. Feeney et al., 2003). Thus, it seems that husbands' emotional support eases anxious wives' sense of threat or danger (allowing them to feel more secure), which in turn protects the wives from postpartum depression.

Following this reasoning, one might argue that a partner's sense of attachment security, which can favorably influence his or her supportive behavior (see Chapter 11, this volume), can also mitigate the link between a target spouse's attachment insecurity and vulnerability to depression; that is, a chronically insecure person may not suffer from depression if he or she lives with a secure partner who provides a reliable safe haven and secure base. Indeed, Volling et al. (1998) found that a husband's security dramatically weakened the link between his wife's attachment insecurity and depression. However, this kind of dyadic process did not explain a husband's depression (Volling et al., 1998), and it has not always been replicated in other studies of married couples (e.g., Carmichael & Reis, 2005; Davila, Bradbury, & Fincham, 1998).

In a sample of couples that included a depressed wife, Whiffen et al. (2001) found that husbands' security predicted a reduction in wives' depressive symptoms 6 months later. In contrast, husbands' avoidant attachment predicted the maintenance of wives' depressive symptoms over the 6-month period. According to Whiffen et al., the lack of warmth, affection, and care provided by an avoidant husband may confirm his depressed wife's feelings of unlovability, thereby maintaining or even exacerbating her attachment anxieties and associated depression. Whiffen (2005) replicated these findings and confirmed the hypothesized dyadic causal pathway in an Internet study of husbands' depression. Path analyses revealed that wives' avoidant attachment led husbands to perceive their wives as less responsive and to report higher levels of attachment anxiety, which in turn predicted increased depression 3 months later. Taken together, these findings highlight the importance of both partners' attachment orientations for an understanding of the links between attachment insecurity and depression: Whereas a secure partner can break the maladaptive cycle of attachment insecurities and depression in his or her mate, an avoidant partner seems to sustain or even exacerbate the maladaptive cycle.

Studies also indicate that personal-history factors that deepen attachment-related doubts heighten the association between attachment insecurities and affective disorders. For example, the link between attachment insecurities and depression is strengthened by a history of childhood physical, psychological, or sexual abuse (e.g., Shapiro & Levendosky, 1999; Styron & Janoff-Bulman, 1997; Whiffen, Judd, & Aube, 1999). The link is also made stronger by stressful life events, physical health problems, and involvement in stormy romantic relationships during adolescence (e.g., Besser et al., 2002; Davila et al., 2004; Hammen et al., 1995). At the same time, these studies also reveal that secure attachment in adulthood can buffer the detrimental effects of these risk factors for depression; that is, childhood abuse, stressful events, health problems, and relationship problems fail to increase the risk of depression among secure people.

TRAUMA AND POSTTRAUMATIC STRESS DISORDER

Traumatic experiences, such as rape, assault, car accidents, floods, war, and a host of other natural and man-made disasters, mobilize internal and external resources for coping with stress, and they place people at risk for short- and long-term mental health and adjustment problems (see M. J. Horowitz, 1982, for a review). In some cases emotional balance is restored shortly after a traumatic event ends, but in other cases there may be profound and prolonged mental health sequelae, including posttraumatic stress disorder (PTSD), which is characterized by repeated reexperiencing of a traumatic event (unwanted intrusion of trauma-related material into thoughts, mental images, and dreams), numbing of responsiveness to or reduced involvement with the external world (trauma-related avoidance), and autonomic, affective, and cognitive indications of hyperarousal (American Psychiatric Association, 1994).

Individual differences in attachment-system functioning play an important role in determining the extent to which PTSD ensues following exposure to trauma. Optimal functioning of the attachment system can allow even a severely threatened person to feel relatively safe and secure, thereby decreasing the likelihood of long-term PTSD. A secure person's internal mental cry for help during distress often results in mobilization of internal representations of security-providing attachment figures and/or actual external sources of support, which in turn sustain optimistic and hopeful beliefs and constructive strategies of affect regulation. In other words, the sense of attachment security acts, at least to an extent, as a protective shield against PTSD.

By the same token, nonoptimal functioning of the attachment system can interfere with restoration of emotional equanimity following traumas, thereby increasing the chances of PTSD. In such cases, a traumatized person's failure to find inner representations of security or external sources of support may interfere with distress regulation. This regulatory failure can initiate a cascade of mental events, including strong feelings of loneliness and rejection, as well as negative working models of self and others, intensification of distress, and reliance on less effective (hyperactivating or deactivating) strategies of affect regulation, which prevents resolution of the trauma and enhances the likelihood of PTSD.

Variations in attachment-system functioning can also affect the specific form that PTSD takes. According to M. J. Horowitz (1982), PTSD is characterized by two kinds of intrapsychic symptoms: intrusion and avoidance. "Intrusion" refers to unwanted and uncontrollable thoughts, images, emotions, and nightmares related to the traumatic event (sometimes called "flashbacks"). "Avoidance" refers to psychic numbing, denial of the significance and consequences of the traumatic event, and behavioral inhibition. Intrusion is generally experienced immediately after the trauma, but the two states can alternate during the posttraumatic period, until successful "working through" of the trauma is achieved (M. J. Horowitz, 1982).

Attachment-related mental processes are important in regulating the intensity and frequency of posttraumatic intrusion and avoidance tendencies. On the one hand, secure attachment can help people work through trauma, reducing the frequency and intensity of both intrusions and avoidance responses. On the other hand, insecure attachment may leave a person insufficiently equipped for working through the trauma. Anxious attachment facilitates reactivation of the traumatic experience and the frustrated cry for help, which encourage what M. J. Horowitz (1982) called "intrusion responses." Avoidant attachment predisposes a traumatized person to deny the trauma and evade direct or symbolic confrontation with trauma reminders, thereby encouraging posttraumatic avoidance responses.

The first systematic attempt to document attachment-style differences in the severity of PTSD symptoms concerned reactions of young adults to Iraqi Scud missile attacks on Israel during the 1991 Gulf War (Mikulincer, Florian, & Weller, 1993). In this study, Israeli undergraduates were approached 2 weeks after the end of the Gulf War and asked to complete a series of self-report measures of attachment style and PTSD symptoms. Compared with participants who had a secure attachment style, participants with an anxious style had more severe PTSD intrusion and avoidance symptoms, and participants with an avoidant attachment style reported more severe posttraumatic avoidance responses.

The association between insecure attachment and PTSD symptom severity has also been observed among adults who were sexually or physically abused as children (P. C. Alexander et al., 1998; Muller & Lemieux, 2000; Muller, Sicoli, & Lemieux, 2000; Roche et al., 1999; Shapiro & Levendosky, 1999; Twaite & Rodriguez-Srednicki, 2004). For example, Twaite and Rodriguez-Srednick found that adults with histories of childhood sexual or physical abuse reacted with more severe PTSD reactions to the terrorist attack on the World Trade Center in New York if they were less securely attached. Attachment insecurities have also been found to contribute to heightened PTSD symptoms among Israeli military veterans who suffered from combat stress reactions during the 1973 Yom Kippur War (Dekel, Solomon, Ginzburg, & Neria, 2004), and among former prisoners of war (POWs) in both the United States and Israel (Dieperink, Leskela, Thuras, & Engdahl, 2001; Z. Solomon et al., 1998; Solomon, & Neria, 2003). In a prospective study of high-exposure survivors of the terrorist attacks on the World Trade Center, Fraley, Fazzari, Bonanno, and Dekel (2006) found that both attachment anxiety and avoidance, as assessed by self-report scales 7 months after the attack, predicted more severe PTSD symptoms and depression 11 months later. Moreover, friends and relatives viewed attachment-anxious survivors as displaying decreased adjustment 7 months after the attacks.

In another study, Kanninen, Punamaki, and Qouta (2003) examined the association between attachment insecurities and PTSD among 176 Palestinian former political prisoners living in the Gaza Strip. The statistical association was observed mainly among political prisoners who had been exposed to high levels of physical torture and ill-treatment. In this group, participants classified as anxious or avoidant in an interview (based on the AAI) reported more severe PTSD symptoms than did participants classified as secure. This difference was not significant among prisoners who had been exposed to high levels of psychological torture involving interpersonal cruelty. It seems that secure attachment acted as a protective safeguard against the development of PTSD following physical torture, but was less effective when the torture was interpersonal and involved the shattering of positive working models. Perhaps this kind of torture creates or activates negative representations of self and others that successfully undermine the protection provided by a previously secure attachment style.

Although these correlational findings are compatible with attachment theory, they do not necessarily reveal a causal connection between attachment-related processes and the formation and course of PTSD: They did not include assessment or manipulation of the cognitive accessibility of attachment-related representations during or following trauma, and attachment style was not measured until after the traumatic experience. Hence, psychological processes other than those related to attachment might explain the observed associations between attachment style and PTSD.

Recently, however, Mikulincer, Shaver, and Horesh (2006) reported two studies that examined the causal role of attachment-related processes in the development of PTSD. One study focused on Israelis' psychological reactions during the 2003 U.S.–Iraq War and examined the effects of global, dispositional attachment orientations measured before the war on the intensity of trauma-related intrusion and avoidance symptoms during the war. These symptoms were assessed daily for 21 days. In addition, each participant's feelings of being comforted, supported, and connected to others (i.e., context-specific feelings of attachment security) were also assessed daily throughout the same period, so that we could examine the extent to which the actual or symbolic mobilization of security-providing figures during the traumatic period moderated the detrimental effects of global attachment anxiety and avoidance on trauma-related symptoms.

Findings indicated that both dispositional and contextual attachment-related processes shaped daily responses to the trauma of war. From a personality perspective, chronically insecure people were found to suffer from more severe, war-related PTSD than did chronically secure people, with anxiously attached people exhibiting more war-related intrusion symptoms, and avoidant people showing more war-related avoidance responses. From a contextual perspective, the sense of attachment security on a given day weakened the severity of war-related intrusion and avoidance responses that day and the next. Moreover, this contextual activation weakened the link between dispositional attachment anxiety and PTSD; that is, the sense of feeling comforted and connected to others on a given day allowed anxiously attached people to react to the trauma of war with fewer mental intrusions than usual. However, this daily activation of attachment security failed to weaken the detrimental effects of avoidant attachment on trauma-related avoidance symptoms. It seems possible, in our view, that avoidant people's deactivating strategies continue to operate even when actual or symbolic attachment figures are available and supportive. These findings highlight the potential healing effects of attachment security, especially for anxiously attached people, and encourage further research on effective interventions for people who are dispositionally avoidant.

Our second study, which focused on Palestinian terrorist attacks on Israeli cities, examined whether global and contextual, attachment-related representations affect implicit responses to trauma (Mikulincer, Shaver, & Horesh, 2006). These responses were assessed in terms of the cognitive accessibility of trauma-related mental representations in a Stroop color-naming task. Cognitive accessibility was operationalized by the time needed to name the color in which a trauma-related word was printed: The higher the latencies for naming the colors of these words, the higher the accessibility of trauma-related thoughts was inferred to be, because such thoughts apparently interfered with color naming. Previous researchers who considered longer reaction times for naming the colors of trauma-related words to reflect implicit PTSD responses have found that individuals suffering from posttraumatic symptoms take longer to name the colors of trauma-related words (for extensive reviews, see Emilien et al., 2000; R. J. McNally, 1998).

Israeli undergraduates, who had previously completed the ECR measure of attachment style, filled out a self-report scale tapping the severity of PTSD symptoms with regard to Palestinian terrorist attacks and were divided into two groups (PTSD, non-PTSD) according to the reported severity of their symptoms. On a later occasion they performed a Stroop color-naming task, which included words connoting terror (e.g., *Hamas, car bomb*), as well as negatively valenced words not related to terror and emotionally neutral words. On each trial, participants were subliminally primed with an attachment security word (the Hebrew word for being loved), a positively valenced but attachment-unrelated word (*success*), or a neutral word (*hat*).

The results replicated previous findings about the accessibility of trauma-related thoughts among people with PTSD symptoms. Participants in the PTSD group produced longer color-naming latencies for terror words (indicating greater automatic accessibility of the words) than did participants in the non-PTSD group. More important, the findings also indicated that the attachment system influenced implicit, trauma-related responses. First, higher scores on the ECR Anxiety and Avoidance scales were associated with longer color-naming latencies for terror words among people with PTSD symptoms. Second, symbolic mobilization of attachment security representations ("being loved") during the Stroop task (security priming) had a soothing effect, lowering the accessibility of trauma-related thoughts among people who usually suffered from PTSD symptoms, and countering the detrimental effects of attachment anxiety on the accessibility of these thoughts. However, security priming failed to reduce the detrimental effects of avoidant attachment. The link between avoidance and longer color-naming responses for terror words was significant in all three priming conditions, suggesting that avoidant people's implicit trauma-related vulnerability remained active even when comforting attachment representations were available.

Overall, the findings support the hypothesis that mobilizing external or internal forms of felt security during traumatic and posttraumatic periods reduces the intensity of PTSD symptoms, which helps to explain why chronically secure people are less likely than their insecure counterparts to develop PTSD. The studies also show that traumatized individuals respond favorably to actual support offered by familiar others in their immediate environment and to the contextual manipulation of their sense of attachment security. Beyond preventing PTSD, attachment security may also contribute to the reconstruction of comforting, health-sustaining beliefs shattered by trauma—an example of what Tedeschi and Calhoun (2004) called "posttraumatic growth." In fact, attachment security has already been associated with cognitive openness and creative exploration of personal experiences (see Chapters 7 and 8, this volume), qualities that Tedeschi and Calhoun view as important contributors to posttraumatic growth.

SUICIDAL TENDENCIES

Suicidal ideation and behavior are relatively common in adolescence and young adulthood. In the United States, suicide is the third leading cause of death among adolescents and young adults, and statistics indicate that the youth suicide rate tripled between the mid-1950s and the mid-1990s (National Center for Health Statistics, 1995). A wide variety of developmental, familial, personality, and contextual factors have been identified as increasing the risk for suicidal ideation and behavior (Orbach, 1997). Among these factors are familial conditions that disrupt attachment-system functioning, such as parental death or parental unavailability, as well as core aspects of attachment insecurity, such as negative models of self and others, hopelessness, perfectionism, self-criticism, and overwhelming mental pain (Orbach, 1997). However, surprisingly few studies have examined the risk of suicide from an attachment perspective.

In a rare theoretical exploration of the role of attachment processes in suicidal behavior, K. S. Adam (1994) proposed a developmental model by which attachment insecurities in infancy and childhood serve as distal risk factors for later suicidal ideation, through their effects on self-representations, emotion regulation, and interpersonal difficulties. More specifically, adverse early attachment experiences and resulting attachment insecurities are theorized to lead to low self-esteem, pessimism, and hopelessness and to hinder an adolescent's ability to develop a stable sense of identity, form satisfying and stable close relationships, and effectively manage stress and distress. (All of these concomitants of attachment insecurity have been discussed in previous chapters of this book.) When this vulnerable state of mind is coupled with an adolescent's current experiences of loss, rejection, or disappointment, the experience is transformed, according to K. S. Adam, into an attachment crisis, accompanied by overwhelming distress and maladaptive defensive reactions that can move a person to self-destruction. K. S. Adam also argued that the sense of attachment security should act as a protective resilience factor during crises and facilitate crisis resolution.

An analysis of the mental states and psychological dynamics that underlie suicide attempts reinforces the hypothesis that attachment insecurities are involved in these destructive acts. In some cases, suicide attempts represent a cry for help, care, and attention, as well as a signal that a person is unable to cope autonomously with hardships and distress (Orbach, 1997). From an attachment perspective, this kind of suicidal behavior is an extreme case of anxious hyperactivation of the attachment system. For anxious individuals, suicide can be a possible means of gaining others' love, compassion, and attention, when other, more adaptive signaling methods have failed to capture the attention of unresponsive and unavailable attachment figures. In other cases, suicide attempts represent a hostile, guilt-inducing reaction to significant others or a protest against social isolation, alienation, and identity diffusion (Orbach, 1997). These kinds of suicide attempts constitute extreme cases of avoidant deactivation of the attachment system, which can lead to not only avoidance of closeness and interdependence but also rejection of other people and even of life itself. In other words, suicidal behavior can be either an extreme form of anxious hyperactivation or an extreme form of avoidant deactivation, hostility, and detachment.

Although no systematic research has examined the etiological role of attachment insecurities in suicidal ideation and behavior, some correlational, cross-sectional studies provide valuable preliminary information about the association between attachment style and suicidality in clinical and nonclinical samples. DeJong (1992) found that undergraduates with a history of serious suicidal thoughts or suicide attempts reported less secure attachment to parents (on the IPPA) than did depressed undergraduates with no history of suicidality and control undergraduates who were not depressed and reported no suicidal tendencies. Furthermore, West, Spreng, Rose, and Adam (1999) and DiFilippo and Overholser (2000) found a link between insecure attachment to parents and suicidal ideation among adolescent psychiatric inpatients. DiFilippo and Overholser also found that the link between attachment insecurity and suicidality was mediated by depression; that is, insecure attachment contributed to depression, which in turn was the best predictor of suicidal thoughts.

Using the AAI, K. S. Adam, Sheldon-Keller, and West (1996) assessed state of mind with respect to attachment among adolescents in psychiatric treatment, and compared adolescents with histories of suicidal ideation and behavior to those without any indication of suicidality. They found a higher prevalence of preoccupied attachment (preoccupied state of mind in the AAI) among suicidal than among nonsuicidal patients. Moreover, suicidal patients displayed higher levels of disorganization in reasoning when discussing an attachment-related trauma (e.g., parental death, childhood abuse) and were more likely to be classified as suffering from unresolved trauma (about losses or abuse).

Similar associations were found in a community sample of expectant parents (Riggs & Jacobvitz, 2002). Participants classified as preoccupied in the AAI or as unable to resolve an attachment-related trauma were more likely than participants classified as secure to report suicidal ideation. Lessard and Moretti (1998) also found that attachment anxiety (assessed with a modified version of the Family Attachment Interview used by Bartholomew and Horowitz, 1991) was associated with more frequent and more severe suicidal ideation, and greater lethality in methods of contemplated suicide in a sample of adolescents in psychiatric treatment. Overall, the findings consistently link attachment insecurities, mainly anxious and disorganized attachment, with suicidal thoughts and acts.

EATING DISORDERS

Eating disorders, including both anorexia nervosa and bulimia nervosa, are prevalent among adolescent and young adult women in modern Western societies. Whereas anorexia is characterized by a compulsive drive for thinness, fears of becoming fat, and attempts to reduce body weight (e.g., through prolonged fastening), bulimia is character- ized by binge eating and attempts to compensate for bingeing by purging (e.g., vomiting) and taking laxatives (American Psychiatric Association, 1994). Eating disorders are thought to develop as a result of biological predispositions, sociocultural influences, developmental challenges, personality factors, and family dynamics, and they show a strong comorbidity with depression and personality disorders (e.g., Bruch, 1973; Zerbe, 1993).

Within attachment theory, dysfunctional eating behavior and attempts to control weight, like other psychiatric disorders, are associated with negative self-representations and problems in the regulation of distress and interpersonal relations (e.g., O'Kearney, 1996; A. Ward, Ramsay, & Treasure, 2000). Consistent with this general proposition, Cole-Detke and Kobak (1996) argued that eating disorders stem from a history of nega- tive interactions with attachment figures and are a behavioral manifestation of avoidant deactivating attempts to divert attention from attachment-related distress. According to these authors, eating- and weight-related concerns are defensive methods of directing attention to external, attachment-unrelated problems and goals and to compensate for feelings of helplessness, insignificance, and vulnerability by exerting control over food intake and body weight. Cole-Detke and Kobak therefore expected a relatively high prev- alence of avoidant attachment among patients with eating disorders.

While agreeing that eating disorders result from frustrating interactions with reject- ing attachment figures, other theorists have argued that these disorders are a behavioral reflection of anxious attachment. Specifically, eating disorders are viewed by these theo- rists as symbolic means to gain proximity, love, and care from unavailable mothers (Orzolek-Kronner, 2002) or to perpetuate an infantile, dependent position by remaining thin and retaining a child-like body (Bruch, 1973; Masterson, 1977; Palazzoli, 1978). According to Masterson (1977), the attachment insecurities of young women with eating disorders are focused on fears of abandonment and rejection and ambivalence concerning autonomy and separation from attachment figures (the core themes of anxious attach- ment), which are resolved by avoiding physical maturity, thereby delaying independent psychological functioning. In our view, both goals—externalizing attachment insecurities and perpetuating anxious dependency—may be implicit in eating disorders depending on a person's preexisting tendencies to deactivate or hyperactivate the attachment system.

The hypothesized involvement of attachment insecurities in eating disorders has received ample empirical support. Kenny and Hart (1992), Chassler (1997), and Orzolek- Kronner (2002) used self-report measures of attachment to parents (e.g., the IPPA or PAQ) and found that female patients with a clinical diagnosis of anorexia or bulimia reported less secure attachment to parents than an age-matched group of healthy women. This difference was also documented by Gutzwiller, Oliver, and Katz (2003), who assessed attachment to parents and eating disorder symptoms (using the Eating Disorder Inventory; EDI) in a sample of undergraduate women. Also, using the Separation Anxiety Test (SAT), Armstrong and Roth (1989) studied 27 women with eating disorders who had been referred to an inpatient unit, and found that 96% of them were characterized by anxious attachment and severe difficulties with separation.

Using the AAI, Cole-Detke and Kobak (1996) found more insecure states of mind among college women scoring high on the EDI (with or without depression) than among women who scored low on both eating disorders and depression. However, whereas an avoidant state of mind was prevalent in women scoring high on eating disorders without depression, an anxious state of mind was prevalent among those who reported having both eating disorders and depression. Ramacciotti et al. (2001) and A. Ward et al. (2001) also reported relatively high avoidance (on the AAI) in small samples of inpatient women diagnosed with eating disorders (N's of 13 and 20, respectively), but Fonagy et al. (1996) found that 13 of 14 inpatients diagnosed with eating disorders in their sample were classified on the AAI as unresolved with respect to trauma or abuse. Interestingly, Candelori and Ciocca (1998) reported that anxious and avoidant states of mind on the AAI were differentially related to particular eating disorders. Whereas patients with anorexia tended to be more avoidant, those with bulimic behaviors of bingeing and purging tended to be more anxiously attached. However, although these differential associations fit with the suppressive, needs-denying nature of deactivating strategies and the chaotic, self-gratifying, and uncontrollable nature of hyperactivating strategies, they were reported in only one small sample of Italian adolescents, so they should be regarded as only suggestive.

Adult attachment studies have also shown that self-reports of attachment anxiety and avoidance in close relationships are associated with eating disorders. Across different countries (England, Israel, Italy, Sweden, the United States) and using different attachment scales, researchers consistently find that outpatient and inpatient women with eating disorders score higher than nondisordered control women on attachment anxiety and/or avoidance (Admoni, 2006; Broberg, Hjalmes, & Nevonen, 2001; Friedberg & Lyddon, 1996; Hochdorf, Latzer, Canetti, & Bachar, 2005; Latzer, Hochdorf, Bachar, & Canetti, 2002; Mallinckrodt, McCreary, & Robertson, 1995; Troisi, Massaroni, & Cuzzolaro, 2005; A. Ward, Ramsay, Turnbull, Benedettini, & Treasure, 2000). Studies have also shown that attachment anxiety and avoidance are associated with more severe eating disorder symptoms and weight concerns in both community and undergraduate samples of women (Brennan & Shaver, 1995; L. Evans & Wertheim, 1998, 2005; Salzman, 1997; Sharpe et al., 1998). Although all of these studies relied on cross-sectional designs that do not permit confident conclusions about the etiological role of attachment insecurities in eating disorders, Burge et al. (1997) found that attachment insecurities (assessed with the IPPA or the AAS) prospectively predicted more severe eating disorder symptoms 12 months later in a sample of female high school students.

In an initial attempt to provide at least some evidence concerning the causal involvement of attachment style in eating disorders, Admoni (2006) conducted two laboratory experiments assessing two frequently observed cognitive aspects of these disorders: heightened preoccupation with food and the body (e.g., Ben Tovim & Walker, 1991), and distorted body image (e.g., Wolszon, 1998). In one study, inpatient women diagnosed with eating disorders and a control group of age-matched healthy women performed a Stroop task, while Admoni measured color-naming latencies (i.e., indicators of cognitive accessibility) for words related to food and body shape. In the other study, a second sample of inpatient women with eating disorders and age-matched, healthy controls performed a computer-based task assessing body image distortions (Harari, Furst, Kiryati, Caspi, & Davidson, 2001). Each participants was presented with a realistic pictorial simulation of life-like weight changes in a picture of herself taken in a previous research session, and was asked to adjust her body shape using a graphical user interface, until the image seemed accurate. In both studies, participants were subliminally primed with either a security-promoting stimulus (the name of a security provider) or the name of a close person or acquaintance who did not fulfill attachment figure functions (e.g., safe haven or secure base). In this way, Admoni (2006) examined whether the contextual activation of attachment security counteracts cognitive components of eating disorders.

In a replication of past findings, Admoni noted heightened access to thoughts about food or body shape (longer latencies in the Stroop color-naming task) and more severe distortions of body image in the eating disordered groups than in the control groups. In addition, attachment anxiety and avoidance (assessed with the ECR) were associated with longer color-naming latencies for words related to food and body shape, and more body image distortions among patients diagnosed with eating disorders, emphasizing the association between attachment insecurities and cognitive manifestations of eating disorders. More important, compared to neutral priming conditions, subliminal priming with security-related names reduced these dysfunctional cognitive responses in patients with eating disorders and dramatically reduced the differences between their performance and that of control women. These findings support a causal interpretation of the linkage between attachment and eating disorders. Combined with previous findings reviewed in this chapter, they suggest a generally healing, soothing, or protective role for attachment security in relation to various forms of psychopathology.

CONDUCT DISORDERS, SUBSTANCE ABUSE, AND CRIMINAL BEHAVIOR

Adult attachment researchers have also examined connections between attachment insecurities and conduct disorders, and problems in social adjustment, such as delinquency, alcoholism, and drug abuse. Interestingly, as we mentioned at the beginning of this chapter and in Chapter 1, Bowlby's original interest in attachment processes began with juvenile delinquency. In a paper entitled "Forty-Four Juvenile Thieves: Their Characters and Home Life," Bowlby (1944) concluded that frustrating and painful experiences with parents result in what he called an "affectionless" character marked by distrust and hostility toward parents and other caregivers, as well as a pervasive lack of empathy and compassion. However, because intense hatred and hostility toward parents may be dangerous or disturbing, the dysfunctional feelings and frustrations may be redirected to other socialization agents, individuals, or institutions, without causing guilt, sorrow, or remorse. In this way, insecure attachment can lead to conduct disorders and socially deviant or criminal behavior.

The link between attachment insecurities and conduct disorders can be conceptualized in terms of dysfunctional uses of secondary attachment strategies. Attachment-anxious individuals can engage in disordered conduct and delinquency as crude means of crying out for attention and care, including from attachment figures (J. P. Allen, Moore, Kuperminc, & Bell, 1998; M T. Greenberg & Speltz, 1988). Avoidant individuals can engage in antisocial behavior as a means of denying the importance of attachment relationships and gaining distance from unresponsive parents (J. P. Allen, Moore, & Kuperminc, 1997; J. P. Allen et al., 2002). Furthermore, avoidant individuals' distrust and hostility can interfere with acceptance of social norms and constraints. Fonagy et al. (1997) described a developmental trajectory in which avoidant children's attempts to gain cognitive and affective distance from frustrating attachment figures reduce their amenability to socialization and interfere with internalization of parental norms and other prosocial codes of behavior.

These paths from attachment insecurities to conduct disorders have also been mentioned in psychodynamic and sociological writings about criminal behavior. For example, Mawson (1980) contended that violent and homicidal behavior often results from a compulsive tendency to gain the attention and care of otherwise unresponsive relationship partners. From a sociological perspective, Hirschi (1969) contended that criminal behavior results from weak ties to the social system, including lack of commitment to conventions and norms, lack of involvement in normative activities, absence of prosocial beliefs, and detachment from parents and schools. The rejection of parental norms and expectations can be based on either affectionless distancing from attachment figures (as in the case of avoidant people) or an angry, vengeful reaction to parental unavailability (in the case of anxiously attached people).

Both avoidant and anxious forms of insecure attachment can also encourage substance abuse. Avoidant individuals, who attempt to detach themselves from psychological distress, can use alcohol and drugs as a means of avoiding painful emotions and self-awareness. Attachment-anxious individuals, who have problems with emotional control, can use alcohol and drugs to pacify or tranquilize their distress and block the uncontrollable spread of anxious ruminations and memories. These defensive functions of substance abuse have been extensively documented in psychological research (e.g., Hull, Young, & Jouriles, 1986).

Attachment studies have turned up cross-sectional associations between adolescents' reports of insecure attachment to parents or peers and involvement in delinquent behaviors, such as theft and assault (e.g., McElhaney, Immele, Smith, & Allen, 2006; Wade & Brannigan, 1998) and approval of norm-violating behavior (Silverberg, Vazsonyi, Schlegel, & Schmidt, 1998). In addition, insecure attachment to parents or peers is associated with higher levels of alcohol consumption, cigarette smoking, and drug abuse in community samples of adolescents (e.g., Bailey & Hubbard, 1990; J. DeFronzo & Pawlak, 1993; Foshee & Bauman, 1994; J. M. Lee & Bell, 2003; Walsh, 1992). This finding has been replicated in a sample of juvenile delinquents (Elgar, Knight, Worrall, & Sherman, 2003) and in a prospective study of adolescent adjustment (Burge et al., 1997). Specifically, insecure attachment in relationships with peers predicted heightened substance use 12 months later. These findings are consistent with studies assessing the quality of parenting or family relationships and finding strong links between enmeshment in the family, low cohesiveness in the family, or "affectionless control" by parents on the one hand, and adolescent children's delinquency and substance abuse on the other (e.g., J. M. Lee & Bell, 2003; Maunder & Hunter, 2001).

Evidence also links insecure states of mind (measured by the AAI) with conduct disorders and deviant behavior. For example, Levinson and Fonagy (2004) compared AAI classifications of 22 imprisoned delinquents with those of 22 patients with personality disorders without a criminal history and 22 healthy controls. They noted a greater prevalence of avoidant attachment and lower levels of reflective function (emotion-related metacognition) in the delinquent group than in the other groups. Moreover, delinquents who had committed violent offenses (e.g., murder, malicious wounding) exhibited greater deficits in reflective function than those who committed nonviolent acts (e.g., theft). In a related study, van IJzendoorn et al. (1997) interviewed 40 male criminal offenders who suffered from mental disorders and found that 95% of the delinquents exhibited insecure states of mind. Similar findings were reported in studies conducted with adolescent psychiatric inpatients (e.g., J. P. Allen et al., 1996; Fonagy et al., 1996; Rosenstein & Horowitz, 1996) and psychopathic incarcerated offenders (e.g., Frodi, Dernevik, Sepa, Philipson, & Bragesjo, 2001).

Although AAI studies indicate more insecure attachment among delinquents, no single insecure AAI classification (avoidant, anxious, or unresolved) has been linked consistently to conduct disorders in both community and clinical samples. Whereas some studies have found that conduct disorders are associated with an avoidant (dismissing) state of mind in the AAI (J. P. Allen et al., 1996; Caspers, Cadoret, Langbehn, Yucuis, &

Troutman, 2005; Riggs & Jacobvitz, 2002; Rosenstein & Horowitz, 1996), others have found an association between these disorders and an anxious (preoccupied) state of mind (J. P. Allen et al., 1998, 2002; Caspers et al., 2005; Fonagy et al., 1996; Marsh, McFarland, Allen, McElhaney, & Land, 2003; McElhaney et al., 2006).

The association between an anxious state of mind and deviant behavior seems to depend on other personal and relational factors. For example, Rosenstein and Horowitz (1996) found that anxious attachment is particularly common among substance abusers diagnosed with depression. Furthermore, J. P. Allen et al. (1998, 2002) and Marsh et al. (2003) found that attachment anxiety was associated with deviant behavior during adolescence and predicted delinquency 2 years later, mainly when mothers did not respond sensitively to their offspring's anxious needs for dependence, guidance, and assistance (low maternal control, high maternal autonomy promotion). In fact, Marsh et al. found that a combination of attachment anxiety and low maternal autonomy promotion predicted depression. Thus, it seems likely that anxious attachment predisposes adolescents to psychopathology, but the specific form of pathology (conduct disorder or depression) depends on non-normative maternal behavior characterized by over- or underpromotion of autonomy.

Using self-report attachment scales, several studies have found that both attachment anxiety and avoidance are related to antisocial tendencies, criminal behavior, and substance abuse in samples of adolescents and young adults (Cooper et al., 1998; Doyle & Markiewicz, 2005; Gwadz, Clatts, Leonard, & Goldsamt, 2004; Muris et al., 2003; Smallbone & Dadds, 2000) and in a nationally representative U.S. sample (Mickelson et al., 1997). Again, the findings do not allow simple conclusions about the relative importance of different forms of attachment insecurity. Some studies find that only avoidance is significantly associated with conduct disorders (Brennan & Shaver, 1995; Burge et al., 1997; Senchak & Leonard, 1992; Vungkhanching et al., 2004); others, that only anxiety is significantly associated with these disorders (Magai, 1999; A. M. McNally, Palfai, Levine, & Moore, 2003; Gwadz et al., 2004). Presumably, the inconsistencies are due to differences in measures, samples, and unmeasured variables.

As with many other attachment studies, most of the ones we review in this section have relied on cross-sectional designs that cannot provide solid information about causal directions and pathways. However, Burge et al. (1997) found that avoidant attachment among high school girls prospectively predicted heightened substance abuse a year later, even after controlling for initial levels of psychiatric symptomatology. A. L. Miller et al. (2002) assessed attachment orientations twice over a 1-year period during adolescence, and found that adolescents who classified themselves as secure at both time points also reported less frequent delinquent behavior than those who classified themselves as insecure at both points, or who changed their attachment classification during the 1-year period.

The link between self-reports of attachment insecurity and deviant behavior has also been documented in special and clinical populations. For example, Andersson and Eisemann (2004) and Schindler et al. (2005) asked patients who were substance abusers and a group of healthy controls to complete self-report attachment scales. These authors found that substance abusers were more anxious and avoidant, on average. Finzi-Dottan et al. (2003) asked a sample of men with a long history of drug abuse to complete Hazan and Shaver's (1987) measure of attachment style, and found that the majority chose insecure styles (73%), mainly the avoidant type, and Ireland and Power (2004) found that avoidant offenders were more likely to be perpetrators of bullying in prison.

Research also reveals some of the motives associated with insecure people's proneness to substance abuse. In studies assessing motives for drinking, anxiously attached people report using alcohol to cope with anxiety, tension, and distress (Brennan & Shaver, 1995; Magai, 1999; McNally et al., 2003). Avoidant people are more likely to say they drink to avoid emotional dependence (Brennan & Shaver, 1995) or to enhance positive mood (Magai, 1999). Cooper et al. (1998) provided some evidence concerning the role of attachment strategies in mediating the association between insecure attachment and deviant behavior. Attachment-anxious people's deviant behavior was mainly explained by intensified feelings of depression and hostility. Avoidant people's deviant behavior was better explained by deactivating strategies that inhibited involvement in social interactions and close relationships.

PERSONALITY DISORDERS

According to the fourth edition of the *Diagnostic and Statistical Manual of Mental Disorders* (DSM-IV; American Psychiatric Association, 1994), personality disorders are characterized by "enduring pattern(s) of inner experience and behavior that deviate markedly from the expectations of the individual's culture, (are) pervasive and inflexible, (have) an onset in adolescence or early adulthood, (are) stable over time, and (lead) to distress or impairment" (p. 629). Whereas some of the disorders are characterized by disturbed patterns of cognition (e.g., schizotypal personality disorder) and others are characterized by dysregulated emotions (e.g., borderline personality disorder), a common central feature of virtually all personality disorders is persistent difficulty with interpersonal relations (Widiger & Frances, 1985). For example, dependent personality disorder is characterized by intolerance of being alone and problems with autonomy; schizoid personality disorder is defined by interpersonal detachment and intolerance of intimacy and dependence; and avoidant personality disorder includes simultaneous desire for, and fear of, close relationships (e.g., Bartholomew, Kwong, & Hart, 2001; Sheldon & West, 1990). This centrality of interpersonal difficulties led Widiger and Frances (1985) to conclude that "personality disorder is essentially a disorder of interpersonal relatedness" (p. 620). In fact, various forms of dysfunctional interpersonal behavior account for 45% of the diagnostic criteria for personality disorders in DSM-IV (Lyddon & Sherry, 2001).

From an attachment perspective, disorders of interpersonal relatedness can be construed as constellations of insecure attachment strategies (Bartholomew et al., 2001; Lyddon & Sherry, 2001; Meyer & Pilkonis, 2005). As shown throughout this book, attachment insecurities create problems in emotion regulation, interfere with the construction of a stable and positive sense of self, disrupt the accomplishment of major developmental tasks, and more or less preclude the maintenance of healthy and satisfying interpersonal relations and close relationships. All of these problems form parts of, or heighten the risks of developing, personality disorders.

This does not mean, however, that attachment insecurities can simply be equated with personality disorders. Attachment theory is a general theory of personality that can explain difficulties in emotion regulation and interpersonal functioning among people with and without personality disorders. In fact, although insecurely attached people have difficulty managing stress and distress, and maintaining satisfying close relationships, they can nevertheless function well within the normal range and do not usually qualify for a clinical diagnosis of personality disorder. Only when these insecurities are combined with certain genetic vulnerabilities or a history of trauma, adversity, abuse, or loss are they likely to develop into full-fledged personality disorders (e.g., Bartholomew et al., 2001; B. Meyer & Pilkonis, 2005). In such cases, one sees extreme, disorganized, or especially dysfunctional attempts to hyperactivate or deactivate the attachment system.

In line with the idea that there is a statistical association between insecure attachment and personality disorder, West, Rose, and Sheldon (1993) found that psychiatric outpatients diagnosed with a personality disorder scored higher on a self-report measure of anxious attachment. In a sample of 40 men confined to a forensic psychiatric hospital, van IJzendoorn et al. (1997) found that the vast majority of patients diagnosed with a personality disorder exhibited an anxious, or preoccupied, state of mind with respect to attachment during the AAI. Additional studies of psychiatric patients also indicate that attachment anxiety and avoidance are associated with diagnosis and severity of personality disorders (Bender, Farber, & Geller, 2001; Bogaerts, Vanheule, & Declercq, 2005; Fossati et al., 2003a; Nakash-Eisikovits, Dutra, & Westen, 2005). Burge et al. (1997) found that attachment anxiety and avoidance during adolescence were significant predictors of heightened personality disorder 1 year later, and Hoermann, Clarkin, Hull, and Fertuck (2004) found that attachment anxiety in a sample of patients diagnosed with personality disorder was an important risk factor in predicting subsequent length of hospitalization.

Although severe disturbances in attachment-system functioning are a key feature of most personality disorders, the specific kind of attachment disturbance differs across different disorders (Bartholomew et al., 2001; Brennan & Shaver, 1998; B. Meyer & Pilkonis, 2005). For example, the major interpersonal difficulties of people suffering from dependent personality disorder are overreliance on others, self-devaluation, fear of being alone, lack of assertiveness, and incapacity for autonomous functioning without social support (Bornstein, 1992). As noted throughout this book, this overly dependent, subassertive behavior is a hallmark of anxious attachment, which in extreme cases virtually paralyzes independent thought, decision making, and action. Attachment anxiety also seems to be involved in histrionic personality disorder, which is characterized by overwhelming, undifferentiated emotional experiences, a desperate need for attention and reassurance, and hyperactive seeking of others' approval (Bartholomew et al., 2001). As Bartholomew et al. noted, however, one cannot simply equate histrionic personality disorder with attachment anxiety, because some histrionic features, such as impulsivity and sensation seeking, are not obviously related to attachment insecurity. A number of correlational studies have found significant associations between attachment anxiety and severity of dependent and histrionic personality disorders in both clinical and community samples (Brennan & Shaver, 1998; Fossati et al., 2003b; Hardy & Barkham, 1994).

Extreme levels of attachment anxiety are also involved in borderline personality disorder (BPD). Two hallmarks of this disorder—affective lability and self-defeating attitudes and behaviors (Bartholomew et al., 2001)—are core features of attachment anxiety (see Chapters 6 and 7, this volume). Anxious attachment-system hyperactivation can also help to explain other important features of BPD, such as unstable and dramatically intense interpersonal relations, feelings of emptiness and loneliness, bursts of rage, chronic fears of abandonment, intolerance of solitude, and an unstable identity and sense of self-worth (American Psychiatric Association, 1994). Moreover, people with BPD symptoms tend to have conflicted, negative models of others, probably because of abuse experienced during childhood; to believe others cannot be trusted; and to perceive themselves as needy, weak, and vulnerable (B. Meyer & Pilkonis, 2005). The involvement of anxious hyperactivating strategies in BPD is also evident in the fact that most symptoms—mood lability, aggression, self-destructive tendencies, and intrusive behavior—tend to be triggered by erroneous appraisals of interpersonal events as indicating rejection, disapproval, or abandonment (Meyer & Pilkonis, 2005).

Whereas dependent, histrionic, and borderline personality disorders are all linked with anxious attachment, they differ in terms of extremity of attachment-system hyperactivation. According to Bartholomew et al. (2001), BPD, in comparison with the other personality disorders, involves more extreme levels of attachment anxiety, more destructive and dysregulated patterns of attachment-system hyperactivation, and more incoherent mental representations of self and others. In addition, BPD can sometimes involve extreme levels of avoidant attachment strategies when people begin to perceive relationships as engulfing or intrusive, yielding a pattern of fearful avoidance that can be viewed as an incoherent mixture of neediness and detachment (Bartholomew et al., 2001).

Studies in clinical samples of patients with BPD that used the AAI have consistently corroborated the theoretical propositions summarized earlier (Barone, 2003; Fonagy et al., 1996; K. N. Levy & Clarkin, 2002; Patrick et al., 1994; Rosenstein & Horowitz, 1996; Stalker & Davies, 1995). Although the sample sizes tend to be small (between 8 and 36 patients), the evidence across studies consistently indicates that an anxious, or preoccupied, state of mind with respect to attachment is the most prevalent attachment pattern among patients with BPD (across different studies, between 44 and 100% of cases) and that fewer than 10% of the patients in each sample were classified as secure. Using the four-way AAI classification system (including the "unresolved" pattern), these studies found a high prevalence of lack of resolution of trauma in patients with BPD. For example, Fonagy et al. (1996) found that 32 of 36 patients diagnosed with BPD were classified in the AAI as unresolved with respect to trauma, and Patrick et al. (1994) found that, although patients with BPD did not seem to have more traumatic histories than depressed patients, they were more likely to be unresolved with respect to trauma. Similarly, Barone (2003) found higher rates of anxious (preoccupied) and unresolved AAI classifications in psychiatric patients diagnosed with BPD than in age- and gender-matched healthy controls.

Conceptually similar findings reported in studies using self-report attachment scales have revealed that higher ratings of anxious and fearful attachment are positively associated with the severity of BPD symptoms in both clinical and community samples (P. C. Alexander, 1993; C. L. Anderson & Alexander, 1996; Bender et al., 2001; Brennan & Shaver, 1998; Dutton et al., 1994; Fossatti et al., 2003b, 2005; Landolt & Dutton, 1997; K. N. Levy, Meehan, Weber, Reynoso, & Clarkin, 2005; B. Meyer, Pilkonis, & Beevers, 2004; B. Meyer, Pilkonis, Proietti, Heape, & Egan, 2001; Nickell, Waudby, & Trull, 2002; Tweed & Dutton, 1998; West, Keller, Links, & Patrick, 1993). In addition, there is evidence that psychiatric patients diagnosed with BPD scored higher than healthy control participants on attachment anxiety and fearful avoidance (Sack, Sperling, Fagen, & Foelsch, 1996; Sperling, Sharp, & Fishler, 1991).

In a study of 91 outpatients diagnosed with BPD, K. N. Levy et al. (2005) found that 53% saw themselves as most similar to the fearful avoidant pattern (based on the Relationship Questionnaire [RQ]), 36% chose the anxious/preoccupied self-description, and only 8% described themselves as secure. Moreover, they found that fearfully avoidant and preoccupied attachment patterns were associated with different kinds of BPD symptoms. Whereas fearfully avoidant attachment was associated with intense anger and aggression, preoccupied attachment was associated with intense fears of separation, loss, or abandonment.

Fearful avoidance is also involved in avoidant personality disorder. People with this disorder crave love, closeness, and intimacy but are so afraid of rejection that they tend to avoid social relations that might potentially lead to rejection or humiliation (Millon & Davis, 1996). Bartholomew et al. (2001) noted, however, that fearful attachment is manifested mainly in close relationships, whereas avoidant personality disorder is related to a wide range of situations evoking timidity, social anxiety, or social avoidance. Several studies of both clinical and community samples provide evidence for a link between avoidant personality disorder and fearful attachment or high scores on both attachment anxiety and avoidance scales (Brennan & Shaver, 1998; Fossati et al., 2003b; Hardy & Barkham, 1994; B. Meyer et al., 2004; Sheldon & West, 1990; West, Rose, & Sheldon-Keller, 1994).

From an attachment perspective, extreme levels of avoidant attachment would also be expected to appear in conjunction with schizoid personality disorder, which is marked by aloofness, lack of interest in interpersonal relations, and maintenance of interpersonal distance (American Psychiatric Association, 1994). However, it is important to differentiate between schizoid and avoidant personality disorders. Although both disorders involve social detachment, avoidant personality disorder includes negative models of self and elevated attachment anxiety, and the detachment response is a defensive reaction against overwhelming fear of rejection. In schizoid personality disorder, there is no evidence of negative models of self or conscious fear of rejection (Bartholomew et al., 2001). Rather, schizoid personality disorder seems to be an extreme case of attachment-system deactivation of the kind Bartholomew (1990) called "dismissing avoidance." Studies support this analysis by linking schizoid personality disorder symptoms with high scores on measures of attachment avoidance or the dismissing style (Brennan & Shaver, 1998; West et al., 1994).

In an attempt to provide a more integrative picture of the links between attachment insecurities and personality disorders, Brennan and Shaver (1998) examined the factor structure of attachment ratings (based on the RQ) and personality disorder scores (on the Personality Disorders Questionnaire) in a large sample of undergraduates. There proved to be two major attachment dimensions (secure vs. fearful and avoidant vs. anxious, which are 45-degree rotations of the familiar avoidance and anxiety dimensions). These two dimensions were aligned with particular personality disorders. The "insecurity" (secure vs. fearful) dimension was linked to general personality pathology, with borderline, avoidant, paranoid, and schizotypal personality disorders loading highest on this dimension. Although lack of security seems to be associated with a general tendency to endorse more problematic personality profiles, the most extreme case of insecurity (the fearful attachment pattern) was associated with worries about being abandoned (BPD), rejected (avoidant personality disorder), and harmed by others (paranoid personality disorder). The second dimension (corresponding to a range of defenses, running from preoccupied to dismissing attachment) was associated with dependent and histrionic personality disorders at one end and schizoid personality disorder at the other end. Overall, Brennan and Shaver's findings imply that adult attachment styles and personality disorders share a common structure, and that specific attachment insecurities are manifested in specific personality disorders.

Following up this research, T. N. Crawford, Livesley, et al. (in press) examined the factor structure of the attachment anxiety and avoidance dimensions (in the ECR) and 18 dimensions of personality disturbances (assessed with the Dimensional Assessment of Personality Problems) in a large community sample of twin pairs. The attachment anxiety dimension loaded on what Livesley (1991) called an "emotional dysregulation" factor of personality disorders. This factor included problems of identity confusion, anxiousness, affective lability, cognitive distortion, submissiveness, oppositionality, self-harm, narcissism, and suspiciousness, all of which seem to be manifestations of attachment-system hyperactivation and reflect the conflicted, tumultuous inner world of severely anxiously attached individuals, including struggles between submissiveness and oppositionality (see

Chapter 9, this volume), and between self-harm and narcissism see Chapter 6, this volume). The attachment avoidance dimension loaded on what Livesley called an "inhibitedness" factor of personality problems, which included restricted expression of emotions, problems with intimacy, social avoidance, and identity problems. As documented throughout this book, these disorders are extreme examples of avoidant deactivating strategies.

These associations were conceptually replicated in another study by T. N. Crawford, Shaver, et al. (2006), in which clusters of personality disorders (assessed by parental reports, self-reports, and psychiatric interviews) and attachment orientations (assessed with brief scales based on the ECR) were assessed at ages 16, 22, and 33 in a nonclinical community sample. The results were consistent across the three waves of measurement. Higher ratings of attachment avoidance were associated with more severe, Cluster A symptoms (paranoid, schizoid, and schizotypal personality disorders). Higher ratings of attachment anxiety were associated with elevated Cluster B (antisocial, borderline, histrionic, and narcissistic personality disorders) and Cluster C (avoidant, dependent, obsessive–compulsive personality disorders) symptoms. Importantly, these associations could not be explained by variations in interpersonal aggression. These findings underscore the importance of distinguishing between avoidant personality disorder and schizoid personality disorder (e.g., Livesley, 1991; Millon, & Davis, 1996; Trull, Widiger, & Frances, 1987), with the avoidant type defined by hyperactivation of attachment needs and strong fears of abandonment and rejection, and the schizoid type by dismissal of personal relationships, and avoidance of closeness and intimacy.

DISSOCIATIVE DISORDERS AND SCHIZOPHRENIA

Attachment theory and research have also focused on relations between attachment insecurities and dissociative disorders, which involve dissociation among states of consciousness, personal memories, and parts of the self (American Psychiatric Association, 1994). Bowlby (1980) claimed early on that avoidant defenses can involve the exclusion of attachment- and threat-related material from consciousness and create "segregated" mental systems that preclude a stable and coherent sense of identity. According to Main and Hesse (1990) and Liotti (1992), these dissociative tendencies are exacerbated by frightened and frightening parental behaviors that cause disorganization of a child's attachment behavior. During interactions with a frightened (including traumatized) or frightening parent, insecure children at times experience parents as caring and available, at other times as frightened, and at still other times as frightening. As a result, they develop multiple incompatible working models of self (as a loved child, a perpetrator of an offense against the frightened parent, or a victim), are unable to distance themselves from the intrusive parent and deactivate the attachment system, and cannot integrate all of their experiences into a coherent, meaningful inner life. Liotti has contended that this kind of difficult attachment experience and the lack of inner coherence and integration heighten the risk for dissociative disorders in adulthood.

In support of this view, Carlson (1998) found that children and adolescents who were classified as disorganized in Ainsworth's Strange Situation at 12 months of age were rated by teachers as exhibiting more dissociative symptoms (than those who had received other attachment classifications in the Strange Situation) in both elementary and high school. Ogawa et al. (1997) found that both avoidant attachment and disorganized attachment in the Strange Situation at 12 months of age were strong predictors of dissociative symptoms at ages 17 and 19 (assessed in a diagnostic interview and with a self-report scale). These findings have been conceptually replicated in studies based on self-reports of adult attachment insecurities. For example, C. L. Anderson and Alexander (1996) found an association between insecure attachment and dissociative symptoms in a sample of adult women who were incest survivors, and Calamari and Pini (2003) replicated this finding in a sample of undergraduate women.

There is also evidence that attachment insecurities are associated with the most extreme and dysfunctional form of psychopathology, schizophrenia. In samples of patients with serious psychopathological disorders, a diagnosis of schizophrenia was associated with insecure states of mind in the AAI (Dozier, 1990; Dozier, Stevenson, Lee, & Velligan, 1991). Dozier et al. also found that avoidant deactivating strategies, as assessed with the AAI, were more notable in patients diagnosed with schizophrenia compared with those diagnosed with affective disorders. A similar pattern of findings was reported by Dozier, Cue, and Barnett (1994) and Tyrrell and Dozier (1997), who found that an avoidant (dismissing) state of mind with respect to attachment was the most common AAI classification among patients with schizophrenia. However, when the four-category classification system was applied to the AAI protocols (i.e., when the category indicating unresolved traumas or abuse was considered), most of the patients with schizophrenia who had been classified as avoidant were classified as unresolved (Tyrrell & Dozier, 1997). Dozier and Lee (1995) also found that interviewers rated patients classified as avoidant in the AAI as suffering from more delusions and hallucinations, and case managers rated these patients as more psychotic. Needless to say, it is not surprising that delusional or hallucination-prone individuals would be classified as having an "incoherent mind" or "incoherent discourse" based on an interview.

Using self-report attachment scales, Mickelson et al. (1997) found that ratings of attachment anxiety and avoidance were associated with more severe schizophrenic symptoms in a nationally representative U.S. survey sample. Moreover, Drayton, Birchwood, and Trower (1998) and Tait, Birchwood, and Trower (2004) found that attachment anxiety and avoidance scores predicted more maladaptive coping responses during recovery from psychosis. (Such responses increase the risk of a subsequent psychotic episode.) In a study of schizotypy (i.e., exhibiting subtle signs of schizophrenia-like mentation in the absence of overt psychosis), Wilson and Constanzo (1996) found that attachment anxiety and avoidance were associated with scores on "schizophrenism" (reflecting the prevalence of bizarre beliefs) and anhedonia (social withdrawal and loss of pleasure). They also found that the association between attachment insecurity and anhedonia was strongest when participants had problems in maintaining attention over long periods of time, suggesting that attentional or other cognitive resources might buffer the association between attachment insecurity and schizotypy.

CONCLUDING REMARKS

Attachment insecurities are clearly prevalent among people with a wide variety of psychological disorders, ranging from mild neuroticism and negative affectivity to severe, disorganizing, and paralyzing personality disorders and schizophrenia. The evidence is compatible with the theoretical idea that attachment security is a resilience resource that reduces the likelihood of psychological disorders and sustains mental health even during times of stress and trauma. In contrast, insecure attachment styles (whether anxious, avoidant, or fearful) are fairly general pathogenic states that increase the risk of psychopathology. Although many of the research findings supporting these ideas are correlational and therefore subject to multiple interpretations, several studies show a prospective connection between earlier attachment style and later vulnerability to disorders. Thus, it is reasonable to believe that insecure attachment predisposes people to psychological disorders.

Perhaps most interesting from a therapeutic standpoint, we have demonstrated that mobilizing internal or external supports for felt security reduces the likelihood and intensity of psychiatric symptoms (e.g., anxiety disorders, PTSD, eating disorders), which helps to explain why dispositionally secure people are less likely than their insecurely attached counterparts to develop mental disorders. The research evidence underscores soothing, healing, therapeutic effects of actual support offered by relationship partners, and the comfort and safety offered by mental representations of supportive experiences and loving/caring attachment figures. This research makes us more optimistic about the utility of clinical interventions that increase clients' sense of attachment security.

The study of attachment-related processes associated with the etiology and course of psychological disorders is an ideal area for interdisciplinary collaboration. Given that attachment theory was originally conceptualized as a theory of social and emotional development, and that attachment-related processes are manifested most directly in family contexts, attachment-oriented research on psychopathology could create useful bridges between personality and social psychology, developmental psychology, clinical psychology, and family psychology. More interdisciplinary research guided by attachment theory should be conducted on the ways in which adaptive and maladaptive strategies of emotion regulation are developed within families. Research should also examine the role of genetic factors, family dynamics, and sociocultural forces in determining the precise links between attachment-related experiences and particular forms of psychopathology.

In the same way that "attachment injuries" have proven useful as a focus for marital therapy (S. M. Johnson & Whiffen, 2003), it would be worthwhile to examine the role of attachment wounds in the development of psychopathology. Attachment theory leads us to expect that major traumatic experiences of attachment figure unavailability (e.g., being abandoned by a parent, exploited by a trusted teacher, or cuckolded by a spouse) will cause a person to feel especially vulnerable to lack of support during subsequent stressful life events, which in turn is likely to exacerbate attachment fears, worries, and defenses, and heighten the risk for psychopathology. As Bowlby (1969/1982) so forcefully argued when criticizing his psychoanalytic colleagues' emphasis on fantasy rather than reality, working models of attachment are "tolerably accurate reflections of a person's actual experiences." Overcoming working models based on attachment injuries and providing countervailing experiences and images of love and support should be major goals of parenting, mentoring, counseling, and psychotherapy. As we discuss in Chapter 14, one of the most important psychotherapeutic tasks is to help clients restore the biologically rooted hope and faith implicit in an infant's cry for help when distressed. Receiving a positive response to this natural human signal is likely to be crucial at every stage in the life cycle.

■ ■ ■

Implications of Attachment Theory and Research for Counseling and Psychotherapy

As we explained in Chapter 1, John Bowlby was a psychoanalyst whose ideas began to take shape before he was formally trained in psychology or psychiatry. They were rooted in observations he made while working in a residential school for troubled children. All through his later professional life, he worked as a clinician at the Tavistock Clinic in London—work that followed his postgraduate education and a 7-year training analysis with a Kleinian psychoanalyst, Joan Riviere. He was not, therefore, an ivory tower, university-based researcher or theorist whose ideas might or might not be stretched to apply to psychotherapy. Although he was very interested in research and made excellent use of it, his main concern, ultimately, was to prevent psychopathology and human suffering—in advance, through education and prevention if possible, or effectively, through appropriate psychotherapy, if prevention was too late.

Bowlby's main collaborator, especially in his later years, Mary Ainsworth, was trained more explicitly for a career in research and university teaching, but she focused from the beginning on what has since come to be called developmental psychopathology. She also coauthored a book about the Rorschach Inkblot Test (a well-known, if controversial, clinical assessment tool) and mentored many clinical psychology graduate students over the years. Following a painful divorce after several years of marriage, she underwent a long and fruitful psychoanalysis, which she valued highly (as indicated in her personal correspondence; Isaacson, 2006).

Both originators of attachment theory therefore had firmly in mind a variety of clinical phenomena, their own experiences in psychotherapy, the societal need for preventive education, and the importance of clinical applications of psychological research. Still, they did not write much about such applications, preferring to discover how attachment works before telling clinicians how to treat its dysfunctional forms. Only in 1988, near the end of his life, did Bowlby summarize his ideas about applying attachment theory clinically. In this chapter we begin with his 1988 book, *A Secure Base* (which he named after Ainsworth's main theoretical construct), and present his theoretical perspective on therapeutic change, the therapeutic relationship, and the therapist's role in emotional healing. We then review empirical evidence regarding changes in working models during therapy and the beneficial effects of a therapist's provision of a safe haven and secure base. Next we focus on attachment-related individual differences and consider the influence of clients' and therapists' attachment orientations on various aspects of therapy—forming and maintaining a working alliance, managing the transference, and dealing with countertransference—including therapy outcomes. Finally, we provide an attachment-theoretical analysis of the therapy supervision process and show how attachment theory and research can help us understand the supervisee–supervisor relationship and ways to supervise effectively.

AN ATTACHMENT THEORETICAL MODEL OF THERAPEUTIC CHANGE

In *A Secure Base*, Bowlby (1988) proposed a model of therapeutic change based on helping a client understand his or her accumulated, and often forgotten or misunderstood, attachment experiences, identify and revise insecure working models by transforming them into more secure models, and learn about ways to achieve both comfortable intimacy and flexible autonomy. Because of the central role played by insecure working models in the genesis of emotional and relational difficulties (as we explained in Chapter 13), Bowlby believed that favorable therapeutic outcomes depend on the extent to which pathogenic mental representations are identified, clarified, questioned, revised, and transformed into more adaptive models.

Bowlby called his book *A Secure Base* partly to acknowledge Ainsworth's important contribution to attachment theory, and partly to indicate that a good therapist's role—providing a secure base for exploration—is similar to the role of a security-providing parent. In the case of a parent, providing a secure base creates the emotional bedrock on which a child can develop knowledge about self and world, and acquire important life skills. In the case of a therapist, providing a secure base allows a client to muster the courage for self-exploration—to delve deeply into partially occluded memories and distorted wishes and feelings, and to develop greater self-understanding, revise working models of self and others, and get back on the path to personal growth. The process of exploration in psychotherapy is bound to be difficult and painful, because the client must confront issues, remember long-forgotten experiences, encounter strong emotions, and explore perplexities that he or she has not been able to face, manage, or understand alone. Only through this difficult process, supported by a skillful and caring therapist, can the client uncover and understand deep-seated fears, well-practiced defenses, and distorted perceptions that interfere with revising working models and create the conditions for a more satisfying and productive life.

Bowlby (1988) discussed five therapeutic tasks that contribute to the revision of insecure working models and the achievement of positive therapeutic outcomes. The first is to provide clients with a safe haven and secure base from which they can begin to explore painful memories and emotions, characteristic but destructive defenses, and maladaptive beliefs and behaviors. This precondition for the entire therapeutic process is based on the concept of attachment–exploration balance proposed by Bowlby (1973) and Ainsworth (1991), and validated by subsequent attachment research on information search and cognitive openness (see Chapter 8, this volume). In the attachment–exploration dynamic, the provision of a secure base by a sensitive and responsive therapist (like a good parent in the lives of young children) allows clients to devote attention and energy to exploration, to take the risks involved in reflecting on painful experiences, and to accept revisions in working models suggested by the therapist. Without such a secure base, clients are likely to be afraid to explore and to disclose thoughts and feelings, instead remaining closed, inauthentic, distrustful, or ambivalent about the therapist's intentions and interpretations. Moreover, a therapist who is unable to provide the client with a sense of security will not be able to create a relationship that the client experiences as refreshingly and therapeutically different from previous relationships, which were likely characterized by criticism, disapproval, disinterest, unpredictability, or abandonment.

The second task is to explore and to understand how the client currently relates to other people, based on particular goals, perceptions, expectations, and fears. The therapist needs to encourage and to assist the client in learning about maladaptive consequences of his or her major pattern of relating to others, whether it be avoidant, anxious, or disorganized; the way the client cognitively construes interpersonal relationships; and the cognitive biases that distort the client's interpretations and memories of interpersonal experiences and relationship partners' actions. As Cobb and Davila (in press) noted, because these cognitive biases are largely unconscious, clients need the help of a therapist's sensitive interventions (e.g., mirroring, interpreting) if they are to become aware of previously unrecognized biases and failed relational strategies. Clients also need a therapist to provide reality-testing tools that reveal the dysfunctional nature and destructive consequences of misguided working models. In most cases, the client will have had a long history of self-destructively misinterpreting his or her own goals, generating the opposite of the emotional outcomes intended, and hurting other people with whom he or she hoped to have mutually rewarding relationships.

The third task is to examine the client's particular relationship with the therapist, which is an example of the client's self-destructive modes of relating to close partners, and one that inevitably includes the transference and projection of established working models onto the therapist and the therapeutic relationship. This task is similar to the core psychoanalytic task of "working through a client's transference" and is based on Bowlby's (1973) notion that working models are automatically projected onto new relationship partners, including the therapist. Bowlby (1988) suggested that clients' examination of their attitudes and feelings toward the therapist, and their patterns of relating to him or her, provides an opportunity to understand how working models are expressed in a particular relationship and how they typically distort the course and experience of that relationship. To some extent, this requires the therapist to avoid falling into the complementary roles required by the client's habitual dramas. Clients' new knowledge about the patterns they repeat and induce in relationship partners, combined with their recognition and reevaluation of personal goals, cognitive appraisals, and emotional reactions as they occur during therapy, can open the door to new and corrective emotional experiences and experimentation, with more secure patterns of relating to the therapist.

The fourth therapeutic task is for clients to reflect on how their working models of self and others are rooted in childhood experiences with primary attachment figures. Accomplishing this difficult and sometimes painful task depends on the therapist's empathic sensitivity and responsiveness while helping and encouraging the client to allow into consciousness, then work through, memories of frustrating and humiliating experiences with inconsistent, rejecting, neglectful, or abusive attachment figures. Clients often need to understand how these experiences shaped their maladaptive beliefs and behaviors before they can revise and update them in beneficial ways.

This exploration of the developmental roots of insecure working models leads to the fifth therapeutic task: helping clients recognize that although their working models may once have been adaptive, or at least may have seemed better than the alternatives when interacting with nonoptimal attachment figures, they are no longer functional. The therapist helps the client to understand how current maladaptive feelings, thoughts, and behaviors relate to early working models of negative attachment experiences and to consider ways in which these beliefs can be revised and updated to fit better with current relational experiences and relationship partners. Through this process, clients can improve their reality-testing skills and create more realistic working models of self and others in the context of current relationships.

Dozier and Tyrrell (1998) summarized these therapeutic tasks in a helpful diagram (Figure 14.1), which includes three processes that contribute to the revision of insecure working models of self and others: (1) the therapist's provision of corrective attachment-related experiences based on the therapist becoming a safe haven and secure base for the client during therapy; (2) the client's exploration of and reflection on current relationships, including the relationship with the therapist; and (3) the client's exploration and reflection on earlier relationships with attachment figures. The two kinds of exploratory ventures—into past relationship experiences and into current experiences, including those with the therapist—affect each other. Exploration of past attachment experiences helps clients become more aware of how they construe and distort current relationships, and exploration of current relationships helps them reflect on earlier attachment experiences. Present distortions inevitably point back to special features of earlier troubled relationships, and past attachment injuries color expectations and strategies in current relationships. Both kinds of therapeutic exploration encourage constructive overhaul of working models, and initiate and sustain a broaden-and-build cycle of attachment security that facilitates therapeutic change and continued personal growth.

Following Bowlby's (1988) principles of therapeutic change, several treatment interventions have been specifically designed to target attachment issues in couples (e.g., S. M. Johnson's [1996, 2003] *emotionally focused couple therapy*) and families (e.g., T. M. Levy & Orlans's [1998] *corrective attachment therapy* and G. S. Diamond & Stern's [2003] *attachment-based family therapy*). These interventions explicitly recognize the trauma induced by rejection, separation, and loss, and the impact these experiences have on couple and family functioning; the self-fulfilling nature of working models; and the likely therapeutic effects of interventions that focus on developing secure emotional connections within a couple or family. Moreover, they underscore the importance of the therapist as a provider of a safe haven and secure base for the exploration and revision of maladaptive working models and dysfunctional patterns of thinking, feeling, emotion regulation techniques, and behavior within a couple or a family.

S. M. Johnson (2003) sees the updating and revision of attachment-related beliefs and behaviors as the primary focus of couple therapy. In her view, couple therapy should produce "an explicit shaping of pivotal attachment responses that redefine a relationship and an addressing of injuries that block relationship repair" (p. 110). Importantly, research indicates that this attachment-based approach to couple therapy is more effective than cognitive-behavioral approaches in reducing relationship distress, even in very troubled, high-risk couples (e.g., Clothier, Manion, Gordon-Walker, & Johnson, 2002; S. M. Johnson & Greenberg, 1985; S. M. Johnson, Hunsley, Greenberg, & Schindler, 1999).

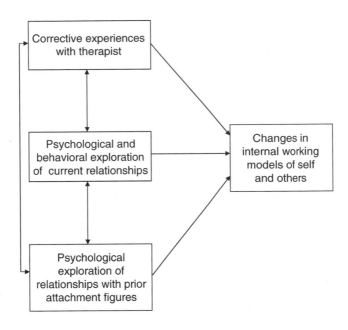

FIGURE 14.1. Dozier and Tyrrell's (1998) figure presenting a schematic representation of Bowlby's (1998) model of therapeutic change. From Dozier and Tyrrell (1998). Copyright 1998 by The Guilford Press. Reprinted by permission of the publisher and authors.

When considering the validity of Bowlby's (1988) model of therapeutic change, one needs to answer three important questions:

1. Can insecure working models of self and others be revised during adulthood?
2. Can these models be challenged effectively in therapy and transformed into more secure ones?
3. Are changes in working models really an important part of achieving beneficial therapeutic outcomes?

With positive answers to these questions we can proceed to ask whether each of Bowlby's five therapeutic tasks actually contributes to the revision of insecure working models, how these tasks are interrelated, and which specific interventions contribute to accomplishing these tasks.

With regard to the possibility of revising and updating working models of self and others during adulthood, the answer is clearly affirmative. As we summarized in Chapter 5, there is good evidence that working models are malleable during adulthood and that corrective emotional experiences with new relationship partners, as well as reflecting on these experiences, can produce beneficial revisions of working models. There is also supportive, although scarce, evidence that therapy can move clients away from insecure and toward secure working models, and that this movement is a good indication of effective treatment. In two independent studies, Blatt, Stayner, Auerbach, and Behrends (1996) and Harpaz-Rotem and Blatt (2005) assessed the severity of psychopathology of seriously disturbed, hospitalized adolescents at the beginning and end of long-term intensive therapy. In addition, Blatt et al. (1996) assessed changes in the structure of descriptions of mother, father, self, and therapist across the course of therapy, and Harpaz-Rotem and Blatt (2005) assessed changes in the description of a significant other whom each patient elected to describe at the beginning and end of treatment. In both studies, improvement over the course of treatment (reduction in severity of psychiatric symptoms) was associated with increases in the coherence of attachment-related representations. Conceptually similar findings were reported by Travis, Bliwise, Binder, and Horne-Moyer (2001), who found significant associations between increases in self-reports of secure attachment (on the Relationship Questionnaire [RQ]) and decreases in the severity of psychiatric symptoms across the course of time-limited dynamic psychotherapy.

Although these preliminary findings are encouraging, we need to be cautious in interpreting them as support for Bowlby's (1988) model of therapeutic change. We do not have good, controlled research that compares the degree of change in working models achieved in therapy with the change that occurs in a wait-list control group. It is therefore too early to conclude that because working models change during therapy, therapy itself brings about the change. More research is also needed on the nature, strength, and temporal course of revisions in insecure working models during therapy and on how particular features of revised models contribute to therapy outcomes in the case of different kinds of emotional and behavioral disorders. Researchers should try to determine whether change in working models is necessary for lasting psychotherapeutic changes in emotional experience and social behavior, and whether therapy can still be effective without change in working models.

So far, there is no published study of the effects of Bowlby's five therapeutic tasks on the revision of insecure working models. Such research would require careful analysis of therapeutic interventions and clients' exploration of and reflection on current and past attachment-related experiences. It would also require recording therapeutic sessions, after first assessing clients' working models and attachment orientations when they entered therapy, and repeatedly reassessing working models and attachment styles across the course of therapy. Luborsky and Crits-Christoph (1998) provided a model of this kind of research, using what they call a "core conflictual relationship theme" (CCRT) approach to coding therapy sessions. They found that it was possible to determine a person's core dysfunctional relational schema and link the therapist's illumination of this schema in particular sessions to the client's increased insight and progress in therapy.

THE ROLE OF THE THERAPIST AS A SECURE BASE

Bowlby (1988) drew an analogy between a psychotherapist and a mother: Just as a sensitive and responsive mother (the kind that Winnicott [1965] called a "good enough mother") induces a sense of attachment security in her child and facilitates the child's exploration of the world by making it clear that support will be available if needed, a "good enough" therapist serves as a safe haven and a secure base from which clients can explore and reflect on painful memories and experiences. Therapists should provide safety, comfort, and unconditional positive regard, and help the client manage the distress associated with exploring and articulating painful memories, thoughts, and feelings. They should also affirm the client's ability to handle distress and problematic life situations, not interfering with exploration by providing inappropriate interpretations, and admiring and applauding the client's efforts and achievements in therapy. In other words, like a good parent, a good therapist ensures the client that the therapist can be relied upon for safety and support, while the client becomes increasingly capable of dealing with distress autonomously. In Bowlby's (1988) words, "The therapist strives to be reliable, attentive, and sympathetically responsive to his patient's exploration, and so far as he can, to see and feel the world through his patients eyes, namely to be empathic" (p. 152).

When the therapeutic relationship develops as intended by the therapist, he or she becomes a genuine attachment figure for the client (i.e., a reliable and relied-upon provider of security and support). Clients typically enter therapy in a state of frustration, anxiety, or demoralization that naturally activates their attachment system and causes them to yearn for support and relief. Attachment needs are easy to direct toward therapists, because therapists, at least when a client believes in their healing powers, are perceived as "stronger and wiser" caregivers, possessing the hallmarks of good attachment figures. Therapists are expected to know better than their clients how to deal with the clients' problems, and they occupy the dominant and caregiving role in the relationship. Therefore, the therapist can easily become a target of the client's proximity seeking and projection of unmet needs for a safe haven and secure base.

Of course, clients' subjective construal of the therapeutic relationship as involving an attachment bond and of the therapist as an attachment figure can also cause the therapist to serve as a target for attachment-related worries, defenses, and hostile projections. These projections sometimes disrupt therapeutic work, but they also provide an opportunity for a therapist to make useful observations and interpretations, and for the client to have corrective emotional experiences and understand him- or herself better.

Borelli and David (2004) noted an additional parallel between therapists and other attachment figures. Like a security-enhancing caregiver who reflects on a young child's experiences and enhances the child's ability to "mentalize" his or her own and other people's experiences (Fonagy, Steele, Steele, Moran, et al., 1991), a therapist reflects on a client's internal states and articulates interpretations in ways the client can understand and model.

> At the same time that the therapist provides the client with a haven during distress and a safe base from which to explore oneself, the therapist should also begin to question why the client may respond in a suboptimally receptive manner within the therapy. For instance, the therapist should work to understand why Client A may be critical or aloof, and why Client B may voice strong veneration and unconditional compliance during the treatment. The therapist should then use this knowledge to guide the client toward self-understanding. (Borelli & David, 2004, p. 267)

There are, however, some important differences between the client–therapist and the child–mother relationship. For example, Farber, Lippert, and Nevas (1995) noted that the client–therapist relationship is more objective and less emotionally involving than the child–mother relationship, and is defined by unique temporal, financial, logistical, and ethical boundaries. Although Farber et al. do not say so, it probably makes a huge difference that parents are usually genetically invested in their children, and that each of their children plays an enormous role in their own sense of significance and self-worth. For a therapist, although each client clearly does and should matter to the therapist's sense of significance and well-being, the investment in any particular client is not likely to be as intense or prolonged as a parent's investment in a child. This difference is likely to be important in allowing the therapist to maintain an objective, therapeutic perspective.

A therapist cannot always be present when needed or wanted by the client—not nearly as often as a good parent can be available during a child's first years of life. Dozier and Tyrrell (1998) also noted that the client–therapist relationship is more difficult than the usual child–mother relationship, because therapists have to compensate for a history of painful attachment experiences, and clients tend to project attachment-related worries and defenses onto their therapist. Clients then tend to react even to a sensitive therapist as if he or she is unavailable or rejecting. Moreover, the exploration process needs to begin almost from the outset of therapy even before a firm secure base has been established (Dozier & Tyrrell, 1998).

In subsequent sections we review evidence concerning the attachment-theoretical perspective on therapy, tackling two major questions: (1) Is it reasonable to conceptualize the client–therapist relationship as an attachment relationship? and (2) Does a therapist's provision of a secure base facilitate therapeutic progress? Beyond examining these issues in the context of counseling and individual psychotherapy, we consider residential treatment and examine the role of client–staff relationships in bringing about therapeutic change. This is an appropriate topic for a chapter based on Bowlby's ideas, because he was working in a residential treatment context (a school for troubled children) when he first began to formulate his theoretical ideas.

The Therapeutic Relationship as Involving an Attachment Bond

Though scarce, and limited by exclusive reliance on self-report methods and cross-sectional designs, there is preliminary evidence that clients tend to use the therapist as a safe haven in times of stress and to react to the therapist's absence with separation protest—two definitional criteria for an attachment bond. (Needless to say, these are classic issues in psychoanalytic psychotherapy more generally.) For example, Geller and Farber (1993) found that clients tend to think about their therapists mainly when painful feelings arise, and Rosenzweig, Farber, and Geller (1996) found that such thoughts produce feelings of comfort, safety, and acceptance. As reviewed in Chapter 3, this volume, these thoughts and feelings are often directed to an attachment figure, but not often to other relationship partners; that is, only mental representations of special people who accomplish attachment functions tend to be activated in times of need and have the effect of increasing security and comfort (Mikulincer, Gillath, & Shaver, 2002). On the basis of these findings, it seems reasonable to conclude that mental representations of a therapist function similarly to mental representations of other attachment figures.

In a study of the "August phenomenon" (i.e., separations that occur because of the usual monthlong summer break in therapy when therapists take vacations), Barchat (1989) observed that such separations are likely to evoke feelings of longing for the therapist, together with anger, sadness, and fear. These responses resemble the mixture of anxiety, anger, and hope for reunion that Bowlby (1969/1982) observed when infants were separated from their primary attachment figures. (As explained in Chapter 1, this volume, he labeled this reaction "protest.") Moreover, Barchat (1989) also found that the intensity of a client's anger and fear were associated with greater difficulties in resuming therapy, which mirrors the strong separation protest reactions displayed by anxious infants in Ainsworth's Strange Situation, when they were reunited with their mother following an unwanted separation. Whether clients in Barchat's study were securely or anxiously attached to their therapist, they reacted with strong emotion during their therapist's absence. (In the Strange Situation, both secure and anxious infants cry and protest when their mothers leave the room, but the secure ones more quickly reestablish a positive mood and return to curious and creative play following reunion.)

In a study of 105 adults who had been involved in therapy for at least 6 months, Parish and Eagle (2003) assessed the extent to which clients construed the therapeutic relationship in line with the definitional criteria for a secure attachment bond. Specifically, clients completed a 45-item self-report scale, Components of Attachment Questionnaire (CAQ), tapping the extent to which they sought proximity to their therapist; felt strong emotions toward the therapist and distress upon separation from him or her; viewed the therapist as a safe haven, a secure base, a stronger and wiser person, an available and sensitive figure, and a unique relationship partner who could not easily be replaced; and relied on mental representations of the therapist for comfort and guidance outside the therapeutic setting. Clients also completed the CAQ with regard to the relationship partner to whom they felt closest (in most cases, a primary attachment figure). In addition, they completed the RQ measure of attachment style.

Although most of the CAQ scores were higher for the primary attachment figure than for the therapist, all of the therapists' scores were above the scale midpoint. Moreover, the therapist was rated higher on the stronger/wiser and availability/sensitivity aspects of attachment than was the primary attachment figure, and the difference between the two figures' scores on the secure base component was statistically insignificant. These findings suggest that clients, at least the ones in Parish and Eagle's (2003) study, view the therapist as a security provider and believe that he or she is even stronger, wiser, and more available and sensitive than their primary attachment figures.

The study also indicated that appraisal of the therapist as a security-enhancing attachment figure was positively associated with duration and frequency of therapy, and the quality of the therapeutic relationship. In addition, higher self-ratings on avoidant attachment were associated with lower ratings of the therapist as a security provider, which is similar to findings reviewed in Chapter 10, this volume, showing that avoidant attachment is associated with partner derogation and relationship dissatisfaction (typical manifestations of negative models of others). In other words, avoidant attachment seems to play a part in psychotherapy and interfere with the formation of a secure attachment relationship, just as it interferes with the formation of strong emotional bonds in other attachment relationships.

Security Provision and Therapeutic Change

Having concluded that the therapist can generally be viewed as a source of security and comfort, we can move to the question of whether good performance by the therapist as a security-providing attachment figure has beneficial effects on therapy outcome. Only three studies have dealt with this important question. In one, Goodwin, Holmes, Cochrane, and Mason (2003) asked clients of mental health services in the United Kingdom to complete a 25-item self-report scale, the Service Attachment Questionnaire (SAQ), tapping (1) feelings of being attended and listened to during therapy, (2) confidence in the continuity and consistency of the therapeutic relationship, (3) confidence in the provision of social support even after discharge, (4) perceptions of therapy as a safe haven rather than a restricting and suffocating environment, (5) feelings of being unconditionally accepted by the staff, and (6) feelings of being valued by the staff.

Goodwin et al. (2003) found that all six subscales loaded highly on a single factor, and that higher SAQ scores were positively associated with clients' reports of mental health improvement and therapy helpfulness; that is, clients who perceived mental health services as a secure base were more satisfied with the outcome of therapy. Although this is compatible with an attachment-theoretical analysis of therapy, it is still fairly weak evidence because of the possibility of cross-measure halo effects. (Satisfied clients may have been satisfied with everything, causing all forms of satisfaction to load on a single factor.)

A prospective study with repeated measures is needed to see how the different forms of satisfaction emerge over time, if in fact they do emerge over time, rather than being a product of other personality factors (e.g., agreeableness, optimism).

In a three-session career counseling study, Litman-Ovadia (2004) asked counselees after the second counseling session to complete a 25-item scale assessing the extent to which their counselor functioned as a secure base (the extent to which he or she was an available, sensitive, supportive, and accepting figure and provided safety and comfort during the counseling process). In addition, counselees completed the ECR attachment style scales before they entered counseling and a scale measuring career exploration (both before and after counseling).

The results replicated Parish and Eagle's (2003) finding that avoidant counselees were less likely to perceive their counselor as a security-enhancing attachment figure. More important, counselees' appraisal of their counselors as security-enhancing attachment figures was a significant predictor of heightened career exploration following counseling (compared to baseline career exploration), even after controlling for counselees' attachment orientations. This appraisal of the therapist as a security-enhancing attachment figure also mitigated the detrimental effects of attachment anxiety and avoidance on career exploration; that is, even insecurely attached counselees who appraised their counselor as a secure base showed an increase in career exploration, and in fact their postcounseling exploration did not differ from that of more secure counselees. Overall, the study provides encouraging evidence for the beneficial effects on counseling outcome of a counselor's provision of a secure base for exploration.

In a study based on data from the multi-site National Institute of Mental Health (NIMH) Treatment for Depression Collaborative Research Program (TDCRP), Zuroff and Blatt (2006) examined the impact on treatment outcome of patients' perceptions of the quality of their relationship with their therapists. One hundred sixty-two seriously depressed outpatients were randomly assigned to one of four 16-week treatments: interpersonal therapy, cognitive-behavioral therapy, imipramine plus clinical management, and placebo plus clinical management. Perceived quality of the therapeutic relationship was measured early in therapy with a self-report scale assessing the therapist's accurate empathy, unconditional positive regard, and genuineness (or congruence). Sample items ask whether the therapist "nearly always knows what I mean" (empathy), "feels a true liking for me" (regard), and "is comfortable and at ease in our relationship" (congruence). Scores on this measure significantly predicted relief from depression and maintenance of therapeutic benefits during an 18-month follow-up period, regardless of the type of therapy administered, and the results were not attributable to patient characteristics or severity of depression. In discussing possible reasons for these effects, Zuroff and Blatt concluded that the experience of a positive therapeutic relationship has a transforming effect on patients' mental representations of the self and others, a conclusion compatible with attachment theory.

Security Provision in a Residential Treatment Setting

An attachment perspective on therapeutic change is important for understanding effective residential treatment of high-risk, difficult adolescents (e.g., H. W. Maier, 1987; Moore, Moretti, & Holland, 1998; Schuengel & van IJzendoorn, 2001). According to H. W. Maier (1987), residential treatment involves corrective emotional experiences based on staff members becoming safe havens and secure bases for emotionally deprived, neglected, or abused adolescents. Under these conditions, adolescents can establish, for the first time in most cases, a secure attachment bond, which allows them to reassess and rebuild their working models and to practice more adaptive patterns of relating to others. The quality of relationships established with staff members is, according to this approach, indicative of adolescents' future personal and social adjustment.

According to H. W. Maier (1987), the most important attachment figure in residential treatment centers is the child care worker (CCW), who is usually a person with no specialized therapeutic training who accompanies adolescents during their daily routine. Moore et al. (1998) also consider CCWs to be the primary therapeutic agents, because, in contrast to other professionals, they are able to integrate the various aspects of an adolescent's life. Like "good enough" parents, CCWs are almost always available when an adolescent needs them, and they serve as models of functional adult behavior. In their daily work, CCWs combine parental functions, therapeutic functions, and social functions, and allow adolescents to participate in a secure attachment relationship (Moore et al., 1998). Interestingly, Schuengel and van IJzendoorn (2001) claimed that institutionalized adolescents' attachment needs are so strong that when CCWs fail to meet them, the adolescents seek alternative security providers, such as maintenance staff or cooks, who do not have a formal therapeutic role but can nevertheless function as available, sensitive, and supportive figures. In any case, security provision by any member of the staff can have beneficial therapeutic consequences. (This is, once again, reminiscent of Bowlby's early role as a care provider for delinquent boys, a role for which he had no formal training.)

Attachment theory is highly relevant to residential treatment, because the vast majority of institutionalized adolescents have a history of negative and frustrating attachment experiences with parents and other adult figures, and they arrive at residential treatment centers with extremely insecure working models (Maier, 1987). Moreover, research has shown that most of them have experienced parental loss, neglect, or abuse and have a variety of attachment-related emotional problems, such as depression, anxiety, and emotional detachment (e.g., J. P. Allen et al., 1996; Bowlby, 1944). Tolmacz (2001) claims that such adolescents have huge attachment injuries, and many suspect there will never be reliable help and support available to them. For such adolescents, forming a relationship with a security-enhancing staff member and developing a secure attachment bond during residential treatment can be an important corrective emotional experience and a "second chance" for building adaptive working models.

Focusing on attachment issues also provides a valuable perspective on the problems that bring adolescents to residential treatment centers. Crittenden (1992), for example, suggests that institutionalized adolescents' hostile and aggressive behaviors are distorted and maladaptive expressions of a desire for proximity and acceptance (see Chapter 13, this volume, for a similar approach to conduct disorders). According to Crittenden, institutionalized adolescents attempt to relate to others in ways that are consistent with their working models and past attachment experiences. Because these experiences have often included inconsistent or ambivalent care, neglect, abuse, or abandonment, aggression and violence can be construed as means of coercing attention and care from unavailable attachment figures (Crittenden, 1992). If CCWs can view these aggressive behaviors as proximity-seeking efforts, they can react in a more empathic and sensitive manner and provide corrective emotional experiences that make the use of aggression and violence as attachment behaviors less necessary (Moore et al., 1998).

Of course, being a staff member who tries to provide a safe haven and secure base for an institutionalized adolescent is difficult; it can be frustrating and exhausting when one is working with an adolescent who seems incapable of forming a stable, secure attachment bond. Adolescents who were extremely neglected or abused by their primary attachment figures are likely to resist forming an attachment bond with staff members, because they cannot allow themselves to trust anyone (B. James, 1994). Moreover, Schuengel and van IJzendoorn (2001), who emphasized the therapeutic importance of establishing secure attachment bonds during residential treatment, claim that not all adolescents who are removed from their homes seek alternative attachment figures, even if staff members offer a safe haven and secure base. Hopes for support from their own parents, feelings of sorrow and anger about being separated from parents, and overwhelming and paralyzing distress can interfere with the formation of a secure attachment bond during residential treatment.

Part of the problem in these cases may be physiological. In a recent study of severely neglected Romanian orphans who were rescued from their orphanages and adopted by loving and economically comfortable parents, Wismer Fries, Ziegler, Kurian, Jacoris, and Pollak (2005) found that despite many improvements in their condition, on average, the orphans continued to have lower levels of vasopressin in their bloodstreams at baseline (compared with normally reared children), and lower levels of oxytocin after having loving interactions with their adoptive parents. Both vasopressin and oxytocin are known to play a role in emotional bonding in mammalian species. Thus, early experiences of neglect and abuse may change a person physiologically, not just psychologically, in ways that make it more difficult to become fully and normally attached. (See C. S. Carter [2005] for a discussion of the role of oxytocin and vasopressin in emotional bonding, and Zeanah, Smyke, Koga, & Carlson [2005] for a description of the attachment behavior of Romanian orphans.) These kinds of physiological barriers to secure attachment should make us cautious, although still hopeful, about how well an attachment approach to institutionalized adolescents can succeed. This kind of therapeutic work is, and always has been, difficult and complicated, and there is no guarantee of success.

Despite the difficulties, there is growing evidence for beneficial effects of forming and maintaining a secure attachment bond with residential staff members. For example, Born, Chevalier, and Humblet (1997), Fritsch and Goodrich (1990), and Shealy (1995) found that institutionalized adolescents who formed more secure relationships with staff members showed better adjustment following residential treatment. Moretti, Holland, and Peterson (1994) evaluated the effectiveness of the "Response Program," which emphasizes secure attachment bonds as the main therapeutic agent in residential treatment of high-risk adolescents, and found that parents and staff members noted a significant decrease in adolescents' conduct disorders during treatment. Adolescents themselves did not report, in the initial stage, any decrease in conduct disorder and even reported an increase in anxiety-related symptoms, but later on, after 12 months of treatment, they also reported a significant decrease in symptoms.

In an effort to provide more systematic evidence on the therapeutic effects of using staff members as a secure base, Gur (2006) conducted a prospective study examining the course of emotional and behavioral problems of 131 Israeli high-risk adolescents during their first year in residential treatment centers. Four meetings were held with each participant, 1 week after beginning treatment and 3, 6, and 12 months later. At Time 1, participants completed the ECR scale and measures of emotional and behavioral adjustment. In the three subsequent waves of measurement, participants completed the adjustment scales and rated the extent to which targeted staff members functioned as a secure base (the extent to which staff members were available, sensitive, responsive, and supportive). The targeted staff members also rated participants' adjustment and their own functioning as a secure base in the second, third, and fourth waves of measurement. In the fourth wave of measurement, adolescents again completed the ECR.

The study replicated the well-established association between attachment insecurities (assessed by the ECR) and adjustment problems at the beginning of residential treatment. However, attachment insecurities did not necessarily interfere with the subsequent perception of staff members as security providers. More important, the study demonstrated that staff members serving as a secure base contributed to positive changes in emotional and behavioral adjustment across the four waves of measurement and notably weakened the detrimental impact of baseline attachment insecurities. These findings were obtained whether the functioning of staff members as a secure base and adjustment was assessed via adolescents' self-reports or staff members' reports. Adolescents who formed more secure attachment bonds with staff members had lower rates of anger, depression, and behavioral problems, as well as higher rates of positive feelings across the study period. The functioning of staff members as a secure base was also associated with positive changes in the adolescents' attachment representations. Adolescents who formed more secure attachment bonds with staff members had lower scores on the ECR insecurity scales after their first year of residential treatment.

Overall, findings to date support the theoretical notion that attachment security can have healing effects even in fairly extreme cases of youngsters who enter residential treatment with insecure attachment representations. Moreover, the findings suggest that security provision should be given top priority in residential treatment, and that such treatment might benefit from the explicit adoption of an attachment approach.

ATTACHMENT AND THERAPEUTIC PROCESSES

Beyond providing a model of therapeutic change and conceptualizing the role of the therapist as a secure base, Bowlby (1988) argued that working models of self and others, by being automatically projected onto new relationships, can affect the client–therapist relationship and help to explain why this relationship at times produces positive therapy outcomes and at other times ends in therapeutic failure. In the same way that attachment orientations shape other kinds of relationships (see Chapters 9–12, this volume), the attachment styles of both clients and therapists can affect the quality of the client–therapist relationship, determine clients' reactions to therapists' interventions and therapists' reactions to clients' disclosures, thereby biasing the therapeutic process. In this section, we focus on three components of the therapeutic process: (1) the working alliance between client and therapist, (2) the client's transference of prior schemas and feelings onto the therapist, and (3) the therapist's countertransference onto the client. We also consider the effects of attachment orientations on therapy outcome.

The Working Alliance

One important aspect of therapy that has been discussed many times and from many different theoretical perspectives is the formation of an alliance between client and therapist (the so-called "working alliance" or therapeutic alliance). The formation of an alliance enables therapist and client to work together collaboratively to reach therapeutic goals (Gelso & Carter, 1985; Greenson, 1967). Every psychotherapist from Freud to the present has probably noticed what Freud called "resistance" to treatment, if not outright rebellion against the therapist's interpretations and influence. According to Bordin (1979) and Gelso and Carter (1985), a working alliance reflects an emotional alignment of client and therapist based on trust, respect, and mutual regard, as well as agreement about the tasks and goals of therapy. This alliance engages the rational, self-observing aspects of the client and the working, therapeutic qualities of the therapist (Bordin, 1979; Horvath & Luborski, 1993). Horvath and Greenberg (1989) constructed a 36-item self-report scale, the Working Alliance Inventory (WAI) to assess clients' and therapists' appraisals of the extent to which they feel they have formed an emotional bond based on trust and mutual regard, and can agree about therapeutic goals and tasks. Research has consistently shown that higher WAI scores early in therapy are good predictors of successful therapeutic outcomes (e.g., Horvath & Greenberg, 1994; Horvath & Symonds, 1991).

Although a good working alliance can be formed in the first phase of therapy and is predictive of therapeutic progress thereafter (Horvath & Greenberg, 1994), the success of therapy also depends on clients' and therapists' abilities to maintain a stable alliance throughout the entire course of therapy and to manage effectively potential or actual ruptures in the alliance (Safran, 1993; Safran & Muran, 1996). Safran and Muran defined these ruptures as negative shifts in the quality of the working alliance due to miscommunications between clients and therapists; clients' feelings of being misunderstood, unloved, rejected, or criticized by their therapists; or clients' angry or distancing reactions to lack of immediate gratification of needs, wishes, or fantasies within therapy. From an attachment perspective, these ruptures are likely to be due to the activation of a client's insecure working models within the therapy setting and the projection of these models onto the therapist. According to Safran (1993), resolution of these ruptures and restoration of a "good enough" working alliance provide the client with corrective emotional experiences, enable the exploration and management of the client's negative feelings, and are crucial for achieving favorable treatment outcomes.

The establishment of a "good enough" working alliance can be viewed as a result of the client's appraisal of the therapist as a security-enhancing attachment figure. The "emotional bond" aspect of the alliance involves the client's feelings of being valued, cared for, and loved by the therapist, as well as his or her sense of trust in the therapist's availability and sensitivity (Horvath & Greenberg, 1994). According to attachment theory (e.g., Bowlby, 1988), all of these feelings emerge whenever a relationship partner, including a therapist, is viewed as an available, sensitive, and supportive attachment figure. Agreement about therapeutic tasks and goals can be greatly facilitated by a client's appraisal of the therapist as a wise caregiver who knows what needs to be done to reduce afflictive emotions and heal damaged relationships. Appraising the therapist as a trustworthy attachment figure help clients to recognize that therapists' interventions and insights are based on good intentions and true concern for clients' welfare. Indeed, two of the studies we reviewed earlier in this chapter (Litman-Ovadia, 2004; Parish & Eagle, 2003) assessed both clients' appraisals of their therapist as a secure base and their ratings of the working alliance (in the WAI), and consistently found a positive association between the two constructs.

Clients' Attachment Styles and the Working Alliance

The attachment perspective on the working alliance also implies that the attachment orientations clients bring with them to therapy are likely to affect the formation and maintenance of an alliance. Secure clients generally find it easy to form a good working alliance. Their positive models of others, core sense of trust in others' availability and good intentions, and propensities to form interdependent, intimate relationships (see Chapters 6 and 9, this volume) all should facilitate the formation of strong emotional bonds with a therapist. Moreover, their reliance on constructive strategies of conflict resolution (see Chapter 9, this volume) should contribute to effective management of ruptures in the alliance. In contrast, insecure people's negative models of others and exaggerated expression of unmet attachment needs or defensive denial of these needs are major impediments to the formation of a working alliance. Insecure clients' propensity to doubt their therapists' regard for them, and their worries and defenses against dependency and intimacy may be present from the first therapy session.

Although anxious clients' desire for merger and consensus may cause them to agree readily with their therapists about the goals and tasks of therapy, their ambivalence toward relationship partners may interfere with forming a strong working alliance in the initial phase of therapy. Moreover, their hunger for attention, care, and love; misinterpretation of others' responses as signs of disapproval, rejection, or criticism; and uncontrollable outbursts of anger (see Chapters 6 and 7, this volume) can increase the frequency and intensity of ruptures in the alliance throughout therapy. As in other close relationships, an anxious client's bond with the therapist can be so emotionally turbulent that it repeatedly interferes with therapeutic work.

The working alliance can also be hindered by avoidant clients' distrust of others, dismissal of attachment needs, and reluctance to engage in interdependent, intimate exchanges (see Chapters 6 and 9, this volume). Avoidant people's desire for self-reliance and uniqueness can also work against accepting a therapist's suggestions about therapeutic goals and tasks, while their reluctance to experience conflict may prevent constructive discussions about client–therapist disagreements and resolution of ruptures in the alliance. Avoidant clients may attempt to maintain emotional distance from the therapist and remain emotionally uninvolved during therapy, which obviously makes it difficult to form a productive alliance.

Studies of the characteristics of clients who find it difficult to form a strong working alliance at the beginning of therapy provide indirect evidence concerning the adverse effects of attachment insecurities. For example, clients who develop weak alliances have been found to feel unsupported and unloved by others, to have poor quality "object relations," problems with the dominance–submission dimension of the interpersonal circumplex, lack of cognitive and affective flexibility, and poor reflective functioning (e.g., Mallinckrodt, 1991; Muran, Segal, Samstag, & Crawford, 1994; E. R. Ryan & Cicchetti, 1985). As we have shown throughout this book, all of these psychological deficits are characteristic of insecurely attached people.

Research has also shown that clients' problems in current relationships with family members—a common interpersonal problem of insecurely attached people (see Chapter 9, this volume)—are significant predictors of problematic therapeutic alliances (Kokotovic & Tracey, 1990; Moras & Strupp, 1982; but see Gaston, Marmar, Thompson, & Gallagher, 1988, who failed to replicate this finding). More important, there is growing evidence that clients' negative mental representations of parental figures (assessed with the Parental Bonding Inventory [PBI]) have adverse effects on their capacity to create a productive working alliance with a therapist, as reported by both clients and therapists (Mallinckrodt; 1991; Mallinckrodt, Coble, & Gantt, 1995).

Assessments of clients' attachment styles have consistently corroborated the hypothesized link between attachment insecurities and problems in the formation of a good working alliance. For example, Dolan, Arnkoff, and Glass (1993) found that therapists of more avoidant clients reported less client–therapist agreement about the goals of therapy (assessed with the WAI) by the third therapeutic session. In contrast, therapists of more secure clients reported more client–therapist agreement about goals and tasks. Similar findings have been obtained when clients themselves complete the WAI and provide their own perspective on the working alliance. Satterfield and Lyddon (1995, 1998),

Kivlighan, Patton, and Foote (1998), and Parish and Eagle (2003) found that more avoidant clients (as assessed with self-report scales) tended to report weaker alliances and more problems in establishing an emotional bond with their therapist during the initial therapy sessions. Moreover, Mallinckrodt, Coble, et al. (1995) found that more anxiously attached clients (as assessed with the Adult Attachment Scale [AAS]) scored lower on self-reports of a good working alliance. However, S. Reis and Grenyer (2004) found no significant association between attachment orientations (based on the RQ) and ratings of working alliance in a sample of clients with major depression.

In an attempt to probe attachment style differences in the way clients relate to their therapists, Mallinckrodt, Gantt, and Coble (1995) constructed a self-report scale (Client Attachment to Therapist Scale, CATS) tapping (1) secure attachment to therapist (perception of the therapist as responsive and consistently emotionally available), (2) fearful avoidant attachment to therapist (distrust of therapist, feeling unsafe or patronized, strong reluctance to self-disclose or become more intimate in therapy), and (3) preoccupied attachment to therapist (longing to be at one with the therapist and worrying about his or her love and approval). In a validation study with 129 outpatients, the secure attachment factor was positively correlated with the bond, task, and goals scores of the WAI. In fact, these correlations (around .80) suggest that secure attachment to the therapist shares a common core with the working alliance (Robbins, 1995). In contrast, fearful avoidant attachment to the therapist was associated with a weaker alliance. Interestingly, no significant association was found between preoccupied attachment and ratings of the working alliance. B. Meyer and Pilkonis (2001) interpreted this result as implying that desires for merger with one's therapist do not guarantee a good alliance or a successful therapy outcome. As they explain, "In their frenetic attempts to avoid rejection, patients with preoccupied attachment may try to submissively please and appease their therapist without engaging in the more risky task of identifying and openly discussing difficult personal problems" (p. 468).

Following this line of research, Mallinckrodt, King, and Coble (1998) found that a client's dysfunctional experiences with parents and difficulties in reflecting on feelings and thoughts interfere with a client's secure attachment to a therapist. Specifically, clients' reports of fear of separation from parents during childhood and their scores on an alexithymia scale (see our discussion of alexithymia in Chapter 7, this volume) were associated with lower levels of secure attachment to a therapist and higher levels of preoccupied and avoidant attachment. In a more recent study, Mallinckrodt, Porter, and Kivlighan (2005) assessed global attachment orientations (with the ECR), attachment to one's therapist (CATS), strength of the working alliance (WAI), and clients' reports of session depth and smoothness. The study participants were 38 clients in time-limited therapy. The investigators found that global ratings of attachment insecurities were associated with less secure attachment to one's therapist, and both kinds of attachment insecurity interfered with the working alliance. Interestingly, less secure attachment to one's therapist was also associated with inhibited exploration of inner experiences during sessions and perception of the therapeutic sessions as less smooth and deep. This association was still significant after controlling for ratings of the working alliance.

Research has also documented the effects of clients' attachment orientations on fluctuations in the working alliance throughout therapy. For example, Eames and Roth (2000) assessed clients' self-reports of attachment style after the first session of cognitive-behavioral therapy, and asked both clients and therapists to complete the WAI after the second, third, fourth, and fifth session. Whereas attachment security was associated with a stronger working alliance from the start and a stably positive alliance across the four assessed sessions (as reported by both clients and therapists), fearful avoidant clients and their therapists reported weaker alliances and more alliance ruptures across the four sessions. Interestingly, although more anxious and avoidant clients showed weaker alliances during initial sessions, they showed a significant improvement in the strength of the alliance over time, as reported by both clients and therapists. According to Eames and Roth, insecure clients' initial worries about a therapist's availability and dependability might have diminished over time due to the therapist's ability to instill a sense of attachment security, which in turn facilitated the formation of a good working alliance as therapy progressed. Thus, the formation of a good working alliance depends on not only clients' attachment style but also therapists' ability to become security providers and calm insecure clients' worries and soften their defenses.

In a related study, Kanninen, Salo, and Punamaki (2000) assessed attachment patterns (in an interview based on the AAI) and working alliance (using the WAI) at the beginning, middle, and end of therapy among 36 Palestinian political ex-prisoners. Whereas securely attached clients formed relatively stable alliances throughout treatment, anxiously attached clients reported a poor alliance in the middle stages but a very strong alliance in later stages of therapy. By contrast, avoidant clients reported a deteriorating alliance toward the end of therapy. According to Kanninen et al., anxious clients' yearning for care and attention might have led them to persist in attempting to establish a close alliance with the therapist even at the end of therapy. This finding is compatible with Eames and Roth's (2000) conclusion that effective therapy can facilitate anxious people's formation of a working alliance in the late stages of therapy. In contrast, avoidant clients may defensively deny problems in the alliance or establish only a superficial relationship with a therapist, while remaining reluctant to connect emotionally. Ruptures and strains in the alliance can appear even near the end of therapy, when issues of separation come to the fore. As reviewed in Chapter 7, this volume, these kinds of problems seem to reactivate memories of attachment-related pain and elicit deactivating defenses.

Overall, there is considerable evidence concerning the obstacles that attachment insecurities place in the way of developing a strong and stable working alliance. The findings also show, however, that skilled therapists can work around these barriers and create a satisfactory alliance with many insecure clients.

Effects of the Therapist's Attachment Style on the Working Alliance

As in other dyadic relationships, the quality of the therapeutic relationship is shaped by both partners' interpersonal dispositions and skills (C. E. Hill, 1992). From an attachment perspective, creating a good working alliance depends on not only the client's willingness and ability to trust the therapist, and view him or her as a "stronger and wiser caregiver," but also the therapist's ability and willingness to occupy the role of security provider. In other words, although the client's working model is important to the formation of a good working alliance, the therapist's effectiveness as a caregiver, which means sensitively providing a safe haven and secure base for the client, is equally important. Moreover, because sensitive caregiving depends on one's sense of attachment security (Chapter 11, this volume), it seems likely that the therapist's contributions to a good working alliance can be disrupted by his or her own attachment insecurities. Whereas a secure therapist should find it easy to occupy the role of security provider and create a good working alliance even with a difficult client, an insecure therapist is likely to complicate the process of alliance formation.

A secure therapist is likely to focus on clients' problems, remain open to new information, and maintain compassion and empathy rather than be overwhelmed by personal distress (Chapter 11, this volume, provides a review of the literature on attachment style and reactions to other people's needs). Being secure allows a therapist to acquire and apply a variety of skills—both simple ones, such as maintaining appropriate eye contact and following a client's personal narrative, and more complex skills such as gradually transforming a professional acquaintanceship into an intimate therapeutic relationship (Mallinckrodt, 2000, 2001). Moreover, habitual reliance on constructive strategies of conflict resolution (see Chapter 9, this volume) can allow therapists with a secure attachment style to handle alliance ruptures more effectively and restore the quality of alliances more easily. In contrast, an insecure therapist is less likely to empathize accurately, to keep personal distress and defenses from interfering with compassion, and to mobilize constructive strategies for managing ruptures in the alliance. In line with research on attachment insecurities and caregiving (see Chapter 11, this volume), avoidant therapists may lack the skills needed to provide sensitive care and promote emotional bonds with clients. Anxiously attached therapists may experience intense distress, a desire to merge or lose boundaries with clients, and difficulty regulating emotions, which can obviously interfere with both objectivity and accurate observation, and empathic sensitivity and responsiveness to a client's needs.

Several studies of therapists' personality traits and mental representations have provided indirect evidence for the beneficial effects of secure attachment on alliance formation and maintenance. For example, W. P. Henry, Schacht, and Strupp (1990) and W. P. Henry and Strupp (1994) found that therapists who have more positive mental representations of close relationships (a core component of attachment security) were more likely to form a strong working alliance. Similarly, Dunkle (1996) found a positive association between therapists' comfort with closeness and clients' ratings of the quality of the working alliance. In an extensive review of therapist factors that affect the working alliance, Ackerman and Hilsenroth (2003) concluded that core traits associated with secure attachment, such as therapist warmth, trustworthiness, and openness, contribute to an effective working alliance.

After directly assessing therapists' attachment orientations, Sauer, Lopez, and Gormley (2003) found that although therapists' attachment anxiety was associated with clients' reports of a better working alliance after the first therapeutic session, this association was gradually reversed by the fourth and seventh sessions; that is, in the long run, anxiously attached therapists had adverse effects on clients' feelings about the working alliance. In a study of 491 psychotherapists with different therapeutic orientations, S. Black, Hardy, Turpin, and Parry (2005) found that securely attached therapists were more likely to report stronger alliances, whereas anxiously attached therapists reported weaker alliances and more therapy-related problems (e.g., "unable to comprehend the essence of my client's problem," "lacking confidence that I have a beneficial effect on the client"). Importantly, these associations were found even after controlling for general personality traits (extraversion, neuroticism) and therapeutic orientation. Similar findings were reported by Rozov (2002), who found that attachment-anxious therapists created poorer alliances in general, and especially poor ones with secure clients. However, Ligiero and Gelso (2002) found no significant association between therapists' attachment styles and quality of working alliances (as rated by therapists and their supervisors), suggesting that sample and other methodological factors remain to be identified.

Tyrrell, Dozier, Teague, and Fallot (1999) examined the joint contribution of clients' and therapists' attachment orientations to the quality of the working alliance and clients' quality of functioning. For this purpose, 54 clients with severe mental disorders and their

21 case managers completed the AAI, clients reported on the alliance (using the WAI), and case managers rated clients' functioning. However, when the AAIs were scored using the typical tripartite classification system, 90% of the case managers were classified as secure and 83% of the clients as insecure. Therefore, due to lack of variability in attachment security, Tyrrell et al. used Kobak's (1993) Q-set system for scoring secondary attachment strategies (deactivation vs. hyperactivation). There were significant interactions between therapists' and clients' reliance on secondary attachment strategies. Therapists who relied on deactivating strategies formed stronger alliances with clients who relied on hyperactivating strategies; therapists who relied on hyperactivating strategies had stronger alliances with clients who relied on deactivating strategies. In addition, the formation of stronger alliances was significantly associated with better client functioning. These findings imply that client–therapist dissimilarity in reliance on secondary attachment strategies, at least when most of the therapists are securely attached, is associated with stronger alliances and more therapeutic gains.

According to Mallinckrodt (2000), Tyrrell et al.'s (1999) findings are an illustration of "countercomplementary attachment proximity strategies," by which a therapist reacts to clients' attitudes toward proximity in ways that collide with their demands and disconfirm their expectations and maladaptive patterns of relatedness. This collision provides an opportunity for corrective emotional experiences that seem to be beneficial for both alliance strength and client functioning. For avoidant clients, who prefer interpersonal distance and tend to elicit emotional detachment from others, corrective emotional experiences can be provided mainly when therapists rely on hyperactivating strategies, tend to increase proximity, and insist on deepening clients' disclosures. For anxiously attached clients, who prefer to remain in an infantile, dependent position, compulsively seek the "savior" who will love and care for them, and tend to elicit compassion and rescue fantasies from others, corrective emotional experiences can be provided mainly when therapists adopt deactivating strategies, maintain optimal distance from clients, and encourage clients to take an autonomous role in dealing with their problems. From this perspective, Tyrrell et al.'s findings imply that these corrective experiences, though provoking uneasiness and anxiety, can heighten clients' trust in the strength and caregiving wisdom of the therapist, because he or she prevents them from reproducing the ineffective and painful patterns of relatedness within therapy.

However, it is important to acknowledge that the vast majority (90%) of the case managers in Tyrrell et al.'s (1999) study were securely attached. Dozier and Tyrrell (1998) argued that when therapists' secondary strategies are accompanied by an insecure state of mind, the beneficial effects of "countercomplementary attachment proximity strategies" no longer hold. They asserted that the clinician must have the strong sense of attachment security necessary to respond to the client in a countercomplementary manner, even if it is uncomfortable for the clinician to do so. Mallinckrodt (2000) suggested that this countercomplementary approach requires considerable interpersonal sensitivity and responsiveness in trying to understand what the client wants to recreate in the therapeutic relationship, and how to break maladaptive patterns without overwhelming the client with anxiety. These skills are rare among insecurely attached people (see Chapter 11, this volume). Mallinckrodt used a creative analogy of control rods in a nuclear reactor to symbolize the extreme sensitivity needed for effective countercomplementary interventions. "If the rods are inserted too far, the energy source (client anxiety) is overcontrolled, all the reactions cease, and the reactor core cools. If the rods are withdrawn too far the energy source becomes uncontained and a 'melt down' ensues" (p. 251).

Dozier and Tyrrell (1998) and Mallinckrodt (2000) concluded that although secure therapists are prone to form strong alliances with every client due to their interpersonal flexibility and caregiving sensitivity, they can form these alliances more easily and rapidly with clients who differ from them in regard to deactivation–hyperactivation. In contrast, insecure therapists are likely to have difficulty forming strong alliances and providing effective therapeutic interventions, even when clients differ from them in secondary attachment strategies. In fact, an insecure therapist might react in a complementary manner to clients' demands, while confirming once again clients' maladaptive patterns and preventing therapeutic change (see relevant findings in the section of this chapter dealing with countertransference).

Transference Reactions

From a psychodynamic perspective, the therapeutic relationship includes not only the working alliance between client and therapist but also less rational and more fantasy-based disruptive processes. One of these processes is the client's transference reactions to the therapist. In his initial writings about transference neurosis, Freud (1905/1953) suggested that unconscious relational representations established during repeated experiences in early relationships with parental figures tend to be reactivated during therapy. Hence, feelings, perceptions, and attitudes that belonged to a past relationship are transferred to the therapist. Freud's initial ideas referred to the transference of Oedipal fantasies to the therapist, but later he extended his ideas to any misperception or misinterpretation of the therapist's traits, intentions, or behaviors derived from clients' earlier experiences with significant others (Luborsky & Crits-Christoph, 1998). Based on this broader conception, Greenson (1967) defined *transference* as "experiencing of feelings, drives, attitudes, fantasies and defenses toward a person in the present which are inappropriate to that person and are a repetition, a displacement of reactions originating in regard to significant people of early childhood" (p. 156). Transference reactions can easily be recognized by a misfit between a therapist's interventions and a client's responses (e.g., the strength of the reaction may seem inappropriate, capricious, or unusually tenacious).

From an attachment perspective, the client's transference reactions reflect the reactivation of conflictual attachment working models during therapy and their projection onto the therapist. Bowlby (1973, p. 206) characterized transference reactions as "forecasts" that clients make about a therapist's traits, intentions, and behaviors based on working models they developed during early attachment experiences. The problem is that in the context of the relationship with the therapist, these "forecasts" are no longer valid and appropriate; they can disrupt the working alliance and prevent therapeutic change, if the therapist fails to identify and deal effectively with them. Therefore, the identification of clients' attachment working models is an important step in understanding their transference reactions and can help therapists foresee the particular kinds of irrational and inappropriate demands and responses that can emerge during therapy.

We believe that attachment patterns can shape the feelings, wishes, and fantasies that clients transfer to a therapist, as well as the intensity, tenacity, and pervasiveness of transference reactions. The sense of attachment security fosters a positive transference that facilitates rather than disrupts the formation of a strong working alliance. Secure clients can transfer to the therapist their positive models of others, which, if not disconfirmed by the therapist's behavior, can strengthen the client–therapist emotional bond and enhance their collaborative work.

However, this positive transference can be moderated by other definitional characteristics of secure attachment. Secure people's cognitive openness and positive attitude toward exploration of new information (see Chapter 9, this volume) can act against automatic, intensive, and pervasive transference of their inner world to the therapist. (We discussed this kind of inhibition of projection of self-traits onto others in Chapter 6.) This kind of transference is likely to be accompanied by a reality-based analysis of information about the therapist and the therapeutic relationship. That is, secure clients may project onto a therapist their positive models of others but still process and reflect on the therapist's reactions, and alter their appraisals and expectations, if their therapist disconfirms their working models.

In contrast, insecure people are likely to transfer to a therapist their negative models of others, to imbue their therapist with the negative traits and intentions that characterized earlier frustrating and rejecting attachment figures, and to re-create earlier conflict-ridden interactions within therapy. Moreover, their cognitive rigidity and defensive impermeability, as well as deficits in their ability to understand and reflect on inner experiences, may amplify the negative effects of transference and prevent a rational, reality-based perspective on the actual therapist and the therapeutic relationship.

Anxiously attached people are likely to transfer their ambivalent working models of others onto their therapists, that is, they are likely to project their longing for love and care onto the therapist, together with their fears of rejection and abandonment, worries about unlovability, and angry reactions to perceived unavailability or lack of responsiveness. According to Woodhouse, Schlosser, Crook, Ligiero, and Gelso (2003), "They tend to vacillate between a desire to cope with a lowered sense of self-worth by wishing to merge with the other (who is perceived as being unrealistically good) and feelings of anger at the other for not being available or understanding enough" (p. 398). As a result, anxious clients' transferences are likely to be characterized by unrealistic hopes, frustration, rage, and perceptions of the therapist as not adequately supportive (Slade, 1999). Avoidant people also possess negative models of others, but their transference is likely to be characterized more by devaluation of the therapist and rejection of his or her interventions. Moreover, their tendency to block open expression of negative feelings and expectations toward a therapist can prevent the analysis of transference reactions and the exploration of dysfunctional working models.

Unfortunately, the likely links between clients' attachment patterns and forms of transference have not received enough empirical attention. Indirect evidence is provided by Honig, Farber, and Geller (1997), who studied how clients' mental representations of parental figures were associated with thoughts about their therapists. Clients were asked to write a short paragraph describing their mothers after the first session of therapy, then 8–12 weeks later write descriptions of the therapist and their feelings toward him or her. Clients with more complex representations of their mothers, which is a well-documented characteristic of securely attached people (Chapter 6, this volume), described their therapists in more differentiated terms, displayed less overlap between parent and therapist representations, and were less likely to include sexual and aggressive content in their mental representations of their therapists. This suggests that secure clients may be able to differentiate between their parents and their therapist. In contrast, insecure clients were more likely to project working models of parents onto the therapist and recreate with him or her unresolved conflicts involving sex and aggression.

The study by Woodhouse et al. (2003) is the single published study providing direct evidence about clients' attachment styles and transference reactions. Following at least five therapy sessions, clients reported their attachment orientation toward their therapists (using the CATS), and therapists completed measures describing clients' positive and negative transference reactions during recent sessions. As expected, more anxiously attached clients were rated as displaying greater transference in general, and higher levels of negative transference (suspiciousness, annoyance) in particular. There was no significant association between avoidant attachment and transference, probably because of avoidant clients' lack of emotional involvement in therapy. Unexpectedly, secure attachment to the therapist was also associated with negative transference reactions. Woodhouse et al. proposed that because secure clients can view the therapist as a secure base, they explore deeper, more negative childhood memories that in turn at times cause a negative reaction to the therapist. According to these authors, negative transference accompanied by secure attachment to a therapist allow clients to gain insight into conflictual patterns of relating and lead to a better therapy outcome. However, this speculative interpretation of unexpected findings is based on a single study. Further research is needed to assess the replicability of the findings and to discover how secure clients make use of negative transference reactions, if in fact they do.

Countertransference

Another irrational process that can damage a therapeutic relationship is countertransference on the part of a therapist toward a client. Countertransference involves a therapist's misinterpretation of a client's needs, or the enactment of behaviors stemming from the therapist's own unresolved conflicts and mental representations of others. Freud (1910/1959) viewed the unconscious reactivation of a therapist's unmet needs and dysfunctional fantasies during therapy as a hindrance to therapeutic work, because the therapist's interventions are determined by his or her inner world rather than a realistic analysis of the client's needs and problems. However, Freud also noted that countertransference can be a joint creation of the client and the therapist, and it sometimes reflects a therapist's unconscious reactions to a client's transference (Gabbard, 2001). As such, countertransference, if accurately detected and acknowledged by a therapist, can be a window on a client's unconscious needs and conflicts, in which case it can provide a lever for therapeutic change. Noticing and handling the transference is obviously a tricky business, however, because the therapist simultaneously has to notice that his or her reactions are irrational or inappropriate and have the strength to do something constructive about them.

The complexity of countertransference is acknowledged in recent psychoanalytic writings (e.g., Gabbard, 2001; Kiesler, 2001). For example, Kiesler differentiated between subjective and objective kinds of countertransference. In the subjective kind, therapists' countertransference reactions result from their own conflicts, anxieties, and defenses, and can be harmful to the therapeutic relationship if they remain undetected. In the objective kind of countertransference, therapists' reactions are triggered by clients' transference of their own conflicts and anxieties, and it can be helpful to therapy if therapists recognize their countertransference feelings, reject clients' unconscious demands or coercive behavioral strategies, analyze these demands and strategies, and provide corrective emotional experiences.

From an attachment perspective, the therapist's sense of attachment security can mitigate countertransference reactions and allow the use of these reactions to understand and respond to a client's unconscious material. As noted throughout this book, secure attachment is associated with emotional and cognitive openness, reflection on inner states, and constructive management of impulses, feelings, and behaviors that tend to interfere with goal pursuit. As a result, securely attached therapists can more easily process what is happening in the "real relationship" with clients, recognize their own countertransference feelings, and prevent the automatic expression of these feelings when expressing them would interfere with effective therapy. In addition, as reviewed earlier in this chapter, secure therapists' interpersonal sensitivity and responsiveness can sometimes facilitate their detection of clients' transference demands and allow them to use countercomplementary strategies (Mallinckrodt, 2000). Rather than playing into and reinforcing the client's dysfunctional transference, a secure therapist may be able to break the transference–countertransference cycle, while still maintaining a good working alliance.

In contrast, attachment insecurities may render therapists more vulnerable to reactivation of their own attachment-related worries and defenses during therapy. Insecure therapists may lack the skills needed to regulate their own distress, to remain fairly accurate in their social perceptions, and to keep their goal-corrected behaviors and interventions on a healthy track (see Chapters 8 and 9, this volume, for examples of these difficulties in nontherapists). This could obviously leave them poorly equipped to detect and manage their countertransference reactions. As a result, their therapeutic interventions are likely at times to be misguided by their own worries, fantasies, and defensive maneuvers, which may cause them to act in a complementary rather than a controlled, countercomplementary way to clients' transference demands. When therapy goes astray in this way, it obviously interferes with a constructive working alliance and may even result in a therapist's unprofessional anger toward or withholding of support for a client, and it can sometimes lead to highly damaging and defensively rationalized sexual relations with a client (Pope, 1994).

In the last decade, attachment research has begun to examine associations between therapists' attachment patterns and countertransference. Ligiero and Gelso (2002) assessed therapists' attachment styles using the RQ, along with supervisors' ratings of the therapists' countertransference reactions in clinical cases they had discussed during supervision. The supervisors completed the Inventory of Countertransference Behavior, which measures both positive countertransference behaviors (e.g., trying to befriend the client, engaging in too much self-disclosure, agreeing too often with the client) and negative countertransference behaviors (e.g., being excessively critical, punitive, or rejecting). There were no significant associations between therapists' attachment orientation and supervisors' ratings of *positive* countertransference behaviors. As expected, however, supervisors rated more securely attached therapists as less likely to engage in negative countertransference behaviors.

Another manifestation of attachment-related processes in countertransference was documented in a study by Marmarosh et al. (2006), in which group therapists completed E. R. Smith et al.'s (1999) measure of group attachment (see Chapter 15, this volume) and reported on their expectations concerning their clients' attitudes about group therapy. More anxiously attached therapists were more likely to expect that patients would hold negative stereotypes and misconceptions about group treatment. In other words, attachment anxiety seemed to bias perceptions of others in ways compatible with the usual worries of attachment-anxious people.

Research has also shown that insecure therapists' countertransference depends on their clients' attachment orientations. For example, Rubino, Barker, Roth, and Fearon (2000) presented to clinical psychology students a variety of videotaped vignettes depicting simulated alliance ruptures with secure, avoidant, or anxious clients. The clinical trainees were asked to respond as if they were interacting with actual clients, and independent raters judged their empathic responses to the vignettes. The results revealed that more anxious therapists (based on the RSQ) responded less empathically to clients' narratives, and this was especially true when clients had secure or avoidant attachment styles. According to Rubino et al., "More anxious therapists might interpret ruptures as an indication of their patients' intention to leave therapy, and their own sensitivity toward abandonment might diminish their ability to be empathic" (p. 416).

In a study of therapists' countertransference reactions during the first therapy session (as rated by the therapists' supervisors), Mohr, Gelso, and Hill (2005) found that supervisors rated avoidant therapists (based on the ECR) as exhibiting more hostile countertransference behaviors (e.g., "therapist was critical of the client during the session"). However, this effect was moderated by clients' attachment patterns: More avoidant therapists exhibited more hostile countertransference behaviors mainly toward anxiously attached clients. Interestingly, more anxiously attached therapists also tended to show heightened hostility only when clients were avoidant; that is, incompatibility of attachment strategies (hyperactivation vs. deactivation) between clients and therapists tended to elicit more hostile countertransference behaviors from the therapists. Possibly this kind of incompatibility works against insecure therapists' attachment strategies, frustrates them, and elicits hostile responses toward frustrating clients. Whereas an anxiously attached client can frustrate an avoidant therapist's attempt to maintain distance, an avoidant, detached client can frustrate an anxious therapist's wish for intimacy and approval. In line with this interpretation, Connors (1997) suggested that anxious therapists are likely to be alarmed by avoidant clients' detachment; hence, they intrude upon these clients with "overly intense efforts to evoke a deeper and more affective relationship" (p. 489). These findings suggest how difficult it may be to maintain the appropriate degree of countercomplementary attachment behavior thought by Dozier and Tyrrell (1998), Mallinckrodt (2000), and Tyrrell et al. (1999) to contribute to good therapeutic outcomes.

Lyddon and Satterfield (1994) also examined the possibility that clients' insecurities and transference demands elicit particular countertransference behavior from therapists. Anxiously attached clients are likely to express excessive distress, vulnerability, and helplessness even during an initial therapy session, and this can cause therapists to become prematurely pulled into excessive emotional involvement and compassion, and an overly intense focus on clients' negative views of self. In contrast, avoidant clients are likely to maintain an emotionally detached position and reject therapeutic interventions that require emotional expression and disclosure of vulnerabilities, thereby causing therapists to use more rational and cognitive techniques that may not get to heart of clients' problems. A therapist who is not sufficiently cognizant of these deactivating strategies may use task-based interventions that do not challenge client defenses but instead reinforce maladaptive relational patterns.

In support of these theoretical possibilities, Lyddon and Satterfield (1994) found that therapists with more anxiously attached clients (as measured by the AAS) were more likely to rate clients' problems as pervasive and due to developmental deficits, and to view the goal of therapy as exploration of core pathological beliefs. It seems that clients' attachment anxiety biased therapists' interventions toward what Guidano (1987) labeled "second-order changes"—interventions that challenge clients' core assumptions about the self and world, and involve intensely painful emotional experiences that must be hashed out during therapy. This sort of distress intensification fits well with anxious people's preferences for emotional drama and hyperactivating attachment strategies.

There is also evidence that therapists use more affective and relationship-oriented interventions with anxiously attached clients, and more cognitive therapeutic methods with avoidant clients. For example, Hardy et al. (1999) content-analyzed transcripts of significant therapy sessions and found that whereas therapists tended to respond to anxiously attached clients by reflecting their emotions and concerns, they reacted to avoidant clients by offering cognitive interpretations. Conceptually similar findings were reported by Rubino et al. (2000), who found therapists to be more deeply involved with anxiously attached clients and to react more empathically to them than to less anxious clients.

There is also important evidence, however, that these countertransference reactions are moderated by therapists' attachment orientations. Dozier et al. (1994) administered the AAI to clients with severe mental disorders and to their therapists. The therapists were interviewed regarding their therapeutic interventions. Whereas secure therapists did not use different interventions for anxious and avoidant clients, insecure clinicians attended more to dependency needs and made more in-depth interpretations when treating clients with an "anxious state of mind with respect to attachment" than when treating avoidant clients. These findings suggest that insecure therapists respond in a complementary way to clients' dysfunctional needs and perhaps perpetuate and reinforce clients' maladaptive attachment strategies. In contrast, secure therapists are less likely to react in a complementary manner, thereby providing a relational context that differs from the relationships that clients probably maintain with other partners and helping clients to reformulate their models and create therapeutic change.

Therapy Outcome

The effects of clients' and therapists' attachment orientations on aspects of the therapy process should be reflected in therapeutic outcomes. Whereas clients' and therapists' attachment security should contribute to good outcomes, attachment insecurities can be expected to impair therapeutic work by interfering with the creation of a good working alliance, distorting the analysis of clients' problematic cognitions and behaviors, and preventing the provision of security and corrective emotional experiences. In fact, negative therapeutic outcomes have been observed even at the level of a single session. Mohr et al. (2005) assessed clients' attachment orientations (using the ECR) and ratings of the smoothness and value of the first therapy session. Insecure clients were less likely to view the first treatment session as smooth and valuable. Moreover, therapists working with insecure clients were also less likely to rate the first session as smooth and comfortable.

Attachment styles may also affect people's willingness or reluctance to seek help from therapists in the first place (see Chapter 7, this volume, for general examples of people's attachment-related attitudes toward help seeking). Lopez et al. (1998) found that undergraduates with an avoidant attachment style, either dismissing or fearful, were less willing than secure undergraduates to seek therapy and had more negative attitudes toward therapy. Along similar lines, Riggs, Jacobvitz, and Hazen (2002), who assessed people's exposure to psychotherapy in a sample of middle-class women, found that women with an avoidant state of mind with respect to attachment (assessed with the AAI) were less likely than secure women ever to have been in therapy.

Insecure people's poor regulation of goal-oriented behavior (difficulties in maintaining a task-oriented focus, persisting with challenging tasks, and inhibiting disrupting thoughts and action tendencies) may also interfere with therapeutic success. These difficulties, which have been shown to interfere with insecure people's compliance with medical treatment regimens (see Chapter 8, this volume), can also contribute to poor compliance in psychotherapy (Cortina, 1999). Dozier (1990) found that an avoidant state of mind (assessed with the AAI) in clients with severe mental disorders was associated with more rejection of treatment providers, less self-disclosure, and poorer use of treatment. In an intervention program for low-SES, high-risk mothers, Korfmacher, Adam, Ogawa, and Egeland (1997) found that mothers classified as insecure on the AAI were less involved in the intervention and accepted fewer treatment suggestions than those who were securely attached. Whereas women with an "unresolved attachment" status seemed to be disoriented during the intervention, avoidant women remained emotionally uninvolved. These findings are compatible with Tasca et al.'s (2006) discovery that self-reported avoidant attachment was associated with dropping out of cognitive-behavioral therapy for eating disorders.

Research has also yielded evidence of an association between clients' attachment styles and therapy outcomes. Cyranowski et al. (2002) assessed clients' attachment orientations prior to therapy and measured the effectiveness of interpersonal psychotherapy in women with recurrent major depression. Although attachment anxiety and avoidance did not distinguish between clients who did and did not show improvement in their mental status by the end of therapy, attachment insecurities were associated with a longer time to relieve depressive symptoms. In related studies, S. Reis and Grenyer (2004) found that self-rated attachment anxiety and avoidance, assessed prior to therapy, predicted more severe depressive symptoms (compared to baseline depression) after six and 16 therapy sessions, and Hardy et al. (2001) found that avoidant clients were less responsive to time-limited cognitive therapy.

In a sample of clients with severe personality disorders, B. Meyer, Pilkonis, Proietti, Heape, and Egan (2001) found that insecure attachment (assessed shortly after clients entered therapy) was associated with a less favorable pattern of anxiety symptoms over 6 months of treatment. Similar findings were reported by Mosheim et al. (2000), who used a prototype methodology to sort clients diagnosed with eating disorders, mood disorders, or anxiety disorders into attachment categories. Insecure attachment was a significant predictor of problems in attaining therapy goals: Patients rated as less comfortable and confident in past and present relationships tended to benefit less from a 7-week course of intensive therapy.

In contrast, Fonagy et al. (1996) found that although secure clients (assessed with the AAI) tended to function better than insecure clients at both admission into and discharge from individual or group psychoanalytic therapy (lasting more than 9 months), avoidant clients exhibited the greatest amount of improvement over the course of treatment. According to B. Meyer and Pilkonis (2001), this finding may be attributable to the special benefits of long-term therapy for avoidant clients: "Those with dismissing attachment may require concentrated or targeted interventions, helping them overcome their characteristic detachment. Once they do connect emotionally with a therapist, however, improvement might be all the more dramatic" (p. 467).

THE SUPERVISION PROCESS AND THERAPISTS' NEED FOR A SECURE BASE

Therapists obviously experience a great deal of stress while conducting therapy with emotionally demanding clients. Like anyone else under stress, they need a safe haven and secure base (outside of their consulting room) in relationships with supervisors, consulting therapists, marital partners, friends, and spiritual advisors (e.g., Hess, 1987; Holloway, 1994). Needless to say, it would be dangerous and destructive for a therapist to reverse roles and attempt to meet his or her attachment needs by relying on clients for comfort, safety, and support—a process that attachment researchers have identified as dysfunctional when it occurs in disturbed parent–child attachment relationships. Recently, Kurtz (2005) provided an extensive review of the needs of therapists who work with severely disordered patients and identified the importance of supervisors' provision of a safe haven and a secure base for clinician supervisees. Using a "chain of security" metaphor, Kurtz argued that therapists benefit from feeling supported, comforted, and empowered by their supervisor, while the therapists themselves attempt to provide security and support to their clients (analogous to the ways in which spousal support helps a parent provide a safe haven and secure base for his or her children [Cohn et al., 1992]).

Attachment theory is also useful for conceptualizing the effects on the therapy supervision process of therapists' and supervisors' attachment orientations. According to Pistole and Watkins (1995), therapists' insecure working models can be reactivated during the supervision process, because supervision entails self-disclosure, reliance on a "stronger and wiser" other, reflection on inner experiences, and discussion of issues related to autonomy and dependency. An avoidant therapist may be reluctant to seek support and assistance from a supervisor; may adopt a defiant, resentful, or disparaging attitude toward the supervisor; and may maintain emotional and cognitive distance from him or her. An anxiously attached therapist is likely to form a clingy, overly dependent relationship with a supervisor, to feel that he or she cannot succeed as a therapist without a great deal of help from the supervisor, and to worry about the supervisor's disapproval or criticism. In either case, the reactivation of insecure working models is likely to impair the supervision process (Neswald-McCalip, 2001). Of course, the supervisor's sense of attachment security and his or her ability to provide a safe have and secure base for supervisees can moderate the detrimental effects of supervisees' insecure attachment. A secure foundation provides a supervisee with sufficient safety so that he or she can feel confident in the supervisor's availability, sensitivity, and responsiveness.

In their work with counseling supervisees, Pistole and Watkins (1995) found that a secure supervisory alliance "serves to ground or hold the supervisee in a secure fashion" (p. 469). The relationship provides supervisees with security or safety by letting them know that "(a) they are not alone in their counseling efforts, (2) their work will be monitored and reviewed across clients, and (3) they have a ready resource or beacon—the supervisor—who will be available in times of need" (p. 469). At present, attachment-oriented research on therapists' relationships with supervisors is scarce. This would be a fruitful area in which to test theory-based supervisory strategies and their effects on both supervisees and clients.

Psychotherapists who work with special populations, such as victims of terrorism, abused children, disaster survivors, dying clients, and severely disturbed patients, sometimes neglect their own needs for care while focusing on the pressing needs of their clients (Figley, 2002). This kind of work can easily result in emotional depletion and professional burnout (Skovholt, Grier, & Hanson, 2001), which is sometimes called "compassion fatigue." This unpleasant and destructive condition is marked by withdrawal and isolation from others, inappropriate emotionality, depersonalization, loss of pleasure in work and perhaps in life more generally, loss of boundaries with patients, and a sense of being overwhelmed (Rainer, 2000). Such emotional deficits are particularly common in attachment-anxious therapists, who have problems regulating their distress while providing care to others. Indeed, Racanelli (2005) found that attachment anxiety was predictive of compassion fatigue among American and Israeli therapists working with victims of terrorism. This finding implies that anxiously attached therapists may be especially in need of good supervision. Paradoxically, however, their attachment insecurities may interfere with the supervision process.

CONCLUDING REMARKS

Attachment theory originated in Bowlby's ideas about the causes of mental disorders and the need for a more scientifically sound approach to psychotherapy. Now that attachment theory has been extended into the adult realm and many measures of attachment-related constructs have been devised and validated, it is possible to explore the realm of psychotherapy itself from an attachment perspective. Bowlby's (1988) own wisdom about therapy, based on both theory and extensive clinical experience, provides a good starting point for anyone wishing to conceptualize psychotherapy and residential treatment from an attachment perspective. Many valuable studies have already been conducted, as indicated in this chapter. But research on the topic (i.e., research on the therapy process, the attachment issues involved in transference and countertransference, and the importance of attachment issues in therapist training and supervision) is relatively new, and many questions need further study. There is some uncertainty about how countercomplementary attachment behaviors can and should be used in therapeutic settings. Almost nothing is known about how to match therapists' and clients' attachment orientations in productive ways, nor is much known about how to help therapists achieve a greater sense of felt security, along with mature social perception and effective social behavior in the therapy setting. Almost every issue discussed in this chapter would benefit from more sophisticated research.

At a conceptual level, it is unclear how differences in the two major lines of adult attachment research (see Chapter 4, this volume)—one based on self-report measures of attachment patterns and the one based on the AAI—can be applied in therapeutic settings. The self-report research tradition leans investigators toward the issues of working models, relational behaviors, and emotion regulation. The AAI tradition leans investigators toward the role of discourse coherence and "mentalizing" in therapy settings. We still know little about how insights from these two research traditions can be combined to optimize psychotherapy. Both basic theory and clinical applications would benefit greatly from examination of both kinds of issues in the same studies of psychotherapy processes and outcomes. It would also be worthwhile to consider how attachment constructs do or do not meld well with specific therapeutic techniques, such as emotion-focused therapy, cognitive-behavioral therapy, and interpersonal therapy. Obegi and Berant's (in press) book on this topic is a valuable place to begin.

Attachment theory arose in a clinical context, took some time to be studied by basic researchers (because of the difficulty of creating good measures, and using them in laboratory experiments and prospective longitudinal studies), and is now ready to be reintegrated into the therapeutic process and clinical research. The reintegration process presents many exciting challenges to clinical researchers.

CHAPTER 15

∎ ∎ ∎

Applications of Attachment Theory and Research in Group and Organizational Settings

As demonstrated in previous chapters, attachment theory has inspired an explosion of research on personality development, close relationships, and the complex interplay between individual- and relationship-level processes in all phases of the lifespan. In recent years, the theory has been extended to organizational settings, and knowledge gained during three decades of attachment research has been applied to people's attitudes, performance, and social relations within large organizations, such as the workplace, the army, and community groups. Hazan and Shaver (1990) were the first to discuss individual differences in attachment-system functioning in organizational settings and (as reviewed in Chapter 8, this volume) their pioneering research set the stage for an examination of associations between attachment style and various aspects of performance in the workplace. Following their lead, attachment researchers have become increasingly interested in organizational processes and have proposed that group dynamics and relations between leaders and followers can be viewed as forms of emotional attachment conceptually similar to the ones children, adolescents, and adults form with parents, friends, romantic partners, and therapists (e.g., Popper & Mayseless, 2003; Rom & Mikulincer, 2003; E. R. Smith et al., 1999). This exciting new research area is likely to receive extensive exploration in coming years.

In this chapter, we review and integrate what is known about the interface between attachment theory and the study of organizational processes. We focus specifically on (1) attachment-style differences in attitudes toward groups and group processes, performance in groups, and the possibility that a group can sometimes serve as a symbolic attachment figure; (2) attachment-related processes underlying leadership, the quality of leader–follower relations, and the beneficial and destructive effects a leader can have on subordinates' performance and emotional well-being; and (3) the contribution of attachment processes to core constructs in organizational psychology, such as organizational citizenship, commitment, and change. Although the application of attachment theory to organizational settings is still in its infancy, preliminary research already confirms the great potential of the theory for illuminating organizational phenomena and enlivening the scientific study of organizational behavior.

ATTACHMENT AND GROUP PROCESSES

In a creative and seminal article, E. R. Smith et al. (1999) argued that "adult attachment theory, which has been prominent in recent years as a theory of interpersonal relationships, may be able to shed light on the processes underlying people's identification with social groups as well" (p. 94). In this section, we follow their lead and provide an attachment-theoretical analysis of group dynamics, showing how attachment theory and research help us understand individual differences in group-related psychological processes and behavior.

Emotional connections with a group or a network of group members can be viewed as attachment bonds (Mayseless & Popper, in press; Rom & Mikulincer, 2003). A person can seek proximity to a group and use the group as a source of comfort, support, and safety in times of need (i.e., a safe haven), and as a secure base for exploration and growth. Research on group identification and intergroup relations show that people generally prefer their own groups, feel comfortable and safe in the midst of their groups, and seek comfort and support from groups, group members, or leaders in times of need (for reviews, see Devine, 1995; Dovidio & Gaertner, 1993; Tajfel, 1982). Moreover, there is research evidence that groups can be attractive and effective sources of support, comfort, and relief during demanding and challenging times (e.g., Hogg, 1992; Mullen & Cooper, 1994). Like individual attachment figures who serve as a secure base, groups also encourage and support exploration and learning of new social, emotional, and cognitive skills (e.g., Forsyth, 1990).

Group cohesion, the best-researched construct in the group dynamics literature (e.g., C. R. Evans & Dion, 1991; Mullen & Cooper, 1994), provides an initial focal point for establishing connections between attachment theory and group processes. "Group cohesion" (or team spirit and solidarity) is defined as the coordination, cooperation, support, and consensus among group members that facilitates learning and effective team performance (Hogg, 1992; Levine & Moreland, 1990). From an attachment perspective, this construct refers to the extent to which a group is appraised as a target for proximity seeking, a safe haven, and a secure base. The higher the group's cohesiveness, the more its typical members feel protected, comforted, supported, and encouraged by the group.

Because of the attachment functions served by groups, group members can construe their group as a symbolic security-enhancing attachment "figure" and form secure attachment bonds with the group as a whole or with the network of individual group members. Moreover, they can project their most accessible working models of self and others onto the group, mainly during threatening, demanding, or challenging group activities, which can in turn bias group-related appraisals, emotions, and behaviors, just as working models color or distort perceptions of dyadic relationship partners (as we discussed in previous chapters). In other words, secure adults are likely to project positive working models onto their group(s) and feel comfortable in proximity to other group members, confident of the group's supportiveness, and emotionally open and secure when engaging in group activities. Less secure individuals may have difficulty construing their groups as available, sensitive, and responsive "attachment figures." However, variations in group cohesion—a property of a group as a whole—can moderate the projection of attachment working models onto the group, with more cohesive groups favoring the formation of a secure attachment to the group despite some members' generally insecure working models. This effect of group cohesion resembles the strong moderating influence that a secure and security-enhancing romantic partner exerts on one's relational cognitions, emotions, and behavior (see Chapter 10, this volume). That is, group-related appraisals, emotions, and actions are likely to reflect the joint action of a group member's attachment style and the cohesiveness of the group in which he or she is embedded.

In the first systematic attempt to apply attachment theory to group processes, E. R. Smith et al. (1999) assumed that people possess working models of themselves as group members (e.g., "I'm a good team player" or "I don't need a group to tell me what to do"), and models of specific groups and groups in general (e.g., "My team is warmly accepting of its members" or "Groups are not dependable"). As in dyadic relationships, these models affect other goals, thoughts, emotions, and behavioral choices. E. R. Smith et al. constructed a 25-item self-report scale to measure attachment anxiety and avoidance with respect to groups, and examined the links between these dimensions and group processes. "Group attachment anxiety" was defined as a sense of being an unworthy group member and worrying about acceptance by one or more groups (e.g., "I often worry my group(s) will not always want me as a member"). "Group avoidant attachment" was defined as viewing closeness to groups as unnecessary or undesirable, and as tending to avoid dependence on groups (e.g., "Often my group(s) want me to be more open about my thoughts and feelings than I feel comfortable being"). (The items were closely modeled on ones included in the dyadically oriented ECR.) E. R. Smith et al. constructed two versions of their scale: one referring to a specific group (e.g., a participant's most important social group, a participant's fraternity/sorority) and the other referring to social groups in general.

Factor analyses confirmed the two-factor structure of the scale in three different samples, and correlational analyses revealed strong similarities between attachment insecurities in close relationships (assessed with a self-report scale) and group attachment insecurities; that is, attachment anxiety in close dyadic relationships was associated with group attachment anxiety, and avoidant attachment in close dyadic relationships was associated with group avoidant attachment. These correlations were statistically significant but only moderate in size, indicating that although group attachment insecurities may be reflections, or special cases, of global insecurities, they are also influenced by other factors, such as past and current experiences in groups. In this way they are like dyadic attachment insecurities in particular relationships—partly a matter of dispositional "traits," and partly a function of a relationship with a particular partner.

More important for the development of a new research domain on attachment to groups, E. R. Smith et al. (1999) found theoretically predictable associations between the two group attachment scales and self-report measures of group engagement, evaluation, and identification. Higher scores on either group attachment anxiety or group avoidant attachment predicted lower engagement in group activities, more negative evaluations of social groups, and lower perceived support from groups. In addition, whereas group attachment anxiety was associated with stronger negative emotions toward groups, group avoidant attachment was associated with lower levels of positive affect toward groups and lower identification with social groups, such as fraternities and sororities. More avoidant study participants were also more likely to be thinking of leaving their fraternity or sorority, which seems parallel to dyadically avoidant individuals' dissatisfaction with their relationships and their openness to "jump ship" in favor of a new, perhaps only short-term relationship. E. R. Smith et al.'s findings indicate that attachment insecurities have negative consequences for group identification and engagement, and make it likely that insecure group members will be ambivalent, uncommitted, or disloyal.

Although this pioneering study provided important preliminary evidence linking attachment insecurities with group processes, it left many questions unanswered. For example, E. R. Smith et al. (1999) asked participants to report their attitudes toward either their most important social group or their fraternity or sorority. But no information was collected about their thoughts, feelings, or behavior during specific interactions with groups or group members (e.g., study groups, athletic teams, or work teams). This is somewhat different from the more established literature on group dynamics (e.g., Forsyth, 1990), which focuses on functional work groups rather than large social groups. Moreover, E. R. Smith et al. (1999) did not collect information about group-level constructs, such as group cohesiveness. Studies on group dynamics have emphasized the importance of a multilevel approach that takes into account both individual- and group-level constructs (e.g., Barry & Stewart, 1997).

In an initial attempt to overcome some of these limitations, Rom and Mikulincer (2003) conducted four studies focusing on a person's attitudes toward small groups, his or her actual performance in group tasks, and the possible moderating role of group cohesion. In one study, participants completed self-report scales tapping (1) the extent to which they appraised task-oriented groups in threatening terms (e.g., "Working with other people in group tasks threatens my self-esteem") or challenging terms (e.g., "Working with other people in group tasks helps me to know myself"); (2) their sense of self-efficacy in group interactions (e.g., "I know how to improve the efficacy of group performance"); and (3) the intensity of positive and negative emotions experienced during group activities. In another study, participants completed scales assessing the importance of "security–love" goals (e.g., "being accepted by group members"), mastery-skill goals (e.g., "learning new skills"), and self-reliance goals (e.g., "maintaining personal freedom while making decisions") during group interactions. In addition, participants were asked to recall three different group interactions and to evaluate their own and other members' performance in each of them.

Rom and Mikulincer (2003) also conducted two naturalistic studies (Studies 3 and 4) with new recruits in the Israel Defense Forces (IDF), whose performance in combat units was evaluated in a 2-day screening session. On the first day, participants completed a self-report attachment style measure. On the second day, they were randomly divided into small groups and performed three group missions (e.g., mounting a rubber boat, assembling a large military tent). Following each mission, they rated their socioemotional functioning—that is, the extent to which they contributed to the positive emotional tone of their group (e.g., "I helped group members express their thoughts and feelings"). They also rated their instrumental performance—the extent to which they contributed to the success of the group mission (e.g., "I contributed to the quality of team performance"). In addition, they rated the cohesiveness of their group (e.g., "In my group, we worked together," "In my group, we helped each other"). In Study 4, external observers also provided ratings of each participant's socioemotional and instrumental functioning during the three group missions, and participants completed an additional measure E. R. Smith et al.'s [1999] scale) at the end of the second screening day to register their anxiety and avoidance toward their group.

Across the four studies, there were theoretically predictable associations between attachment insecurities, negative group-related appraisals and emotions, and poor group functioning. Higher ratings of attachment anxiety were associated with appraising group interactions as a threat, lower self-efficacy in dealing with group tasks, more negative emotional reactions during group activities, more negative memories of group interactions, and higher identification with security–love goals. In addition, more attachment-anxious participants performed relatively poorly in group missions (as assessed by both self-reports and observers' ratings). More avoidant individuals were less likely to appraise the group activities as challenging and engaging, and less likely to perceive other group members' qualities as positive. In addition, avoidant attachment was associated with more negative emotional reactions during group activities, more negative memories of specific group interactions, higher identification with self-reliance goals, and lower levels of both instrumental and socioemotional functioning during group missions (again, as assessed by both self-reports and observers' ratings).

With regard to attachment-anxious recruits, Rom and Mikulincer's (2003) findings revealed what seemed to be a direct projection of their anxious working models of self and their hyperactivating strategies onto group activities. First, anxiously attached individuals' self-assessments of their poor performance as group members paralleled their generally negative working models of themselves as unworthy, vulnerable, and helpless (Chapter 6, this volume). Second, their appraisal of group activities as threatening, and their strong negative emotional reactions to group interactions, parallel the well-documented dyadic-level hyperactivating strategies that intensify distress (Chapter 7, this volume). Third, anxiously attached individuals' pursuit of love–security goals in group interactions and their impaired instrumental functioning during group missions parallel their usual search for external sources of support, comfort, and safety, and the consequent diversion of attention from instrumental task performance. In summary, these group-related appraisals, emotions, and behaviors mirror the ways attachment-anxious people relate to close dyadic relationship partners.

With regard to avoidant attachment, Rom and Mikulincer's (2003) findings reflect both the extension of deactivating strategies to group activities and the possible breakdown of these strategies during group tasks. Deactivating defenses can easily account for avoidant people's negative appraisals of group members, their dismissal of the potential benefits of group interactions, their pursuit of self-reliance goals during group tasks, and their failure to foster closeness and consensus among group members. However, the failure of avoidant people to suppress negative memories of group interactions, to block distressing feelings during group activities, and to function well instrumentally during group missions suggests a breakdown of deactivating defenses under pressure.

In Chapters 7 and 13, we showed that although avoidant deactivating defenses can sometimes succeed in blocking out stressors and negative emotional reactions, there are situations in which these strategies fail to eliminate painful perceptions of current stressors (e.g., giving birth to a child with a serious heart defect), and thoughts and memories of rejection, disapproval, and criticism. The avoidant mind, when operating under a high cognitive or emotional "load" can become overwhelmed with negative emotions and self-conceptions that interfere with effective functioning. Group activities, at least in a military context, seem to create such a load. During group activities, avoidant people are required to acknowledge and cooperate with other group members; they simply cannot dismiss or deny the interdependent nature of the group's tasks. Moreover, they are unable to distance themselves from their group without provoking conflicts with other group members. These conflicts are likely to arouse attachment-related worries and discomforts that interfere noticeably with performance in a military group, which is ironic, because an avoidant demeanor might seem to fit military stereotypes of the "tough," unemotional, uncommunicative male.

Rom and Mikulincer (2003) also found that group cohesion improved the socioemotional and instrumental functioning of group members and reduced the detrimental effects of attachment anxiety on instrumental functioning during group missions. From an attachment perspective, a cohesive group can be viewed as providing a group-specific sense of approval and security, which makes anxious hyperactivating strategies less necessary and enables an attachment-anxious person to engage more single-mindedly in instrumental tasks. A sense of group cohesion can signal that closeness, support, and consensus, prominent goals of attachment-anxious people, have been achieved, thereby freeing resources for task performance. In line with this interpretation of the results, Rom and Mikulincer found that a cohesive group could attenuate globally attachment-anxious people's group-specific attachment anxiety.

Interestingly, group cohesion failed to improve the functioning of avoidant military recruits (Rom & Mikulincer, 2003). Some of the findings even suggested that a cohesive group exacerbated avoidant people's poor instrumental functioning. As reviewed in previous chapters (Chapters 7, 9, and 13, this volume), avoidant people are resistant to symbolic activation of attachment security representations or to the actual presence of supportive others. This imperviousness seems to hold up even during group activities. Interdependent group interactions may be so threatening or distasteful to avoidant people that they fail to benefit from a potentially available group-specific sense of security. Alternatively, group cohesion, which implies a very high level of interdependence among group members, may exacerbate rather than calm avoidant people's attachment-related fears and discomfort. High group cohesion may threaten avoidant people's sense of complete self-reliance.

Rom and Mikulincer (2003) also replicated E. R. Smith et al.'s (1999) discovery of a strong association between dyadic and group-specific attachment styles. Dyadic attachment anxiety, which we have portrayed throughout this book as a long-standing personal disposition, was associated with group attachment anxiety, and dyadic avoidant attachment was associated with group avoidant attachment. However, Rom and Mikulincer (2003) also showed that group processes and dynamics affected the "transference" of one's dyadic attachment style to the group level. First, group cohesion significantly attenuated group-level attachment insecurities, whether anxious or avoidant, and weakened the transference of dyadic attachment anxiety to the group context. This finding supports the proposition that group cohesion enhances group members' sense of security. Second, dyadic avoidance actually contributed to group-specific attachment *anxiety*. We interpret this finding as an indication that military group activities are so threatening for avoidant people that they are unable to suppress attachment-related anxiety, which impairs their instrumental performance.

Attachment-related impediments to group functioning have also been observed in the context of group psychotherapy (E. C. Chen & Mallinckrodt, 2002; Mallinckrodt & Chen, 2004; Shechtman & Rybko, 2004). For example, E. C. Chen and Mallinckrodt (2002) and Mallinckrodt and Chen (2004) assessed group attraction and perception of other group members' interpersonal traits in American university students participating in 10–12 group counseling sessions intended to facilitate interpersonal growth. Attachment style (assessed with the ECR) was measured before the group counseling sessions began, and the other measures were collected at midpoint (fifth or sixth session) and termination of the counseling process. Findings revealed that more avoidant participants were less attracted to their group and less accurate in appraising other group members' interpersonal traits (compared with aggregate ratings provided by all other group members). Once again, this outcome parallels findings from studies of dyadic relationships, in which avoidant couple members typically report poor impressions of their partner and relationship (Chapters 6 and 10, this volume).

In another study of socioemotional functioning during group counseling, Shechtman and Rybko (2004) asked 436 Israeli university students to complete the RQ before beginning a series of 12 or 13 two-hour sessions of group counseling. Participants were randomly assigned to groups of 10–25 participants, in which they were expected, with the help of a counselor, to share personal information, listen empathically to others, and help other group members deal with interpersonal problems. The transcripts of the first counseling session were analyzed, and two judges rated each participant's level of self-disclosure during the session. In addition, at the end of the last session, participants rated their self-disclosure, group intimacy, and empathy toward other group members. Counselors also provided ratings of each participant's self-disclosure, intimacy, empathy, and constructive work during the counseling process. Both avoidant- and attachment-anxious participants were rated after the first group session as sharing less intimate personal information than that shared by secure participants. In addition, whereas avoidant participants scored lower than secure ones on self-disclosure, intimacy, and empathy at the end of the counseling process (based on either self- or counselor reports), counselors rated anxiously attached participants as working less constructively than secure ones during group sessions.

Overall, the studies conducted so far support the application of attachment theory and research to the study of groups. The findings indicate that attachment anxiety and avoidance encourage negative attitudes toward groups and impair people's instrumental and socioemotional functioning in group contexts. These findings have been replicated in social groups (e.g., fraternities and sororities), small work teams, and group counseling settings. However, these studies do not distinguish, on the one hand, between relatively small, face-to-face groups in which there is a direct dyadic relationship among pairs of members and, on the other hand, large groups or organizations in which more symbolic bonds exist (e.g., identification with one's nation). Future research should determine whether the attachment system operates in a similar manner in more symbolic groups and organizations, and how the need for proximity is manifested in these groups. It is also worth noting that the studies we just reviewed did not take into account the likelihood that attachment-related processes in group contexts interact with other behavioral systems, such as affiliation or exploration, and other needs, such as the need to belong and need for companionship, that operate in these contexts.

There is also some evidence that the sense of security fostered by a cohesive group can have healing, ameliorative effects on attachment-anxious people. This finding supports McCluskey's (2002) contention that "failures in early attachment relationships can be revisited within the context of therapeutic groups and that groups can provide the context for supporting authentic connection with one's own affect and encourage resonance with the affect of other people" (p. 140). More research is needed on the psychological and interpersonal processes through which groups might help insecure adults revise their working models of self and others.

Research is also needed on the possible effects of various group compositions based on group members' attachment styles (i.e., the relative proportions of secure, anxious, and avoidant group members). Do homogeneous groups of securely attached members function better than heterogeneous groups of secure and insecure members? Perhaps so. Throughout this book we have described many situations in which security proves to be adaptive. But there might also be cases in which the inclusion of anxious and avoidant people has beneficial effects on group functioning. Anxious individuals may be good "threat detectors," who can rapidly inform other group members about potential problems in accomplishing group tasks. Avoidant people may react quickly when there is insufficient time for group discussion and consensus formation. If so, the benefits may still depend on the presence of some secure individuals who can coordinate the group members; maintain cooperation, consensus, and solidarity; and respect and encourage others' autonomy and creativity. Future research should test these ideas, which may have practical value for composing work teams that optimize the contributions of all members.

ATTACHMENT AND LEADERSHIP

Attachment theory is also useful in conceptualizing leader–follower relations. In an elaboration and extension of Freud's (1930/1961) metaphor of the leader as a father, Popper and Mayseless (2003) applied attachment theory to leader–follower relationships, proposing a close correspondence between leaders (e.g., managers, political and religious authorities, teachers, supervisors, and military officers) and attachment figures. "Leaders, like parents, are figures whose role includes guiding, directing, taking charge, and taking care of others less powerful than they and whose fate is highly dependent on them" (p. 42); that is, leaders can adopt the role of "stronger and wiser" caregiver, and provide a safe haven and secure base for their followers. Like security-enhancing attachment figures, effective leaders are likely to be available, sensitive, and responsive to their followers' needs; provide advice, guidance, and emotional and instrumental resources to group members; develop followers' autonomy, initiative, and creativity; build followers' sense of self-worth, competence, and mastery; support their desire to take on new challenges and acquire new skills; affirm their ability to deal with challenges; admire and applaud their successes; and encourage their personal growth (Bass, 1985; House & Howell, 1992; Howell, 1988; Shamir, House, & Arthur, 1993; Zaleznick, 1992). In other words, leaders can be sensitive and responsive caregivers ("good shepherds") who provide their followers with a sense of security and a solid platform for autonomous growth (Mayseless & Popper, in press).

From an attachment perspective, followers occupy the role of the dependent, needy, and vulnerable "child" when they seek a leader's support and guidance. According to Popper and Mayseless (2003), this search for a "stronger and wiser" leader reflects activation of the attachment system and formation of a symbolic attachment bond with the leader. In their view, just as attachment needs and behaviors are activated by threat appraisals (Bowlby, 1969/1982), desire for a strong leader tends to arise in times of personal or collective crisis, trauma, or uncertainty (e.g., Mayseless & Popper, in press; Popper, 2001; Shamir, 1999). During such demanding and challenging periods, followers want to feel close to a leader who can protect them and provide advice and guidance. The followers' position need not be conceptualized as infantile or regressive, however. Bowlby (1969/1982) strongly criticized his psychoanalytic predecessors who viewed attachment as an example of excessive dependency or childishness, viewing it instead as a natural tendency of primates, including human beings. Attachment provides both a safe haven and a secure base for personal growth toward mature autonomy. Like Bowlby, several leadership theorists view followers' desire for a "stronger and wiser" attachment figure–leader as a prerequisite for personal growth and self-actualization (e.g., Bass, 1985; Howell, 1988; Shamir et al., 1993). Just as students with caring teachers become increasingly independent learners and performers, and as well-parented children become high-functioning adults, organizational followers can become better, stronger, and wiser adults, and in some cases leaders in their own right under the guidance and good judgment of an effective leader.

An attachment perspective on leader–follower relations helps us to understand the effects of a leader on followers' development and functioning. A sensitive and responsive leader, like other security-enhancing attachment figures, can support a broaden-and-build cycle of attachment security in followers. As discussed and documented in Chapter 3, this volume, this cycle involves a cascade of mental processes that facilitate personal adjustment and growth, including feelings of being esteemed and accepted, increased confidence in one's coping abilities and interpersonal skills, greater reliance on constructive methods of managing stress, and increased application of mental resources to creative exploration and skills acquisition. According to Popper and Mayseless (2003), creating a sense of attachment security and exploratory courage in followers is an effective leader's main method of empowering them and increasing their self-esteem, competence, autonomy, creativity, and overall well-being. Moreover, providing a sense of security is the key to the corrective, therapeutic changes a good leader can sometimes effect in maladjusted or troubled followers. Like a therapist who provides a secure base for exploring personal and interpersonal problems (see Chapter 14, this volume), a leader (e.g., a teacher, manager, rabbi, general, or president) can provide a secure base for initiating and sustaining adaptive changes in personal and social behavior (M. A. Hill, 1984; Rosenthal & Jacobson, 1968).

As in other cases of attachment figure insensitivity or unavailability, a leader's inability or unwillingness to respond sensitively to followers' needs can heighten followers' anxiety, demoralization, or rebellion ("protest"). Of course, as we have indicated throughout this book, followers' insecurities can amplify their sense of vulnerability and need, reinforce doubts about their worth and efficacy, and direct their attention to worries and their energy to defenses, thus interfering with adjustment and growth. Moreover, an unavailable or insensitive leader can provoke hyperactivating or deactivating attachment strategies in followers that either increase childish, anxious dependence on a destructive (e.g., totalitarian) figure or compulsively self-reliant rejection of the leader's guidance. In both cases, these secondary attachment strategies can radically alter the relationship between leader and follower, and transform what began as the promise of a safe haven and secure base into a destructive, conflicted, irrationally hostile relationship that is self-defeating for both leader and followers. (Nazi Germany under Hitler and the Soviet Union under Stalin come to mind as dramatic examples, as do the downfalls of many earlier regimes and empires throughout history.) From an attachment perspective, the key factor in a leader's failure to empower followers is the development of an insecure attachment bond, because of the leader's lack of sensitivity and responsiveness to followers' genuine and legitimate needs. Also important are followers' distrust, ambivalence, and rejection of the leader's distorted approach to "caregiving."

Attachment theory and research also suggest that leaders' and followers' attachment styles are likely to be important for understanding leadership and the quality of leader–follower relations. Secure leaders can confidently and skillfully adopt the role of "stronger and wiser" caregiver (Franklin Roosevelt, with his "fireside chats" and the admonition not to succumb to "fear of fear itself," is an example among American presidents; the Dalai Lama, whose *Ethics for a New Millennium* (1999) epitomizes an open, tolerant approach to relations between individuals, cultures, religions, and governments, is an example among religious and cultural leaders). This approach to leadership infuses a sense of courage, hope, and dedication in followers, whereas an insecure approach to leadership encourages anxiety, anger, disorganization, dishonesty, and despair. Moreover, followers who are attached to a security-enhancing leader are more likely to trust him or her, rely on the leader's advice and guidance, and organize themselves effectively to carry out the group's functions. This is likely to result in increased success of the group and an enhanced sense of competence and value in the group members.

Because accepting the role of leader transforms an individual, at least for a time, into an attachment figure and calls for effective caregiving behavior, the positive effects of a leader's attachment security can be partially explained by the interplay between the leader's attachment and caregiving systems (Bowlby, 1969/1982; Collins, Guichard, et al., 2006; Gillath, Shaver, & Mikulincer, 2005; Kunce & Shaver, 1994). As discussed and empirically supported in Chapter 11, this volume, secure individuals, when functioning as parents, partners, or helpers, can focus fully and accurately on others' needs, without being deflected by personal distress or cynical lack of empathy. Their positive models of self and others are likely to sustain sensitive, responsive, and effective caregiving. In contrast, insecure people, either anxious or avoidant, have difficulty organizing and delivering sensitive and responsive acts of care toward close relationship partners and other needy human beings. Therefore, secure individuals are well equipped to occupy the role of security-enhancing leader, whereas insecure individuals are likely to have difficulty meeting followers' needs for a safe haven and secure base.

Attachment-anxious people's self-preoccupied focus on personal threats and unsatisfied attachment needs can draw mental resources away from attending and responding empathically to followers' needs. They may seek the role of leader as a means of satisfying unmet needs for attention, closeness, and acceptance rather than as a means of meeting followers' needs and promoting their healthy development. Moreover, anxious leaders can intrude upon followers and promote dependence even when followers do not need immediate assistance or help. Nervous but narcissistic teachers who draw too much attention to themselves, monopolize the "air space" and cause their students to feel helpless rather than increasingly capable are examples. American president Bill Clinton's overly ambitious and premature efforts to reform the American health care system and solve the problem of gays in the military (not to mention his inability to ignore a worshipful intern's thong underwear) are examples in the political realm. According to Keller (2003), attachment-anxious leaders' attitudes "may inadvertently undermine followers' sense of competence as followers come to doubt their abilities and rely heavily on the leader" (p. 150). Such leaders may also create reactance or resistance that makes achievement of their goals (education, international understanding, universal health care, equal treatment for gays and straights) unlikely.

In addition, an attachment-anxious person's negative models of self can create doubts about his or her efficacy as a leader, which arouses followers' anxiety and demoralization. (We see a parallel here to what happened in the United States when President Jimmy Carter, a well-intentioned, ethical person, demoralized citizens to the point that they lost trust, lowered their expectations, and rudderless and adrift [Shaver, 1980].) From an attachment perspective, anxiously attached people, who habitually present themselves as weak and vulnerable, are not likely to be perceived by followers as capable of occupying the role of leader in times of crisis. Instead, followers are likely to respond with disapproval, criticism, and rejection.

Avoidant leaders' lack of comfort with closeness and interdependence, and their negative models of others, are likely to interfere with empathic perception of followers' needs and concerns. (Whichever royal personage first said "Let them eat cake" [in response to hearing that the peasants had no bread] would be an example, as would President Nixon's dismissive comment that "the American people are children.") Avoidant leaders are likely to view leadership as another opportunity to reinforce their inflated view of themselves as strong, tough, and independent, and to win followers' admiration and applause. In addition, because they often maintain what they think is a safe distance from the experience and expression of emotions, avoidant leaders are likely to concentrate on the task at hand rather than getting involved with followers' emotional needs. Avoidant leaders may therefore complete important functional tasks (making money, running a large company), yet fail to provide emotional support, empower their followers, and create optimal conditions for their followers' growth and self-actualization.

An interesting example of a person who, at least from a distance and based on news reports, seems to be high on avoidant attachment is the current U.S. Vice President Dick Cheney. He is known throughout the journalistic and comedy worlds for his tight-lipped mumble, grouchy cynicism, extreme conservatism, and exceptional secretiveness, yet he makes millions of dollars a year more than the President because of his previous life as a successful CEO of a giant energy corporation, Halliburton. While we were working on this book, his image became momentarily very visible on satirical comedy shows after he accidentally shot one of his hunting companions in the face, then failed to report it for as long as possible.

The liberal newsletter, *MoveOn Bulletin* (2002), described Cheney's propensity to maintain a low profile:

> For months, he rarely appeared at all, emerging only to sell his political ideas on CNN or to dismiss allegations of corporate wrongdoing. Even now, Cheney mostly stays in a "secure location," ready to spring into action if President Bush is attacked. Unlike most politicians, Cheney actually enjoys working in the background. By his own account, he doesn't relish campaigning, and he's hardly a natural spokesman.

As *New Yorker* writer Jane Mayer (2004) explained: "As Defense Secretary, Cheney developed a contempt for Congress, which, a friend said, he came to regard as 'a bunch of annoying gnats.' " This is an example of a "negative model of others" expressed at the group level.

That kind of dismissive language may not be unusual for the Vice President. As described by Dewar and Milbank (2004) in the *Washington Post*:

> A chance meeting with Sen. Patrick J. Leahy, the ranking Democrat on the Judiciary Committee, became an argument about Cheney's ties to Halliburton Co., an international energy services corporation, and President Bush's judicial nominees. The exchange ended when Cheney offered some crass advice. "Fuck yourself," said the man who is a heartbeat from the presidency.

Compare this with Harwood's (2003) description of the facilitating leader who

> uses his own cohesion, vitality, and ideals for the protection and benefit of all members of the group. He uses empathic introspection in order to be aware of each member's subjectivity for the growth and benefit of each individual as well as the group. . . . The facilitating leader has a quiet . . . charisma [that] leads to growth and spontaneity for each individual member. (p. 127)

Followers' attachment insecurities can also create problems for the leader–follower relationship. In Chapters 6 and 7, we discussed insecurely attached individuals' negative appraisals of close relationship partners in particular and fellow human beings in general; their reluctance to seek support and comfort from attachment figures; and their inability or unwillingness to cultivate supportive relationships and benefit from them during periods of stress. Their lack of synchrony and interdependence with dyadic partners can easily become transformed into distrust of a leader, criticism or rejection of the leader's efforts to provide a safe haven and secure base, and dissatisfaction with the leader's performance. Not surprisingly, the conjunction of insecure followers and an insecure leader can have disastrous consequences, running from compliance with demagogues, such as Senator Joseph McCarthy and the frightened anti-Communists who believed his every paranoid accusation, and "The Gang of Four" that sparked the incredibly irrational and destructive Cultural Revolution in China.

In a creative but speculative theoretical article, Keller (2003) claimed that the combination of an avoidant leader and anxious followers or of an anxious leader and avoidant followers is the most dangerous. As in marital relationships, these configurations can create destructive pursuit–distancing or demand–withdrawal patterns of interdependent behavior (Chapter 10, this volume). An anxious person's dependency needs frustrate an avoidant person's wish for distance, and an avoidant person's inattention and rejection of proximity bids exacerbate an anxious person's fear of rejection and doubts about self-worth. Interestingly, Keller suggested that a combination of avoidant leader and avoidant follower can be more benign: "The avoidant follower may be grateful to be left alone without intrusions from the leader, while the avoidant leader may admire the follower's independence" (p. 152). Keller also suggested than an anxious leader and an anxious follower can sometimes coexist, because each can meet the other's need for attention, dependency, and proximity. However, marital research indicates instead that the pairing of two anxious partners can create destructive, narcissistic pursuit–pursuit patterns of relating that can result in mutual frustration and even violence (Chapter 10, this volume).

Keller's (2003) interesting ideas still await empirical examination. To date, research has focused on leaders' or followers' attachment styles, but not on the ways in which various configurations of attachment styles affect the quality of leader–follower relations. In the following sections we review evidence on the contribution of a leader's attachment style to his or her performance and reception by followers. We also review the few studies that have examined the independent contributions of leaders' and followers' attachment styles to the quality of their interactions and joint outcomes.

Patterns of Leadership

Initial evidence regarding the possible association between attachment style and leadership was provided by Mikulincer and Florian (1995) in a study of young Israeli military recruits' reactions to combat training. These authors assessed recruits' attachment styles (using self-report scales) at the beginning of 4 months of intensive combat training, then at the end of training asked recruits to provide leadership nominations. Each recruit nominated three other recruits from his unit based on leadership qualities ("Which recruits have what is needed to be good military officers?"). As it turned out, securely attached recruits were perceived as having the qualities needed for leadership, and attachment-anxious recruits were not. This result was replicated in a larger study of 402 Israeli soldiers undergoing 3 months of combat training, this time even after statistical control for other personality traits, such as locus of control and trait anxiety (Popper, Amit, Gal, Mishkal-Sinai, & Lisak, 2004).

Other studies have revealed theoretically predictable associations between leaders' attachment orientations and their style of leadership. For example, Popper, Mayseless, and Castelnovo (2000) focused in three studies on the distinction between transactional and transformational leadership (e.g., Bass, 1985; Zaleznik, 1992). Transactional leaders are ones who encourage followers to perform the tasks they are assigned by offering them immediate rewards for performance; transformational leaders are more interested in empowering followers and promoting their growth and self-actualization. Bass and

Avolio (1990) delineated four characteristics of transformational leadership: (1) idealized influence—the leader places followers' needs ahead of his or her own needs, avoids using authority for personal gains, and exhibits high moral standards; (2) inspirational motivation—the leader inspires trust and respect and engages followers by communicating a vision of a better future and showing commitment to pursuit of this vision; (3) individualized consideration—the leader treats each follower as a special person and mentors him or her on a path to self-actualization; (4) intellectual stimulation—the leader inspires followers to explore new ideas and approaches, learn new skills, and emphasizes creativity and innovation in problem solving.

In their first study, Popper et al. (2000) asked instructors of officer cadet courses in the Israeli Army to rate attachment style and the extent to which each cadet exhibited the four qualities of a transformational leader. In the second study, the instructors rated each cadet's transformational leadership qualities, and the cadets themselves rated their own attachment style. In the third study, the transformational leadership qualities of Israeli squad commanders in infantry units were evaluated by their soldiers, and the commanders rated their own attachment style. In all three studies, a secure attachment style was associated with transformational leadership qualities; that is, more secure cadets were rated by their instructors (Studies 1–2) or more secure commanders were rated by their followers (Study 3) as exhibiting more idealized influence, inspirational motivation, individualized consideration, and intellectual stimulation. In addition, attachment insecurities (both anxiety and avoidance) were associated with lower levels of transformational leadership. It therefore seems, as expected, that secure individuals have the potential to become transformational leaders who set their followers on a path to autonomy, creativity, growth, and self-expansion.

Popper (2002) and Davidovitz, Mikulincer, Shaver, Ijzak, and Popper (2006, Studies 1 and 2) assessed associations between attachment style and another taxonomy of leadership styles: personalized versus socialized (e.g., House & Howell, 1992; Howell, 1988). Personalized leaders put their own interests ahead of their followers' needs and exhibit a dictatorial style of leadership that includes belittling followers and ascribing maximum importance to themselves. Socialized leaders use power to serve and empower others, align their vision with followers' needs and aspirations, and respect the followers' rights and feelings. In Popper's (2002) study, instructors of officer cadet courses in the Israeli army rated each cadet's style of leadership, and the cadets reported on their own attachment style. In Davidovitz et al.'s (2006) studies, Israeli military officers and managers in the public or private sector rated their attachment style using the ECR scales and also characterized their style of leadership.

Across the studies, avoidant attachment was associated with lower levels of socialized leadership and higher levels of personalized leadership. In addition, Davidovitz et al. (2006, Studies 1 and 2) found that attachment-anxious leaders were more likely than less anxious leaders to endorse a personalized style of leadership; that is, attachment insecurities seem to interfere with a nurturant, other-focused leadership style and favor more narcissistic forms of leadership. This narcissistic tendency may explain Johnston's (2000) finding that insecurely attached managers were less likely than secure ones to delegate responsibility and power to subordinates and more likely to create centralized authority structures.

Insecure people's narcissistic approach to leadership was also noted in Davidovitz et al.'s (2006, Study 1) assessment of motives for leadership. Based on semistructured interviews with well-known Israeli political, economic, and military leaders, Davidovitz et al. constructed a self-report scale tapping five different motives to lead: (1) self-serving or self-enhancing motives related to self-protection and social admiration ("I want to win respect and esteem"); (2) prosocial motives, such as advancing social goals and contributing to others' welfare ("I want to bring about changes in my organization"); (3) need for control, and the use of leadership to satisfy this need ("I want things to be done according to my plans"); (4) task-oriented motives and the successful accomplishment of instrumental tasks ("I like the challenge of getting people to perform a task"); and (5) desire for freedom, self-reliance, and avoidance of dependence on others ("I want to get more freedom of action in my organization"). There were significant cross-sectional associations between the different motives and leaders' ECR scores. Attachment anxiety was associated with self-enhancing motives for leadership, control-related motives, and self-reliance motives. Avoidant attachment was associated with self-reliance motives and weaker prosocial motives. Overall, the findings support the hypothesis that leaders' attachment insecurities go hand in hand with self-focused motives to lead rather than other-focused (prosocial) motives.

Davidovitz et al. (2006, Studies 1 and 2) also examined attachment-style differences in perceptions of self-efficacy in performing leadership tasks. They constructed a self-report scale to assess the extent to which participants believed they could cope effectively with situations involving followers' emotional needs and leader–follower emotional bonds (emotion-focused situations) and situations calling for the achievement of instrumental goals or completion of group tasks (task-focused situations). Attachment anxiety was associated with lower perceived self-efficacy in task-focused situations, and avoidance, with lower perceived self-efficacy in emotion-focused situations.

Taken together, these new findings begin to paint portraits of the kinds of leadership associated with each kind of attachment insecurity (anxiety or avoidance). More anxious leaders tend to focus on their own needs and to adopt a dictatorial style of leadership that includes belittling followers and at the same time harbor doubts about their own ability to help followers complete instrumental tasks. More avoidant leaders tend to view leadership as an opportunity to bolster their self-reliance and avoid dependence on others, while ignoring the nurturant and caring aspects of the leadership role and harboring doubts about their ability to handle followers' emotional needs. These leadership styles are obviously parallel to the attachment-related behavior patterns we have found, in earlier chapters, to arise in close dyadic relationships, suggesting that the effects of attachment styles are pervasive and similar across different kinds of relationships.

The Quality of Leader–Follower Relationships and the Behavior of Followers

In two separate studies, Davidovitz et al. (2006, Studies 2 and 3) examined the effects of a leader's attachment style on the quality of leader–follower relations. These studies, conducted in the Israeli Army, also provide preliminary evidence regarding the biases that followers' attachment styles impose on their perceptions of their leaders. In one study, 549 Israeli soldiers in regular military service, from 60 different military units participating in a leadership workshop, rated themselves on attachment anxiety and avoidance using the ECR scales. They also rated the cohesiveness of their military unit and their own instrumental and socioemotional functioning within this unit (using scales similar to the ones employed by Rom & Mikulincer [2003] described earlier in this chapter). Soldiers also rated their direct officer's pattern of leadership (personalized vs. socialized) and the officer's effectiveness as a leader. The 60 direct officers completed the ECR, providing a description of their own attachment orientations. Thus, Davidovitz et al. (2006) were able to examine the effects of leaders' and followers' attachment styles on the followers' perceptions of the leader, the cohesiveness of their group, and the followers' instrumental and socioemotional functioning within their unit.

The results revealed that followers' perceptions of their leader matched the leader's self-reports, indicating considerable convergent validity. More avoidant officers were rated by their followers as having a relatively personalized leadership style, meaning that these officers were less able to deal effectively with their followers' emotional needs. Also, they rated more anxious officers as less able to bring about the successful completion of group tasks. Thus, both insecurely attached officers and their soldiers noticed the same problematic patterns of leadership. However, there were also some interesting and predictable *biases* in the soldiers' appraisals of their officers' leadership: The more avoidant a soldier, the more he appraised his officer as a personalized rather than a socialized leader, and the more critical were his appraisals of the officer's ability to lead in both task- and emotion-focused situations. This pattern of appraisals fits well with avoidant individuals' well-documented negative mental representations, or working models, of others (Chapter 6, this volume). Interestingly, the analyses revealed no significant interaction between soldiers' and officers' attachment scores, implying that avoidant soldiers tend to generate more negative than average appraisals of their leaders, even when the leaders are secure and exhibit a more socialized pattern of leadership that is noticed and acknowledge by less avoidant soldiers.

Replicating Rom and Mikulincer's (2003) findings, soldiers' avoidance was associated with impaired instrumental and socioemotional functioning in their unit. Moreover, the study revealed negative influences of a leader's avoidance on his followers' functioning in the group: Officer's avoidance had a detrimental effect on group cohesion and on soldiers' socioemotional functioning. These negative effects were mediated by avoidant officers' lack of a socialized leadership style and lack of efficacy in dealing with soldiers' emotional needs. It seems likely, therefore, and in line with theory, that a leader's avoidance is associated with low nurturance and supportiveness, which adversely affects followers' socioemotional functioning and group cohesion. An avoidant leader alienates and demoralizes followers, reduces their enthusiasm for each other and their group tasks, and leaves them feeling dissatisfied—perhaps not too different from an avoidant spouse's effect on his or her partner's feelings.

Davidovitz et al. (2006) also found that the effects of officers' avoidance did not interact with their soldier-followers' avoidance. The two effects were independent and contributed jointly (additively) to the soldiers' functioning. This means that the poorest functioning was observed when soldiers high on avoidance were paired with an officer who was also high on avoidance. This clearly contradicts Keller's (2003) speculative idea that avoidant leaders and avoidant followers might coexist comfortably, with good results for group performance. At least in a military context, this specific pairing of leader and followers has serious negative consequences for followers' performance and well-being.

With regard to a leader's attachment anxiety, the findings revealed a complex pattern of effects on followers' functioning. On one hand, officers' attachment anxiety had a negative effect on soldiers' instrumental functioning, which was mediated by anxious officers' lack of efficacy in dealing with task-focused situations. It seems likely that a leader's attachment anxiety interferes with efficient and successful completion of group tasks, which in turn erodes followers' confidence in their own instrumental functioning. In other words, an anxious leader's doubts about his own functioning are echoed in his followers' doubts about task completion.

On the other hand, Davidovitz et al. (2006, Study 2) found an unexpected positive effect of officers' attachment anxiety on group cohesion and on soldiers' socioemotional functioning. It seems possible, therefore, that an anxious leader's emphasis on emotional closeness and interdependence helps followers become emotionally involved and interpersonally close. It is also possible that followers' attempts to maintain group cohesion, consensus, and morale may be a defensive reaction of the group to the anxieties, worries, and uncertainties of an attachment-anxious leader. In any case, followers' good socioemotional functioning under these conditions seems to be achieved at the expense of deficits in instrumental functioning. Perhaps an anxiously attached leader diverts followers' attention and resources toward socioemotional issues and away from instrumental task completion.

In another study, Davidovitz et al. (2006, Study 3) approached 541 Israeli military recruits and their 72 direct officers at the beginning of a 4-month period of intensive combat training and asked them to report on their attachment styles (using Hazan & Shaver's [1987] prototype ratings). At the same time, soldiers completed a self-report scale measuring their baseline mental heath (Mental Health Inventory). After 2 months, soldiers reported on their mental health again and provided appraisals of their officer as a provider of security (i.e., the officer's ability and willingness to be available in times of need, and to accept and care for his or her soldiers rather than rejecting and criticizing them). Two months later (4 months after combat training began), soldiers once again evaluated their mental health. In this way, Davidovitz et al. (2006) assessed the effects of leaders' and followers' attachment styles on a novel leadership construct derived directly from attachment theory—a leader's ability to serve as a security-providing figure—while tracking changes in followers' mental health during a highly stressful period. During such a period, it was expected that an officer's attachment security and his functioning as a security provider would be important for soldiers' emotional well-being.

The more avoidant an officer was, the less his soldiers viewed him as accepting and available, and the more they felt rejected and criticized by him. It is interesting to see how well this finding generalizes across different measures of leadership (Popper, 2002; Popper et al., 2000). Regardless of the measures used, avoidant leaders are observed to dismiss or ignore the nurturant and caring aspects of leadership, and fail to provide a safe haven and secure base for their followers. Davidovitz et al. (2006) also found that more avoidant soldiers tended to appraise their officer as more rejecting and unavailable, again demonstrating their pervasive negative models of others (Chapter 6, this volume) and the negative biases imposed by these models on perception of a leader.

Also of great significance, a leader's attachment style seems to bring about undesirable changes in followers' mental health during combat training. At the beginning of training, baseline mental health was an exclusive reflection of soldiers' own attachment anxiety: The higher their anxiety, the worse their mental health (in line with findings in nonmilitary samples summarized in Chapter 13, this volume). At the time of the baseline assessment, leaders' attachment style had no significant effect on followers' well-being, as could be expected given that the soldiers hardly knew their officers at this point. However, leaders' attachment insecurities influenced changes in soldiers' mental health over the weeks of training (taking the baseline assessment into account). The higher the officer's avoidance score, the more his soldiers' mental health deteriorated over 2 and 4 months of intensive combat training. Analyses also revealed that the detrimental effect of a leader's avoidance was mediated by his functioning as a security provider; that is, an officer's avoidance impaired his functioning as a security-providing attachment figure, which in turn had negative effects on his soldiers' mental health during combat training.

These findings resonate with the repeatedly observed detrimental effects of parents' attachment insecurities on their offsprings' mental health during childhood (e.g., Cowan, Cohn, Cowan, & Pearson, 1996; Crowell et al., 1991; DeKlyen, 1996; Marchand, Schedler, & Wagstaff, 2004; Whiffen, Kerr, & Kallos-Lilly, 2005) and adolescence (e.g., Bosquet & Egeland, 2001; Kobak & Ferentz-Gillies, 1995). Like insecure parents, avoidant officers' poor-quality caregiving impairs soldiers' adjustment during stressful combat training. Hence, Davidovitz et al.'s (2006) findings support the metaphor of leaders as parents and highlight the importance of leader's secure attachment for the maintenance of followers' mental health and emotional well-being. Moreover, these leader–follower studies are not susceptible to the usual doubts about the social, as opposed to exclusively genetic, effects of parents on their children. The different kinds of military leaders obviously had no genetic influences on their followers.

It is also important to realize that soldiers' attachment scores significantly moderated the effects of officers' avoidant attachment on changes in mental health. Officers' avoidance brought about a significant deterioration of soldiers' mental health during the initial 2 months of combat training mainly among insecurely attached soldiers, whether they were relatively anxious, avoidant, or both. (This supports our perspective in Chapter 13, where we portrayed attachment insecurity as a general vulnerability factor for poor mental health rather than viewing each form of insecurity as leading to a specific kind of mental disorder.) More secure soldiers were able to maintain a relatively stable and high level of mental health despite being under the command of an avoidant officer; that is, soldiers who had either internalized a secure base earlier in development or were able to bring one with them mentally from home were able to escape the detrimental effects of an avoidant officer's lack of nurturance and poor socialized leadership skills.

Notably, this buffering effect of followers' security was evident mainly when mental health was assessed only 2 months after combat training began. After 4 months of combat training, an officer's avoidance had negative effects on soldiers' mental health regardless of the soldiers' attachment style. In other words, as time passed and problems continued, the negative effects of an officer's avoidant style on soldiers' mental health overrode the initial buffering effects of soldiers' dispositional attachment security. It is important to remember that these findings were obtained during a highly stressful period in which soldiers were under the complete control of their officer and in a situation where their physical welfare depended on their obedience to the officer's commands. We need to examine in future studies how leaders' and followers' attachment orientations interact in less extreme and demanding situations, and in other kinds of organizational contexts (e.g., manager–subordinate relations in a workplace). For us, the findings help explain why, even in societies and subcultures where most children grow up with secure attachment styles, when stressful conditions and poor leadership cross some threshold, and almost everyone feels endangered, strained, and insecure, "bad things can happen to good people" (to paraphrase the title of Rabbi Harold Kuschner's famous 1981 book).

Overall, these studies highlight the detrimental effects of a leader's attachment insecurities on the quality of leader–follower relations and followers' emotional and instrumental functioning. Moreover, they suggest a dynamic interplay between leaders' and followers' attachment orientations. However, we should keep in mind that these are studies of men in military contexts. Future studies should attempt to replicate and extend the findings to other organizational settings and should include women. More systematic and longitudinal research is also needed to identify and examine leader–follower processes in more detail. Future studies should address a host of unanswered questions, such as whether and how securely attached followers can defend against the deleterious effects of an insecure leader; whether and how a group as a whole can protect its members from such deleterious effects; whether and how insecurely attached followers can neurotically resist, to their own detriment, a secure leader's beneficial influences; and whether and how a secure leader can provide corrective experiences and move insecure followers toward increased security and personal growth. A deeper understanding of these processes can help management schools and organizational psychologists create better leadership development programs and better interventions aimed at improving poor leader–follower relations.

Research should also identify the personal, interpersonal, and sociocultural factors that cause followers to accept the authority of insecure leaders and to comply with their destructive, narcissistic influences. In addition, future studies should explore the attachment-related techniques that self-serving leaders use to manipulate insecurely attached followers and convince them to commit destructive acts against themselves or others (e.g., the mass suicides in Jonestown, the disaster that befell a devoted religious cult in Waco, Texas, and the homicidal and suicidal terrorist attacks of September 11, 2001, not to mention genocide in Germany, Cambodia, the Balkans, Rwanda, Darfur, and countless other places throughout the world and all through human history).

Attachment insecurity is evident in Stern's (2003) description of the ways in which people are recruited to the role of violent terrorist—an important topic at present. Recruiters target people who are chronically insecure because of prior abuse, trauma, or humiliation, then bring them progressively into line with the aims of terrorist groups or religious cults by alternately heightening their sense of insecurity (by reactivating the trauma and humiliation, and exacerbating the sense of helplessness), then reducing it through group solidarity exercises, praise from cult leaders, and applause for feats of violence against threatening enemies. In this way, hapless followers can identify with the grandiosity of a destructively charismatic leader who promises security, safety, and permanent approval (martyrdom) to compensate for their sense of meaninglessness, futility, and vulnerability. It is easy to disapprove of the martyrs' behavior, especially when one is a target, but it is also possible to understand why they do what they do. Whether a person is viewed as a hero or a maniac is often a matter of one's political and religious affiliation or the outcome of a long battle. (The victors write the prevailing historical accounts.) Still, the enormous danger of this kind of attachment dynamic for humankind is evident to anyone who thinks very deeply about it.

ATTACHMENT AND ORGANIZATIONAL BEHAVIOR

Besides explaining certain aspects of the quality of social interactions within an organization (between group members, between leaders and followers, between ideologies and self-sacrifice), attachment theory helps us to understand the attitudes that both leaders and followers, and managers and subordinates, have toward their organization. As we discussed in Chapter 8, attachment style affects a person's attitudes toward two kinds of organizations—schools and workplaces. Secure people tend to have more positive attitudes toward these organizations, to be more satisfied with school and work activities, and to have fewer school- and work-related problems than their insecure peers. These attachment style correlates may reflect fairly broad orientations toward organizations and organizational processes; hence . they are important for the field of organizational psychology, which has already devoted considerable attention to issues such as organizational commitment and citizenship behavior.

Becoming a committed and productive member of an organization (e.g., a social club, an academic department, or a commercial firm) involves exploration and reorganization of one's role identities and personal priorities (e.g., "How will people treat me when they learn that I'm working for this prestigious law firm?" or "What kind of person will I be if I join this neo-Nazi political party?"). It also requires flexible adaptation to organizational rules, norms, expectations, and demands, as well as acceptance of responsibility and expenditure of effort to accomplish organizational goals. In most cases, organizational membership requires extensive communication, coordination, and negotiation with other members, as well as becoming increasingly interdependent with them, and engaging in work and leisure activities, while remembering their needs for autonomy, privacy, and personal space. Attachment security is likely to be associated with the acquisition and use of the necessary self-regulatory and interpersonal skills (Chapters 8 and 9, this volume). If so, security is likely to be associated with positive experiences in organizations and positive attitudes toward them. In contrast, insecure people's deficits in self-regulation, interpersonal coordination, and prosocial orientation can create obstacles to becoming a committed and productive member of an organization.

Unfortunately, beyond the studies we reviewed in Chapter 8 dealing with satisfaction and problems in schools and workplaces, and a single study on preferences for different employment contracts (Krausz et al., 2001), attachment researchers have not systematically examined attachment style differences in organizational attitudes and behaviors. In the following paragraphs, we present some new, previously unpublished findings about the effects of attachment orientations on organizational citizenship behavior, organizational commitment, and reactions to organizational change. These findings, although preliminary, are compatible with the hypothesis that attachment insecurities interfere with people's efforts to become committed and productive organization members. The findings therefore indicate the potential importance of attachment theory for advancing research and practice in organizational psychology.

One important construct in organizational psychology is organizational citizenship behaviors (OCB)—organizational actions that assist "in the maintenance and enhancement of the social and psychological context that supports task performance" (Organ, 1997, p. 91). Although these behaviors are not explicit organizational requirements and are not directly rewarded by formal organizational reward systems, they play an important part in enhancing organizational effectiveness and sustainability (e.g., King, George, & Hebl, 2005; LePine, Erez, & Johnson, 2002). Based on a meta-analysis of studies examining the structure of the OCB construct, LePine et al. (2002) concluded that it reflects a broad prosocial orientation manifested in five kinds of organizational behavior: cooperative and helpful behavior toward other organization members ("altruism"), inhibition of proclivities and behaviors that might damage organizational efforts and interfere with the accomplishment of organizational tasks ("conscientiousness"), not complaining about mundane organizational issues ("sportsmanship"), respect for other organization members' needs and rights ("courtesy"), and personal involvement in matters of concern for the organization ("civic virtue").

All of these organizational citizenship behaviors can be disrupted, derailed, or overshadowed by attachment insecurities. For example, avoidant people's negative models of others and lack of empathy and prosocial values (Chapters 6 and 11, this volume) interfere with the altruism and courtesy components of OCB. Their tendency to remain defensively detached and personally uninvolved during interdependent activities (Chapter 9, this volume) interferes with civic virtue. In addition, attachment-anxious people's problems with self-control and self-regulation, and their tendency to appraise personal and interpersonal problems in catastrophic terms (Chapters 7 and 8, this volume), are likely to disrupt conscientiousness and sportsmanship, and their egoistic focus on unmet needs for closeness and acceptance (Chapter 9, this volume) are likely to cause disregard for other organization members' rights and needs. Indeed, Desivilya, Sabag, and Ashton (2007) found that higher attachment anxiety and avoidance scores (based on a brief version of the ECR) were significantly associated with lower scores on a self-report measure of OCBs. These early findings suggest that insecurely attached people are insufficiently cooperative and helpful in organizational settings, and that attachment style differences are relevant to organizational effectiveness and sustainability.

Additional unpublished findings of our own suggest that insecurely attached people have problems committing themselves to an organization, engaging in productive organizational behavior, and coping with organizational changes. In one correlational study of a sample of 142 Israeli workers in a high-tech company, we asked participants to complete the ECR, along with scales measuring organizational commitment, intent to quit, and organizational spontaneity. Workers' supervisors also evaluated workers' commitment and spontaneity using the same scales. Organizational commitment was assessed with six items from J. P. Meyer, Allen, and Smith's (1993) scale (e.g., "I really feel a sense of belonging to my organization," "I am proud to belong to this organization"). Intent to quit was measured with two items: "I often think about quitting this organization" and "I intend to search for a position with another employer within the next year." Organizational spontaneity was assessed with five items from Lynch, Eisenberger, and Armeli's (1999) measure (e.g., "I encourage others to try new and more effective ways of doing their job," "I continue to look for new ways to improve the effectiveness of my work").

As can be seen in Table 15.1, more anxious and avoidant people scored lower on organizational commitment and organizational spontaneity, and these characteristics of insecurely attached people were evident in both self-reports and supervisors' evaluations. In addition, avoidant attachment, but not attachment anxiety, was associated with intending to quit the organization, probably reflecting avoidant people's predisposition to leave activities and relationships as soon as they experience strain, threat, or challenge (Chapters 8 and 10, this volume). Again, these findings suggest that attachment insecurities are a risk factor interfering with organizational involvement. Insecure employees' lack of organizational commitment may explain Krausz et al.'s (2001) finding that less secure workers were more likely to prefer external contracts (being hired and paid by an external agency, while temporarily working for a client company) rather than having a more stable committed relationship with their company (being directly hired and paid by a company for a predetermined period).

In another study, we examined attachment style differences in reactions to organizational change. With increasing globalization and rapid technological changes in industrial and service sectors of the economy, planned or "episodic" organizational change (e.g., merging, downsizing) seem to be common and sometimes inevitable ways to retain or enhance an organization's competitive position. Nevertheless, organizational change is a major stressor for organization members. It can challenge their understanding of the organization and its goals, and cause them to question their future value to the organization. It may mean that they have to acquire new skills quickly or risk losing their income.

Of course, organizational change, like almost everything else, elicits different reactions from different people. Some may crave permanence and stability, dread change, and have problems exploring a new organizational environment and adapting to new organizational demands. Others may welcome change, confidently explore new opportunities, and flexibly adjust to changing circumstances. Understanding the causes of these different reactions may help managers identify workers who facilitate or obstruct change.

TABLE 15.1. Pearson Correlations and Standardized Regression Coefficients (β) Showing Associations between Attachment Dimensions and Organizational Variables

Organizational variables	ECR anxiety		ECR avoidance	
	r	β	r	β
Workers' self-reports				
Organizational commitment	−.29**	−.31**	−.27**	−.29**
Organizational spontaneity	−.28**	−.29**	−.25**	−.26**
Intention to quit	.19	.19	.29**	.30**
Workers' supervisors ratings				
Organizational commitment	−.24**	−.25**	−.30**	−.31**
Organizational spontaneity	−.23**	−.25**	−.26**	−.27**
Intention to quit	.10	.11	.35**	.36**

Note. N = 142.
**p < .01.

As we discussed in Chapter 8, attachment insecurities are negatively associated with cognitive openness, novelty seeking, exploratory tendencies, and flexible adjustment to new ideas and new social roles and demands. Moreover, insecurely attached people tend to adopt dysfunctional strategies for dealing with external or internal sources of stress and distress, either intensifying the distress or avoiding constructive problem solving (Chapter 7, this volume). As a result, insecurities may arouse resistance to organizational change and interfere with adjustment to changing organizational circumstances. In contrast, people who possesses a solid, authentic sense of safety, security, and self-efficacy are more able to deal more effectively with changing circumstances, open themselves to the new opportunities offered by these circumstances, and facilitate organizational change.

To take an initial look at possible attachment style differences in reactions to organizational change, we asked 125 Israeli nurses in a private health organization to complete the ECR scales, along with Judge, Thoresen, Pucik, and Welbourne's (1999) measure of coping with organizational change, which assesses both negative reactions to change (e.g., "The changes in this organization cause me stress") and facility in adapting to change (e.g., "When dramatic changes happen in this organization, I feel I can handle them with ease"). In addition, participants were asked to think about an immediate downsizing of health services in their organization, and to report positive and negative feelings elicited by thoughts of organizational change. Attachment insecurities were associated with resistance to organizational change (see Table 15.2). Specifically, more attachment-anxious and avoidant nurses reported more negative reactions and more problems in adjusting to organizational change, as well as more negative feelings when thinking about a specific change in their organization. It therefore seems likely that studying attachment insecurities will help us to understand resistance to organizational change. In today's rapidly changing work environment, this is an important topic for research.

CONCLUDING REMARKS

In this chapter we have shown how attachment theory contributes to organizational science. Individual differences in attachment security, and in kinds of insecurity (anxiety and avoidance), are associated with group- and organization-related cognitions, emotions, behaviors, patterns of leadership, quality of leader–follower relations, organizational citizenship, organizational commitment, and resistance to organizational change. Moreover,

TABLE 15.2. Pearson Correlations and Standardized Regression Coefficients (β) Showing Associations between Attachment Dimensions and Responses to Organizational Change

Reactions to organizational change	ECR anxiety		ECR avoidance	
	r	β	r	β
Judge et al.'s (1999) scale				
Negative reactions to change	.40**	.46**	.33**	.39**
Facility in adapting to change	−.45**	−.48**	−.23**	−.29**
Thought exercise				
Negative feelings	.47**	.51**	.24**	.31**
Positive feelings	.10	.12	−.20	−.16

Note. N = 125.
**p < .01.

cohesive groups and socialized, transformational leaders tend to function as symbolic attachment figures, bolstering members' and followers' senses of safety, security, and permanence, activating and supporting a broaden-and-build cycle of attachment security, and facilitating personal and organizational effectiveness and personal growth.

This application of attachment theory to organizational issues encourages us to believe that important psychodynamic issues, such as conflicts related to love, dependence, and security, and the defenses that arise when a person struggles to master or cope with these conflicts, underlie group processes and leader–follower relationships. The theory may also help us to understand the developmental roots of transformational and destructively self-serving leaders, as well as followers' compliance with destructive leaders. Because attachment theory is both an evolutionary psychological theory and a theory of personality development, it suggests that organizational theorists and researchers should pay attention to both the biological and developmental roots of people's organizational behavior and the ways in which it is shaped by interactions with attachment figures during infancy and childhood. As Bowlby (1969/1982) intended, attachment theory creates important bridges between still-useful psychoanalytic ideas about the human mind and macro-level perspectives on human behavior in groups and organizations.

We hope that the ideas and findings presented in this chapter stimulate researchers to apply Bowlby's theory to the study of other organizational processes (e.g., negotiation, bargaining, empowerment, managerial decision making) and broader societal, economic, and political issues (e.g., intergroup relations, terrorism and war, financial decision making, market dynamics, consumption, media campaigns, and voting behavior). We also hope that future research will examine the contribution to group and organizational processes of normative and individual-difference aspects of other behavioral systems (e.g., exploration, caregiving, sex, and affiliation). Bowlby's ideas about the attachment behavioral system can be extended to provide guides to the investigation of other behavioral systems, each of which involves additional areas of striving, conflict, and defense. Moving beyond the almost exclusive emphasis on the attachment behavioral system, which has characterized the field of attachment research so far, including our own work, would yield a much broader integration of motivation, personality, and organizational psychology. When more fully developed, this integration might yield a deeper understanding of broad sociocultural phenomena and useful leads for parents, clinicians, educators, and organizational leaders who wish to create a more kind, tolerant, harmonious, creative, and peaceful society based on attachment security.

The application of attachment theory, which grew out of the study of parent–child relationships, to larger social and organizational settings is controversial. One of the sources of tension between developmental psychologists, who study attachment phenomena primarily within families (using behavioral observations and clinical-style interviews), and social–personality psychologists like ourselves, who study a broader range of relationships and social environments, is that the theory and its associated measures expand into research domains where concepts such as attitudes, leadership, cohesiveness, and alienation become relevant, and the notion of a particular kind of biologically based dyadic relationship becomes less central. We know from participating in many professional meetings and debates that the extended use of attachment theory, which we favor and find intellectually exciting, seems to child-developmental attachment researchers to be a dangerous adventure into general personality or social psychology, where the uniqueness and special value of the theory are likely to be underappreciated and inadvertently contaminated.

This has always been a source of tension in psychoanalytic psychology. Freud began his work with a mixture of neurology and individual psychotherapy, and ended up writing about religion (*The Future of an Illusion*, 1927/1975), preliterate groups (*Totem and Taboo*, 1913/1956), art and artists, and modern warfare. There is still no agreement among professionals about the value or danger of this kind of expansive theorizing. We confess to being enthusiastic fans of both Freud in particular and expansive theorizing in general. Academic psychologists often talk, especially in methods classes, about ideas being cheap, and good data collection and analyses techniques being more important parts of the research process. Our own view is that data and methods have been proliferating faster than good ideas. The two scientific ideologies, one favoring theory and the other favoring methodological rigor, can coexist and cooperate by allowing ideas to hatch and be clarified and extended before they are prematurely pruned or eviscerated by methods. When it comes to the important field of organizational and group psychology, we can use both dazzling new ideas and pristine methods.

PART V

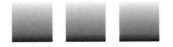

EPILOGUE

CHAPTER 16

Reflections on Attachment Security

Throughout this book we have tried to be faithful to the large scientific literature on secure and insecure attachment. This has required keeping our personal impressions and speculative flights of fancy to a minimum, a requirement of scientific work that we happily accept and embrace. Nevertheless, one cannot ponder a theoretical tradition and a set of related psychological questions for 15–20 years without considering their personal significance and broader implications for human welfare—concerns that carry us beyond specific studies and the current reach of attachment theory. Studying attachment security has been an important part of both our personal journeys. One of us (MM) moved from studies of helplessness and depression to research on security and resilience; the other (PRS) moved from studies of loneliness and isolation to research on secure love. While collaborating on the ideas and studies described in this book, we became good friends who have encouraged each other's courage and creativity, allowing us to move, in more than one sense, from loneliness and isolation to security, resilience, and deeper insight. We want to understand better, with deeper probing, "what it all means."

In this final chapter, we allow our imaginations freer rein. While keeping the empirical literature in mind, we ask some larger, more expansive questions: What is it about attachment security (the lasting effect of being loved, well cared for, and emotionally supported) that has such a remarkably wide range of beneficial effects? If we were to distill what has been learned from attachment research about the human mind and its social roots, how would the essence compare, not just with other scientific theories, but with major ethical, philosophical, and religious perspectives? Is it possible that a person can be "too secure" and thereby overly dull, complacent, and self-satisfied? Is it possible that attachment theorists have "deified" the secure child and the secure adult to an extent that is dangerous for people trying to apply the theory to themselves or their children? How can a person seeking optimal development (self-actualization) and deepest maturity benefit from a sense of security without losing the vital edge of challenge, critical questioning, and change? If security is so important, and if most children and adults in most modern societies are secure (which is what existing research suggests), why is the world not a happier, safer, and more loving place?

We have had many conversations about these matters while working on this book. Here, we attempt to articulate what we have learned, groping toward a philosophy to supplement our scientific theory. We do this not only to mark the end of this particular collaborative project but also to encourage readers who are so inclined to probe the deeper implications of attachment theory and research.

SECURE ATTACHMENT AND RESILIENCE

Throughout this book, we have seen that close relationships with available, sensitive, and supportive attachment figures—good parents and loving spouses, for example—help people to become happier and more resilient in the face of adversity. Some of the same benefits flow from good relationships with skilled psychotherapists, good mentors and coaches, and transformational leaders. People with a secure attachment style enjoy deep, pervasive, stable, and well-integrated feelings of self-acceptance, self-esteem, and self-efficacy, but without being arrogant, selfish, or narrow-minded. Their coping strategies are generally effective, and they regulate their emotions successfully. Their moods and outlook are often optimistic and hopeful even when fate delivers agonizing blows (an inevitable part of human existence), and they rebound relatively quickly without having to shut out or distort reality (see Chapters 6, 7, and 13, this volume). As Bowlby (1980) noted early on, they cope well with the loss of relationship partners and other distressing or traumatic events, without having to deny their suffering or suppress authentic emotions, including anger, fear, and sadness. Their emotions flow freely, but without causing disorganization or disorientation; they can look suffering, disappointment, aging, and change directly in the face, without losing their balance or becoming lastingly demoralized. They "work through" losses and traumas, reorganize mental representations of attachment figures, and make sense of painful experiences, while moving on to new challenges and relationships.

One way to frame these findings is in terms of Kobasa's (1982) concept of "hardiness." Hardy people are stress-resistant—committed to what they are doing, confident they can influence their surroundings and outcomes, and able to regard major life events and transformations as challenges to be mastered rather than threats to be passively and bitterly endured or energetically denied. Throughout this book we have noted secure people's commitment to their personal identities, careers, close relationships, social groups, and organizations (without being ego- or ethnocentric); their sense of control, mastery, and personal agency; and their cognitive and emotional openness to a wide range of experiences. Equipped with these qualities, secure people appraise potentially stressful events as manageable, as problems to be solved or overcome realistically, and they both rely on their effective coping skills and turn to others for comfort and support if necessary. They are neither compulsively self-reliant nor compulsively dependent. They can think and talk about distressing experiences coherently, without becoming enmeshed in or overwhelmed by painful memories, old injuries, and hostile feelings, and without having to suppress, repress, or deny injuries and aggravations. They can face aging and death with relative equanimity, enjoying life and love while it lasts and expecting symbolic immortality when physical mortality inevitably takes its toll (Chapter 7, this volume).

In an effort to understand how relationships with security-enhancing attachment figures increase a person's resilience, we (Mikulincer & Shaver, 2004) tentatively proposed that "internalization" of and identification with such figures allows a person to develop effective self-soothing techniques based on what we call "security-based self-representations" (Chapter 6, this volume). Following a well-established thread in psychoanalytic theory, running from Freud to the present, we proposed that people who have had many comforting and encouraging interactions with supportive attachment figures view themselves as reassuringly similar to those skillful, loving models. They can call up memories of the way they feel, or felt, in those people's reassuring and encouraging presence when they are threatened by stress or demoralization (see Figure 16.1 for a schematic summary of these ideas). Elements of both sides of the attachment–caregiving dynamic are woven into the fabric of their conscious and unconscious minds.

The first step in this internalization process is to use soothing interactions with an actual attachment figure to form mental representations of this comforting person, and of oneself interacting with him or her. The second step involves weaving these representations into one's memory networks, especially into one's working model of self. The attachment figure and his or her soothing, supportive reactions become integrated into one's own self-caregiving and self-compassion "subroutines" (Neff, 2003), and the self-with-attachment-figure representation becomes a stable, integrated component of one's actual self. The third step is to reactivate these representations in times of stress or need as a natural part of searching (mentally) for attachment-related sources of comfort and support. Originally, this search is for an actual flesh-and-blood attachment figure, but increasingly, as a consequence of generally favorable social experiences, the search turns up self-sustaining mental representations and coping techniques, without there being an immediate need for an actual attachment figure. In a sense, some parts of the self are sensitive and caring toward other parts, and the latter parts are represented and experienced as secure, calm, and able to cope with threats. With practice, the entire system of representations and self-regulatory efforts becomes fully and seamlessly integrated into one's personality, making past links to attachment figures less conscious, and perhaps even invisible. This is the way in which autonomy emerges from a history of reliable attachments and dependencies.

Activation of security-based self-representations in the face of threats is an important part of the broaden-and-build cycle of attachment security we have referred to repeatedly in previous chapters. People who possess such self-representations find it easier to remain mindful of whatever is actually happening to them and around them, to analyze problems (including other people's needs) more accurately and quickly, to mobilize effective coping strategies, and to endure inevitable periods of upheaval, loss, or trauma. This is the process by which esteem from others gradually becomes authentic self-esteem.

Security-based mental representations and self-soothing routines help to explain another aspect of the secure person's resilience: mobilization of positive emotions even in the midst of stressful experiences. Both theoretical and empirical research indicate that the capacity to sustain positive feelings in the face of adversity facilitates coping, minimizes distress, and renders people less vulnerable to the effects of stress (e.g., Bonanno, 2004; Fredrickson, 2001; Zautra, Smith, Affleck, & Tennen, 2001). This maintenance of positive feelings is important not only for oneself, but also for high-functioning close relationships. Gottman (1994), for example, found that good marriages depend on at least a 5-to-1 ratio of positive-to-negative interactions, and that high-functioning couples, despite having the usual, inevitable conflicts and disagreements, intersperse jokes, jibes, and signs of empathy and affection in the midst of conflict discussions, whereas distressed and unraveling couples repeatedly and quickly fall into a rigid tit-for-tat series of negative exchanges, similar to an irrational but unstoppable war between nations. This difference

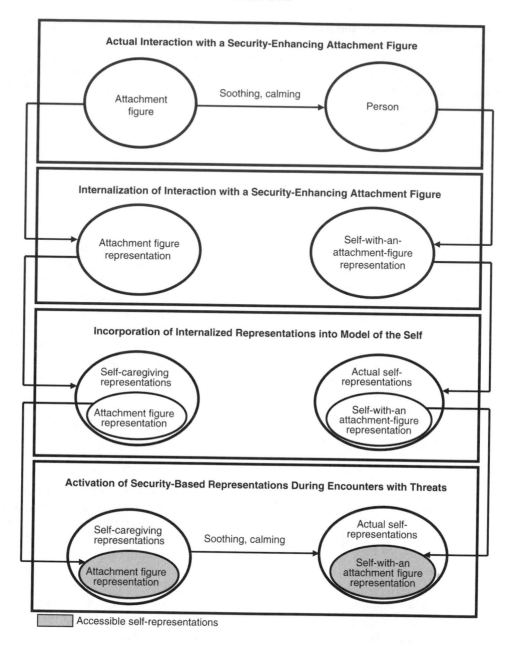

FIGURE 16.1. Mikulincer and Shaver's (2004) schematic representation of the formation and activation of security-based self-representations. From Mikulincer and Shaver (2004). Copyright 2004 by The Guilford Press. Reprinted by permission.

in emotional patterning is an excellent predictor of marital stability versus divorce. Positive emotions speed recovery from stressful life events by interrupting the flow of negative emotions and counteracting distress-related autonomic arousal and destructive blood chemistry (Fredrickson, 2001). We found in our research that activation of security-based self-representations had immediate, positive emotional effects that resemble the relief, comfort, and gratitude produced by interactions with loving, caring, and supportive attachment figures (Mikulincer & Shaver, 2004; see also Neff, 2003). As a result, individuals with a secure attachment style are able to remain calm, confident, hopeful, and open to others' needs, which is beneficial both to them and to their relationship partners.

In his analysis of alternative paths to resilience, Bonanno (2004) reviewed research showing that defensive self-enhancement and repressive coping can sometimes produce positive outcomes following painful experiences. He and other researchers have therefore questioned the need for grieving or for social support following environmental disasters and military hostilities. Although securely attached people are able to use "avoidant" defensive strategies when these seem likely to be effective in the short run (Chapter 7, this volume), they do not usually rely on defensive self-aggrandizement, problem avoidance, or mental repression in the long run.

As we have shown throughout this book, such strategies are more characteristic of avoidant people, who cope with threats by maintaining a facade of imperturbability and extreme self-reliance. It is possible that such defenses equip avoidant people with a degree of resilience (which is theoretically why the defenses were adopted in the first place), but research shows that these coping strategies break down under intense and prolonged stress (Chapters 7 and 13, this volume). Moreover, unlike secure people, who can flexibly choose a coping strategy that fits the demands of a situation, avoidant individuals are rigid in their choice of strategies and fail to adjust when circumstances favor active problem solving, reliance on social support, or reorganization of goals and plans. Even Bonanno (2005) champions elasticity, or behavioral flexibility, as a key feature of resilience and successful adaptation. We are confident that this desirable quality is more characteristic of secure than of avoidant people.

OPTIMIZING THE PERFORMANCE OF OTHER BEHAVIORAL SYSTEMS

The research reviewed in this book indicates that relationships with loving, caring, and sensitive attachment figures, and the resulting sense of attachment security, enhance the functioning of other behavioral systems such as exploration, affiliation, caregiving, and sex. As shown in Chapter 8, security-enhancing interactions with attachment figures facilitate confident and relaxed exploration of new ideas, places, people, and social roles. They encourage the acquisition of new skills and the broadening of personal perspectives, and they foster creative, flexible adjustment to changing life circumstances. The interplay between attachment security and creative exploration provides people with a sense of mastery and competence, and contributes to the successful accomplishment of important life tasks.

Secure adults are sensitive and responsive caregivers who allow their relationship partners (e.g., friends, spouses, children, coworkers, employees, students, elderly parents) to cope with threats and challenges autonomously if they are so inclined, but they also offer well-timed and appropriately delivered support and guidance, if needed (Chapter 12, this volume). This sensitive and responsive care can also be seen in the ways secure therapists and organizational leaders empower their clients and followers, placing them on a path to personal growth and collective well-being (Chapters 14 and 15, this volume).

Similarly, people with a secure attachment style find it easy to get psychologically close to others, to coordinate their needs and actions with those of other people, and to enjoy membership in groups and organizations (Chapters 9 and 15, this volume). Securely attached people also view sex as a mutually enjoyable way to foster intimacy and affection in the context of a stable relationship (Chapter 12, this volume). They are not usually sexually anxious, out to prove themselves sexually, rigid in their sexual demands or behavior, or inclined to manipulate or "use" their sexual partners.

It is still unclear how best to conceptualize the relations among the different behavioral systems. Bowlby and Ainsworth began their theorizing by portraying attachment security as part of a relational "secure base for exploration," which suggests that the attachment system is primary, comes first in development, and forms either a solid or shaky foundation for the other behavioral systems. One reason for thinking this is that attachment behavior and attachment styles show up early in infant development (Chapter 5, this volume), whereas caregiving (e.g., as first indicated, for example, by empathy in 3-year-olds; Kestenbaum et al., 1989) and affiliative interactions with peers appear next, and sex—at least full genital sexuality—appears later. We can also view the early importance of the attachment system in terms of its evolved biological function, ensuring protection (i.e., survival), which is obviously necessary for exploring one's surroundings, gradually distancing oneself to some extent from attachment figures (i.e., protectors), and autonomously confronting novelty, ambiguity, and uncertainty with confidence that support and comfort will be available, if needed. Survival is also the first condition for eventually reaching the age of sexual reproduction and parenting, which are necessary for continuing and evolving a particular genetic heritage.

Once a child has a functioning attachment system and has begun to adapt to the local caregiving environment (i.e., once a fairly stable attachment style has developed), the child's caregiving and affiliation systems come online to deal with sibling and peer relationships and to allow the child to be influenced by enculturation and moral socialization. Given that children with different attachment styles act and experience social relationships somewhat differently, the operating parameters of the caregiving and affiliation systems may be shaped in predictably different directions. Also important are imitation and modeling of primary caregivers, which create similarities between a child's attachment system (shaped by the parents) and his or her caregiving and affiliation systems (modeled on those of the parents). Once the attachment, affiliation, and caregiving systems have developed in tandem and accommodated each other, they are available to influence adolescent and adult sexual relationships. Hence, when we study sexual motives and behavior in college and adult samples, the operating parameters of the sexual system are predictable to some extent from the operating parameters of the attachment system.

There is, however, second way to think about the interrelations among the attachment, exploration, affiliation, caregiving, and sexual systems: They may all be affected by individual differences in temperament or personality. As we have explained throughout this volume, several studies have examined whether global attachment styles, or attachment style dimensions, are totally redundant with one or more of the "Big Five" personality traits: openness to experience, conscientiousness, extroversion, agreeableness, and neuroticism. The evidence so far suggests that they are not. In both contemporaneous and longitudinal research designs, attachment measures have frequently outperformed global personality measures in predicting exploration, affiliation, caregiving, and sexual behavior. In addition, several researchers have controlled for neuroticism, general anxiety, self-esteem, or interpersonal trust and still obtained predicted effects of attachment anxiety and avoidance. Attachment effects are never fully, and usually not even partially, explained by alternative personality constructs. In a recent study using fMRI, we (Gillath,

Bunge, et al., 2005) even found different patterns of regional brain activation associated with neuroticism and attachment anxiety.

Still, the positive correlation between neuroticism and attachment anxiety is substantial (Chapter 13, this volume), and the negative correlations between avoidant attachment, agreeableness, and extraversion are often statistically significant, if not large (Chapter 9, this volume). Graziano and Tobin (2002) found that agreeableness is positively associated with compassion and altruism in some of the same ways that avoidant attachment is negatively associated with those prosocial states. It nevertheless seems unlikely, given the relatively modest correlation between avoidance and agreeableness, that the attachment effects are redundant with the agreeableness effects. Moreover, and this is very important to us, nothing in the conceptualization of the "Big Five" traits would have generated the huge research program, carried out over the past 25 years and summarized in this book, inspired by attachment theory. Attachment theory is more dynamic and more coherently rooted in evolutionary biology and developmental psychology. The "Big Five" trait model is, by comparison, merely descriptive, not at all dynamic, and not theoretically rooted in evolutionary biology. Thus, attachment theory and its associated measures are scientifically fruitful whether or not attachment styles turn out to overlap to some extent, and for reasons not yet fully understood, with global personality traits.

Whatever kinds of qualities they assess, attachment style measures may be influenced by genes. In the case of the "Big Five" personality traits, about half of the individual-difference variance is attributable to genetic factors (Bouchard & Loehlin, 2001). To date, only a handful of behavior genetic studies of attachment in infancy and adulthood have been published and, although their findings are inconsistent, some suggest a role for genetic, temperamental factors in shaping patterns of attachment across the lifespan (Chapter 5, this volume). It is possible, therefore, that similarities and differences in what is tapped by the Strange Situation, the AAI, and self-report measures of adult attachment style can eventually be better understood by discovering the extent to which they have similar or different genetic roots. There may also be common genetic influences on the variance shared by global personality traits, measures of attachment style, and measures of exploration, affiliation, caregiving, and sexual behaviors. Also interesting is the possibility that social experiences, such as receiving maternal affection, change gene expression in ways that shape the development of personality characteristics (e.g., Meaney, 2004).

A third, even more complex approach to the observed relations among behavioral systems includes not only developmental and genetic sources of shared variance but also possible recursive influences of exploration, affiliation, caregiving, and sexual experiences on attachment security. Even if the operating parameters of these systems are shaped by common genetic factors and variations in attachment security, each is also molded by specific life circumstances that facilitate or block its smooth functioning. For example, growing up in a family that emphasizes empathy, compassion, and benevolence may contribute to optimal development of the caregiving system; being discriminated against by social groups who reject one's bids for affiliation and acceptance may reduce a person's sense of security and personal worth; and being subjected to partner violence or sexual abuse may damage a person's sexual functioning. Even fairly mild disapproval of early childhood precursors of sexuality (e.g., the masturbation that young children often engage in without knowing what genitals are for) might contribute to attachment insecurity (something that, to the best of our knowledge, has not been discussed in the attachment literature). And often the disapproval is more than mild. Sex therapist Stella Resnick (1997) provides examples, including the following:

Our grandparents and great grandparents were likely to have been raised in a Victorian atmosphere, and they in turn had a strong impact on the sexual attitudes of the mothers and fathers who raised us. A single man in his late thirties . . . told me that when his father was a little boy his mother locked him in a closet for several hours after catching him masturbating. Tom felt that he could trace his own sexual [problems] to that particular sexual trauma endured by his father. Every time a situation with a woman started to get sexual, Tom would get anxious and awkward. . . . That's how powerfully these multi-generational patterns are locked into our bodies. Tom's father was punished and shamed as a child for sex and he, in turn, punished and shamed his son, making him sexually insecure. (p. 226)

To make matters more complex, as we explained in Chapter 5, adult attachment styles are not mere reflections of early parent–infant interactions and working model prototypes; they are also affected by many later social experiences. Hence, changes in the functioning of the other behavioral systems (e.g., failure to learn new skills and then doubting one's competence and value; volunteering to help others and becoming more self-confident as a result) and experiences in close relationships (e.g., having sexual problems or caring poorly for a romantic partner, thereby contributing to low relationship satisfaction or partner infidelity) can feed back on attachment security.

At present we know little about the extent to which other behavioral systems affect the attachment system. However, Gillath's (2003) experimental studies provide initial evidence for effects of sexual arousal on attachment security and caregiving inclinations. In four studies, heterosexual adults were subliminally primed with either neutral pictures or photographs of naked members of the opposite sex and asked to report on their willingness to self-disclose, become psychologically intimate, deal constructively with interpersonal conflicts, and sacrifice for a partner. The results indicated that priming the sexual system moved people, on average, in the direction of greater self-disclosure and intimacy—tendencies usually associated with attachment security. Moreover, subliminal sexual priming, compared with neutral priming, produced a stronger tendency to sacrifice for a partner and more constructive handling of conflicts, presumably reflecting a more loving, caring, and supportive attitude toward close relationship partners.

We can imagine that priming people with a sense of caring (i.e., priming the caregiving system) might also increase momentary attachment security, at least slightly—for example, by strengthening a person's sense of connectedness. We have preliminary evidence for such effects when anxious people become more secure as a result of volunteering to help others (Gillath, Shaver, Mikulincer, Nitzberg, et al., 2005). We need more research that identifies the mediators of these effects, but Gillath's (2003) findings suggest that, at least in adults, different behavioral systems are intertwined, such that activation of one has effects on the others, and individual differences in one tend to be correlated with individual differences in the others.

In attempting to integrate the three alternative approaches to explaining relations among the behavioral systems, we consider three converging sources of shared variance among the systems. First, an influence of genetically determined temperament may create individual differences in broad personality traits, which in turn contribute to the optimal or suboptimal functioning of several or all behavioral systems. Second, there is a developmental source, by which early parent–child interactions and attachment working model prototypes affect the functioning of systems that emerge later in development. Third, at least in adulthood, there are personal and interpersonal experiences that impinge on the exploration, affiliation, caregiving, and sexual systems, and feed back on the attachment system. There is already considerable evidence for the temperamental and developmental sources (discussed throughout this book), but the last source of shared variance—reciprocal influences among the systems—remains to be studied further. We also need more research on possible interactions among the three kinds of influences.

ATTACHMENT SECURITY AND EGO TRANSFORMATION

From a classical psychodynamic perspective, the sense of attachment security is an ego resource that supports reality-attuned, effective transactions with other people, promotes personal and social adjustment, and facilitates goal pursuit and need gratification. However, secure attachment not only supports "ego" functioning (which contemporary personality and social psychologists prefer to discuss in terms of self-regulation, coping, and adjustment), but also prepares a person to transcend the ego—that is, to grow beyond the limits of "normal" adjustment, to find new meanings beyond personal accomplishments and possessions, and to achieve a deeper form of maturity and well-being. As we explained in previous chapters, attachment security promotes ego-transcendence by freeing a person to a great extent from anxiety and defensiveness and encouraging a calmer, more mindful, more generous attitude toward self and others.

In our view, mental representations related to secure relationships and current feelings of attachment security reduce what Higgins (1998) called a *prevention* (i.e., avoidance) motivational orientation—a stance focused on the need for safety and security, and the avoidance of negative, painful experiences. Dropping this prevention orientation and embracing a *promotion* (i.e., approach) orientation makes it less necessary to employ defenses such as egoistic self-enhancement, false consensus and uniqueness biases, cognitive rigidity and closed-mindedness, and hostile defenses of one's own cultural or religious worldview. Securely attached people generally feel sufficiently safe and protected, without having to activate defenses. Moreover, they can interact with other people in a confident and open way, without worrying about being abandoned, engulfed, or controlled by someone else. This means that for relatively secure people, life can be more than survival, social acceptance, lack of pain, and accumulation of possessions and achievements (not that there is anything wrong with these goals in themselves, but by classical religious and philosophical standards, they are relatively low on the list of standards for a life well lived). A life grounded in security can also include tackling greater challenges, contributing to others' welfare, self-expansion, and actualization of talents, which is likely to require abandoning or revising previous adjustments, role identities, and life circumstances.

The view that attachment security is related both to mental health and to lack of defensiveness challenges social psychological theories that equate defensiveness (especially defensive self-enhancement) with mental health, and equate lack of defensiveness with psychopathology (e.g., S. E. Taylor & Brown, 1988). We (Mikulincer & Shaver, 2005a) have proposed an alternative, two-level model of psychological defenses. At the primary level, we view security-enhancing interactions with attachment figures as natural building blocks of a secure, solid, and stable psychological foundation. At this level, representations of attachment security act as resilience resources that maintain emotional equanimity and effective functioning, without reality-distorting defenses. Securely attached people can do without illusory beliefs about complete control, power, or freedom; they can find safety and protection in security-enhancing mental representations, and in the love and care of actual and internalized attachment figures.

A secondary level of defenses is required when a person fails to form secure attachments and is unable to build a secure psychological foundation that permits clear and open mindfulness of internal and external events. For an insecurely attached person, many everyday experiences threaten the sense of safety and raise doubts about one's tenuous hold on life, identity, and knowledge of the world. At this level, a prevention orientation and the use of biased, distorting defenses can sometimes compensate for the absence of attachment security, create a semblance or facade of self-esteem and self-efficacy, and contribute a degree of adjustment. For a person who is insecure at the primary level, defensiveness at the secondary level may contribute positively to mental health, whereas lack of defensiveness, or a breakdown of defenses, may increase the risk of psychopathology; that is, contrary to S. E. Taylor and Brown's (1988) view, the equation of mental health with self-enhancing defensiveness seems to fit relatively insecure people better than secure ones (see also Shedler, Mayman, & Manis, 1993).

The notion of a secondary level of defenses is equally applicable to avoidant and anxious people. Although defensiveness is most evident in avoidant people, who engage frequently in defensive self-enhancement and repressive coping, the alternative anxious, hyperactivating strategies can also serve defensive functions and may provide a degree of adjustment. For attachment-anxious people, distress intensification, worrying, ruminating on threats, and openly expressing vulnerability and neediness may have two beneficial effects. First, it sometimes brings about the desired attention, care, and love from others, which is theoretically the reason the anxious strategy developed in the first place: It often worked, which put the person on an extinction-resistant partial reinforcement schedule supporting hyperactivation despite all the times it did not work. But there may also be a second, less obvious, benefit: The hubbub and distraction generated by strident, impulsive expressions of pain, need, and anger may sometimes direct attention and energy away from a deeper problem—sensing oneself as not very substantial and not worthy of anyone's care. Agitating and grabbing someone's attention is at least likely to make *something* happen, and even if that something is unpleasant, it may feel better than nothing, better than social isolation. (This reminds us of an acquaintance who said that when she is alone, she begins to feel herself dissolve, evaporate, or disintegrate "like molecules dispersing quietly into the air"—a much scarier condition than arguing with her unfaithful, unreliable lover.)

We suspect that after a person has practiced this form of defensiveness for years, it is somewhat calming and reassuring—much more so than existential terror or dread—even though agitation, rumination, and anger do not seem, to more secure people, to be sensible or effective ways to cope or communicate. We suspect, although this remains to be studied, that giving attachment-anxious people an opportunity to express their helplessness, self-doubts, and worries might have a cathartic and calming effect (for a while), whereas asking them to reflect on their strengths and capacity for independence and autonomy might make them uncomfortable. (In at least one existing study, a manipulation intended to create a positive mood—and that did create a more a positive mood and enhanced creativity in secure people—induced cognitive constriction and lowered creativity in attachment-anxious people [Mikulincer & Sheffi, 2000].)

The seemingly beneficial effects of avoidant and anxious defenses are achieved, however, at a considerable cost: cognitive and emotional rigidity, distorted perception of social reality, interpersonal and intergroup friction and conflict, and destructive leadership and unnecessary self-sacrifice. These negative side effects do not arise if one uses defenses at the first, or primary, level. At this level, attachment security promotes mental health, while allowing accurate social perception; a compassionate, loving attitude toward others, even those who are different from oneself; cognitive openness and flexibility; and a confident approach to challenges and new experiences. It supports prosocial, transformational leadership and productive membership in groups and organizations. These protective effects of attachment security interfere with neither stable love and active engagement with the world nor personal growth. And they benefit other people rather than injuring or destroying them.

Beyond reducing defenses, attachment security allows a calmer, less frantic approach to goal pursuit and need gratification. Security-enhancing interactions with good attachment figures strengthen a person's sense that problems are solvable, obstacles can be overcome, and goals can be attained even if one does not have complete control or power over events (which, of course, is usually the case). We suspect that such interactions instill faith in "stronger and wiser" forces, originally experienced in the guise of parental caregivers but later transferred and extended to other close relationship partners, and symbolic or abstract figures and forces (e.g., a social group, God, the Tao, the Dharma, synchronicity, good karma).

These generators of felt security can seem, subjectively, to guide, assist, and take care of us while we tackle important life projects. This is, in our opinion, the positive side of religion that Freud (1927/1975) failed to emphasize in *The Future of an Illusion*. He was thinking of the Old Testament's angry God (a powerful father figure, like Freud's actual father) rather than the more forgiving, uplifting supernatural forces also common in many religions (e.g., the loving, fertile mother goddess; the empathic "son" Jesus; the kind and enlightened Buddha). Hope and faith of a certain kind allow secure people to forgo anxious efforts to gain complete control over events, to be more tolerant of temporary failures and setbacks, to let go of unattainable goals, and to trust that life will bring more positive than negative experiences over time (perhaps in Gottman's (1994) 5-to-1 ratio, which may be what secure people have usually experienced in their actual lives). This attitude is nicely expressed in a Taoist poem quoted by Burtt (1957):

> The sage puts himself last,
> And finds himself in the foremost place;
> Regards his body as accidental,
> And his body is thereby preserved.
> Is it not because he does not live for Self
> That his Self achieves perfection? (p. 191)

This relaxed, trusting, open attitude does not require that secure people be fatalistic or possess an external locus of control. Rather, security-enhancing interactions with attachment figures who were helpful, engaged in mutual dialogue, and encouraged exploration and autonomy foster a fruitful integration of proactive, autonomous behavior and acceptance of "stronger and wiser" forces (which can be conceptualized in many different ways).

During interactions with security-providing attachment figures, people experience a sense of agency, control, and power, because their emotional and verbal signals and behaviors alter an attachment figures' behavior, and result in getting attached persons' problems solved and their needs met. At the same time, these interactions cause people to realize and accept that their welfare depends on a "stronger and wiser" other's wisdom and good intentions. As such, security-enhancing interactions provide people with both a sense that they are forceful, effective agents who can alter the course of life *and* the realization that they are sometimes dependent on larger, more powerful or encompassing but generally benevolent forces. The resulting sense of security extends to a vague sense that (in the poetic words of the 14th-century English mystic, Dame Julian of Norwich, 1670/ 2003) "All shall be well, and all shall be well, and all manner of things shall be well."

This pervading residue of security-enhancing experiences is probably what causes many secure people to have a positive image of God (if they are religious theists) or a more abstract feeling that life is meaningful and their actions cumulate in ways that contribute to the general good and to their own symbolic immortality (Florian & Mikulincer, 1998; Kirkpatrick, 2005). This positive feeling, like the cosmic background radiation pervading the physical universe, is everywhere. It is a form of "good karma" that permeates a person's mental and physical space like an echo of the "Big Bang." In the case of secure attachment, however, the warm glow is an echo of many past experiences in loving relationships, not of a single event. This positive aura allows a person to engage life fully in a calm, trusting, and optimistic way.

But how exactly does this work? First, security allows a person to devote resources to growth-promoting, self-expanding activities that transcend "adjustment." Rather than being perpetually on guard so as not to be injured in one way or another, securely attached people can explore new experiences, new territories, and new social groups, without worrying a great deal about protection and safety. Second, secure people can focus undistorted attention on existential concerns about aging, death, and freedom; relate deeply to others; and find meaning in life. Although dealing with these issues sometimes destabilizes almost everyone, the more secure among us rebalance themselves, evolve psychologically, and achieve a deeper appreciation of life, the natural world, and other people. Third, attachment security encourages social responsibility, compassionate love, and multifaceted, mutually enriching I–Thou relationships (Buber, 1958). It is no accident that humanistic psychologists and philosophers, such as Rogers, Maslow, and Buber, as well as transformational religious and political leaders (Buddha, Jesus, Gandhi, Martin Luther King, Jr.), stressed the importance of "unconditional positive regard" (Carl Rogers), Being-love (Maslow), compassionately taking on others' suffering (Jesus, Buddha), and ending racism and other forms of egocentrism (King). This generous love is characteristic of secure, socially engaged, self-actualized people.

ATTACHMENT SECURITY, GROWTH PROCESSES, AND THE FULLY FUNCTIONING PERSON

As mentioned, attachment theory's broader implications extend into the intellectual and ethical territory of humanistic psychology, although accompanied by more research evidence than was available to early humanistic psychologists. One of the most fleshed-out humanistic theories was Carl Rogers's (1961) conception of the fully functioning person, which he described in terms of several admirable qualities.

The first is *openness to experience*—the capacity to listen to one's feelings, notice what is going on within oneself, and reflect on thoughts and feelings. This is closely related to the Buddhist concept of mindfulness, which has recently become important in cognitive approaches to psychotherapy (e.g., Germer, Siegel, & Fulton, 2005). Openness to experience means being open to and curious about new information, new kinds of experiences, and both positive and negative feelings and ideas. The fully functioning person is cognizant of and curious about his or her experiences and those of other people, and can engage in coherent conversations about them (as shown, in the case of securely attached adults, in the AAI [Hesse, 1999]). In Carl Rogers's (1961) words, a fully functioning person "is more open to his feelings of fear and discouragement and pain. He is also more open to his feelings of courage, tenderness, and awe. He is free to live his feelings subjectively, as they exist in him, and also free to be aware of these feelings" (p. 188). Carl Rogers thought, as do we, that this kind of undefended openness is a beneficial outcome of having been unconditionally loved.

As shown in Chapters 6 and 7, this volume, securely attached people are able to experience their thoughts and feelings deeply; they open themselves to new insights and information, even if these are threatening; and they engage in dialogue with relationship partners, even if it creates tension and conflict or arouses negative feelings. This openness makes defenses less necessary, fosters a realistic view of self and others, and creates new paths to personal development and fulfillment. It allows deeper engagement with relationship partners.

Another characteristic of the fully functioning person, according to Carl Rogers (1961), is *existential living*—enjoying the flow of experience and living fully at every moment. It means being "a participant in and an observer of the ongoing process of organismic experience, rather than being in control of it" (p. 188). This approach to life involves spontaneity, cognitive flexibility, and an ability to adapt one's beliefs about self and world to accommodate incoming information. As we explained in Chapter 8, attachment research indicates that security facilitates cognitive openness and adaptive revision of knowledge structures in response to new information, without arousing much fear of disapproval, criticism, or rejection. Attachment security also contributes to two other aspects of existential living—savoring good moments and capitalizing on positive emotions, evident in diary and laboratory studies documenting secure people's enjoyment of daily activities and social interactions, as well as cognitive expansion following inductions of positive affect (Chapters 7–9, this volume).

Two other core characteristics of a fully functioning person are *organismic trusting*—trusting one's feelings, thoughts, and sensations, and making decisions based on what one feels is right rather than being driven by external forces—and *experiential freedom*—being free to choose among alternative courses of action and taking responsibility for one's choices. According to Carl Rogers (1961), these qualities indicate that a person has a strong sense of inner coherence, personal responsibility, and self-determination. As discussed throughout this volume, interactions with loving, caring, and sensitive attachment figures increase confidence in the acceptability and serviceability of one's personality, talents, and skills, and allow an individual to maintain a sense of consistency and clarity in experiences and choose actions thoughtfully even under threatening conditions. This sense of personal coherence and strength contributes to a sense of personal direction and meaning, and the ability to resist contrary opinions, social pressures, and paranoid conspiracy theories about events at the personal, local, national, and international levels.

The fifth characteristic of a fully functioning person, according to Carl Rogers (1961), is *creativity*—the ability to produce new and effective thoughts, actions, and objects, and willingness to contribute to other people's growth and actualization. This characteristic is related to full engagement in projects of all kinds, a sense of generativity, and steady endorsement of prosocial values and goals that cause a person to care about others' welfare and about the protection and improvement of physical and social surroundings. As shown in Chapters 8 and 11, this volume, securely attached people are able to engage in creative exploration and to participate fully in the wider world, while remaining sensitive and responsive to others' needs. They are more likely than their avoidant peers to volunteer in their communities and to help a suffering stranger in our laboratory experiments.

In a compact description of the fully functioning person, Carl Rogers (1961) wrote:

> To be part of this process means that one is involved in the frequently frightening and frequently satisfying experience of more sensitive living, with greater range, greater variety, greater richness. It seems to me that clients who have moved significantly in therapy live more intimately with their feelings of ecstasy; that anger is more clearly felt, but so also is love; that fear is an experience they know more deeply, but so is courage. And the reason they can thus live fully in a wider range is that they have this underlying confidence in themselves as trustworthy instruments for encountering life. (pp. 195–196)

Evidence amassed by attachment researchers suggests that security-enhancing interactions with loving attachment figures, including effective psychotherapists (like Carl Rogers), provide people with the "confidence in themselves as trustworthy instruments for encountering life," which is compatible with Rogers's idea that such confidence emerges in the context of another person's "unconditional positive regard." Security-providing attachment figures provide this kind of regard, and more. Rogers was sketchy in characterizing unconditional positive regard, but it has been mapped in greater detail by attachment researchers. The good attachment figure's love and support is not really "unconditional" in the sense of being always the same regardless of conditions. Instead it is responsive to a person's specific, actual needs. Instead of being always silently present and passively glowing, like a low-wattage light bulb, it is more like situation-specific "emotion coaching," as Gottman and Declaire (1998) explained (based on Gottman's empirical studies of parent–child interactions).

The qualities of securely attached people resemble those that Allport (1961) discussed in terms of "psychological growth" or the transformation of "adequate" or "normal" adjustment into full maturity. In his view, a fully mature person (1) engages in and enjoys activities that are not directly linked to immediate need gratification, ego defenses, or adjustment pressures; (2) relates to others in a warm, tolerant, and intimate manner; (3) possesses fundamental emotional security and self-acceptance; (4) holds realistic views of self and social reality; (5) maintains positive relations with self and others, and deeply understands one's own and others' experiences; and (6) authentically explores and questions the meaning of life and the purpose of whatever he or she is doing. These are all qualities that emerge from the cascade of experiences and events produced by the broaden-and-build cycle of attachment security (Chapter 3, this volume): a solid sense of personal safety and inherent value, in which one opens oneself to warm and intimate relations with others, and confidently engages in exploration, self-expansion, and beneficial creativity.

This is the chain of personal qualities that unfolds naturally when infants, children, adolescents, or adults develop in the context of loving, caring, accepting, sensitive, and responsive attachment figures. However, when the broaden-and-build cycle of security is broken, people may react with frustration, protest, angry demands, and aggression on the one hand, or defensive detachment, narcissistic self-aggrandizement, and lack of attention to inner experiences on the other. In such cases, tension reduction, need gratification, and ego defenses remain the most important aims, and hyperactivating or deactivating emotion regulation strategies are invoked as familiar ways to achieve a degree of adjustment and control. An insecure person is likely to be so preoccupied or overwhelmed by neediness and vulnerability, or by defensive attempts to manage these states, that he or she is unable to devote resources to unfettered psychological growth.

THE EXISTENTIAL MEANING
OF ATTACHMENT SECURITY

Attachment security allows a developing adolescent or adult to come to terms with basic existential concerns. In his book *Existential Psychotherapy*, Yalom (1980) discussed four of the most important existential concerns: death, freedom, isolation, and meaninglessness. Every person with normal cognitive capacities feels the disturbing mismatch between awareness of eventual death and the intense desire to keep on living. As we mentioned in Chapter 7, this mismatch is the focus of "terror management theory," which we view as highly compatible with attachment theory, because the latter portrays the perception of threats (to life and well-being) as the attachment system's major "trigger." In fact, the attachment system is thought to have evolved to protect immature and troubled human beings from predation, injury, and death.

The existential concern with freedom arises from our awareness that despite a strong wish for control and self-determination, we usually cannot be certain that our important decisions are correct. There are no absolute truths, values, or norms directing our choices and actions. To some extent, as individuals and societies, we are making life up as we go along. The existential concern with isolation results from the awareness that we will never be able to share fully our subjective experiences with others, and never be able to appreciate fully or understand other people's subjectivity despite our intense desires for connection, solidarity, and intimacy. The existential concern with meaninglessness "stems from the dilemma of a meaning-seeking creature who is thrown into a universe that has no meaning" (Yalom, 1980, p. 9). (Even people who think they know the meaning of life and the universe realize that most other people in the world do not agree with them, which is a cause for considerable discomfort.)

These concerns can provoke intense, in some cases almost paralyzing anxiety, so many people erect defenses to keep them out of awareness most of the time. Otherwise, it would be difficult to get on with daily life. However, according to Yalom (1980), with whom we heartily agree, denial of these givens of existence obstructs growth, encourages cognitive rigidity and social conformity, and contributes to hostility and aggression (see Greenberg, Koole, & Pyszczynski's [2004] *Handbook of Experimental Existential Psychology* for a detailed examination of these issues).

In Chapter 7, we showed that securely attached people can be aware of the inevitability of death, without having to cling to rigid cultural worldviews or myths designed to protect them from acknowledging their ultimate fate. Their courageous attitude toward death rests on a solid sense of value, connectedness, continuity, and influence—Lifton's (1979) "symbolic immortality"—that in turn stems from interactions with loving, caring, and sensitive attachment figures and with people, such as their children, friends, and students or employees, who have benefited from their loving care. These deep social connections give secure people an opportunity to be part of a larger symbolic entity (e.g., couple, family, group, profession, organization, church or synagogue, community) that transcends their biological limitations, and expands the boundaries and capacities of their admittedly small and limited selves (A. Aron et al., 2001). Social connections and a sense of contributing to other people's lives reduce one's sense of insignificance and fear of losing one's personal identity after death, which is one of the major forms of death anxiety (Florian & Kravetz, 1983). Secure people feel confident they will continue to exist in the thoughts, memories, and accomplishments of their relationship partners and both real and symbolic offspring. In addition, loving romantic and marital relationships offer people an opportunity to experience passionate love, which can include what Maslow (1971) called "peak experiences" or, at least, the more common but still very important feelings of being fully alive and recognized as special.

Lifton and Olson (1974) proposed that relationships with loving and sensitive caregivers are a source of symbolic immortality, which weakens the connection between aloneness and death. It is commonly said that "everyone dies alone," but this is wrong in at least two respects. First, many people die in the presence of loved ones whose support and touch clearly matter. Second, the mind of a secure person is not necessarily ever alone in the sense of being without comforting mental representations, conscious and unconscious, of connections with others. For many religious people, there is also a sense of connection with God, saints, deceased relatives, and so on. Research has shown that these mental representations reduce a person's reliance on the more objectionable (egocentric and ethnocentric) forms of "terror management" (Florian & Mikulincer, 1998). As Lifton and Olson (1974) noted, "Life for the baby means being connected to the source of care and support. Powerful fears and anxiety appear when the child is left alone, separated from the source of nurture. This image of separation is related to an image of death" (p. 46). Secure people, who feel more connected even when physically isolated, can transcend this equation of death and separation, at least to an important extent. They are therefore better able to remain calm and creatively engaged despite their awareness of eventual death.

Attachment security may provide protection from three threatening conceptions of death. The first such conception portrays death as an ultimate and irreversible separation; hence, fears of separation and abandonment exacerbate death concerns (Kalish, 1985; Mikulincer, Florian, Birnbaum, et al., 2002). Second, according to Rank (1945), death is symbolically equivalent to union, fusion, and loss of individuation and differentiation from others. Therefore, fear of losing one's personal identity, distinctness, possessions, and achievements may compound the terror of death. Third, death represents the greatest unknown, and many people are afraid of it because of the impenetrable mystery of what happens to one's mind (or spirit) after death. All three of these troubling conceptions of death can be defanged to some extent by attachment security. As we have shown throughout this volume, secure people differ from anxious ones in being better able to endure separations. Moreover, secure people differ from avoidant ones in being less afraid of losing their self-reliance, autonomy, and personal identity; more tolerant of uncertainty, ambiguity, and confusion; and more capable of accepting and exploring the unknown. Thus, secure people are less likely to be burdened by death-related concerns and more able to accept death as an inevitable part of life.

When we had the pleasure of discussing psychological research with the Dalai Lama and some of his followers in Dharamsala, India, in 2004, he said that, far from being afraid of death, he had spent a great deal of time and mental energy meditating on it (as it is described in *The Tibetan Book of the Dead*) and was looking forward to seeing what it is like. He seemed to us similar to a talented and well-trained athlete (e.g., skier or rock climber)—eager to be challenged, educated, and tested, expecting the experience to be exhilarating and ultimately rewarding.

The existential conflict between our desire for freedom and self-determination on the one hand, and our sense of groundlessness and uncertainty about the correctness of our choices on the other can also be ameliorated to some extent by attachment security. Security-enhancing relationships with attachment figures offer people a sense of certainty, or at least high likelihood, that important partners will accept, love, comfort, and support them even if they make occasional mistakes or unfortunate choices. Supportive relationships make it easier for people to take a *leap of faith* (a concept often attributed to Kierkegaard, 1846/1992, but which is not found in his writings in exactly that form or with its contemporary sense). What writers like Yalom mean by borrowing the term is that such a leap sustains joyful exploration, passionate commitment, and acceptance of responsibility for one's actions despite existential uncertainty about the correctness or optimality of these actions (compared with missed alternatives).

Although we would not go so far as to call an open, risk-taking, creative, and engaged life "absurd," as some existentialist writers have done (following Kierkegaard, who meant that life presents problems that cannot be solved through rationality alone), a leap of faith is evident in several of the findings reviewed in this book, showing that secure people openly disclose their personal thoughts and feelings to relationship partners, even if they lead to disagreements; expose their vulnerability and need for support, even if doing so leaves them open to disapproval; open their cognitive schemas to new information, even though doing so entails uncertainty and reorganization; explore challenging and changing life circumstances and new experiences; and commit themselves to the personal choices they make in their career and close relationships.

Kierkegaard was quite serious when he described some religious choices as "absurd," because he was talking about a leap of faith (or *to* faith) in the God of the Old Testament, who inexplicably attacked his faithful follower Job and instructed Abraham to kill his son Isaac. At least when viewed psychologically, Kierkegaard's feelings about life and God seemed to be darkly colored by his childhood interactions with his very troubled, guilty, and depressed father, and his own proneness to depression and despair. His is not the only kind of leap of faith available, however. Faith in "stronger and wiser" inner and outer forces that love, accept, guide, and support one throughout life can occur without Kierkegaardian *sturm und drang*, or depression, and this kind of faith in the general goodness of the world can help a person with the freedom-related concerns discussed by Yalom. On one hand, securely attached people do not urgently need to defend or justify their decisions and actions (to reduce what Festinger [1957] called cognitive dissonance), or deny a degree of uncertainty about the correctness of their decisions. A defensive approach to justifying one's decisions is more characteristic of avoidant people, who feel that their identity and personal value are contingent on the unimpeachable correctness of their decisions. Furthermore, secure people do not need to evade freedom and self-determination by conforming to prescribed societal and cultural expectancies, norms, and values. This is more characteristic of attachment-anxious people, who worry that they may be disapproved of or abandoned if they make shameful mistakes. Thus, secure people, more than insecure ones, can take what we consider to be a healthy leap of faith and commit themselves fully to their choices, and at the same time be open to the possibility that some of their decisions will be wrong.

An example of this kind of leap appears in Nobel Prize–winner Eric Kandel's (2006) autobiography, *In Search of Memory: The Emergence of a New Science of Mind*. In explaining how he chose to work on the large neurons of the sea snail *Aplysia*—a choice that eventually allowed him to make some of the most important discoveries in neurobiology—despite his colleagues' dire warnings, he said:

> I liked the idea of big cells and, despite the risks involved, I was convinced that *Aplysia* was the right system and that I had the tools to study behavior in the snail effectively. [Also], I had learned something in marrying Denise [his wife, to whom he has now been happily married for 50 years]. I had been reluctant and fearful of marriage, even to Denise, whom I loved much more than any other woman I had ever thought of marrying. But Denise was confident

that our marriage would work, so I took a *leap of faith* [our italics] and went ahead. I learned from that experience that there are many situations in which one cannot decide on the basis of cold facts alone—because facts are insufficient. One ultimately has to trust one's unconscious, one's instincts, one's creative urge. I did this again in choosing *Aplysia*. (p. 149)

Secure relationships with attachment figures, and the internal representations and emotional residues of these relationships, can also reduce people's concerns with existential isolation. Security-enhancing relationships and mental representations instill confidence that other people often perceive our needs and communications correctly, empathically understand our dilemmas and struggles, and affirm the validity of our experiences. At the same time, such relationships allow us to be more tolerant of attachment figures' momentary unavailability, empathic failures, and occasional lack of responsiveness, because we gradually become confident of their overall goodwill and, in effect, take a leap of faith in their approachability. As a result, secure people can feel connected to others, without denying or distorting the unbridgeable gap that sometimes exists between their own and other people's subjectivity. Their sense of connectedness is sufficiently solid and deep that they can live comfortably with periods of disconnection, solitude, or perplexity.

By comparison, avoidant people tend to resolve the inevitable gap between different subjectivities by remaining disinterested and disengaged, attempting not to think about or hope for connection, and denigrating other people's engagement and enthusiasm. (As we mentioned in Chapter 9, diary studies reveal that avoidant people are alienated and bored during daily social interactions, which is probably a consequence of their own disengagement and lack of interest.) Anxious people feel the inevitable separateness that results from ultimately distinct subjectivities, but try to deny the gap by imagining false similarities between themselves and their interaction partners, striving to merge psychologically with their mates or children, and imagining perfect love with fictional or media characters. Frequently, however, reality intervenes and foils the wish for total merger.

In their introduction to the *Handbook of Experimental Existential Psychology*, Pyszczynski et al. (2004, p. 7) claim that "the problem of meaninglessness is the result of the first three basic concerns: In a world where the only true certainty is death, where meaning and value are subjective human creations rather than absolute truths, and where one can never fully share one's experiences with others, what meaning does life have?" The answer, based on attachment research, is that secure people are not terrified by death, do not require certainty, and have sufficiently good communication with at least some close relationship partners that immersion in a life of shared activities, personal growth, creative contributions to the world, and mutual intimacy is meaningful.

The perspective of atheistic existential philosophy (which was quite different from Kierkegaard's religious existentialism)—that God is dead, we are alone, life is unpredictable and meaningless, and no current social order will last forever—was a product of Western science's challenge to traditional religions combined with two incredibly devastating and bloody world wars. It emerged from a sense of helplessness and hopelessness that rarely plagues secure people under normal circumstances. Secure people's stance is also "existential" in the sense that it acknowledges human finitude, fallibility, and lack of complete control over events. But their view of existence is not generally darkened by helplessness, hopelessness, or incoherence. They can view events and experiences fairly objectively, while taking pleasure and comfort in the endless possibilities for creativity, shared goals, and real accomplishments. Existentialism of the depressive sort has become much less attractive as the distance from economic depression and two world wars has widened, although there is still plenty to be gloomy about, if a person prefers gloom. In large parts of the world where hopelessness is still common for other reasons (economic and political disintegration or stagnation, hunger, disease, poor education, ethnic and religious warfare), fundamentalism is more likely to take hold than is existentialism. These horrible life conditions obviously make psychological security difficult to sustain.

Nevertheless, even under punishing conditions, there may still be measurable distinctions between secure and insecure people. As we have seen in previous chapters, relatively secure adults are able to give coherent, evidence-based accounts of their experiences. They can reflect sensibly on their inner and outer worlds, open themselves to alternative perspectives, and adjust their beliefs and actions in light of new information. Their general sense that "all will be well" (their kind of leap of faith) allows for negotiation, change, uncertainty, and unpredictability, with a minimum of static rumination and existential dread. Less secure people are more vulnerable to the idea that life is meaningless and nothing has value, or that it is meaningful but based on an absolute and unchangeable single truth or dogma. As every educated person knows too well, these tendencies, when extreme, incline a person to violence, suicide, or both. Thus, the only hope for peace and improved economic conditions is for relatively secure people to use their skills and hopeful faith to assist others and educate them away from deadly despair. This is the kind of challenging but optimistic project that should appeal to today's secure people.

Although we are undoubtedly oversimplifying and painting a somewhat idealistic portrait of security (as discussed in a subsequent section of this chapter), a large body of research implies that altering human practices, so that more children experience security-enhancing support from attachment figures, will allow these children, as they grow up and become adults, to confront core existential concerns with greater resilience and more constructive strategies. Enhanced security makes it possible, at least to a worthwhile extent, to achieve an integration of what sometimes seem like irreconcilable opposites: a joyful, creative, loving life in the presence of frequent threats and the certainty of eventual death; warm, satisfying intimacy despite ultimately distinct subjectivities; freedom to choose in the presence of constant change and inevitable mistakes; and expansive, optimistic creation of stories, music, books, art objects, marriages, children, families, social organizations, and societies, side by side with scientists' best guess that life is, at least compared with the promises of previous religious myths, time-limited and objectively "meaningless" until we freely and creatively endow it with meaning.

ATTACHMENT AND I–THOU FORMS OF LOVE

Secure attachment bonds are by definition dialogical creations: The needy infant expresses his or her subjectivity to the mother (or another attachment figure) by crying or clinging, thereby "asking" this person to pay attention and provide comfort, encouragement, and protection. The good caregiver empathically and effectively responds to these signals, while respecting and reaffirming the infant's subjectivity and nascent independent will. This strengthens the child's sense of personal value, efficacy, and connection to the world and other people. In adulthood, secure people can express their subjective experiences in friendships, romantic relationships, and group interactions, and reciprocate their friends', romantic partners', and children's acts of love and care (see Chapters 9–12, this volume); that is, secure adults are able to occupy the role of security-providing attachment figure, while respecting the subjectivity and autonomy of their relationship partners. In this way, attachment security helps people establish what Buber (1958) called I–Thou relationships—in which each partner openly and confidently expresses his or her subjectivity, while validating the other's subjective experiences. Loved, supported, respected, and appreciated by their attachment figures, securely attached people are well equipped to love, support, respect, and joyfully appreciate the subjectivity of others.

How do primal, egotistic needs for safety and security get transformed into mutual respect and genuine concern for others' welfare? The transformation implies a "dynamic of security" in which one can be both a recipient of security and an active transmitter of it. By the processes of identification and internalization, discussed earlier in this chapter, a person who perceives his or her attachment figure as sensitive and caring tends to view him- or herself as also sensitive and caring. This identification process and the incorporation of attachment figures' qualities into one's self-concept may be crucial for secure people's sensitive, empathic, and altruistic attitudes and behavior toward others who are in need. It may explain their sensitive parenting; their ability to provide a secure base for their offspring, peers, and coworkers; and their willingness to contribute in prosocial ways to local and wider communities.

This process is implied by many religious sayings and practices. The Golden Rule, for example, which enjoins people to treat others as they would like to be treated, is easier to follow if one knows what it is like to be treated well, accurately empathizes with other people, and provides what others need, without feeling cheated or entitled to effusive praise. Interestingly, religious "models" (Oman & Thoresen, 2003) are generally portrayed in scriptures and religious stories as security-providing attachment figures for their followers, who in turn are enjoined to treat others as the model treats them. Jesus, for example, is described by John (13:35) as saying, "By this all will know that you are my disciples, if you have love for one another." Luke (6:30–36) describes Jesus as giving the following specific instructions: "Give to everyone who asks of you. And from him who takes away your goods do not ask them back. And just as you want men to do to you, you also do to them. . . . Love your enemies, do good, and lend, hoping for nothing in return."

In Buddhism, a common form of compassion meditation involves remembering vividly how one feels when someone provides unconditional love (one's mother is often suggested, but someone else can be substituted if she was not a supportive attachment figure), then turn that process, in one's mind (and eventually in one's behavior as well), toward other targets. Chödrön (2003) describes this process as follows:

> To begin, we start just where we are. We connect with the place where we currently feel loving-kindness, compassion, joy, or equanimity, however limited they may be. . . . We aspire that we and our loved ones can enjoy the quality we are practicing. Then we gradually extend that aspiration to a widening circle of relationships. . . . "May I be free from suffering and the root of suffering. May you be free from suffering and the root of suffering. May all beings be free of suffering and the root of suffering." (pp. 66–67)

This is similar to the security inductions we (Mikulincer & Shaver, 2001; Mikulincer et al., 2005) used to reduce outgroup prejudice and to foster compassion, altruism, gratitude, and forgiveness, even though we had not yet read or heard about the Buddhist version of the same technique. We began with reminders of others who had provided our study participants with love and kindness; then we checked to see whether greater tolerance and compassion emerged as a result—and they did! Our manipulations were based on attachment theory rather than Buddhism, but the two approaches are surprisingly similar in this and other respects.

Constructively dealing with existential concerns—death, freedom, and isolation— may make it easier to adopt a compassionate, responsible, and respectful attitude toward other people (and even toward all "sentient beings," as Buddhists say). By acknowledging the inevitability of suffering, aging, and death, secure people find it fairly easy to understand the common concerns of all human beings. They can identify with other people's vulnerabilities, weaknesses, and needs, because everyone wants and deserves support, comfort, and protection. In contrast, denial of death may have implications for one's reaction to needy and vulnerable others, because their suffering is a reminder of one's own vulnerability and finitude. Denial of death may cause a person to turn away from others who are in need or in pain, instead of reacting to them with effective compassion. This is what characterized avoidant people in our studies of compassion and altruism (Chapter 12, this volume).

By acknowledging the ambiguities, uncertainties, and mistakes inherent in human decisions and actions, secure people are more likely to take responsibility for their choices and actions, knowing that sometimes they will make mistakes. They are also more likely to forgive others who make mistakes. Moreover, because secure people tend to be aware of the web of interconnections and shared responsibilities inherent in social life, they may be especially able to reflect on the ways their decisions and behavior affect other people. Avoidant people's defensive conviction that their decisions and actions cannot be wrong (or had better not be wrong), and attachment-anxious people's wish that someone else would embrace them and guide them through life, militate against taking responsibility for one's actions and paying attention to the needs of others.

Secure individuals' ability to recognize the unbridgeable gap between their own and their relationship partners' experiences, while maintaining a dialogue and being genuinely curious about and interested in others' needs and experiences, also helps them love other people and support their exploratory ventures. As we discussed in Chapter 6, attachment security reduces blind projection of one's own experiences, traits, and preferences onto others. Anxious individuals tend to project onto their relationship partners their own unmet needs for safety and protection, and assume detailed interpersonal similarities where important differences exist. Avoidant people tend to project onto a relationship partner their own undesirable traits, which gives them an added reason to dismiss or disparage others and maintain distance from them. In terms of object relations theory (e.g., Joseph, 1989), secure people are freer of defensive projection (of the avoidant kind) and projective identification (of the anxious kind). They can perceive and treat others as "whole subjects" rather than imaginary "part objects" who exist solely to satisfy their own needs. In this way, secure people are better equipped to form mature I–Thou relationships.

Such relationships allow us to see that our relationship partners are more complicated and more valuable than our projections, which means we can expand and extend ourselves by engaging in authentic dialogue with them (A. Aron & Aron, 2006). Hollis (1998) provided a good description of the self-expansion that occurs in this kind of dialogical relationship:

> When relationship is not driven by need, but by caring for the other as other, then we are free to experience him or her. When we let go of our projections . . . we are free to love. When we are free to love, we are present to the mystery embodied by the other. Without such mystery we are prisoners of childhood, trapped in the trivial. Blake said he could see eternity in the grain of sand; so we lesser mortals may glimpse the eternal in and through our beloved. This other, paradoxically, is a sacred vehicle toward ourselves, not because we use the other to serve our own narcissistic ends, but because he or she serves our deepest end by remaining wholly other. (p. 64)

ATTACHMENT THEORY AND BUDDHISM

As indicated in previous sections, and by our occasional use of the term "mindfulness" in previous chapters, attachment theory is strikingly similar to Buddhist psychology, at least when attachment theory is extended to the philosophical level we are considering in this chapter. As already mentioned briefly, in 2004, we participated in a weeklong discussion with the Dalai Lama, several psychologists and neuroscientists, and an audience of Tibetan Buddhist monks and interested spectators. We had been studying attachment security, compassion, and altruism, and noted parallels between our approach and the Buddhist literature. The parallels include fostering compassion by "priming attachment security" (in our words), as well as focusing on the issue of security. Here, we continue to rely on Chödrön's writings (2003), because her translations are already slanted in the direction of contemporary psychological language. First, Buddhism, like attachment theory, emphasizes the importance of security:

> Our mind is always seeking zones of safety. We're in this zone of safety and that's what we consider life, getting it all together, security. Death is losing that. We fear losing our illusion of security—that's what makes us so anxious. . . . The mind is always seeking zones of safety, and these zones of safety are continually falling apart. . . . That's the essence of samsara—the cycle of suffering that comes from continuing to seek happiness in all the wrong places. (pp. 23–24)

This is similar to attachment researchers' notion that there are various strategies for coping with threats, and some of them are more successful than others. But Chödrön seems to believe that everyone has an anxious, grasping mind, whereas attachment research suggests that this is a relative matter. People who have been treated well by their attachment figures are less afraid of death, more open cognitively and emotionally, less easily thrown off course, less grasping and preoccupied with attachment, and more secure. In other words, security is not always, or simply, an illusion.

Second, Buddhism recognizes the centrality of giving and receiving love to the development of a healthy mind:

> The essential practice is to cultivate maitri, or loving-kindness. The Shambala teachings speak of "placing our fearful mind in the cradle of loving-kindness." Another image for maitri is that of a mother bird who protects and cares for her young until they are strong enough to fly away. People sometimes ask, 'Who am I in this image—the mother or the chick?' The answer is *both*. . . . Without loving-kindness for ourselves, it is difficult, if not impossible, to genuinely feel it for others. (Chödrön, 2003, pp. 9–10; italics in original)

This is similar to our ideas about secure self-representations, including representations of self with a loving attachment figure and self as one's own caregiver. But attachment theory points to the social origins of these self-soothing processes, and attachment research shows that it is much harder for some people than for others to apply *maitri* to themselves and others.

Third, during meditation, one of the goals is to achieve and maintain a state of deep relaxation and natural, gentle breathing, combined with alert attention (not drowsiness or mental laxity; B. A. Wallace, 2006). Another goal is to be open to whatever arises, without "grasping" or "suppressing," and to be attentive and curious about what arises but without becoming lost in it. As Chödrön (2003) explains:

It's helpful to remind yourself that meditation is about opening and relaxing to whatever arises, without picking and choosing. It's definitely not meant to repress anything, and it's not intended to encourage grasping, either. . . . To the degree that we're willing to see our enmeshment or grasping and our repressing clearly, they begin to wear themselves out. . . . That's what we're doing in meditation: Up come all these thoughts, but rather than squelch them or obsess about them, we acknowledge them and let them fade. (pp. 35, 47–48)

This is remarkably similar to the idea in attachment theory that the major forms of insecurity are avoidance (repression, squelching) and anxiety (grasping, obsessing), with security being, in a sense, a "middle way." It is interesting that the forms of insecurity emphasized by the two "theories" (Buddhism and attachment theory) are so similar.

At first we thought there was one big difference between attachment theory and Buddhist psychology, at least as portrayed in Chödrön's writings. Attachment theory focuses on social processes as the foundation of security, whereas English-language books about Buddhist meditation make the process seem pretty solitary and asocial. During our discussions in Dharamsala, however, it was pointed out that one of the simplest and most frequently spoken Buddhist prayers is "I take *refuge* in the Buddha, the Dharma, and the Sangha," which means (in our terms) the mental representation of the Buddha as a loving, compassionate, and wise teacher; the Buddha's teachings (Dharma); and the community of fellow Buddhists (sangha). In other words, the key concept is "taking refuge," which is similar to Bowlby and Ainsworth's notion of using an attachment figure as a "safe haven." The social nature of Buddhism is also evident in the Dalai Lama's writings (e.g., *The Heart of Compassion*, 2002). When explaining what Buddhism calls "the Triple Gem" he writes: "Which object of refuge will never deceive us? There are three: the rare and supreme Buddha, the Dharma, and the Sangha. . . . The Buddha is the protector and is like a doctor; the precious Dharma is like the medicine; and the spiritual sangha is like a nurse, taking care of us like a good friend" (pp. 17–22).

Seeing the similarity between central ideas in attachment theory and Buddhism, as well as other religions (as implied by our quotations from the Bible), and the similarities between attachment theory and previous ideas in existential philosophy and humanistic psychology, causes us to suspect that the thrust of attachment theory is a set of ideas that appears repeatedly—throughout human history in general, and in the history of psychology in particular. Once one sees the form these ideas take in Buddhism, for example, it becomes more evident that they probably have been discovered and rediscovered by anyone who has ever taken mental healing and optimal human development seriously (see Mitchell [1998] for many beautiful and inspiring examples). In the same way, for example, that Buddhism suggests deep relaxation combined with an open, nongrasping, and nonsuppressing mind, Freud (1917/1963) developed the psychoanalytic technique of having a client lie on a couch and free-associate, attempting to let his or her mind remain open and loosely associative without resisting or defending. Later, when behaviorists thought they were rejecting psychoanalysis in favor of something more scientific, they invented systematic desensitization (e.g., Wolpe, 1969)—a procedure in which deep muscle relaxation is combined with gradual imagination of objects or situations a client fears, in hopes that he or she will stop being preoccupied with or defending against them and instead remain calm in their presence. Around the same time, Carl Rogers (1961) was promoting a technique in which the therapist provided unconditional positive regard, so that the client could become less defensive and more open to "organismic experiencing."

The potential advantages of attachment theory, when seen in the context of all the previous psychological, religious, and philosophical approaches that resemble it, are that it is rooted in an evolutionary biological conception of the human mind and is increasingly supported by research evidence. Our hope is that as the evidence mounts, we will be able to retain and integrate the valid insights of previous thinkers, while providing more detail about psychological and neural mechanisms, and clearer implications for parenting, education, organizational leadership, psychotherapy, and social policy.

THE PERILS OF DEIFYING SECURE ATTACHMENT

Having explored the very positive implications of attachment security, it is time to consider the dangers of overidealizing it. Although the results of the hundreds of studies reviewed here certainly make attachment security seem important and desirable, there are other key determinants of a good life besides this one. Many of the secure people identified by our measures are well-adjusted but presumably far from Carl Rogers's (1961) conception of the fully functioning person or Maslow's (1968) conception of self-actualization. Due to innate factors (e.g., intelligence, temperament), life history, and other environmental, societal, economic, and cultural factors, these securely attached people tend to live comfortably in accordance with social norms and expectancies rather than their own subjective experiences and insights. At least from our vantage point, many of them seem pretty ordinary rather than exceptionally creative or accomplished. Just as attachment insecurities do not, by themselves, produce psychopathology (Chapter 13, this volume), attachment security does not, by itself, necessarily produce exceptional psychological growth, authentic confrontation with the givens of existence, or deep I–Thou relationships. Psychological growth results from multiple converging processes, and attachment security is just the psychological foundation on which other growth-promoting processes can build, because many worries and defenses that would otherwise interfere with growth have been reduced or rendered unnecessary. For example, attachment security can increase the likelihood of psychological growth in adults who were fortunate enough to grow up in families or societies that valued and reinforced existential living, openness to experience, and creativity. However, security-enhancing interactions with loving and sensitive caregivers can also occur within families that value tradition, conformity, and stasis, which probably enhance adjustment without fostering all of the qualities of Carl Rogers's (1961) fully functioning person. (We admit that this is a Western conception of "fully functioning," with which we happen to agree. But it is not by any means the only conception.)

We do not want to deify secure attachment, because surely there is more to life than security. But we do believe that other desirable outcomes are facilitated by attachment security. In the same sense that identity foreclosure (fastening onto a conventional identity too quickly and easily, without exploration or struggle; Marcia, 1980) can provide a person with an identity, which Erikson (1950/1993) viewed as one of the most important steps in adolescent and adult development, without ensuring optimal development, secure attachment may lead no further than complacency if it is not stretched to include exploration, broad learning, and self-expansion. Throughout this book we have emphasized the insufficiency of anxious people's mere search for security. Such people are often willing to forgo exploration, autonomy, and growth as long as they can find a reliable safe haven. In such cases, the hope for security is not a hope for psychological growth but rather a desire to escape the challenges of growth, while remaining immature and dependent.

Without the support of other psychological growth factors, secure attachment might lead to a middle- or upper-SES gated community or retirement home—in other words, the cushy "good life." In such cases, a secure person might be able to love and work productively (thereby meeting the Freudian criteria for adequate adjustment), be quite satisfied with personal possessions and achievements, feel good about social relations and family life, yet see no reason for challenges or changes. This kind of "good life," made possible and sustained by secure attachment, might be common in societies or subcultures that place a high value on stability, conformity, and personal possessions (as seems to be the case in modern Western societies). This kind of complacency puts a damper on psychological growth of the kind discussed by Carl Rogers, Maslow, and Yalom. Many of our students, when we first present the basics of attachment theory, assume that securely attached people must be boring conformists who accept what they have and forgo the quest for a more creative but demanding existence.

The same reasoning is evident in biographies and theoretical analyses of creative geniuses who seem to have reached the summit of creativity despite, or even because of, anxiety, insecurity, and maybe even bouts of madness or self-destruction (prototypical examples are Van Gogh and Modigliani). According to this view, attachment security and the "good life" actually work against creativity, because they eliminate the anxiety, emotional turmoil, vulnerability, or grandiosity that fuel creative work. However, just as secure attachment should not be viewed as sufficient for creativity, it also should not be viewed as necessarily impeding it. In fact, creative work is not just a matter of inspiration and escape from the comfortable "good life"; it often requires commitment, coherent cognitive organization, and behavioral self-regulation to translate creativity into valuable creative products, and these qualities are generally associated with attachment security and are diminished by attachment-related anxieties, worries, and defenses (Chapter 8, this volume). Moreover, although we can find many examples of suffering and maladjusted artists (many of whom might have accomplished even more and lived longer if they had been more secure; Kramer, 2005), we can also find many examples of well-adjusted artists who have many of the qualities we have identified as associated with security (Picasso and Monet might be examples among painters; John Bowlby is a good example among psychological theorists). These people are not "normal" in the sense of being common (they could not be, while also being exceptionally talented and extremely dedicated to their careers), but they displayed prolonged creativity, while also having generally good relations with their children, friends, colleagues, students, and romantic partners.

The lives of many creative geniuses have been filled with obstacles, losses, traumatic experiences, and other sources of inner pain that gave them an opportunity to touch, taste, and smell the frightening aspects of human existence. Almost by definition, to do something exceptional requires competing or arguing with other people (e.g., as Bowlby did with his fellow psychoanalysts, and as Ainsworth did with her colleagues, many of whom were dyed-in-the-wool behaviorists or laboratory experimentalists, who thought naturalistic observations of children viewed from a psychodynamic perspective would lead nowhere). At the same time, much of their strength and ability to push on stemmed from supportive relationships with at least one parent, a supportive sibling, a spouse, or a security-enhancing mentor. (Ainsworth, for example, had a good relationship with her father, inspiring mentors, including Blatz and Bowlby, and an effective psychotherapist, yet it took her quite a while to emerge from a troubled marriage to become a sturdy, extremely accomplished, and self-confident scientist and mentor.) Without some islands of love and security, painful experiences and self-doubts can paralyze, overwhelm, and disorganize a person in ways that interfere with creativity.

In a challenging Jungian analysis of attachment theory and attachment researchers (ourselves included), A. Aron and Aron (2006) noted some additional perils of the deification of secure attachment. They claimed that attachment theorists have an idyllic view of the perfect child, which the Arons equate with the Jungian archetype of the Divine Child, "the redeemer of mankind, the eventual innocent sacrifice for the sins of ruined adults . . . the wise, heroic, compassionate adult we need" (p. 375). This archetype stresses the innate perfection of the child (i.e., the pure biological wisdom of the attachment system) and the obligation of parents to provide the perfect environment in which the Divine Child can flourish (rather than the insensitive and inconsistent treatment that produces attachment insecurities or disorganization). The danger described by the Arons is that attachment theory's emphasis on the perfect natural child may unintentionally cause parents to reject, neglect, or even abandon children who are born with minor imperfections (e.g., difficult temperament, physical or mental disabilities). Moreover, being afraid of the imagined damage they could inflict on their perfect child, parents might avoid exposing the child to challenging life circumstances or awareness of the terrifying givens of human existence, thereby coupling secure attachment with the kind of "good life" that reduces the chances of psychological growth:

> Identification of oneself or of others with an archetype such as the Divine Child invariably leads to dangerous inflation or deflation—worship or crucifixion. Moreover, something important, the potential wholeness of life, is left out of the perfectly secure life. We would not wish onto any child the terror, rage, despair, hate, and other scars that come from having been neglected, not seen, rejected, betrayed, or abused. But they are part of a universal, archetypal experience. (p. 377)

This again brings to mind the starting point of Buddhism, the first "noble truth": There is suffering or dissatisfaction (the human mind is never simply at rest, and everything inside and outside the mind is constantly changing). It would not be very realistic or sensible to deny this fundamental fact of human existence.

We acknowledge the potential problems that A. Aron and Aron (2006) noted in connection with the Divine Child archetype, but we also believe that attachment research has gone beyond the image of a perfect child. First, as we discussed in Chapter 5, attachment theory and research recognize that the child's innate characteristics influence parent–child relations, and require that parental sensitivity and responsiveness take the child's uniqueness into account. Moreover, these days, a great deal of research on infancy and attachment is directed at "imperfect" children with special physical and mental needs (like the ones Berant et al. [2001a, 2001b] studied, who were born with congenital heart defects; see Chapter 7, this volume), and therapeutic interventions have been designed to aid parents who care for these children. Neither infants nor their parents, nor any actual societies, are close to perfect, and whenever changes are made to improve conditions, they have unintended side effects, foiling any hope of stable perfection. Reality—both physical and social—is highly complex, multidimensional, and full of contradictions, interactions among diverse forces, and constant variability. There is no danger of ever achieving perfection.

Second, attachment theory emphasizes not only the safe haven function of parenting but also the secure base function, which assumes that parental support, validation, and encouragement lead the way for children's exploration, risk taking, and engagement in growth-promoting activities. There is no assumption that the child is complete or perfect at the start, or that he or she will end up perfect by the parents' or anyone else's assessment. (Many critics have been bothered by the fact that the people Maslow [1968] described as self-actualized had flaws, like Abraham Lincoln and Eleanor Roosevelt. But Maslow never said that self-actualized people were perfect; he thought they were models of what was possible at the high end of the continuum.) A secure base can help children become creative, honest, and perceptive adults, who confront their uniqueness and the existential universals of human life, including the existence of their own Jungian "shadows" (dark, hidden aspects), failures, injuries, and weaknesses. In fact, this is one of the basic tasks in attachment-based therapy—providing a secure base that supports exploration of painful and threatening experiences (see Chapter 14, this volume). The task of living and developing is never finished until death, however. Perfection is never achieved, and the kind of security we have been describing is a launching pad for continued development, not a final, dusty psychological trophy.

In one respect, however, we can agree with the thrust of A. Aron and Aron's (2006) "Divine Child" criticism of attachment theory. The theory tends to downplay or remain quiet about aggression and dominance, manifestations of one of the two major "instincts" that Freudian psychoanalysis featured (*eros* and *thanatos*). In some ways, the relative silence regarding aggression on the part of attachment theorists can be viewed as an attempt by Bowlby to suggest that aggression and anger, contra Freud, are not innate necessities, but rather reactions to inadequate care ("protests," in his terms). Certainly he and Ainsworth noticed that infants react with anger to unexpected separations from their attachment figures. Moreover, Bowlby began his study of "maternal deprivation" in part because he wished to understand the angry, hostile, and destructive behavior of juvenile delinquents. He assumed, however, that this kind of behavior is not a normal or necessary part of development but is instead an outgrowth of insecurity. While agreeing with his analysis of much of criminal and delinquent behavior, we cannot help wondering whether aggression and dominance get too little attention when they are attributed solely to insecurity. In the same way that Bowlby traced attachment to its evolutionary roots, it might make sense to reconsider the evolutionary roots of aggression and dominance, possibly adding a behavioral system to Bowlby's list: attachment, exploration, caregiving, affiliation, sex—and *aggression/dominance*. The existence of a behavioral system along these lines would make good biological sense, and its exploration is an important task for future research and theorizing.

According to A. Aron and Aron (2006), another peril of the Divine Child archetype is the exaggerated emphasis in attachment theory on early childhood experiences as determinants of adult personality, and the consequent dismissal of the "second half of life" as an important developmental stage. This glorification of childhood may keep adults from capitalizing on the possibilities for psychological growth during the second half of life. It may make them hopeless prisoners of their early experiences and discourage adaptive changes on the part of people who suffered attachment injuries during childhood and adolescence. However, although Bowlby (1969/1982) put strong emphasis on the formative influence of early experiences, he also emphasized the continual accommodation and updating of working models across the lifespan. Moreover, attachment studies have consistently shown changes and discontinuities in attachment patterns from infancy to adulthood (see Chapter 5, this volume), and attachment-related psychotherapy is based on the notion of "earned security" (Berlin & Cassidy, 1999), the ability of adults who grew up insecure to become secure as adults. It is true, however, that attachment theorists and researchers should devote more attention to the second half of life, including its later phases (aging toward death), and should figure out how continuous and earned security contribute to personal growth during this developmental period.

More research is also needed on the potentially adaptive consequences of anxious and avoidant attachment. If we want to avoid characterizing attachment insecurities as simply "bad" and keep from adopting a hostile stance toward insecurely attached people, we should remember Ainsworth's (1991) insight that anxious and avoidant attachment are *adaptive* responses to certain kinds of caregiving. Moreover, we need to examine whether and how these adaptive responses might sometimes contribute positively to a person's or community's welfare. In Chapter 14, we raised the possibility that anxious and avoidant people can play beneficial roles in the defense, maintenance, and enhancement of their communities. It is possible that our criticism, in this chapter, of the idea that creative geniuses are often troubled, was extreme in ignoring the fact that many of them *have* been troubled, and their troubles sometimes contributed to their depth of insight into depression, grief, and existential dread. Unfortunately, there is still no attachment-oriented research on these possibilities, so we cannot draw confident conclusions about them.

Finally, we need to remember that the personality, or attachment style, differences we have emphasized in this book—because they are emphasized in the literature we were reviewing—always interact with situations and current conditions. Most studies to date have compared people who share the same, mainly normal, life conditions (e.g., attending the same university, enjoying decent housing and nourishment, and living in modern, industrialized societies). Less is known about how secure people respond to major crises, such as hurricanes, epidemics, and wars, or nagging harassment and stresses due to racism or poverty. Although we have included studies connected with the anxiety of war, being a prisoner of war, having a child with a serious, life-threatening illness, and suffering from various emotional disorders, most of the existing research was done on normal, reasonably healthy people living under generally favorable conditions. Thus, little is known about how relatively secure people in oppressed groups, or relatively secure soldiers in an ongoing war that is killing their comrades, balance their usual loving-kindness and generosity with their wish to destroy their oppressors or enemies. These are matters about which we know very little, despite living in a world full of oppression and violence.

CONCLUDING REMARKS

Just as parents have to gradually relinquish control of their children and wish them well as they head out into the wider world to meet their fate, author-scientists eventually have to let go of their creations and see what contributions they make to their field. Our main motive in writing this book is to provide other scholars, especially young ones, with a single source that summarizes the large literature on adult attachment, especially the literature generated by social and personality psychologists. Much has been learned over the past 20–25 years about adult attachment, but it has become difficult for young scholars, or senior scholars in other disciplines or subfields of psychology, including clinical and applied subfields, to dig into the mushrooming literature and understand the terminology, measures, and research methods they encounter. We hope this volume provides a useful point of entry for interested students, scholars, clinicians, and teachers.

It has been challenging and rewarding for us to read and organize the vast literature on attachment, and to hold long conversations and exchange countless e-mail messages about it. We have even greater respect and gratitude than before for our many colleagues, who have invested their intelligence and creativity, and expended immense amounts of energy in the study of adult attachment. May their insights and discoveries continue to blossom and bear fruit.

APPENDICES

APPENDIX A

■ ■ ■

Adult Attachment Questionnaire (AAQ)

Please indicate how you typically feel toward romantic (dating) partners *in general*. Keep in mind that there are no right or wrong answers. Use the 7-point scale provided below and darken the appropriate number for each item on the Scantron answer sheet or place it on the line in front of the item. [*Note*. Researchers need to provide the answer sheet or modify the questionnaire to include it.]

1	2	3	4	5	6	7
I strongly disagree						I strongly agree

1. I find it relatively easy to get close to others.
2. I'm not very comfortable having to depend on other people.
3. I'm comfortable having others depend on me.
4. I rarely worry about being abandoned by others.
5. I don't like people getting too close to me.
6. I'm somewhat uncomfortable being too close to others.
7. I find it difficult to trust others completely.
8. I'm nervous whenever anyone gets too close to me.
9. Others often want me to be more intimate than I feel comfortable being.
10. Others often are reluctant to get as close as I would like.
11. I often worry that my partner(s) don't really love me.
12. I rarely worry about my partner(s) leaving me.
13. I often want to merge completely with others, and this desire sometimes scares them away.
14. I'm confident others would never hurt me by suddenly ending our relationship.
15. I usually want more closeness and intimacy than others do.
16. The thought of being left by others rarely enters my mind.
17. I'm confident that my partner(s) love me just as much as I love them.

Note. Items 1, 3, 4, 12, 14, 16, and 17 must be reverse-keyed prior to computing the following scores:

1. The *Avoidant Attachment* score is computed by averaging items 1–3 and 5–9. Higher scores reflect greater avoidance.
2. The *Attachment Anxiety* (sometimes called Ambivalence) score is computed by averaging items 4 and 10–17. Higher scores reflect greater anxiety/ambivalence.

When referencing the AAQ, please cite the following article:

Simpson, J. A., Rholes, S. W., & Phillips, D. (1996). Conflict in close relationships: An attachment perspective. *Journal of Personality and Social Psychology, 71,* 899–914.

APPENDIX B

■ ■ ■

Adult Attachment Scale (AAS)

Please read each of the following statements and rate the extent to which it describes your feelings about romantic relationships. Please think about all of your relationships (past and present) and respond in terms of how you generally feel in these relationships. If you have never been involved in a romantic relationship, answer in terms of how you think you would feel.

Please use the scale below by placing a number between 1 and 5 in the space provided to the right of each statement.

1 ———————— 2 ———————— 3 ———————— 4 ———————— 5

Not at all
characteristic
of me

Very
characteristic
of me

1. I find it relatively easy to get close to people. _____
2. I find it difficult to allow myself to depend on others. _____
3. I often worry that romantic partners don't really love me. _____
4. I find that others are reluctant to get as close as I would like. _____
5. I am comfortable depending on others. _____
6. I *don't* worry about people getting too close to me. _____
7. I find that people are never there when you need them. _____
8. I am somewhat *un*comfortable being close to others. _____
9. I often worry that romantic partners won't want to stay with me. _____
10. When I show my feelings for others, I'm afraid they will not feel the same about me. _____
11. I often wonder whether romantic partners really care about me. _____
12. I am comfortable developing close relationships with others. _____
13. I am *un*comfortable when anyone gets too emotionally close to me. _____
14. I know that people will be there when I need them. _____

15. I want to get close to people, but I worry about being hurt.   _____
16. I find it difficult to trust others completely.   _____
17. Romantic partners often want me to be emotionally closer than I feel
    comfortable being.   _____
18. I am not sure that I can always depend on people to be there when I need them. _____

Note. Items 1, 5, 6, 12, and 14 must be reverse-keyed prior to computing the following scores:

1. The *Discomfort with Dependency* score is computed by averaging items 2, 5, 7, 14, 16, and 18. Higher scores reflect greater discomfort depending on others.
2. The *Discomfort with Closeness* score is computed by averaging items 1, 6, 8, 12, 13, and 17. Higher scores reflect greater discomfort with closeness and intimacy.
3. The *Anxiety* score is computed by averaging items 3, 4, 9, 10, 11, and 15. Higher scores reflect stronger fear of being rejected or unloved.

When referencing this version of the AAS, please cite the following article:

Collins, N. L. (1996). Working models of attachment: Implications for explanation, emotion, and behavior. *Journal of Personality and Social Psychology, 71*, 810–832.

APPENDIX C

Attachment Style Questionnaire (ASQ)

Show how much you agree or disagree with each of the following items by rating them on this scale: 1 = totally disagree; 2 = strongly disagree; 3 = slightly disagree; 4 = slightly agree; 5 = strongly agree; or 6 = totally agree.

___ 1. Overall, I am a worthwhile person.
___ 2. I am easier to get to know than most people.
___ 3. I feel confident that other people will be there for me when I need them.
___ 4. I prefer to depend on myself rather than other people.
___ 5. I prefer to keep to myself.
___ 6. To ask for help is to admit that you're a failure.
___ 7. People's worth should be judged by what they achieve.
___ 8. Achieving things is more important than building relationships.
___ 9. Doing your best is more important that getting on with others.
___ 10. If you've got a job to do, you should do it no matter who gets hurt.
___ 11. It's important to me that others like me.
___ 12. It's important to me to avoid doing things that others won't like.
___ 13. I find it hard to make a decision unless I know what other people think.
___ 14. My relationships with others are generally superficial.
___ 15. Sometimes I think I am no good at all.
___ 16. I find it hard to trust other people.
___ 17. I find it difficult to depend on others.
___ 18. I find that others are reluctant to get as close as I would like.
___ 19. I find it relatively easy to get close to other people.
___ 20. I find easy to trust others.
___ 21. I feel comfortable depending on other people.
___ 22. I worry that others won't care about me as much as I care about them.
___ 23. I worry about people getting to close.

___ 24. I worry that I won't measure up to other people.

___ 25. I have mixed feelings about being close to others.

___ 26. While I want to get close to others, I feel uneasy about it.

___ 27. I wonder why people would want to be involved with me.

___ 28. It's very important to me to have a close relationship.

___ 29. I worry a lot about my relationships.

___ 30. I wonder how I would cope without someone to love me.

___ 31. I feel confident about relating to others.

___ 32. I often feel left out or alone.

___ 33. I often worry that I do not really fit with other people.

___ 34. Other people have their own problems, so I don't bother them with mine.

___ 35. When I talk over my problems with others, I generally feel ashamed or foolish.

___ 36. I am too busy with other activities to put much time into relationships.

___ 37. If something is bothering me, others are generally aware and concerned.

___ 38. I am confident that other people will like and respect me.

___ 39. I get frustrated when others are not available when I need them.

___ 40. Other people often disappoint me.

Note. Items 20, 21, and 33 must be reverse-keyed prior to computing the following scores:

1. The *Confidence* score is computed by averaging items 1–3, 19, 31, 33, 37, and 38. Higher scores reflect greater confidence.

2. The *Discomfort with Closeness* score is computed by averaging items 4, 5, 16, 17, 20, 21, 23, 25, 26, and 34. Higher scores reflect greater discomfort with closeness.

3. The *Relationships as Secondary* score is computed by averaging items 6–10, 14, and 36. Higher scores reflect a stronger tendency to appraise relationships as secondary.

4. The *Need for Approval* score is computed by averaging items 11–13, 15, 24, 27, and 35. Higher scores reflect greater need for approval.

5. The *Preoccupation* score is computed by averaging items 18, 22, 28–30, 32, 39, and 40. Higher scores reflect greater preoccupation with relationships.

In addition to yielding the above five scores, ASQ items can be used to form scores for attachment anxiety and avoidant attachment. In this case, items 3, 19–21, 31, 37, and 38 must be reverse-keyed prior to computing the following two scores:

1. The *Avoidant Attachment* score is computed by averaging items 3–5, 8–10, 14, 16, 17, 19–21, 23, 25, 34, and 37. Higher scores reflect more avoidant attachment.

2. The *Attachment Anxiety* score is computed by averaging items 11, 13, 15, 18, 22, 24, 27, 29–33, and 38. Higher scores reflect greater attachment anxiety.

When referencing the ASQ, please cite the following chapter:

Feeney, J. A., Noller, P., & Hanrahan, M. (1994). Assessing adult attachment. In M. B. Sperling & W. H. Berman (Eds.), *Attachment in adults: Clinical and developmental perspectives* (pp. 128–152). New York: Guilford Press.

APPENDIX D

Relationship Style Questionnaire (RSQ)

Please read each of the following statements and rate the extent to which you believe each statement best describes your feelings about *close relationships*. Write the number in the space provided, using the following rating scale:

1	2	3	4	5
Not at all like me		Somewhat like me		Very much like me

__ 1. I find it difficult to depend on other people.

__ 2. It is very important to me to feel independent.

__ 3. I find it easy to get emotionally close to others.

__ 4. I want to merge completely with another person.

__ 5. I worry that I will be hurt if I allow myself to become too close to others.

__ 6. I am comfortable without close emotional relationships.

__ 7. I am not sure that I can always depend on others to be there when I need them.

__ 8. I want to be completely emotionally intimate with others.

__ 9. I worry about being alone.

__ 10. I am comfortable depending on other people.

__ 11. I often worry that romantic partners don't really love me.

__ 12. I find it difficult to trust others completely.

__ 13. I worry about others getting too close to me.

__ 14. I want emotionally close relationships.

__ 15. I am comfortable having other people depend on me.

__ 16. I worry that others don't value me as much as I value them.

__ 17. People are never there when you need them.

__ 18. My desire to merge completely sometimes scares people away.

495

___ 19. It is very important to me to feel self-sufficient.

___ 20. I am nervous when anyone gets too close to me.

___ 21. I often worry that romantic partners won't want to stay with me.

___ 22. I prefer not to have other people depend on me.

___ 23. I worry about being abandoned.

___ 24. I am somewhat uncomfortable being close to others.

___ 25. I find that others are reluctant to get as close as I would like.

___ 26. I prefer not to depend on others.

___ 27. I know that others will be there when I need them.

___ 28. I worry about having others not accept me.

___ 29. Romantic partners often want me to be closer than I feel comfortable being.

___ 30. I find it relatively easy to get close to others.

Note. Items 6, 9, and 28 must be reverse-keyed prior to computing the following four attachment style scores:

1. The *Secure Style* score is computed by averaging items 3, 9, 10, 15, and 28. Higher scores reflect more secure attachment.
2. The *Preoccupied (Anxious) Style* score is computed by averaging items 6, 8, 16, and 25. Higher scores reflect more preoccupied attachment.
3. The *Dismissing Avoidance Style* score is computed by averaging items 2, 6, 19, 22, and 26. Higher scores reflect more dismissing avoidance.
4. The *Fearful Avoidance Style* score is computed by averaging items 1, 5, 12, and 24. Higher scores reflect more fearful avoidance.

In addition to the four attachment style scores, scores for the three Hazan and Shaver (1987) attachment styles can be obtained by going back to their original Adult Attachment Style measure (shown in this book in Chapter 1) and matching up the statements. Additionally, scores on attachment anxiety (model of self) and avoidant attachment (model of others) can be computed (1) by conducting a factor analysis of the items (specifying a two-factor solution) or (2) by using the scores from the four attachment styles to create linear combinations representing the anxiety and avoidance dimensions. Kurdek (2002) offered a useful guide for scoring the RSQ dimensionally.

When referencing the RSQ, please cite the following chapter:

Griffin, D. W., & Bartholomew, K. (1994). The metaphysics of measurement: The case of adult attachment. In K. Bartholomew & D. Perlman (Eds.), *Advances in personal relationships: Attachment processes in adulthood* (Vol. 5, pp. 17–52). London: Kingsley.

APPENDIX E

███ ███ ███

Experiences in Close Relationships Scale (ECR)

The following statements concern how you generally feel in close relationships (e.g., with romantic partners, close friends, or family members). Respond to each statement by indicating how much you agree or disagree with it. Write the number in the space provided, using the following rating scale:

1	2	3	4	5	6	7
Disagree strongly	Disagree	Disagree slightly	Neutral/ mixed	Agree slightly	Agree	Agree strongly

___ 1. I prefer not to show others how I feel deep down.
___ 2. I worry about being rejected or abandoned.
___ 3. I am very comfortable being close to other people.
___ 4. I worry a lot about my relationships.
___ 5. Just when someone starts to get close to me I find myself pulling away.
___ 6. I worry that others won't care about me as much as I care about them.
___ 7. I get uncomfortable when someone wants to be very close to me.
___ 8. I worry a fair amount about losing my close relationship partners.
___ 9. I don't feel comfortable opening up to others.
___ 10. I often wish that close relationship partners' feelings for me were as strong as my feelings for them.
___ 11. I want to get close to others, but I keep pulling back.
___ 12. I want to get very close to others, and this sometimes scares them away.
___ 13. I am nervous when another person gets too close to me.
___ 14. I worry about being alone.
___ 15. I feel comfortable sharing my private thoughts and feelings with others.
___ 16. My desire to be very close sometimes scares people away.
___ 17. I try to avoid getting too close to others.
___ 18. I need a lot of reassurance that close relationship partners really care about me.

___ 19. I find it relatively easy to get close to others.

___ 20. Sometimes I feel that I try to force others to show more feeling, more commitment to our relationship than they otherwise would.

___ 21. I find it difficult to allow myself to depend on close relationship partners.

___ 22. I do not often worry about being abandoned.

___ 23. I prefer not to be too close to others.

___ 24. If I can't get a relationship partner to show interest in me, I get upset or angry.

___ 25. I tell my close relationship partners just about everything.

___ 26. I find that my partners don't want to get as close as I would like.

___ 27. I usually discuss my problems and concerns with close others.

___ 28. When I don't have close others around, I feel somewhat anxious and insecure.

___ 29. I feel comfortable depending on others.

___ 30. I get frustrated when my close relationship partners are not around as much as I would like.

___ 31. I don't mind asking close others for comfort, advice, or help.

___ 32. I get frustrated if relationship partners are not available when I need them.

___ 33. It helps to turn to close others in times of need.

___ 34. When other people disapprove of me, I feel really bad about myself.

___ 35. I turn to close relationship partners for many things, including comfort and reassurance.

___ 36. I resent it when my relationship partners spend time away from me.

Note. Items 3, 15, 19, 22, 25, 27, 29, 31, 33, and 35 must be reverse-keyed prior to computing the following scores.

1. The *Avoidant Attachment* score is computed by averaging the 18 odd-numbered (1, 3, 5, etc.) items. Higher scores reflect greater avoidance.
2. The *Attachment Anxiety* score is computed by averaging the 18 even-numbered items (2, 4, 6, etc.). Higher scores reflect greater anxiety.

When referencing the ECR, please cite the following chapter:

Brennan, K. A., Clark, C. L., & Shaver, P. R. (1998). Self-report measurement of adult romantic attachment: An integrative overview. In J. A. Simpson & W. S. Rholes (Eds.), *Attachment theory and close relationships* (pp. 46–76). New York: Guilford Press.

Note. Do not use the formula in the appendix of Brennan et al's (1998) chapter to *classify* people into type categories based on their dimensional scores. Use the dimensional scores themselves in correlational or regression analyses. (The classification equation is misleading.)

APPENDIX F

The ECR-R Items

[The ECR-R uses instructions similar to those for the ECR, but replaces some of the ECR items with new ones based on analyses described by Fraley, Waller, and Brennan (2000).]

Avoidance Items
1. I prefer not to show a partner how I feel deep down.
2. I feel comfortable sharing my private thoughts and feelings with my partner.*
3. I find it difficult to allow myself to depend on romantic partners.
4. I am very comfortable being close to romantic partners.*
5. I don't feel comfortable opening up to romantic partners.
6. I prefer not to be too close to romantic partners.
7. I get uncomfortable when a romantic partner wants to be very close.
8. I find it relatively easy to get close to my partner.*
9. It's not difficult for me to get close to my partner.*
10. I usually discuss my problems and concerns with my partner.*
11. It helps to turn to my romantic partner in times of need.*
12. I tell my partner just about everything.*
13. I talk things over with my partner.*
14. I am nervous when partners get too close to me.
15. I feel comfortable depending on romantic partners.*
16. I find it easy to depend on romantic partners.*
17. It's easy for me to be affectionate with my partner.*
18. My partner really understands me and my needs.*

Anxiety Items
1. I'm afraid that I will lose my partner's love.
2. I often worry that my partner will not want to stay with me.
3. I often worry that my partner doesn't really love me.
4. I worry that romantic partners won't care about me as much as I care about them.
5. I often wish that my partner's feelings for me were as strong as my feelings for him or her.
6. I worry a lot about my relationships.

7. When my partner is out of sight, I worry that he or she might become interested in someone else.
8. When I show my feelings for romantic partners, I'm afraid they will not feel the same about me.
9. I rarely worry about my partner leaving me.*
10. My romantic partner makes me doubt myself.
11. I do not often worry about being abandoned.*
12. I find that my partner(s) don't want to get as close as I would like.
13. Sometimes romantic partners change their feelings about me for no apparent reason.
14. My desire to be very close sometimes scares people away.
15. I'm afraid that once a romantic partner gets to know me, he or she won't like who I really am.
16. It makes me mad that I don't get the affection and support I need from my partner.
17. I worry that I won't measure up to other people.
18. My partner only seems to notice me when I'm angry.

Note. * Denotes items that are reverse-keyed.

When referencing the ECR-R, please cite the following article:

Fraley, R. C., Waller, N. G., & Brennan, K. A. (2000). An item response theory analysis of self-report measures of adult attachment. *Journal of Personality and Social Psychology, 78*, 350–365.

APPENDIX G

▪ ▪ ▪

Caregiving Questionnaire

For each statement, write the number that indicates how descriptive the statement is of you. Write the number in the space provided, using the following rating scale:

1	2	3	4	5	6
Not at all descriptive of me					Very descriptive of me

___ 1. I sometimes push my partner away when s/he reaches out for a needed hug or kiss.

___ 2. I can always tell when my partner needs comforting, even when s/he doesn't ask for it.

___ 3. I always respect my partner's ability to make his/her own decisions and solve his/her own problems.

___ 4. When my partner cries or is distressed, my first impulse is to hold or touch him/her.

___ 5. I help my partner without becoming overinvolved in his/her problems.

___ 6. Too often, I don't realize when my partner is upset or worried about something.

___ 7. When my partner is troubled or upset, I move closer to provide support and comfort.

___ 8. I'm good at knowing when my partner needs my help or support and when s/he would rather handle things alone.

___ 9. I feel comfortable holding my partner when s/he needs physical signs of support and reassurance.

___ 10. I'm not very good at "tuning in" to my partner's needs and feelings.

___ 11. I tend to get overinvolved in my partner's problems and difficulties.

___ 12. I don't like it when my partner is needy and clings to me.

___ 13. I often end up telling my partner what to do when s/he is trying to make a decision.

___ 14. I sometimes miss the subtle signs that show how my partner is feeling,

___ 15. When necessary I can say "no" to my partner's requests for help without feeling guilty.

___ 16. I tend to be too domineering when trying to help my partner.

___ 17. When it's important, I take care of my own needs before I try to take care of my partner's.

___ 18. I am very attentive to my partner's nonverbal signals for help and support.

___ 19. I can easily keep myself from becoming overly concerned about or overly protective of my partner.

___ 20. I'm very good about recognizing my partner's needs and feelings, even when they're different from my own.

___ 21. I can help my partner work out his/her problems without "taking control."

___ 22. I sometimes draw away from my partner's attempts to get a reassuring hug from me.

___ 23. I am always supportive of my partner's *own efforts* to solve his/her problems.

___ 24. I tend to take on my partner's problems—and then feel burdened by them.

___ 25. When my partner seems to want or need a hug, I'm glad to provide it.

___ 26. When I help my partner with something, I tend to want to do things "my way."

___ 27. I frequently get too "wrapped up" in my partner's problems and needs.

___ 28. I sometimes "miss" or "misread" my partner's signals for help and understanding.

___ 29. When my partner is crying or emotionally upset, I sometimes feel like withdrawing.

___ 30. When my partner tells me about a problem, I sometimes go too far in criticizing his/her own attempts to deal with it.

___ 31. I create problems by taking on my partner's troubles as if they were my own

___ 32. When helping my partner solve a problem, I am much more "cooperative" than "controlling."

Note. Items 1, 3, 5, 6, 10, 12, 14, 15, 17, 19, 21, 22, 23, 28, 29, and 32 must be reverse-keyed prior to computing the following scores:

1. The *Proximity Maintenance* score is computed by averaging items 1, 4, 7, 9, 12, 22, 25, and 29. Higher scores reflect a stronger tendency to approach and comfort a relationship partner in times of need.

2. The *Sensitivity* score is computed by averaging items 2, 6, 8, 10, 14, 18, 20, and 28. Higher scores reflect greater sensitivity to a relationship partner's needs.

3. The *Controlling Caregiving* score is computed by averaging items 3, 13, 16, 21, 23, 26, 30, and 32. Higher scores reflect a more controlling, domineering approach to providing care or assistance.

4. The *Compulsive Caregiving* score is computed by averaging items 5, 11, 15, 17, 19, 24, 27, and 31. Higher scores reflect greater overinvolvement in a partner's problem-solving efforts.

When referencing the Caregiving Questionnaire, please cite the following chapter:

Kunce, L. J., & Shaver, P. R. (1994). An attachment-theoretical approach to caregiving in romantic relationships. In K. Bartholomew & D. Perlman (Eds.), *Advances in personal relationships: Attachment processes in adulthood* (Vol. 5, pp. 205–237). London: Kingsley.

References

Abramson, L. Y., Metalsky, G. I., & Alloy, L. B. (1989). Hopelessness depression: A theory-based subtype of depression. *Psychological Review, 96*, 358–372.

Ackerman, S. J., & Hilsenroth, M. J. (2003). A review of therapist characteristics and techniques positively impacting the therapeutic alliance. *Clinical Psychology Review, 23*, 1–33.

Adam, E. K., Gunnar, M. R., & Tanaka, A. (2004). Adult attachment, parent emotion, and observed parenting behavior: Mediator and moderator models. *Child Development, 75*, 110–122.

Adam, K. S. (1994). Suicidal behavior and attachment: A developmental model. In M. B. Sperling & W. H. Berman (Eds.), *Attachment in adults: Clinical and developmental perspectives* (pp. 275–298). New York: Guilford Press.

Adam, K. S., Sheldon-Keller, A. E., & West, M. (1996). Attachment organization and history of suicidal behavior in clinical adolescents. *Journal of Consulting and Clinical Psychology, 64*, 264–272.

Admoni, S. (2006). *Attachment security and eating disorders*. Unpublished doctoral dissertation, Bar-Ilan University, Ramat Gan, Israel.

Adshead, G., & Bluglass, K. (2005). Attachment representations in mothers with abnormal illness behavior by proxy. *British Journal of Psychiatry, 187*, 328–333.

Ainsworth, M. D. S. (1940). *An evaluation of adjustment based on the concept of security*. Unpublished doctoral dissertation, University of Toronto, Ontario, Canada.

Ainsworth, M. D. S. (1967). *Infancy in Uganda: Infant care and the growth of love*. Baltimore: Johns Hopkins University Press.

Ainsworth, M. D. S. (1973). The development of infant–mother attachment. In B. M. Caldwell & H. N. Ricciuti (Eds.), *Review of child development research* (Vol. 3, pp. 1–94). Chicago: University of Chicago Press.

Ainsworth, M. D. S. (1982). Attachment: Retrospect and prospect. In C. M. Parkes & J. Stevenson-Hinde (Eds.), *The place of attachment in human behavior* (pp. 3–30). New York: Basic Books.

Ainsworth, M. D. S. (1991). Attachment and other affectional bonds across the life cycle. In C. M. Parkes, J. Stevenson-Hinde, & P. Marris (Eds.), *Attachment across the life cycle* (pp. 33–51). New York: Routledge.

Ainsworth, M. D. S., Bell, S. M. V., & Stayton, D. J. (1973). Individual differences in the Strange Situation behavior of one-year-olds. In L. S. Stone, H. T. Smith, & L. B. Murphy (Eds.), *The competent infant* (pp. 17–52). New York: Basic Books.

Ainsworth, M. D. S., Blehar, M. C., Waters, E., & Wall, S. (1978). *Patterns of attachment: Assessed in the Strange Situation and at home*. Hillsdale, NJ: Erlbaum.

Ainsworth, M. D. S., & Bowlby, J. (1991). An ethological approach to personality development. *American Psychologist, 46*, 333–341.

Ainsworth, M. D., & Wittig, B. A. (1969). Attachment and exploratory behavior of one-year-olds in a strange situation. In B. M. Foss (Ed.), *Determinants of infant behavior* (Vol. 4, pp. 113–136). London: Methuen.

Alexander, P. C. (1993). The differential effects of abuse characteristics and attachment in the prediction of long-term effects of sexual abuse. *Journal of Interpersonal Violence, 8*, 346–362.

Alexander, P. C., Anderson, C. L., Brand, B., Schaeffer, C. M., Grelling, B. Z., & Kretz, L. (1998). Adult attachment and long-term effects in survivors of incest. *Child Abuse and Neglect, 22,* 45–81.

Alexander, R., Feeney, J., Hohaus, L., & Noller, P. (2001). Attachment style and coping resources as predictors of coping strategies in the transition to parenthood. *Personal Relationships, 8,* 137–152.

Alexandrov, E. O., Cowan, P. A., & Cowan, C. P. (2005). Couple attachment and the quality of marital relationships: Method and concept in the validation of the new couple attachment interview and coding system. *Attachment and Human Development, 7,* 123–152.

Allen, E. S., & Baucom, D. H. (2004). Adult attachment and patterns of extradyadic involvement. *Family Process, 43,* 467–488.

Allen, J. P., & Hauser, S. T. (1996). Autonomy and relatedness in adolescent–family interactions as predictors of young adults' states of mind regarding attachment. *Development and Psychopathology, 8,* 793–809.

Allen, J. P., Hauser, S. T., & Borman-Spurrell, E. (1996). Attachment theory as a framework for understanding sequelae of severe adolescent psychopathology: An 11-year follow-up study. *Journal of Consulting and Clinical Psychology, 64,* 254–263.

Allen, J. P., & Land, D. J. (1999). Attachment in adolescence. In J. Cassidy & P. R. Shaver (Eds.), *Handbook of attachment: Theory, research, and clinical applications* (pp. 319–335). New York: Guilford Press.

Allen, J. P., Marsh, P., McFarland, C., McElhaney, K.-B., Land, D. J., Jodl, K. M., et al. (2002). Attachment and autonomy as predictors of the development of social skills and delinquency during mid-adolescence. *Journal of Consulting and Clinical Psychology, 70,* 56–66.

Allen, J. P., McElhaney, K.-B., Kuperminc, G. P., & Jodl, K. M. (2004). Stability and change in attachment security across adolescence. *Child Development, 75,* 1792–1805.

Allen, J. P., Moore, C., & Kuperminc, G. P. (1997). Developmental approaches to understanding adolescent deviance. In S. S. Luthar, J. A. Burack, D. Cicchetti, & J. R. Weisz (Eds.), *Developmental psychopathology: Perspectives on adjustment, risk, and disorder* (pp. 548–567). New York: Cambridge University Press.

Allen, J. P., Moore, C., Kuperminc, G. P., & Bell, K. (1998). Attachment and adolescent psychosocial functioning. *Child Development, 69,* 1406–1419.

Allen, K. M. Blascovich, J., Tomaka, J., & Kelsey, R. M. (1991). Presence of human friends and pet dogs as moderators of autonomic responses to stress in women. *Journal of Personality and Social Psychology, 61,* 582–589.

Allison, C. J., Bartholomew, K., Mayseless, O., & Dutton, D. G. (2005). *Love as a battlefield: Attachment and relationship dynamics in couples identified for male partner violence.* Unpublished manuscript, Simon Fraser University, Vancouver, Canada.

Allport, G. W. (1954). *The nature of prejudice.* Reading, MA: Addison-Wesley.

Allport, G. W. (1961). *Pattern and growth in personality.* New York: Holt, Rinehart & Winston.

Alonso-Arbiol, I., Shaver, P. R., & Yarnoz, S. (2002). Insecure attachment, gender roles, and interpersonal dependency in the Basque Country. *Personal Relationships, 9,* 479–490.

Altman, I., & Taylor, D. (1973). *Social penetration: The development of interpersonal relationships.* New York: Holt, Rinehart & Winston.

American Psychiatric Association. (1994). *Diagnostic and statistical manual of mental disorders* (4th ed.). Washington, DC: Author.

Amir, M., Horesh, N., & Lin-Stein, T. (1999). Infertility and adjustment in women: The effects of attachment style and social support. *Journal of Clinical Psychology in Medical Settings, 6,* 463–479.

Anders, S. L., & Tucker, J. S. (2000). Adult attachment style, interpersonal communication competence, and social support. *Personal Relationships, 7,* 379–389.

Andersen, S. M., & Chen, S. (2002). The relational self: An interpersonal social-cognitive theory. *Psychological Review, 109,* 619–645.

Andersen, S. M., & Glassman, N. S. (1996). Responding to significant others when they are not there: Effects on interpersonal inference, motivation, and affect. In R. M. Sorrentino & E. T. Higgins (Eds.), *Handbook of motivation and cognition: Vol. 3. The interpersonal context* (pp. 262–321). New York: Guilford Press.

Anderson, J. (1994). *Cognitive psychology.* New York: Academic Press.

Anderson, C. L., & Alexander, P. C. (1996). The relationship between attachment and dissociation in adult survivors of incest. *Psychiatry: Interpersonal and Biological Processes, 59,* 240–254.

Andersson, P., & Eisemann, M. (2004). Parental rearing and substance related disorders: A multi-factorial controlled study in a Swedish sample. *Clinical Psychology and Psychotherapy, 11,* 392–400.

Andersson, P., & Perris, C. (2000). Attachment styles and dysfunctional assumptions in adults. *Clinical Psychology and Psychotherapy, 7,* 47–53.

Antonucci, T. C., Akiyama, H., & Takahashi, K. (2004). Attachment and close relationships across the life span. *Attachment and Human Development, 6,* 353–370.

Appelfeld, A. (2004). *The story of a life* (A. Halter, Trans.). New York: Schocken Books.

Arend, R., Gove, F. L., & Sroufe, L. A. (1979). Continuity of individual adaptation from infancy to kindergarten: A predictive study of ego-resiliency and curiosity in preschoolers. *Child Development, 50,* 950–959.

Armsden, G. C., & Greenberg, M. T. (1987). The inventory of parent and peer attachment: Relationship to well-being in adolescence. *Journal of Youth and Adolescence, 16,* 427–454.

Armsden, G. C., McCauley, E., Greenberg, M. T., Burke, P. M., & Mitchell, J. (1990). Parent and peer attachment in early adolescent depression. *Journal of Abnormal Child Psychology, 18,* 683–697.

Armstrong, J. G., & Roth, D. M. (1989). Attachment and separation difficulties in eating disorders: A preliminary investigation. *International Journal of Eating Disorders, 8,* 141–155.

Arndt, J., Schimel, J., Greenberg, J., & Pyszczynski, T. (2002). The intrinsic self and defensiveness: Evidence that activating the intrinsic self reduces self-handicapping and conformity. *Personality and Social Psychology Bulletin, 28,* 671–683.

Aron, A., & Aron, E. N. (2006). Romantic relationships from the perspectives of the self-expansion model and attachment theory. In M. Mikulincer & G. S. Goodman (Eds.), *Dynamics of romantic love: Attachment, caregiving, and sex* (pp. 359–382). New York: Guilford Press.

Aron, A., Aron, E. N., & Allen, J. (1998). Motivations for unreciprocated love. *Personality and Social Psychology Bulletin, 24,* 787–796.

Aron, A., Aron, E. N., & Norman, C. (2001). Self-expansion model of motivation and cognition in close relationships and beyond. In G. J. O. Fletcher & M. S. Clark (Eds.), *Blackwell handbook of social psychology: Interpersonal processes* (pp. 478–501). Malden, MA: Blackwell.

Aron, L. (1996). *Meetings of minds.* Hillsdale, NJ: Analytic Press.

Asendorpf, J. B., Banse, R., Wilpers, S., & Neyer, F. J. (1997). Relationship-specific attachment scales for adults and their validation with network and diary procedures. *Diagnostica, 43,* 289–313.

Asendorpf, J. B., & Wilpers, S. (2000). Attachment security and available support: Closely linked relationship qualities. *Journal of Social and Personal Relationships, 17,* 115–138.

Aspelmeier, J. E., & Kerns, K. A. (2003). Love and school: Attachment/exploration dynamics in college. *Journal of Social and Personal Relationships, 20,* 5–30.

Aspinwall, L. G., & Staudinger, U. M. (Eds.). (2003). *A psychology of human strengths: Fundamental questions and future directions for a positive psychology.* Washington, DC: American Psychological Association.

Atkinson, J. W. (1957). Motivational determinants of risk-taking behavior. *Psychological Review, 64,* 359–372.

Atkinson, L., Niccols, A., Paglia, A., Coolbear, J., Parker, K. C. H., Poulton, L., et al. (2000). A meta-analysis of time between maternal sensitivity and attachment assessments: Implications for internal working models in infancy/toddlerhood. *Journal of Social and Personal Relationships, 17,* 791–810.

Atkinson, L., Paglia, A., Coolbear, J., Niccols, A., Parker, K. C. H., & Guger, S. (2000). Attachment security: A meta-analysis of maternal mental health correlates. *Clinical Psychology Review, 20,* 1019–1040.

Averill, J. R. (1982). *Anger and aggression: An essay on emotion.* New York: Springer-Verlag.

Aviezer, O., Sagi, A., Resnick, G., & Gini, M. (2002). School competence in young adolescence: Links to early attachment relationships beyond concurrent self-perceived competence and representations of relationships. *International Journal of Behavioral Development, 26,* 397–409.

Avihou, N. (2006). *Attachment orientations and dreaming: An examination of the unconscious components of the attachment system.* Unpublished doctoral dissertation, Bar-Ilan University, Ramat Gan, Israel.

Ayduk, O., Downey, G., & Kim, M. (2001). Rejection sensitivity and depressive symptoms in women. *Personality and Social Psychology Bulletin, 27,* 868–877.

Babcock, J. C., Jacobson, N. S., Gottman, J. M., & Yerington, T. P. (2000). Attachment, emotional regulation, and the function of marital violence: Differences between secure, preoccupied, and dismissing violent and nonviolent husbands. *Journal of Family Violence, 15,* 391–409.

Baccus, J. R., Baldwin, M. W., & Packer, D. J. (2004). Increasing implicit self-esteem through classical conditioning. *Psychological Science, 15,* 498–502.

Backstrom, M., & Holmes, B. M. (2001). Measuring adult attachment: A construct validation of two self-report instruments. *Scandinavian Journal of Psychology, 42,* 79–86.

Bailey, S. L., & Hubbard, R. L. (1990). Developmental variation in the context of marijuana initiation among adolescents. *Journal of Health and Social Behavior, 31,* 58–70.

Bajor, J. K., & Baltes, B. B. (2003). The relationship between selection optimization with compensation, conscientiousness, motivation, and performance. *Journal of Vocational Behavior, 63,* 347–367.

Baker, E., & Beech, A. R. (2004). Dissociation and variability of adult attachment dimensions and early maladaptive schemas in sexual and violent offenders. *Journal of Interpersonal Violence, 19,* 1119–1136.

Baker, R. W., & Siryk, B. (1984). Measuring adjustment to college. *Journal of Counseling Psychology, 31,* 179–189.

Bakermans-Kranenburg, M. J., & van IJzendoorn, M. H. (1993). A psychometric study of the Adult Attachment Interview: Reliability and discriminant validity. *Developmental Psychology, 29,* 870–879.

Bakermans-Kranenburg, M. J., & van IJzendoorn, M. H. (2004). No association of the dopamine D4 receptor (DRD4) and -521 C/T promoter polymorphisms with infant attachment disorganization. *Attachment and Human Development, 6,* 211–218.

Bakermans-Kranenburg, M. J., van IJzendoorn, M. H., Bokhorst, C. L., & Schuengel, C. (2004). The importance of shared environment in infant–father attachment: A behavioral genetic study of the attachment Q-sort. *Journal of Family Psychology, 18,* 545–549.

Bakermans-Kranenburg, M. J., van IJzendoorn, M. H., & Juffer, F. (2003). Less is more: Meta-analyses of sensitivity and attachment interventions in early childhood. *Psychological Bulletin, 129,* 195–215.

Bakermans-Kranenburg, M. J., van IJzendoorn, M. H., & Juffer, F. (2005). Disorganized infant attachment and preventive interventions: A review and meta-analysis. *Infant Mental Health Journal, 26,* 191–216.

Bakker, W., Van Oudenhoven, J. P., & Van Der Zee,

K. I. (2004). Attachment styles, personality, and Dutch emigrants' intercultural adjustment. *European Journal of Personality, 18,* 387–404.

Baldwin, M. W. (1992). Relational schemas and the processing of social information. *Psychological Bulletin, 112,* 461–484.

Baldwin, M. W., & Fehr, B. (1995). On the instability of attachment style ratings. *Personal Relationships, 2,* 247–261.

Baldwin, M. W., Fehr, B., Keedian, E., Seidel, M., & Thompson, D. W. (1993). An exploration of the relational schemata underlying attachment styles: Self-report and lexical decision approaches. *Personality and Social Psychology Bulletin, 19,* 746–754.

Baldwin, M. W., & Kay, A. C. (2003). Adult attachment and the inhibition of rejection. *Journal of Social and Clinical Psychology, 22,* 275–293.

Baldwin, M. W., Keelan, J. P. R., Fehr, B., Enns, V., & Koh Rangarajoo, E. (1996). Social-cognitive conceptualization of attachment working models: Availability and accessibility effects. *Journal of Personality and Social Psychology, 71,* 94–109.

Baldwin, M. W., & Meunier, J. (1999). The cued activation of attachment relational schemas. *Social Cognition, 17,* 209–227.

Banai, E., Mikulincer, M., & Shaver, P. R. (2005). "Selfobject" needs in Kohut's self psychology: Links with attachment, self-cohesion, affect regulation, and adjustment. *Psychoanalytic Psychology, 22,* 224–260.

Banai, E., Weller, A., & Mikulincer, M. (1998). Interjudge agreement in evaluation of adult attachment style: The impact of acquaintanceship. *British Journal of Social Psychology, 37,* 95–109.

Bandura, A. (1977). *Social learning theory.* New York: General Learning Press.

Banse, R. (2004). Adult attachment and marital satisfaction: Evidence for dyadic configuration effects. *Journal of Social and Personal Relationships, 21,* 273–282.

Barabi, L., Mikulincer, M., & Shaver, P. R. (2006). *An attachment perspective on the Oedipus complex.* Unpublished manuscript, Bar-Ilan University, Ramat-Gan, Israel.

Barchat, D. (1989, June). *Representations and separations in therapy: The August phenomenon.* Paper presented at the meeting of the Society for Psychotherapy Research, Toronto, Canada.

Bargh, J. A. (1989). Conditional automaticity: Varieties of automatic influence in social perception and cognition. In J. S. Uleman & J. A. Bargh (Eds.), *Unintended thought* (pp. 3–51). New York: Guilford Press.

Bargh, J. A. (1990). Auto-motives: Preconscious determinants of social interaction. In E. T. Higgins & R. M. Sorrentino (Eds.), *Handbook of motivation and cognition: Foundations of social behavior* (Vol. 2, pp. 93–130). New York: Guilford Press.

Bargh, J. A., Chen, M., & Burrows, L. (1996). Automaticity of social behavior: Direct effects of trait construct and stereotype activation on action. *Journal of Personality and Social Psychology, 71,* 230–244.

Bar-Haim, Y., Sutton, D., Fox, N. A., & Marvin, R. S.

(2000). Stability and change of attachment at 14, 24, and 58 months of age: Behavior, representation, and life events. *Journal of Child Psychology and Psychiatry, 41,* 381–388.

Barkow, J. H., Cosmides, L., & Tooby, J. (Eds.). (1992). *The adapted mind: Evolutionary psychology and the generation of culture.* New York: Oxford University Press.

Barlow, D. H. (1986). Causes of sexual dysfunction: The role of anxiety and cognitive interference. *Journal of Consulting and Clinical Psychology, 54,* 140–148.

Bar-On, N. (2005). *Attachment anxiety and explicit and implicit manifestations of relational ambivalence.* Unpublished doctoral dissertation, Bar-Ilan University, Ramat Gan, Israel.

Barone, L. (2003). Developmental protective and risk factors in borderline personality disorder: A study using the Adult Attachment Interview. *Attachment and Human Development, 5,* 64–77.

Barrett, P. M., & Holmes, J. (2001). Attachment relationships as predictors of cognitive interpretation and response bias in late adolescence. *Journal of Child and Family Studies, 10,* 51–64.

Barry, B., & Stewart, G. L. (1997). Composition, process, and performance in self-managed groups: The role of personality. *Journal of Applied Psychology, 82,* 62–78.

Bartholomew, K. (1990). Avoidance of intimacy: An attachment perspective. *Journal of Social and Personal Relationships, 7,* 147–178.

Bartholomew, K., & Allison, C. J. (2006). An attachment perspective on abusive dynamics in intimate relationships. In M. Mikulincer & G. S. Goodman (Eds.), *Dynamics of romantic love* (pp. 102–127). New York: Guilford Press.

Bartholomew, K., & Horowitz, L. M. (1991). Attachment styles among young adults: A test of a four-category model. *Journal of Personality and Social Psychology, 61,* 226–244.

Bartholomew, K., Kwong, M. J., & Hart, S.D. (2001). Attachment. In J. W. Livesley (Ed.), *Handbook of personality disorders: Theory, research, and treatment* (pp. 196–230). New York: Guilford Press.

Bartholomew, K., & Perlman, D. (Eds.). (1994). *Advances in personal relationships: Attachment processes in adulthood* (Vol. 5). London: Jessica Kingsley.

Bartholomew, K., & Shaver, P. R. (1998). Methods of assessing adult attachment: Do they converge? In J. A. Simpson & W. S. Rholes (Eds.), *Attachment theory and close relationships* (pp. 25–45). New York: Guilford Press.

Bartz, J. A., & Lydon, J. E. (2004). Close relationships and the working self-concept: Implicit and explicit effects of priming attachment on agency and communion. *Personality and Social Psychology Bulletin, 30,* 1389–1401.

Bartz, J. A., & Lydon, J. E. (2006). Navigating the interdependence dilemma: Attachment goals and the use of communal norms with potential close others. *Journal of Personality and Social Psychology, 91,* 77–96.

Bass, B. M. (1985). *Leadership and performance beyond expectations.* New York: Free Press.

Bass, B. M., & Avolio, B. J. (1990). The implications of transactional and transformational leadership for individual, team, and organizational development. In R. W. Woodman & W. A. Passmore (Eds.), *Research in organizational change and development* (pp. 231–272). Greenwich, CT: JAI Press.

Batgos, J., & Leadbeater, B. J. (1994). Parental attachment, peer relations, and dysphoria in adolescence. In M. B. Sperling & W. H. Berman (Eds.), *Attachment in adults: Clinical and developmental perspectives* (pp. 155–178). New York: Guilford Press.

Batson, C. D. (1976). Religion as prosocial: Agent or double agent? *Journal for the Scientific Study of Religion, 15,* 29–45.

Batson, C. D. (1991). The altruism question: Toward a social-psychological answer. Hillsdale, NJ: Erlbaum.

Batson, C. D., Schoenrade, P. A., & Ventis, W. L. (1993). *Religion and the individual: A social-psychological perspective.* New York: Oxford University Press.

Baumeister, R. F., Wotman, S. R., & Stillwell, A. M. (1993). Unrequited love: On heartbreak, anger, guilt, scriptlessness, and humiliation. *Journal of Personality and Social Psychology, 64,* 377–394.

Beck, A. (1976). *Cognitive therapy and the emotional disorders.* New York: International Universities Press.

Beck, R., & McDonald, A. (2004). Attachment to God: The Attachment to God Inventory, tests of working model correspondence, and an exploration of faith group differences. *Journal of Psychology and Theology, 32,* 92–103.

Becker, T. E., Billings, R. S., Eveleth, D. M., & Gilbert, N. W. (1997). Validity of scores on three attachment style scales: Exploratory and confirmatory evidence. *Educational and Psychological Measurement, 57,* 477–493.

Becker-Stoll, F., Delius, A., & Scheitenberger, S. (2001). Adolescents' nonverbal emotional expressions during negotiation of a disagreement with their mothers: An attachment approach. *International Journal of Behavioral Development, 25,* 344–353.

Beckwith, L., Cohen, S. E., & Hamilton, C. E. (1999). Maternal sensitivity during infancy and subsequent life events relate to attachment representation at early adulthood. *Developmental Psychology, 35,* 693–700.

Beinstein Miller, J. (1996). Social flexibility and anxious attachment. *Personal Relationships, 3,* 241–256.

Beinstein Miller, J. (1999). Attachment style and memory for attachment-related events. *Journal of Social and Personal Relationships, 16,* 773–801.

Beinstein Miller, J. (2001). Attachment models and memory for conversation. *Journal of Social and Personal Relationships, 18,* 404–422.

Beinstein Miller, J., & Noirot, M. (1999). Attachment memories, models, and information processing. *Journal of Social and Personal Relationships, 16,* 147–173.

Beitel, M., & Cecero, J. J. (2003). Predicting psychological mindedness from personality style and attachment security. *Journal of Clinical Psychology, 59,* 163–172.

Bell, K. L. (1998). Family expressiveness and attachment. *Social Development, 7,* 37–53.

Belsky, J. (1988). Infant day care and socioemotional development: The United States. *Journal of Child Psychology and Psychiatry, 29,* 397–406.

Belsky, J. (1996). Parent, infant, and social–contextual antecedents of father–son attachment security. *Developmental Psychology, 32,* 905–913.

Belsky, J. (1997). Theory testing, effect-size evaluation, and differential susceptibility to rearing influence: The case of mothering and attachment. *Child Development, 68,* 598–600.

Belsky, J. (1999). Modern evolutionary theory and patterns of attachment. In J. Cassidy & P. R. Shaver (Eds.), *Handbook of attachment: Theory, research, and clinical applications* (pp. 141–161). New York: Guilford Press.

Belsky, J. (2002). Developmental origins of attachment styles. *Attachment and Human Development, 4,* 166–170.

Belsky, J. (2005). Attachment theory and research in ecological perspective: Insights from the Pennsylvania Infant and Family Development Project and the NICHD Study of Early Child Care. In K. E. Grossmann, K. Grossmann, & E. Waters (Eds.), *Attachment from infancy to adulthood: The major longitudinal studies* (pp. 71–97). New York: Guilford Press.

Belsky, J., Campbell, S. B., Cohn, J. F., & Moore, G. (1996). Instability of infant–parent attachment security. *Developmental Psychology, 32,* 921–924.

Belsky, J., Fish, M., & Isabella, R. A. (1991). Continuity and discontinuity in infant negative and positive emotionality: Family antecedents and attachment consequences. *Developmental Psychology, 27,* 421–431.

Belsky, J., & Isabella, R. A. (1988). Maternal, infant, and social–contextual determinants of attachment security. In J. Belsky & T. Nezworski (Eds.), *Clinical implications of attachment* (pp. 41–94). Hillsdale, NJ: Erlbaum.

Belsky, J., Rosenberger, K., & Crnic, K. (1995). The origins of attachment security: "Classical" and contextual determinants. In S. Goldberg, R. Muir, & J. Kerr (Eds.), *Attachment theory: Social, developmental, and clinical perspectives* (pp. 153–183). Hillsdale, NJ: Analytic Press.

Belsky, J., & Rovine, M. J. (1987). Temperament and attachment security in the strange situation: An empirical rapprochement. *Child Development, 58,* 787–795.

Belsky, J., & Rovine, M. J. (1988). Nonmaternal care in the first year of life and the security of infant–parent attachment. *Child Development, 59,* 157–167.

Belsky, J., Spritz, B., & Crnic, K. (1996). Infant attachment security and affective–cognitive information processing at age 3. *Psychological Science, 7,* 111–114.

Belsky, J., Steinberg, L., & Draper, P. (1991). Childhood experience, interpersonal development, and reproductive strategy: An evolutionary theory of socialization. *Child Development, 62,* 647–670.

Bem, S. L. (1981). Gender schema theory: A cognitive account of sex typing. *Psychological Review, 88,* 354–364.

Ben Ari, A., & Lavee, Y. (2005). Dyadic characteristics of individual attributes: Attachment, neuroticism, and their relation to marital quality and closeness. *American Journal of Orthopsychiatry, 75,* 621–631.

Bender, D. S., Farber, B. A., & Geller, J. D. (2001). Cluster B personality traits and attachment. *Journal of the American Academy of Psychoanalysis and Dynamic Psychiatry, 29,* 551–563.

Benjamin, J. (1992). Recognition and destruction: An outline of intersubjectivity. In N. J. Skolnick & S. C. Warshaw (Eds.), *Relational perspectives in psychoanalysis* (pp. 43–69). Hillsdale, NJ: Analytic Press.

Benjamin, L. S. (1974). Structural analysis of social behavior (SASB). *Psychological Review, 81,* 392–425.

Benjamin, L. S. (1994). SASB: A bridge between personality theory and clinical psychology. *Psychological Inquiry, 5,* 273–316.

Benoit, D., & Parker, K. C. H. (1994). Stability and transmission of attachment across three generations. *Child Development, 65,* 1444–1456.

Benson, M. J., Harris, P. B., & Rogers, C. S. (1992). Identity consequences of attachment to mothers and fathers among late adolescents. *Journal of Research on Adolescence, 2,* 187–204.

Benson, P., & Spilka, B. (1973). God image as a function of self-esteem and locus of control. *Journal for the Scientific Study of Religion, 12,* 297–310.

Ben Tovim, D. I., & Walker, M. K. (1991). Further evidence for the Stroop test as a quantitative measure of psychopathology in eating disorders. *International Journal of Eating Disorders, 10,* 609–613.

Ben-Zeev, A. (1999). Mercy, pity, and compassion. In A. Brien (Ed.), *The quality of mercy* (pp. 132–145). Amsterdam: Rodopi.

Berant, E., Mikulincer, M., & Florian, V. (2001a). The association of mothers' attachment style and their psychological reactions to the diagnosis of infant's congenital heart disease. *Journal of Social and Clinical Psychology, 20,* 208–232.

Berant, E., Mikulincer, M., & Florian, V. (2001b). Attachment style and mental health: A 1-year follow-up study of mothers of infants with congenital heart disease. *Personality and Social Psychology Bulletin, 27,* 956–968.

Berant, E., Mikulincer, M., & Florian, V. (2003). Marital satisfaction among mothers of infants with congenital heart disease: The contribution of illness severity, attachment style, and the coping process. *Anxiety, Stress, and Coping, 16,* 397–415.

Berant, E., Mikulincer, M., & Shaver, P. R. (in press). Attachment style, mental health, and intergenerational transmission of emotional problems: A seven-year study of mothers of children with congenital heart disease. *Journal of Personality.*

Berant, E., Mikulincer, M., Shaver, P. R., & Segal, Y. (2005). Rorschach correlates of self-reported attachment dimensions: Dynamic manifestations of hyperactivating and deactivating strategies. *Journal of Personality Assessment, 84,* 70–81.

Berglas, S., & Jones, E. E. (1978). Drug choice as a self-handicapping strategy in response to noncontingent success. *Journal of Personality and Social Psychology, 36,* 405–417.

Berlin, L. J., & Cassidy, J. (1999). Relations among relationships: Contributions from attachment theory and research. In J. Cassidy & P. R. Shaver (Eds.), *Handbook of attachment: Theory, research, and clinical applications* (pp. 688–712). New York: Guilford Press.

Berlin, L. J., Cassidy, J., & Belsky, J. (1995). Loneliness in young children and infant–mother attachment: A longitudinal study. *Merrill–Palmer Quarterly, 41,* 91–103.

Berman, W. H., Marcus, L., & Berman, E. R. (1994). Attachment in marital relations. In M. B. Sperling & W. H. Berman (Eds.), *Attachment in adults: Clinical and developmental perspectives* (pp. 204–231). New York: Guilford Press.

Berman, W. H., & Sperling, M. B. (1991). Parental attachment and emotional distress in the transition to college. *Journal of Youth and Adolescence, 20,* 427–440.

Bernier, A., & Dozier, M. (2002). Assessing adult attachment: Empirical sophistication and conceptual bases. *Attachment and Human Development, 4,* 171–179.

Bernier, A., Larose, S., Boivin, M., & Soucy, N. (2004). Attachment state of mind: Implications for adjustment to college. *Journal of Adolescent Research, 19,* 783–806.

Bernier, A., Larose, S., & Whipple, N. (2005). Leaving home for college: A potentially stressful event for adolescents with preoccupied attachment patterns. *Attachment and Human Development, 7,* 171–185.

Berscheid, E. (1984). Interpersonal attraction. In G. Lindzey & E. Aronson (Eds.), *Handbook of social psychology* (3rd ed., Vol. 2, pp. 413–484). Reading, MA: Addison-Wesley.

Berscheid, E., & Regan, P. (2004). *The psychology of interpersonal relationships.* New York: Prentice-Hall.

Besser, A., & Priel, B. (2003). A multisource approach to self-critical vulnerability to depression: The moderating role of attachment. *Journal of Personality, 71,* 515–555.

Besser, A., & Priel, B. (2005). The apple does not fall far from the tree: Attachment styles and personality vulnerabilities to depression in three generations of women. *Personality and Social Psychology Bulletin, 31,* 1052–1073.

Besser, A., Priel, B., & Wiznitzer, A. (2002). Childbearing depressive symptomatology in high-risk pregnancies: The roles of working models and social support. *Personal Relationships, 9,* 395–413.

Bifulco, A., Figueiredo, B., Guedeney, N., Gorman, L. L., Hayes, S., & Muzik, M. (2004). Maternal attachment style and depression associated with childbirth: Preliminary results from a European and US cross-cultural study. *British Journal of Psychiatry, 184,* 31–37.

Bifulco, A., Lillie, A., Ball, B., & Moran, P. (1998). *Attachment Style Interview (ASI)—Training manual*. London: Royal Holloway, University of London.

Bifulco, A., Moran, P. M., Ball, C., & Bernazzani, O. (2002). Adult attachment style: I. Its relationship to clinical depression. *Social Psychiatry and Psychiatric Epidemiology, 37,* 50–59.

Bifulco, A., Moran, P. M., Ball, C., & Lillie, A. (2002). Adult attachment style: II. Its relationship to psychosocial depressive-vulnerability. *Social Psychiatry and Psychiatric Epidemiology, 37,* 60–67.

Bippus, A. M., & Rollin, E. (2003). Attachment style differences in relational maintenance and conflict behaviors: Friends' perceptions. *Communication Reports, 16,* 113–123.

Birgegard, A., & Granqvist, P. (2004). The correspondence between attachment to parents and God: Three experiments using subliminal separation cues. *Personality and Social Psychology Bulletin, 30,* 1122–1135.

Biringen, Z., Brown, D., Donaldson, L., Green, S., Krcmarik, S., & Lovas, G. (2000). Adult Attachment Interview: Linkages with dimensions of emotional availability for mothers and their prekindergarteners. *Attachment and Human Development, 2,* 188–202.

Birnbaum, G. E. (2007). Attachment orientations, sexual functioning, and relationship satisfaction in a community sample of women. *Journal of Social and Personal Relationships, 24,* 21–35.

Birnbaum, G. E., & Gillath, O. (2006). Measuring subgoals of the sexual behavioral system: What is sex good for? *Journal of Social and Personal Relationships, 23,* 675–701.

Birnbaum, G. E., Orr, I., Mikulincer, M., & Florian, V. (1997). When marriage breaks up: Does attachment style contribute to coping and mental health? *Journal of Social and Personal Relationships, 14,* 643–654.

Birnbaum, G. E., Reis, H. T., Mikulincer, M., Gillath, O., & Orpaz, A. (2006). When sex is more than just sex: Attachment orientations, sexual experience, and relationship quality. *Journal of Personality and Social Psychology, 91,* 929–943.

Black, K. A., & McCartney, K. (1997). Adolescent females' security with parents predicts the quality of peer interactions. *Social Development, 6,* 91–110.

Black, S., Hardy, G., Turpin, G., & Parry, G. (2005). Self-reported attachment styles and therapeutic orientation of therapists and their relationship with reported general alliance quality and problems in therapy. *Psychology and Psychotherapy, 78,* 363–377.

Blain, M. D., Thompson, J. M., & Whiffen, V. E. (1993). Attachment and perceived social support in late adolescence: The interaction between working models of self and others. *Journal of Adolescent Research, 8,* 226–241.

Blatt, S. J. (1974). Levels of object representation in anaclitic and introjective depression. *Psychoanalytic Study of the Child, 29,* 107–157.

Blatt, S. J., & Behrends, R. S. (1987). Internalization, separation–individuation, and the nature of thera-peutic action. *International Journal of Psychoanalysis, 68,* 279–297.

Blatt, S. J., Stayner, D. A., Auerbach, J. S., & Behrends, R. S. (1996). Change in object and self-representations in long-term, intensive, inpatient treatment of seriously disturbed adolescents and young adults. *Psychiatry, 59,* 82–107.

Blatt, S. J., Wein, S. J., Chevron, E. S., & Quinlan, D. M. (1992). Parental representations and depression in normal young adults. *Journal of Abnormal Psychology, 88,* 388–397.

Blazina, C., & Watkins, J. C. (2000). Separation/individuation, parental attachment, and male gender role conflict: Attitudes toward the feminine and the fragile masculine self. *Psychology of Men and Masculinity, 1,* 126–132.

Block, J. (1961). Ego identity, role variability, and adjustment. *Journal of Consulting Psychology, 25,* 392–397.

Blustein, D. L. (1997). A context-rich perspective of career exploration across the life roles. *Career Development Quarterly, 45,* 260–274.

Blustein, D. L., Fama, L. D., White, S. F., Ketterson, T. U., Schaefer, B. M., Schwam, M. F., et al. (2001). A qualitative analysis of counseling case material: Listening to our clients. *Counseling Psychologist, 29,* 240–258.

Blustein, D. L., Walbridge, M. M., Friedlander, M. L., & Palladino, D. E. (1991). Contributions of psychological separation and parental attachment to the career development process. *Journal of Counseling Psychology, 38,* 39–50.

Bogaert, A. F., & Sadava, S. (2002). Adult attachment and sexual behavior. *Personal Relationships, 9,* 191–204.

Bogaerts, S., Vanheule, S., & DeClercq, F. (2005). Recalled parental bonding, adult attachment style, and personality disorders in child molesters: A comparative study. *Journal of Forensic Psychiatry and Psychology, 16,* 445–458.

Bokhorst, C. L., Bakermans-Kranenburg, M. J., Fearon, R., van IJzendoorn, M. H., Fonagy, P., & Schuengel, C. (2003). The importance of shared environment in mother–infant attachment security: A behavioral genetic study. *Child Development, 74,* 1769–1782.

Bollas, C. (1987). *The shadow of the object*. New York: Columbia University Press.

Bombar, M. L., & Littig, L. W., Jr. (1996). Babytalk as a communication of intimate attachment: An initial study in adult romances and friendships. *Personal Relationships, 3,* 137–158.

Bonanno, G. (2001). Grief and emotion: A social–functional perspective. In M. Stroebe, W. Stroebe, R. O. Hansson, & H. A. W. Schut (Eds.), *Handbook of bereavement research: Consequences, coping, and care* (pp. 493–515). Washington, DC: American Psychological Association.

Bonanno, G. (2004). Loss, trauma, and human resilience: Have we underestimated the human capacity to thrive after extremely aversive events? *American Psychologist, 59,* 20–28.

Bonanno, G. (2005). Clarifying and extending the construct of adult resilience. *American Psychologist, 60,* 265–267.

Bond, S. B., & Bond, M. (2004). Attachment styles and violence within couples. *Journal of Nervous and Mental Disease, 192*, 857–863.

Bookwala, J. (2003). Being "single and unattached": The role of adult attachment styles. *Journal of Applied Social Psychology, 33*, 1564–1570.

Bookwala, J., & Zdaniuk, B. (1998). Adult attachment styles and aggressive behavior within dating relationships. *Journal of Social and Personal Relationships, 15*, 175–190.

Boon, S. D., & Griffin, D. W. (1996). The construction of risk in relationships: The role of framing in decisions about intimate relationships. *Personal Relationships, 3*, 293–306.

Bordin, E. S. (1979). The generalizability of the psychoanalytic concept of the working alliance. *Psychotherapy, 16*, 252–260.

Borelli, J. L., & David, D. H. (2004). Attachment theory and research as a guide to psychotherapy practice. *Imagination, Cognition and Personality, 23*, 257–287.

Born, M., Chevalier, V., & Humblet, I. (1997). Resilience, desistance, and delinquent career of adolescent offenders. *Journal of Adolescence, 20*, 679–694.

Bornstein, R. F. (1992). The dependent personality: Developmental, social, and clinical perspectives. *Psychological Bulletin, 112*, 3–23.

Bosquet, M., & Egeland, B. (2001). Associations among maternal depressive symptomatology, state of mind, and parent and child behaviors: Implications for attachment-based interventions. *Attachment and Human Development, 3*, 173–199.

Bouchard, T. J., & Loehlin, J. C. (2001). Genes, evolution, and personality. *Behavior Genetics, 31*, 243–273.

Bouthillier, D., Julien, D., Dubé, M., Bélanger, I., & Hamelin, M. (2002). Predictive validity of adult attachment measures in relation to emotion regulation behaviors in marital interactions. *Journal of Adult Development, 9*, 291–305.

Bowlby, J. (1944). Forty-four juvenile thieves: Their characters and home life. *International Journal of Psychoanalysis, 25*, 19–52, 107–127.

Bowlby, J. (1951). *Maternal care and mental health.* Geneva, Switzerland: World Health Organization.

Bowlby, J. (1956). The growth of independence in the young child. *Royal Society of Health Journal, 76*, 587–591.

Bowlby, J. (1958). The nature of the child's tie to his mother. *International Journal of Psychoanalysis, 39*, 350–373.

Bowlby, J. (1960a). Separation anxiety. *International Journal of Psycho-Analysis, 41*, 89–113.

Bowlby, J. (1960b). Grief and mourning in infancy and early childhood. *Psychoanalytic Study of the Child, 15*, 9–52.

Bowlby, J. (1973). *Attachment and loss: Vol. 2. Separation: Anxiety and anger.* New York: Basic Books.

Bowlby, J. (1979). *The making and breaking of affectional bonds.* London: Tavistock.

Bowlby, J. (1980). *Attachment and loss: Vol. 3. Sadness and depression.* New York: Basic Books.

Bowlby, J. (1969/1982). *Attachment and loss: Vol. 1.*

Attachment (2nd ed.). New York: Basic Books. (Original work published 1969)

Bowlby, J. (1988). *A secure base: Clinical applications of attachment theory.* London: Routledge.

Bowlby, J. (1990). *Charles Darwin: A new life.* New York: Norton.

Brack, G., Gay, M. F., & Matheny, K. B. (1993). Relationships between attachment and coping resources among late adolescents. *Journal of College Student Development, 34*, 212–215.

Bradbury, T. N., Fincham, F. D., & Beach, S. R. H. (2000). Research on the nature and determinants of marital satisfaction: A decade in review. *Journal of Marriage and the Family, 62*, 964–980.

Bradford, E., & Lyddon, W. J. (1993). Current parental attachment: Its relation to perceived psychological distress and relationship satisfaction in college students. *Journal of College Student Development, 34*, 256–260.

Bradford, S. A., Feeney, J. A., & Campbell, L. (2002). Links between attachment orientations and dispositional and diary-based measures of disclosure in dating couples: A study of actor and partner effects. *Personal Relationships, 9*, 491–506.

Brassard, A., Shaver, P. R., & Lussier, Y. (2007). *Attachment, sexual experience, and sexual pressure in romantic relationships: A dyadic approach.* Manuscript under review.

Brehm, S. S. (1992). *Intimate relationships.* New York: McGraw-Hill.

Brennan, K. A., & Bosson, J. K. (1998). Attachment-style differences in attitudes toward and reactions to feedback from romantic partners: An exploration of the relational bases of self-esteem. *Personality and Social Psychology Bulletin, 24*, 699–714.

Brennan, K. A., & Carnelley, K. B. (1999). Using meaning to mend holes in the nomological net of excessive reassurance-seeking and depression. *Psychological Inquiry, 10*, 282–285.

Brennan, K. A., Clark, C. L., & Shaver, P. R. (1998). Self-report measurement of adult romantic attachment: An integrative overview. In J. A. Simpson & W. S. Rholes (Eds.), *Attachment theory and close relationships* (pp. 46–76). New York: Guilford Press.

Brennan, K. A., & Morris, K. A. (1997). Attachment styles, self-esteem, and patterns of seeking feedback from romantic partners. *Personality and Social Psychology Bulletin, 23*, 23–31.

Brennan, K. A., & Shaver, P. R. (1993). Attachment styles and parental divorce. *Journal of Divorce and Remarriage, 21*, 161–175.

Brennan, K. A., & Shaver, P. R. (1995). Dimensions of adult attachment, affect regulation, and romantic relationship functioning. *Personality and Social Psychology Bulletin, 21*, 267–283.

Brennan, K. A., & Shaver, P. R. (1998). Attachment styles and personality disorders: Their connections to each other and to parental divorce, parental death, and perceptions of parental caregiving. *Journal of Personality, 66*, 835–878.

Brennan, K. A., Shaver, P. R., & Tobey, A. E. (1991). Attachment styles, gender, and parental problem drinking. *Journal of Social and Personal Relationships, 8*, 451–466.

Brennan, K. A., Wu, S., & Loev, J. (1998). Adult romantic attachment and individual differences in attitudes toward physical contact in the context of adult romantic relationships. In J. A. Simpson & W. S. Rholes (Eds.), *Attachment theory and close relationships* (pp. 394–428). New York: Guilford Press.

Bretherton, I. (1985). Attachment theory: Retrospect and prospect. *Monographs of the Society for Research in Child Development, 50*, 3–35.

Bretherton, I. (1992). The origins of attachment theory: John Bowlby and Mary Ainsworth. *Developmental Psychology, 28*, 759–775.

Brewer, M. B. (1999). The psychology of prejudice: Ingroup love or outgroup hate? *Journal of Social Issues, 55*, 429–444.

Bringle, R. G., & Bagby, G. J. (1992). Self-esteem and perceived quality of romantic and family relationships in young adults. *Journal of Research in Personality, 26*, 340–356.

Britton, P. C., & Fuendeling, J. M. (2005). The relations among varieties of adult attachment and the components of empathy. *Journal of Social Psychology, 145*, 519–530.

Broberg, A. G., Hjalmers, I., & Nevonen, L. (2001). Eating disorders, attachment, and interpersonal difficulties: A comparison between 18- to 24-year-old patients and normal controls. *European Eating Disorders Review, 9*, 381–396.

Broemer, P., & Blumle, M. (2003). Self-views in close relationships: The influence of attachment styles. *British Journal of Social Psychology, 42*, 445–460.

Brown, G. W., & Harris, T. O. (1993). Aetiology of anxiety and depressive disorders in an inner-city population: I. Early adversity. *Psychological Medicine, 23*, 143–154.

Brown, S. (1988). *Treating adult children of alcoholics: A developmental perspective*. New York: Wiley.

Bruch, H. (1973). *Eating disorders: Obesity, anorexia nervosa, and the person within*. New York: Basic Books.

Brumbaugh, C. C., & Fraley, R. C. (2006). Transference and attachment: How do attachment patterns get carried forward from one relationship to the next? *Personality and Social Psychology Bulletin, 32*, 552–560.

Brussoni, M. J., Jang, K. L., Livesley, W., & MacBeth, T. M. (2000). Genetic and environmental influences on adult attachment styles. *Personal Relationships, 7*, 283–289.

Bruner, J. S. (1973). *Beyond the information given: Studies in the psychology of knowing*. New York: Norton.

Buber, M. (1958). *I and Thou* (2nd ed.). New York: Scribner.

Buchheim, A., & Mergenthaler, E. (2000). The relationship among attachment representation, emotion-abstraction patterns, and narrative style: A computer-based text analysis of the Adult Attachment Interview. *Psychotherapy Research, 10*, 390–407.

Buelow, S. A., Lyddon, W. J., & Johnson, J. T. (2002). Client attachment and coping resources. *Counseling Psychology Quarterly, 15*, 145–152.

Burge, D., Hammen, C., Davila, J., Daley, S. E., Paley, B., Herzberg, D., et al. (1997). Attachment cognitions and college and work functioning two years later in late adolescent women. *Journal of Youth and Adolescence, 26*, 285–301.

Burk, L. R., & Burkhart, B. R. (2003). Disorganized attachment as a diathesis for sexual deviance: Developmental experience and the motivation for sexual offending. *Aggression and Violent Behavior, 8*, 487–511.

Burlingham, D., & Freud, A. (1944). *Infants without families*. London: Allen & Unwin.

Burtt, E. A. (1957). *Man seeks the divine: A study in the history and comparison of religions*. New York: Harper.

Bus, A. G., & van IJzendoorn, M. H. (1988). Attachment and early reading: A longitudinal study. *Journal of Genetic Psychology, 149*, 199–210.

Bus, A. G., & van IJzendoorn, M. H. (1992). Patterns of attachment in frequently and infrequently reading mother–child dyads. *Journal of Genetic Psychology, 153*, 395–403.

Buss, D. M. (1998). Sexual strategies theory: Historical origins and current status. *Journal of Sex Research, 35*, 19–31.

Buss, D. M., & Kenrick, D. T. (1998). Evolutionary social psychology. In D. T. Gilbert, S. T. Fiske, & G. Lindzey (Eds.), *Handbook of social psychology* (Vol. 2, pp. 982–1026). New York: McGraw-Hill.

Buunk, B. P. (1997). Personality, birth order, and attachment styles as related to various types of jealousy. *Personality and Individual Differences, 23*, 997–1006.

Bylsma, W. H., Cozzarelli, C., & Sumer, N. (1997). Relation between adult attachment styles and global self-esteem. *Basic and Applied Social Psychology, 19*, 1–16.

Byrd, K. R., & Boe, A. (2001). The correspondence between attachment dimensions and prayer in college students. *International Journal for the Psychology of Religion, 11*, 9–24.

Byrne, D. (1971). *The attraction paradigm*. New York: Academic Press.

Cafferty, T. P., Davis, K. E., Medway, F. J., O'Hearn, R. E., & Chappell, K. D. (1994). Reunion dynamics among couples separated during Operation Desert Storm: An attachment theory analysis. In K. Bartholomew & D. Perlman (Eds.), *Advances in personal relationships: Attachment processes in adulthood* (Vol. 5, pp. 309–330). London: Jessica Kingsley.

Calabrese, M. L., Farber, B. A., & Westen, D. (2005). The relationship of adult attachment constructs to object relational patterns of representing self and others. *Journal of the American Academy of Psychoanalysis and Dynamic Psychiatry, 33*, 513–530.

Calamari, E., & Pini, M. (2003). Dissociative experiences and anger proneness in late adolescent females with different attachment styles. *Adolescence, 38*, 287–303.

Campbell, L., Simpson, J. A., Boldry, J., & Kashy, D. A. (2005). Perceptions of conflict and support in romantic relationships: The role of attachment anxiety. *Journal of Personality and Social Psychology, 88*, 510–531.

Candelori, C., & Ciocca, A. (1998). Attachment and eating disorders. In P. Bria, A. Ciocca, & S. de Risio (Eds.), *Psychotherapeutic issues in eating disorders: Models, methods, and results* (pp. 139–153). Rome: Societa Editrice Universo.

Cannon, W. B. (1939). *The wisdom of the body* (2nd ed.). New York: Simon. (First edition published 1932)

Cantor, N., & Kihlstrom, J. F. (1987). *Personality and social intelligence.* Englewood Cliffs, NJ: Prentice-Hall.

Carlson, E. A. (1998). A prospective longitudinal study of attachment disorganization/disorientation. *Child Development, 69,* 1107–1128.

Carlson, E. A., Sroufe, L. A., & Egeland, B. (2004). The construction of experience: A longitudinal study of representation and behavior. *Child Development, 75,* 66–83.

Carmichael, C. L., & Reis, H. T. (2005). Attachment, sleep quality, and depressed affect. *Health Psychology, 24,* 526–531.

Carnelley, K. B., & Janoff-Bulman, R. (1992). Optimism about love relationships: General vs. specific lessons from one's personal experiences. *Journal of Social and Personal Relationships, 9,* 5–20.

Carnelley, K. B., Pietromonaco, P. R., & Jaffe, K. (1994). Depression, working models of others, and relationship functioning. *Journal of Personality and Social Psychology, 66,* 127–140.

Carnelley, K. B., Pietromonaco, P. R., & Jaffe, K. (1996). Attachment, caregiving, and relationship functioning in couples: Effects of self and partner. *Personal Relationships, 3,* 257–277.

Carnelley, K. B., & Ruscher, J. B. (2000). Adult attachment and exploratory behavior in leisure. *Journal of Social Behavior and Personality, 15,* 153–165.

Carnelley, K. B., Ruscher, J. B., & Shaw, S. K. (1999). Meta-accuracy about potential relationship partners' models of others. *Personal Relationships, 6,* 95–109.

Carpenter, B. D. (2001). Attachment bonds between adult daughters and their older mothers: Associations with contemporary caregiving. *Journals of Gerontology: Series B, Psychological Sciences and Social Sciences, 56,* 257–266.

Carpenter, E. M., & Kirkpatrick, L. A. (1996). Attachment style and presence of a romantic partner as moderators of psychophysiological responses to a stressful laboratory situation. *Personal Relationships, 3,* 351–367.

Carranza, L. V., & Kilmann, P. R. (2000). Links between perceived parent characteristics and attachment variables for young women from intact families. *Adolescence, 35,* 295–312.

Carter, B., & McGoldrick, M. (Eds.). (1988). *The changing family life cycle: A framework for family therapy.* New York: Gardner Press.

Carter, C. S. (2005). Biological perspectives on social attachment and bonding. In C. S. Carter, L. Ahnert, K. E. Grossmann, S. B. Hrdy, M. E. Lamb, S. W. Porges, et al. (Eds.), *Attachment and bonding: A new synthesis* (pp. 85–100). Cambridge, MA: MIT Press.

Carter, C. S., Ahnert, L., Grossmann, K. E., Hrdy, S.

B., Lamb, M. E., Porges, S. W., et al. (Eds.). (2005). *Attachment and bonding: A new synthesis.* Cambridge, MA: MIT Press.

Carvallo, M., & Gabriel, S. (2006). No man is an island: The need to belong and dismissing avoidant attachment style. *Personality and Social Psychology Bulletin, 32,* 697–709.

Carver, C. S. (1997). Adult attachment and personality: Converging evidence and a new measure. *Personality and Social Psychology Bulletin, 23,* 865–883.

Carver, C. S., & Scheier, M. F. (1981). *Attention and self-regulation: A control-theory approach to human behavior.* New York: Springer-Verlag.

Carver, C. S., & Scheier, M. F. (1990). Origins and functions of positive and negative affect: A control-process view. *Psychological Review, 97,* 19–35.

Carver, C. S., & Scheier, M. F. (1998). *On the self-regulation of behavior.* New York: Cambridge University Press.

Carver, C. S., & White, T. L. (1994). Behavioral inhibition, behavioral activation, and affective responses to impending reward and punishment: The BIS/BAS scales. *Journal of Personality and Social Psychology, 67,* 319–333.

Cash, T. F., Theriault, J., & Annis, N. M. (2004). Body image in an interpersonal context: Adult attachment, fear of intimacy, and social anxiety. *Journal of Social and Clinical Psychology, 23,* 89–103.

Caspers, K. M., Cadoret, R. J., Langbehn, D., Yucuis, R., & Troutman, B. (2005). Contributions of attachment style and perceived social support to lifetime use of illicit substances. *Addictive Behaviors, 30,* 1007–1011.

Caspi-Berkowitz, N. (2003). *Mortality salience effects on the willingness to sacrifice one's life: The moderating role of attachment orientations.* Unpublished doctoral dissertation, Bar-Ilan University, Ramat Gan, Israel.

Cassidy, J. (1994). Emotion regulation: Influences of attachment relationships. *Monographs of the Society for Research in Child Development, 59,* 228–283.

Cassidy, J. (1995). Attachment and generalized anxiety disorder. In D. Cicchetti & S. L. Toth (Eds.), *Emotion, cognition, and representation* (pp. 343–370). Rochester, NY: University of Rochester Press.

Cassidy, J. (1999). The nature of the child's ties. In J. Cassidy & P. R. Shaver (Eds.), *Handbook of attachment: Theory, research, and clinical applications* (pp. 3–20). New York: Guilford Press.

Cassidy, J., & Berlin, L. J. (1994). The insecure/ambivalent pattern of attachment: Theory and research. *Child Development, 65,* 971–981.

Cassidy, J., & Kobak, R. R. (1988). Avoidance and its relationship with other defensive processes. In J. Belsky & T. Nezworski (Eds.), *Clinical implications of attachment* (pp. 300–323). Hillsdale, NJ: Erlbaum.

Cassidy, J., & Shaver, P. R. (Eds.). (1999). *Handbook of attachment: Theory, research, and clinical applications.* New York: Guilford Press.

Cassidy, J., Ziv, Y., Mehta, T. G., & Feeney, B. C. (2003). Feedback seeking in children and adolescents: Associations with self-perceptions, attachment representations, and depression. *Child Development, 74,* 612–628.

Cattell, R. B. (1957). *Personality and motivation: Structure and measurement.* New York: Harcourt, Brace, Jovanovich.

Cavell, T. A., Jones, D. C., Runyan, R., Constantin-Page, L. P., & Velasquez, J. M. (1993). Perceptions of attachment and the adjustment of adolescents with alcoholic fathers. *Journal of Family Psychology, 7,* 204–212.

Cawthorpe, D., West, M., & Wilkes, T. (2004). Attachment and depression: The relationship between the felt security of attachment and clinical depression among hospitalized female adolescents. *Canadian Child and Adolescent Psychiatry Review, 13,* 31–35.

Ceglian, C. P., & Gardner, S. (1999). Attachment style: A risk for multiple marriages? *Journal of Divorce and Remarriage, 31,* 125–139.

Ceglian, C. P., & Gardner, S. (2000). Attachment style and the "wicked stepmother" spiral. *Journal of Divorce and Remarriage, 34,* 111–129.

Chappell, K. D., & Davis, K. E. (1998). Attachment, partner choice, and perception of romantic partners: An experimental test of the attachment-security hypothesis. *Personal Relationships, 5,* 327–342.

Chartrand, T. L., & Bargh, J. A. (2002). Nonconscious motivations: Their activation, operation, and consequences. In A. Tesser & D. A. Stapel (Eds.), *Self and motivation: Emerging psychological perspectives* (pp. 13–41). Washington, DC: American Psychological Association.

Chassler, L. (1997). Understanding anorexia nervosa and bulimia nervosa from an attachment perspective. *Clinical Social Work Journal, 25,* 407–423.

Cheek, J. M., & Buss, A. H. (1981). Shyness and sociability. *Journal of Personality and Social Psychology, 41,* 330–339.

Chen, E. C., & Mallinckrodt, B. (2002). Attachment, group attraction, and self–other agreement in interpersonal circumplex problems and perceptions of group members. *Group Dynamics, 6,* 311–324.

Chen, M., & Bargh, J. A. (1999). Consequences of automatic evaluation: Immediate behavioral predispositions to approach or avoid the stimulus. *Personality and Social Psychology Bulletin, 25,* 215–224.

Chödrön, P. (2003). *Comfortable with uncertainty.* Boston: Shambhala.

Chotai, J., Jonasson, M., Hagglof, B., & Adolfsson, R. (2005). Adolescent attachment styles and their relation to the temperament and character traits of personality in a general population. *European Psychiatry, 20,* 251–259.

Christensen, A. (1988). Dysfunctional interaction patterns in couples. In P. Noller & M. A. Fitzpatrick (Eds.), *Perspectives in marital interaction* (pp. 31–52). Philadelphia: Multilingual Matters.

Christensen, A., & Heavey, C. L. (1990). Gender and social structure in the demand/withdraw pattern of marital conflict. *Journal of Personality and Social Psychology, 59,* 73–81.

Cicirelli, V. G. (1993). Attachment and obligation as daughters' motives for caregiving behavior and subsequent effect on subjective burden. *Psychology and Aging, 8,* 144–155.

Cicirelli, V. G. (1995). A measure of caregiving daughters' attachment to elderly mothers. *Journal of Family Psychology, 9,* 89–94.

Ciechanowski, P. S., Katon, W. J., & Russo, J. E. (2005). The association of depression and perceptions of interpersonal relationships in patients with diabetes. *Journal of Psychosomatic Research, 58,* 139–144.

Ciechanowski, P. S., Katon, W. J., Russo, J. E., & Dwight-Johnson, M. M. (2002). Association of attachment style to lifetime medically unexplained symptoms in patients with hepatitis C. *Psychosomatics, 43,* 206–212.

Ciechanowski, P. S., Katon, W. J., Russo, J. E., & Walker, E. A. (2001). The patient–provider relationship: Attachment theory and adherence to treatment in diabetes. *American Journal of Psychiatry, 158,* 29–35.

Ciechanowski, P. S., Russo, J. E., Katon, W. J., VonKorff, M., Ludman, E., Lin, E., et al. (2004). Influence of patient attachment style on self-care and outcomes in diabetes. *Psychosomatic Medicine, 66,* 720–728.

Ciechanowski, P. S., Russo, J. E., Katon, W. J., & Walker, E. A. (2004). Attachment theory in health care: The influence of relationship style on medical students' specialty choice. *Medical Education, 38,* 262–270.

Ciechanowski, P. S., Sullivan, M., Jensen, M., Romano, J., & Summers, H. (2003). The relationship of attachment style to depression, catastrophizing, and health care utilization in patients with chronic pain. *Pain, 104,* 627–637.

Ciechanowski, P. S., Walker, E. A., Katon, W. J., & Russo, J. E. (2002). Attachment theory: A model for health care utilization and somatization. *Psychosomatic Medicine, 64,* 660–667.

Ciesla, J. A., Roberts, J. E., & Hewitt, R. G. (2004). Adult attachment and high-risk sexual behavior among HIV-positive patients. *Journal of Applied Social Psychology, 34,* 108–124.

Clark, L. A., & Watson, D. (1991). Tripartite model of anxiety and depression: Psychometric evidence and taxonomic implications. *Journal of Abnormal Psychology, 100,* 316–336.

Clark, M. S., Fitness, J., & Brissette, I. (2001). Understanding people's perceptions of relationships is crucial to understanding their emotional lives. In G. Fletcher & M. Clark (Eds.), *Blackwell handbook of social psychology: Interpersonal processes* (pp. 253–278). Oxford, UK: Blackwell.

Clark, M. S., Reis, H. T., Tsai, F. F., & Brissette, I. (2005). *The willingness to express emotions in relationships.* Unpublished manuscript. Yale University, New Haven, CT.

Clothier, P., Manion, I., Gordon-Walker, J., & Johnson, S. M. (2002). Emotionally-focused interventions for couple with chronically ill children: A two-year follow-up. *Journal of Marital and Family Therapy, 28,* 391–398.

Coan, J. A., Schaefer, H. S., & Davidson, R. J. (2006).

Lending a hand: Social regulation of the neural response to threat. *Psychological Science, 17,* 1032–1039.

Cobb, R. J., & Davila, J. (in press). Internal working models and change. In J. Obegi & E. Berant (Eds.), *Clinical applications of adult attachment.* New York: Guilford Press.

Cobb, R. J., Davila, J., & Bradbury, T. N. (2001). Attachment security and marital satisfaction: The role of positive perceptions and social support. *Personality and Social Psychology Bulletin, 27,* 1131–1143.

Cohen, D. L., & Belsky, J. (2006). *Avoidant romantic attachment and female orgasm: Testing an emotion-regulation hypothesis.* Unpublished manuscript, Birkbeck University of London, London, UK.

Cohen, J. (2004). Parasocial break-up from favorite television characters: The role of attachment styles and relationship intensity. *Journal of Social and Personal Relationships, 21,* 187–202.

Cohen, O., Birnbaum, G. E., Meyuchas, R., Levinger, Z., Florian, V., & Mikulincer, M. (2005). Attachment orientations and spouse support in adults with type 2 diabetes. *Psychology, Health, and Medicine, 10,* 161–165.

Cohen, O., & Finzi-Dottan, R. (2005). Parent–child relationships during the divorce process: From attachment theory and intergenerational perspective. *Contemporary Family Therapy: An International Journal, 27,* 81–99.

Cohen, S., Gottlieb, B. H., & Underwood, L. G. (2000). Social relationships and health. In S. Cohen, L. G. Underwood, & B. H. Gottlieb (Eds.), *Social support measurement and intervention* (pp. 3–25). New York: Oxford University Press.

Cohen, S., & McKay, G. (1984). Social support, stress, and the buffering hypothesis: A theoretical analysis. In A. Baum, S. E. Taylor, & J. E. Singer (Eds.), *Handbook of psychology and health* (pp. 253–267). Hillsdale, NJ: Erlbaum.

Cohen, S., & Wills, T. A. (1985). Stress, social support, and the buffering hypothesis. *Psychological Bulletin, 98,* 310–357.

Cohn, D. A., Cowan, P. A., Cowan, C. P., & Pearson, J. (1992). Mothers' and fathers' working models of childhood attachment relationships, parenting styles, and child behavior. *Development and Psychopathology, 4,* 417–431.

Cohn, D. A., Silver, D. H., Cowan, C. P., Cowan, P. A., & Pearson, J. (1992). Working models of childhood attachment and couple relationships. *Journal of Family Issues, 13,* 432–449.

Cole-Detke, H., & Kobak, R. (1996). Attachment processes in eating disorder and depression. *Journal of Consulting and Clinical Psychology, 64,* 282–290.

Colin, V. L. (1996). *Human attachment.* New York: McGraw-Hill.

Collins, N. L. (1996). Working models of attachment: Implications for explanation, emotion, and behavior. *Journal of Personality and Social Psychology, 71,* 810–832.

Collins, N. L., Cooper, M., Albino, A., & Allard, L. (2002). Psychosocial vulnerability from adolescence to adulthood: A prospective study of attach-ment style differences in relationship functioning and partner choice. *Journal of Personality, 70,* 965–1008.

Collins, N. L., & Feeney, B. C. (2000). A safe haven: An attachment theory perspective on support seeking and caregiving in intimate relationships. *Journal of Personality and Social Psychology, 78,* 1053–1073.

Collins, N. L., & Feeney, B. C. (2004). Working models of attachment shape perceptions of social support: Evidence from experimental and observational studies. *Journal of Personality and Social Psychology, 87,* 363–383.

Collins, N. L., & Feeney, B. C. (2005). *Attachment processes in daily interaction: Feeling supported and feeling secure.* Unpublished manuscript, University of California, Santa Barbara.

Collins, N. L., Ford, M. B., Guichard, A. C., & Allard, L. M. (2006). Working models of attachment and attribution processes in intimate relationships. *Personality and Social Psychology Bulletin, 32,* 201–219.

Collins, N. L., Ford, M. B., Guichard, A. C., & Feeney, B. C. (2005). *Responding to need in intimate relationships: The role of attachment security.* Unpublished manuscript, University of California, Santa Barbara.

Collins, N. L., Guichard, A. C., Ford, M. B., & Feeney, B. C. (2004). Working models of attachment: New developments and emerging themes. In W. S. Rholes & J. A. Simpson (Eds.), *Adult attachment: Theory, research, and clinical implications* (pp. 196–239). New York: Guilford Press.

Collins, N. L., Guichard, A. C., Ford, M. B., & Feeney, B. C. (2006). Responding to need in intimate relationships: Normative processes and individual differences. In M. Mikulincer & G. S. Goodman (Eds.), *Dynamics of romantic love: Attachment, caregiving, and sex* (pp. 149–189). New York: Guilford Press.

Collins, N. L., & Read, S. J. (1990). Adult attachment, working models, and relationship quality in dating couples. *Journal of Personality and Social Psychology, 58,* 644–663.

Collins, N. L., & Read, S. J. (1994). Cognitive representations of attachment: The structure and function of working models. In K. Bartholomew & D. Perlman (Eds.), *Advances in personal relationships: Attachment processes in adulthood* (Vol. 5, pp. 53–92). London: Jessica Kingsley.

Connors, M. E. (1997). The renunciation of love: Dismissive attachment and its treatment. *Psychoanalytic Psychology, 14,* 475–493.

Conte, H. P., & Plutchik, R. (1981). A circumplex model for interpersonal personality traits. *Journal of Personality and Social Psychology, 40,* 701–711.

Cook, W. L. (2000). Understanding attachment security in family context. *Journal of Personality and Social Psychology, 78,* 285–294.

Cooley, C. H. (1902). *Human nature and the social order.* New York: Schocken Books.

Cooley, E. L. (2005). Attachment style and decoding of nonverbal clues. *North American Journal of Psychology, 7,* 25–33.

Cooper, M. L., Pioli, M., Levitt, A., Talley, A.,

Micheas, L., & Collins, N. L. (2006). Attachment styles, sex motives, and sexual behavior: Evidence for gender specific expressions of attachment dynamics. In M. Mikulincer & G. S. Goodman (Eds.), *Dynamics of romantic love: Attachment, caregiving, and sex* (pp. 243–274). New York: Guilford Press.

Cooper, M. L., Shaver, P. R., & Collins, N. L. (1998). Attachment styles, emotion regulation, and adjustment in adolescence. *Journal of Personality and Social Psychology, 74*, 1380–1397.

Corcoran, K. O., & Mallinckrodt, B. (2000). Adult attachment, self-efficacy, perspective taking, and conflict resolution. *Journal of Counseling and Development, 78*, 473–483.

Cortina, M. (1999). Causality, adaptation, and meaning: A perspective from attachment theory and research. *Psychoanalytic Dialogues, 9*, 557–596.

Costa, N. M., & Weems, C. F. (2005). Maternal and child anxiety: Do attachment beliefs or children's perceptions of maternal control mediate their association? *Social Development, 14*, 574–590.

Cotterell, J. L. (1992). The relation of attachments and support to adolescent well-being and school adjustment. *Journal of Adolescent Research, 7*, 28–42.

Cowan, P. A., Cohn, D. A., Cowan, C. P., & Pearson, J. L. (1996). Parents' attachment histories and children's externalizing and internalizing behaviors: Exploring family systems models of linkage. *Journal of Consulting and Clinical Psychology, 64*, 53–63.

Cozzarelli, C., Hoekstra, S. J., & Bylsma, W. H. (2000). General versus specific mental models of attachment: Are they associated with different outcomes? *Personality and Social Psychology Bulletin, 26*, 605–618.

Cozzarelli, C., Karafa, J. A., Collins, N. L., & Tagler, M. J. (2003). Stability and change in adult attachment styles: Associations with personal vulnerabilities, life events, and global construals of self and others. *Journal of Social and Clinical Psychology, 22*, 315–346.

Cozzarelli, C., Sumer, N., & Major, B. (1998). Mental models of attachment and coping with abortion. *Journal of Personality and Social Psychology, 74*, 453–467.

Craik, K. (1943). *The nature of explanation.* Cambridge, UK: Cambridge University Press.

Crandell, L. E., Fitzgerald, H. E., & Whipple, E. E. (1997). Dyadic synchrony in parent–child interactions: A link with maternal representations of attachment relationships. *Infant Mental Health Journal, 18*, 247–264.

Crawford, M., & Gartner, R. (1992). *Women killing: Intimate femicide in Ontario, 1974–1990.* Toronto: Women's Directorate, Ministry of Social Services.

Crawford, T. N., Livesley, W. J., Jang, K. L., Shaver, P. R., Cohen, P., & Ganiban, J. (in press). Insecure attachment and personality disorder: A twin study of adults. *European Journal of Personality.*

Crawford, T. N., Shaver, P. R., Cohen, P., Pilkonis, P. A., Gillath, O., & Kasen, S. (2006). Self-reported attachment, interpersonal aggression, and personality disorder in a prospective community sample of adolescents and adults. *Journal of Personality Disorders, 20*, 331–351.

Creasey, G. (2002a). Associations between working models of attachment and conflict management behavior in romantic couples. *Journal of Counseling Psychology, 49*, 365–375.

Creasey, G. (2002b). Psychological distress in college-aged women: Links with unresolved/preoccupied attachment status and the mediating role of negative mood regulation expectancies. *Attachment and Human Development, 4*, 261–277.

Creasey, G., & Hesson-McInnis, M. (2001). Affective responses, cognitive appraisals, and conflict tactics in late adolescent romantic relationships: Associations with attachment orientations. *Journal of Counseling Psychology, 48*, 85–96.

Creasey, G., Kershaw, K., & Boston, A. (1999). Conflict management with friends and romantic partners: The role of attachment and negative mood regulation expectancies. *Journal of Youth and Adolescence, 28*, 523–543.

Creasey, G., & Ladd, A. (2004). Negative mood regulation expectancies and conflict behaviors in late adolescent college student romantic relationships: The moderating role of generalized attachment representations. *Journal of Research on Adolescence, 14*, 235–255.

Creasey, G., & Ladd, A. (2005). Generalized and specific attachment representations: Unique and interactive roles in predicting conflict behaviors in close relationships. *Personality and Social Psychology Bulletin, 31*, 1026–1038.

Crispi, E. L., Schiaffino, K., & Berman, W. H. (1997). The contribution of attachment to burden in adult children of institutionalized parents with dementia. *Gerontologist, 37*, 52–60.

Crittenden, P. M. (1992). Children's strategies for coping with adverse home environments: An interpretation using attachment theory. *Child Abuse and Neglect, 16*, 329–343.

Crittenden, P. M., Partridge, M. F., & Claussen, A. H. (1991). Family patterns of relationship in normative and dysfunctional families. *Development and Psychopathology, 3*, 491–512.

Crockenberg, S. B. (1981). Infant irritability, mother responsiveness, and social support influences on the security of infant–mother attachment. *Child Development, 52*, 857–865.

Cronbach, L. J., & Meehl, P. E. (1955). Construct validity in psychological tests. *Psychological Bulletin, 52*, 281–302.

Crowell, J. A., & Feldman, S. (1989). Assessment of mothers' working models of relationships: Some clinical implications. *Infant Mental Health Journal, 10*, 173–184.

Crowell, J. A., & Feldman, S. (1991). Mothers' working models of attachment relationships and mother and child behavior during separation and reunion. *Developmental Psychology, 27*, 597–605.

Crowell, J. A., Fraley, R. C., & Shaver, P. R. (1999). Measurement of adult attachment. In J. Cassidy & P. R. Shaver (Eds.), *Handbook of attachment: Theory, research, and clinical applications* (pp. 434–465). New York: Guilford Press.

Crowell, J. A., O'Connor, E., Wollmers, G., Sprafkin, J., & Rao, U. (1991). Mothers' conceptualizations of parent–child relationships: Relation to mother–child interaction and child behavior problems. *Development and Psychopathology, 3,* 431–444.

Crowell, J. A., & Owens, G. (1996). *Current Relationship Interview and scoring system.* Unpublished manuscript, State University of New York, Stony Brook.

Crowell, J. A., & Treboux, D. (1995). A review of adult attachment measures: Implications for theory and research. *Social Development, 4,* 294–327.

Crowell, J. A., & Treboux, D. (2001). Attachment security in adult partnerships. In C. Clulow (Ed.), *Adult attachment and couple psychotherapy: The "secure base" in practice and research* (pp. 28–42). London: Brunner-Routledge.

Crowell, J. A., Treboux, D., Gao, Y., Fyffe, C., Pan, H., & Waters, E. (2002). Assessing secure base behavior in adulthood: Development of a measure, links to adult attachment representations, and relations to couples' communication and reports of relationships. *Developmental Psychology, 38,* 679–693.

Crowell, J. A., Treboux, D., & Waters, E. (1999). The Adult Attachment Interview and the Relationship Questionnaire: Relations to reports of mothers and partners. *Personal Relationships, 6,* 1–18.

Crowell, J. A., Treboux, D., & Waters, E. (2002). Stability of attachment representations: The transition to marriage. *Developmental Psychology, 38,* 467–479.

Cummings, E. M., & Cicchetti, D. (1990). Toward a transactional model of relations between attachment and depression. In M. T. Greenberg, D. Cicchetti, & E. M. Cummings (Eds.), *Attachment in the preschool years: Theory, research, and intervention* (pp. 339–372). Chicago: University of Chicago Press.

Cutrona, C. E., Cole, V., Colangelo, N., Assouline, S. G., & Russell, D. W. (1994). Perceived parental social support and academic achievement: An attachment theory perspective. *Journal of Personality and Social Psychology, 66,* 369–378.

Cyranowski, J. M., & Andersen, B. L. (1998). Schemas, sexuality, and romantic attachment. *Journal of Personality and Social Psychology, 74,* 1364–1379.

Cyranowski, J. M., Bookwala, J., Feske, U., Houck, P., Pilkonis, P., Kostelnik, B., et al. (2002). Adult attachment profiles, interpersonal difficulties, and response to interpersonal psychotherapy in women with recurrent major depression. *Journal of Social and Clinical Psychology, 21,* 191–217.

Dalai Lama. (1999). *Ethics for a new millennium.* New York: Riverhead Books.

Dalai Lama. (2001). *An open heart: Practicing compassion in everyday life.* (N. Vreeland, Ed.). Boston: Little, Brown.

Dalai Lama. (2002). *The heart of compassion.* Boston: Little, Brown.

Davidovitz, R., Mikulincer, M., Shaver, P. R., Ijzak, R., & Popper, M. (2006). *An attachment perspective on leadership and the leader–follower relationship.* Unpublished manuscript, Bar-Ilan University, Ramat-Gan, Israel.

Davila, J. (2001). Refining the association between excessive reassurance seeking and depressive symptoms: The role of related interpersonal constructs. *Journal of Social and Clinical Psychology, 20,* 538–559.

Davila, J., & Bradbury, T. N. (2001). Attachment insecurity and the distinction between unhappy spouses who do and do not divorce. *Journal of Family Psychology, 15,* 371–393.

Davila, J., Bradbury, T. N., & Fincham, F. (1998). Negative affectivity as a mediator of the association between adult attachment and marital satisfaction. *Personal Relationships, 5,* 467–484.

Davila, J., Burge, D., & Hammen, C. (1997). Why does attachment style change? *Journal of Personality and Social Psychology, 73,* 826–838.

Davila, J., & Cobb, R. J. (2003). Predicting change in self-reported and interviewer-assessed adult attachment: Tests of the individual difference and life stress models of attachment change. *Personality and Social Psychology Bulletin, 29,* 859–870.

Davila, J., & Cobb, R. J. (2004). Predictors of changes in attachment security during adulthood. In W. S. Rholes & J. A. Simpson (Eds.), *Adult attachment: Theory, research, and clinical implications* (pp. 133–156). New York: Guilford Press.

Davila, J., Hammen, C., Burge, D., Daley, S. E., & Paley, B. (1996). Cognitive/interpersonal correlates of adult interpersonal problem-solving strategies. *Cognitive Therapy and Research, 20,* 465–480.

Davila, J., Karney, B. R., & Bradbury, T. N. (1999). Attachment change processes in the early years of marriage. *Journal of Personality and Social Psychology, 76,* 783–802.

Davila, J., & Sargent, E. (2003). The meaning of life (events) predicts changes in attachment security. *Personality and Social Psychology Bulletin, 29,* 1383–1395.

Davila, J., Steinberg, S. J., Kachadourian, L., Cobb, R., & Fincham, F. (2004). Romantic involvement and depressive symptoms in early and late adolescence: The role of a preoccupied relational style. *Personal Relationships, 11,* 161–178.

Davis, D. (2006). Attachment-related pathways to sexual coercion. In M. Mikulincer & G. S. Goodman (Eds.), *Dynamics of romantic love: Attachment, caregiving, and sex* (pp. 293–336). New York: Guilford Press.

Davis, D., Carlen, L., & Gallio, J. (2006, May). *Attachment, rape supportive attitudes, and perceived validity of claims in three rape scenarios.* Paper presented in the Annual Conference on the American Psychological Society, New York.

Davis, D., Follette, W. C., & Vernon, M. L. (2001, March). *Adult attachment style and the experience of unwanted sex.* Paper presented in the Annual Western Psychological Association Conference, Maui, HI.

Davis, D., Shaver, P. R., & Vernon, M. L. (2003). Physical, emotional, and behavioral reactions to breaking up: The roles of gender, age, emotional involvement, and attachment style. *Personality and Social Psychology Bulletin, 29,* 871–884.

Davis, D., Shaver, P. R., & Vernon, M. L. (2004). Attachment style and subjective motivations for sex. *Personality and Social Psychology Bulletin, 30,* 1076–1090.

Davis, D., Shaver, P. R., Widaman, K. F., Vernon, M. L., Follette, W. C., & Beitz, K. (2006). "I can't get no satisfaction": Insecure attachment, inhibited sexual communication, and sexual dissatisfaction. *Personal Relationships, 13,* 465–483.

Davis, D., & Vernon, M. L. (2002). Sculpting the body beautiful: Attachment style, neuroticism, and use of cosmetic surgeries. *Sex Roles, 47,* 129–138.

Davis, K. E., Ace, A., & Andra, M. (2002). Stalking perpetrators and psychological maltreatment of partners: Anger–jealousy, attachment insecurity, need for control, and break-up context. In K. E. Davis & I. H. Frieze (Eds.), *Stalking: Perspectives on victims and perpetrators* (pp. 237–264). New York: Springer.

Davis, M. H., Morris, M. M., & Kraus, L. A. (1998). Relationship-specific and global perceptions of social support: Associations with well-being and attachment. *Journal of Personality and Social Psychology, 74,* 468–481.

DeBerard, M. S., Spielmans, G. I., & Julka, D. L. (2004). Predictors of academic achievement and retention among college freshmen: A longitudinal study. *College Student Journal, 38,* 66–80.

Deci, E. L., La Guardia, J. G., Moller, A. C., Scheiner, M. J., & Ryan, R. M. (2006). On the benefits of giving as well as receiving autonomy support: Mutuality in close friendships. *Personality and Social Psychology Bulletin, 32,* 313–327.

DeFranc, W., & Mahalik, J. R. (2002). Masculine gender role conflict and stress in relation to parental attachment and separation. *Psychology of Men and Masculinity, 3,* 51–60.

DeFronzo, R., Panzarella, C., & Butler, A. C. (2001). Attachment, support seeking, and adaptive inferential feedback: Implications for psychological health. *Cognitive and Behavioral Practice, 8,* 48–52.

DeFronzo, J., & Pawlak, R. (1993). Effects of social bonds and childhood experiences on alcohol abuse and smoking. *Journal of Social Psychology, 133,* 635–642.

de Haas, M. A., Bakermans-Kranenburg, M. J., & van IJzendoorn, M. H. (1994). The Adult Attachment Interview and questionnaires for attachment style, temperament, and memories of parental behavior. *Journal of Genetic Psychology, 155,* 471–486.

de Jong, M. L. (1992). Attachment, individuation, and risk of suicide in late adolescence. *Journal of Youth and Adolescence, 21,* 357–373.

Dekel, R., Solomon, Z., Ginzburg, K., & Neria, Y. (2004). Long-term adjustment among Israeli war veterans: The role of attachment style. *Anxiety, Stress and Coping: An International Journal, 17,* 141–152.

DeKlyen, M. (1996). Disruptive behavior disorder and intergenerational attachment patterns: A comparison of clinic-referred and normally functioning preschoolers and their mothers. *Journal of Consulting and Clinical Psychology, 64,* 357–365.

Deniz, M., Hamarta, E., & Ari, R. (2005). An investigation of social skills and loneliness levels of university students with respect to their attachment styles in a sample of Turkish students. *Social Behavior and Personality, 33,* 19–32.

DeOliveira, C. A., Moran, G., & Pederson, D. R. (2005). Understanding the link between maternal adult attachment classifications and thoughts and feelings about emotions. *Attachment and Human Development, 7,* 153–170.

Desivilya, H. S., Sabag, Y., & Ashton, E. (2007). *Prosocial tendencies in organizations: The role of attachment styles and organizational justice in shaping organizational citizenship.* Manuscript under review.

Devine, P. G. (1995). Prejudice and out-group perception. In A. Tesser (Ed.), *Advanced social psychology* (pp. 466–524). New York: McGraw-Hill.

Dewar, H., & Milbank, D. (2004, June 25). Cheney dismisses critic with obscenity: Clash with Leahy about Halliburton. *Washington Post,* p. A04.

de Wolff, M., & van IJzendoorn, M. H. (1997). Sensitivity and attachment: A meta-analysis on parental antecedents of infant attachment. *Child Development, 68,* 571–591.

Diamond, D., & Doane, J. A. (1994). Disturbed attachment and negative affective style: An intergenerational spiral. *British Journal of Psychiatry, 164,* 770–781.

Diamond, G. S., & Stern, R. S. (2003). Attachment-based family therapy for depressed adolescents: Repairing attachment failures. In S. M. Johnson & V. E. Whiffen (Eds.), *Attachment processes in couple and family therapy* (pp. 191–212). New York: Guilford Press.

Diamond, L. M. (2003). What does sexual orientation orient?: A biobehavioral model distinguishing romantic love and sexual desire. *Psychological Review, 110,* 173–192.

Diamond, L. M. (2006). How do I love thee?: Implications of attachment theory for understanding same-sex love and desire. In M. Mikulincer & G. S. Goodman (Eds.), *Dynamics of romantic love: Attachment, caregiving, and sex* (pp. 275–292). New York: Guilford Press.

Diamond, L. M., & Hicks, A. M. (2005). Attachment style, current relationship security, and negative emotions: The mediating role of physiological regulation. *Journal of Social and Personal Relationships, 22,* 499–518.

Diamond, L. M., Hicks, A. M., & Otter-Henderson, K. (2006). Physiological evidence for repressive coping among avoidantly attached adults. *Journal of Social and Personal Relationships, 23,* 205–229.

Dickinson, K. A., & Pincus, A. L. (2003). Interpersonal analysis of grandiose and vulnerable narcissism. *Journal of Personality Disorders, 17,* 188–207.

Dickstein, S., Seifer, R., Albus, K. E., & Magee, K. D. (2004). Attachment patterns across multiple family relationships in adulthood: Associations with maternal depression. *Development and Psychopathology, 16,* 735–751.

Dickstein, S., Seifer, R., St Andre, M., & Schiller, M. (2001). Marital Attachment Interview: Adult attachment assessment of marriage. *Journal of Social and Personal Relationships, 18,* 651–672.

Didion, J. (2005). *The year of magical thinking.* New York: Knopf.

Diehl, M., Elnick, A. B., Bourbeau, L. S., & Labouvie-Vief, G. (1998). Adult attachment styles: Their relations to family context and personality. *Journal of Personality and Social Psychology, 74,* 1656–1669.

Dieperink, M., Leskela, J., Thuras, P., & Engdahl, B. (2001). Attachment style classification and posttraumatic stress disorder in former prisoners of war. *American Journal of Orthopsychiatry, 71,* 374–378.

DiFilippo, J. M., & Overholser, J. C. (2000). Suicidal ideation in adolescent psychiatric inpatients as associated with depression and attachment relationships. *Journal of Clinical Child Psychology, 29,* 155–166.

DiFilippo, J. M., & Overholser, J. C. (2002). Depression, adult attachment, and recollections of parental caring during childhood. *Journal of Nervous and Mental Disease, 190,* 663–669.

Diller, G. (2006). *The contribution of attachment security to religious quest orientation among Israeli Jews.* Unpublished doctoral dissertation, Bar-Ilan University, Ramat Gan, Israel.

DiTommaso, E., Brannen-McNulty, C., Ross, L., & Burgess, M. (2003). Attachment styles, social skills, and loneliness in young adults. *Personality and Individual Differences, 35,* 303–312.

Doherty, N. A., & Feeney, J. A. (2004). The composition of attachment networks throughout the adult years. *Personal Relationships, 11,* 469–488.

Doherty, R. W., Hatfield, E., Thompson, K., & Choo, P. (1994). Cultural and ethnic influences on love and attachment. *Personal Relationships, 1,* 391–398.

Doi, S. C., & Thelen, M. H. (1993). The Fear-of-Intimacy Scale: Replication and extension. *Psychological Assessment, 5,* 377–383.

Dolan, R. T., Arnkoff, D. B., & Glass, C. R. (1993). Client attachment style and the psychotherapist's interpersonal stance. *Psychotherapy, 30,* 408–412.

Donahue, E. M., Robins, R. W., Roberts, B. W., & John, O. P. (1993). The divided self: Concurrent and longitudinal effects of psychological adjustment and social roles on self-concept differentiation. *Journal of Personality and Social Psychology, 64,* 834–846.

Dovidio, J. F., & Gaertner, S. L. (1993). Stereotypes and evaluative intergroup bias. In D. M. Mackie & D. L. Hamilton (Eds.), *Affect, cognition, and stereotyping* (pp. 167–193). San Diego: Academic Press.

Downey, G., & Feldman, S. I. (1996). Implications of rejection sensitivity for intimate relationships. *Journal of Personality and Social Psychology, 70,* 1327–1343.

Doyle, A. B., & Markiewicz, D. (2005). Parenting, marital conflict, and adjustment from early- to mid-adolescence: Mediated by adolescent attachment style? *Journal of Youth and Adolescence, 34,* 97–110.

Dozier, M. (1990). Attachment organization and treatment use for adults with serious psychopathological disorders. *Development and Psychopathology, 2,* 47–60.

Dozier, M., Cue, K. L., & Barnett, L. (1994). Clini-

cians as caregivers: Role of attachment organization in treatment. *Journal of Consulting and Clinical Psychology, 62,* 793–800.

Dozier, M., & Kobak, R. (1992). Psychophysiology in attachment interviews: Converging evidence for deactivating strategies. *Child Development, 63,* 1473–1480.

Dozier, M., & Lee, S. W. (1995). Discrepancies between self- and other-report of psychiatric symptomatology: Effects of dismissing attachment strategies. *Development and Psychopathology, 7,* 217–226.

Dozier, M., Stevenson, A. L., Lee, S. W., & Velligan, D. I. (1991). Attachment organization and familial overinvolvement for adults with serious psychopathological disorders. *Development and Psychopathology, 3,* 475–489.

Dozier, M., Stovall, K. C., & Albus, K. E. (1999). Attachment and psychopathology in adulthood. In J. Cassidy & P. R. Shaver (Eds.), *Handbook of attachment: Theory, research, and clinical applications* (pp. 497–519). New York: Guilford Press.

Dozier, M., Stovall, K., Albus, K. E., & Bates, B. (2001). Attachment for infants in foster care: The role of caregiver state of mind. *Child Development, 72,* 1467–1477.

Dozier, M., & Tyrrell, C. (1998). The role of attachment in therapeutic relationships. In J. A. Simpson & W. S. Rholes (Eds.), *Attachment theory and close relationships* (pp. 221–248). New York: Guilford Press.

Drach-Zahavy, A. (2004). Toward a multidimensional construct of social support: Implications of provider's self-reliance and request characteristics. *Journal of Applied Social Psychology, 34,* 1395–1420.

Drayton, M., Birchwood, M., & Trower, P. (1998). Early attachment experience and recovery from psychosis. *British Journal of Clinical Psychology, 37,* 269–284.

Ducharme, J., Doyle, A. B., & Markiewicz, D. (2002). Attachment security with mother and father: Associations with adolescents' reports of interpersonal behavior with parents and peers. *Journal of Social and Personal Relationships, 19,* 203–231.

Duemmler, S. L., & Kobak, R. (2001). The development of commitment and attachment in dating relationships: Attachment security as relationship construct. *Journal of Adolescence, 24,* 401–415.

Duggan, E., & Brennan, K. A. (1994). Social avoidance and its relation to Bartholomew's adult attachment typology. *Journal of Social and Personal Relationships, 11,* 147–153.

Dunkle, J. H. (1996). *The contribution of therapists' personal and professional characteristics to the strength of the therapeutic alliance.* Unpublished doctoral dissertation, State University of New York, Albany.

Dutton, D. G., & Browning, J. J. (1988). Concern for power, fear of intimacy, and wife abuse. In G. T. Hotaling, D. Finkelhor, J. T. Kirpatrick, & M. Straus (Eds.), *New directions in family violence research* (pp. 163–175). Beverly Hills, CA: Sage.

Dutton, D. G., Saunders, K., Starzomski, A., &

Bartholomew, K. (1994). Intimacy-anger and insecure attachment as precursors of abuse in intimate relationships. *Journal of Applied Social Psychology, 24*, 1367–1386.

Eagle, M. (1997). Attachment and psychoanalysis. *British Journal of Medical Psychology, 70*, 217–229.

Eames, V., & Roth, A. (2000). Patient attachment orientation and the early working alliance: A study of patient and therapist reports of alliance quality and ruptures. *Psychotherapy Research, 10*, 421–434.

Easterbrooks, M. (1989). Quality of attachment to mother and to father: Effects of perinatal risk status. *Child Development, 60*, 825–830.

Eberly, M. B., & Montemayor, R. (1998). Doing good deeds: An examination of adolescent prosocial behavior in the context of parent–adolescent relationships. *Journal of Adolescent Research, 13*, 403–432.

Eberly, M. B., & Montemayor, R. (1999). Adolescent affection and helpfulness toward parents: A 2-year follow-up. *Journal of Early Adolescence, 19*, 226–248.

Edelstein, R. S., Alexander, K. W., Shaver, P. R., Schaaf, J. M., Quas, J. A., Lovas, G. S., & Goodman, G. S. (2004). Adult attachment style and parental responsiveness during a stressful event. *Attachment and Human Development, 6*, 31–52.

Edelstein, R. S., Ghetti, S., Quas, J. A., Goodman, G. S., Alexander, K. W., Redlich, A. D., & Cordon, I. M. (2005). Individual differences in emotional memory: Adult attachment and long-term memory for child sexual abuse. *Personality and Social Psychology Bulletin, 31*, 1537–1548.

Edens, J. L., Larkin, K. T., & Abel, J. L. (1992). The effect of social support and physical touch on cardiovascular reactions to mental stress. *Journal of Psychosomatic Research, 36*, 371–381.

Edwards, E. P., Eiden, R. D., & Leonard, K. E. (2004). Impact of fathers' alcoholism and associated risk factors on parent–infant attachment stability from 12 to 18 months. *Infant Mental Health Journal, 25*, 556–579.

Egeland, B., & Farber, E. A. (1984). Infant–mother attachment: Factors related to its development and changes over time. *Child Development, 55*, 753–771.

Egeland, B., & Sroufe, L. A. (1981). Attachment and early maltreatment. *Child Development, 52*, 44–52.

Eiden, R. D., Teti, D. M., & Corns, K. M. (1995). Maternal working models of attachment, marital adjustment, and the parent–child relationship. *Child Development, 66*, 1504–1518.

Eisenberger, N. I., Lieberman, M. D., & Williams, K. D. (2003). Does rejection hurt?: An fMRI study of social exclusion. *Science, 302*, 290–292.

Ekman, P., & Friesen, W. Y. (1975). *Unmasking the face: A guide to recognizing emotions from facial clues*. Oxford, UK: Prentice-Hall.

El-Guebaly, N., West, M., Maticka-Tyndale, E., & Pool, M. (1993). Attachment among adult children of alcoholics. *Addiction, 88*, 1405–1411.

Elgar, F. J., Knight, J., Worrall, G. J., & Sherman, G.

(2003). Attachment characteristics and behavioural problems in rural and urban juvenile delinquents. *Child Psychiatry and Human Development, 34*, 35–48.

Elicker, J., Englund, M., & Sroufe, L. A. (1992). Predicting peer competence and peer relationships in childhood from early parent–child relationships. In R. D. Parke & G. W. Ladd (Eds.), *Family-peer relationships: Modes of linkage* (pp. 77–106). Hillsdale, NJ: Erlbaum

Elizur, Y., & Mintzer, A. (2001). A framework for the formation of gay male identity: Processes associated with adult attachment style and support from family and friends. *Archives of Sexual Behavior, 30*, 143–167.

Elizur, Y., & Mintzer, A. (2003). Gay males' intimate relationship quality: The roles of attachment security, gay identity, social support, and income. *Personal Relationships, 10*, 411–435.

Elliot, A. J., & Church, M. A. (1997). A hierarchical model of approach and avoidance achievement motivation. *Journal of Personality and Social Psychology, 72*, 218–232.

Elliot, A. J., & McGregor, H. A. (2001). A 2 x 2 achievement goal framework. *Journal of Personality and Social Psychology, 80*, 501–519.

Elliot, A. J., & Reis, H. T. (2003). Attachment and exploration in adulthood. *Journal of Personality and Social Psychology, 85*, 317–331.

Emilien, G., Penasse, C., Charles, G., Martin, D., Lasseaux, L., & Waltregny, A. (2000). Post-traumatic stress disorder: Hypotheses from clinical neuropsychology and psychopharmacology research. *International Journal of Psychiatry in Clinical Practice, 4*, 3–18.

Emmons, R. A. (1992). Abstract versus concrete goals: Personal striving level, physical illness, and psychological well-being. *Journal of Personality and Social Psychology, 62*, 292–300.

Emmons, R. A. (1997). Motives and goals. In R. Hogan, J. Johnson, & S. Briggs (Eds.), *Handbook of personality psychology* (pp. 485–512). New York: Academic Press.

Eng, W., Heimberg, R. G., Hart, T. A., Schneier, F. R., & Liebowitz, M. R. (2001). Attachment in individuals with social anxiety disorder: The relationship among adult attachment styles, social anxiety, and depression. *Emotion, 1*, 365–380.

Engels, C. M. E., Finkenauer, C., Meeus, W., & Dekovic, M. (2001). Parental attachment and adolescents' emotional adjustment: The associations with social skills and relational competence. *Journal of Counseling Psychology, 48*, 428–439.

Enns, M. W., Cox, B. J., & Clara, I. (2002). Parental bonding and adult psychopathology: Results from the US national comorbidity survey. *Psychological Medicine, 32*, 997–1008.

Epstein, S. (1983). *Scoring and interpretation of Mother–Father–Peer Scale*. Unpublished manuscript, University of Massachusetts, Amherst.

Epstein, S., & Meier, P. (1989). Constructive thinking: A broad coping variable with specific components. *Journal of Personality and Social Psychology, 57*, 332–350.

Ercolani, M., Farinelli, M., Trombini, E., &

Bortolotti, M. (2004). Gastroesophageal reflux disease: Attachment style and parental bonding. *Perceptual and Motor Skills, 99*, 211–222.

Erikson, E. H. (1959). *Identity and the life cycle*. New York: International Universities Press.

Erikson, E. H. (1968). *Identity: Youth and crisis*. New York: Norton.

Erikson, E. H. (1993). *Childhood and society*. New York: Norton. (Original work published 1950)

Ernst, J. M., & Cacioppo, J. T. (1999). Lonely hearts: Psychological perspectives on loneliness. *Applied and Preventive Psychology, 8*, 1–22.

Evans, C. R., & Dion, K. L. (1991). Group cohesion and group performance: A meta-analysis. *Small Group Research, 22*, 175–186.

Evans, L., & Wertheim, E. H. (1998). Intimacy patterns and relationship satisfaction of women with eating problems and the mediating effects of depression, trait anxiety and social anxiety. *Journal of Psychosomatic Research, 44*, 355–365.

Evans, L., & Wertheim, E. H. (2005). Attachment styles in adult intimate relationships: Comparing women with bulimia nervosa symptoms, women with depression, and women with no clinical symptoms. *European Eating Disorders Review, 13*, 285–293.

Exner, J. E., Jr. (1993). *The Rorschach: A comprehensive system: Vol. 1. Basic foundations* (3rd ed.). Oxford, UK: Wiley.

Fairbairn, W. R. D. (1954). *An object-relationships theory of the personality*. New York: Basic Books.

Faravelli, C., Webb, T., Ambronetti, A., Fonnesu, F., & Sesarego, A. (1985). Prevalence of traumatic early life events in 31 agoraphobic patients with panic attacks. *American Journal of Psychiatry, 142*, 1493–1494.

Farber, B. A., Lippert, R. A., & Nevas, D. B. (1995). The therapist as attachment figure. *Psychotherapy, 32*, 204–212.

Fass, M. E., & Tubman, J. G. (2002). The influence of parental and peer attachment on college students' academic achievement. *Psychology in the Schools, 39*, 561–574.

Feeney, B. C. (2004). A secure base: Responsive support of goal strivings and exploration in adult intimate relationships. *Journal of Personality and Social Psychology, 87*, 631–648.

Feeney, B. C. (2005). *Individual differences in secure base support provision: The role of attachment style, relationship characteristics, and underlying motivations*. Unpublished manuscript, Carnegie Mellon University, Pittsburgh, PA.

Feeney, B. C., & Cassidy, J. (2003). Reconstructive memory related to adolescent–parent conflict interactions: The influence of attachment-related representations on immediate perceptions and changes in perceptions over time. *Journal of Personality and Social Psychology, 85*, 945–955.

Feeney, B. C., & Collins, N. L. (2001). Predictors of caregiving in adult intimate relationships: An attachment theoretical perspective. *Journal of Personality and Social Psychology, 80*, 972–994.

Feeney, B. C., & Collins, N. L. (2003). Motivations for caregiving in adult intimate relationships: Influences on caregiving behavior and relationship functioning. *Personality and Social Psychology Bulletin, 29*, 950–968.

Feeney, B. C., & Collins, N. L. (2004). Interpersonal safe haven and secure base caregiving processes in adulthood. In W. S. Rholes & J. A. Simpson (Eds.), *Adult attachment: Theory, research, and clinical implications* (pp. 300–338). New York: Guilford Press.

Feeney, B. C., & Kirkpatrick, L. A. (1996). Effects of adult attachment and presence of romantic partners on physiological responses to stress. *Journal of Personality and Social Psychology, 70*, 255–270.

Feeney, J. A. (1994). Attachment style, communication patterns, and satisfaction across the life cycle of marriage. *Personal Relationships, 1*, 333–348.

Feeney, J. A. (1995a). Adult attachment and emotional control. *Personal Relationships, 2*, 143–159.

Feeney, J. A. (1995b). Adult attachment, coping style, and health locus of control as predictors of health behavior. *Australian Journal of Psychology, 47*, 171–177.

Feeney, J. A. (1996). Attachment, caregiving, and marital satisfaction. *Personal Relationships, 3*, 401–416.

Feeney, J. A. (1998). Adult attachment and relationship-centered anxiety: Responses to physical and emotional distancing. In J. A. Simpson & W. S. Rholes (Eds.), *Attachment theory and close relationships* (pp. 189–219). New York: Guilford Press.

Feeney, J. A. (1999a). Adult attachment, emotional control, and marital satisfaction. *Personal Relationships, 6*, 169–185.

Feeney, J. A. (1999b). Issues of closeness and distance in dating relationships: Effects of sex and attachment style. *Journal of Social and Personal Relationships, 16*, 571–590.

Feeney, J. A. (1999c). Adult romantic attachment and couple relationships. In J. Cassidy & P. R. Shaver (Eds.), *Handbook of attachment: Theory, research, and clinical applications* (pp. 355–377). New York: Guilford Press.

Feeney, J. A. (2002a). Attachment, marital interaction, and relationship satisfaction: A diary study. *Personal Relationships, 9*, 39–55.

Feeney, J. A. (2002b). Early parenting and parental attachment: Links with offspring's attachment and perceptions of social support. *Journal of Family Studies, 8*, 5–23.

Feeney, J. A. (2003). *The systemic nature of couple relationships: An attachment perspective*. In P. Erdman & T. Caffery (Eds.), *Attachment and family systems: Conceptual, empirical, and therapeutic relatedness* (pp. 139–164). New York: Brunner-Routledge.

Feeney, J. A. (2004a). Transfer of attachment from parents to romantic partners: Effects of individual and relationship variables. *Journal of Family Studies, 10*, 220–238.

Feeney, J. A. (2004b). Hurt feelings in couple relationships: Towards integrative models of the negative effects of hurtful events. *Journal of Social and Personal Relationships, 21*, 487–508.

Feeney, J. A. (2005). Hurt feelings in couple relationships: Exploring the role of attachment and perceptions of personal injury. *Personal Relationships, 12,* 253–271.

Feeney, J. A. (2006). Parental attachment and conflict behavior: Implications for offspring's attachment, loneliness, and relationship satisfaction. *Personal Relationships, 13,* 19–36.

Feeney, J. A., Alexander, R., Noller, P., & Hohaus, L. (2003). Attachment insecurity, depression, and the transition to parenthood. *Personal Relationships, 10,* 475–493.

Feeney, J. A., & Hohaus, L. (2001). Attachment and spousal caregiving. *Personal Relationships, 8,* 21–39.

Feeney, J. A., Hohaus, L., Noller, P., & Alexander, R. (2001). *Becoming parents: Exploring the bonds between mothers, fathers, and their infants.* Cambridge, UK: Cambridge University Press.

Feeney, J. A., & Humphreys, T. (1996). *Parental, sibling and romantic relationships: Exploring the functions of attachment bonds.* Paper presented at the fifth Australian Research Conference, Brisbane, Australia.

Feeney, J. A., Kelly, L., Gallois, C., Peterson, C., & Terry, D. J. (1999). Attachment style, assertive communication, and safer-sex behavior. *Journal of Applied Social Psychology, 29,* 1964–1983.

Feeney, J. A., & Noller, P. (1990). Attachment style as a predictor of adult romantic relationships. *Journal of Personality and Social Psychology, 58,* 281–291.

Feeney, J. A., & Noller, P. (1991). Attachment style and verbal descriptions of romantic partners. *Journal of Social and Personal Relationships, 8,* 187–215.

Feeney, J. A., & Noller, P. (1992). Attachment style and romantic love: Relationship dissolution. *Australian Journal of Psychology, 44,* 69–74.

Feeney, J. A., & Noller, P. (1996). *Adult attachment.* Thousand Oaks, CA: Sage.

Feeney, J. A., Noller, P., & Callan, V. J. (1994). Attachment style, communication, and satisfaction in the early years of marriage. In K. Bartholomew & D. Perlman (Eds.), *Advances in personal relationships: Attachment processes in adulthood* (Vol. 5, pp. 269–308). London: Jessica Kingsley.

Feeney, J. A., Noller, P., & Hanrahan, M. (1994). Assessing adult attachment. In M. B. Sperling & W. H. Berman (Eds.), *Attachment in adults: Clinical and developmental perspectives* (pp. 128–152). New York: Guilford Press.

Feeney, J. A., Noller, P., & Patty, J. (1993). Adolescents' interactions with the opposite sex: Influence of attachment style and gender. *Journal of Adolescence, 16,* 169–186.

Feeney, J. A., Passmore, N. L., & Peterson, C. (in press). Adoption, attachment and relationship concerns: A study of adult adoptees. *Personal Relationships.*

Feeney, J. A., Peterson, C., Gallois, C., & Terry, D. J. (2000). Attachment style as a predictor of sexual attitudes and behavior in late adolescence. *Psychology and Health, 14,* 1105–1122.

Feeney, J. A., & Ryan, S. M. (1994). Attachment style and affect regulation: Relationships with health behavior and family experiences of illness in a student sample. *Health Psychology, 13,* 334–345.

Feldman, G., & Hayes, A. (2005). Preparing for problems: A measure of mental anticipatory processes. *Journal of Research in Personality, 39,* 487–516.

Felsman, D. E., & Blustein, D. L. (1999). The role of peer relatedness in late adolescent career development. *Journal of Vocational Behavior, 54,* 279–295.

Festinger, L. (1957). A theory of cognitive dissonance. Evanston, IL: Row & Peterson.

Field, N. P., Nichols, C., Holen, A., & Horowitz, M. J. (1999). The relation of continuing attachment to adjustment in conjugal bereavement. *Journal of Consulting and Clinical Psychology, 67,* 212–218.

Field, N. P., & Sundin, E. C. (2001). Attachment style in adjustment to conjugal bereavement. *Journal of Social and Personal Relationships, 18,* 347–361.

Figley, C. R. (2002). Compassion fatigue and the psychotherapist's chronic lack of self-care. *Journal of Clinical Psychology, 58,* 1433–1441.

Finch, J. F., Okun, M. A., Pool, G. J., & Ruehlman, L. S. (1999). A comparison of the influence of conflictual and supportive social interactions on psychological distress. *Journal of Personality, 67,* 581–622.

Fincham, F. D. (2000). The kiss of the porcupines: From attributing responsibility to forgiving. *Personal Relationships, 7,* 1–23.

Fincham, F. D., & Beach, S. R. (1999). Marital conflict: Implications for working with couples. *Annual Review of Psychology, 50,* 47–77.

Finkel, D., & Matheny, A. P. (2000). Genetic and environmental influences on a measure of infant attachment security. *Twin Research, 3,* 242–250.

Finzi-Dottan, R., Cohen, O., Iwaniec, D., Sapir, Y., & Weizman, A. (2003). The drug-user husband and his wife: Attachment styles, family cohesion, and adaptability. *Substance Use and Misuse, 38,* 271–292.

Fischer, A. R., & Good, G. E. (1998). Perceptions of parent–child relationships and masculine role conflicts of college men. *Journal of Counseling Psychology, 45,* 346–352.

Fischer, K. W., Shaver, P. R., & Carnochan, P. (1990). How emotions develop and how they organize development. *Cognition and Emotion, 4,* 81–127.

Fisher, H. E. (1998). Lust, attraction, and attachment in mammalian reproduction. *Human Nature, 9,* 23–52.

Fisher, H. E., Aron, A., Mashek, D., Li, H., & Brown, L. L. (2002). Defining the brain systems of lust, romantic attraction, and attachment. *Archives of Sexual Behavior, 31,* 413–419.

Fishtein, J., Pietromonaco, P. R., & Feldman-Barrett, L. (1999). The contribution of attachment style and relationship conflict to the complexity of relationship knowledge. *Social Cognition, 17,* 228–244.

Fiske, S. T., & Taylor, S. E. (1991). *Social cognition.* New York: McGraw Hill.

Fitzpatrick, M. A., Fey, J., Segrin, C., & Schiff, J. L. (1993). Internal working models of relationships and marital communication. *Journal of Language and Social Psychology, 12,* 103–131.

Florian, V., & Kravetz, S. (1983). Fear of personal death: Attribution, structure, and relation to religious belief. *Journal of Personality and Social Psychology, 44,* 600–607.

Florian, V., & Mikulincer, M. (1998). Symbolic immortality and the management of the terror of death: The moderating role of attachment style. *Journal of Personality and Social Psychology, 74,* 725–734.

Florian, V., Mikulincer, M., & Bucholtz, I. (1995). Effects of adult attachment style on the perception and search for social support. *Journal of Psychology: Interdisciplinary and Applied, 129,* 665–676.

Florian, V., Mikulincer, M., & Hirschberger, G. (2002). The anxiety buffering function of close relationships: Evidence that relationship commitment acts as a terror management mechanism. *Journal of Personality and Social Psychology, 82,* 527–542.

Follingstad, D. R., Bradley, R. G., Helff, C. M., & Laughlin, J. E. (2002). A model for predicting dating violence: Anxious attachment, angry temperament, and need for relationship control. *Violence and Victims, 17,* 35–48.

Fonagy, P. (1996). The significance of the development of metacognitive control over mental representations in parenting and infant development. *Journal of Clinical Psychoanalysis, 5,* 67–86.

Fonagy, P., Leigh, T., Steele, M., Steele, H., Kennedy, R., Mattoon, G., et al. (1996). The relation of attachment status, psychiatric classification, and response to psychotherapy. *Journal of Consulting and Clinical Psychology, 64,* 22–31.

Fonagy, P., Steele, H., & Steele, M. (1991). Maternal representations of attachment during pregnancy predict the organization of infant–mother attachment at one year of age. *Child Development, 62,* 891–905.

Fonagy, P., Steele, M., Steele, H., Moran, G. S., & Higgitt, P. (1991). The capacity for understanding mental states: The reflective self in parent and child and its significance for security of attachment. *Infant Mental Health Journal, 12,* 201–218.

Fonagy, P., Target, M., Steele, H., & Steele, M. (1998). *Reflective-functioning manual for application to adult attachment interviews.* London: University College.

Fonagy, P., Target, M., Steele, M., Steele, H., Leigh, T., Levinson, A., & Kennedy., R. (1997). Morality, disruptive behavior, borderline personality disorder, crime, and their relationship to security of attachment. In L. Atkinson & K. J. Zucker (Eds.), *Attachment and psychopathology* (pp. 223–274). New York: Guilford Press.

Forgas, J. P. (1995). Mood and judgment: The affect infusion model (AIM). *Psychological Bulletin, 117,* 39–66.

Forsyth, D. R. (1990). *Group dynamics* (2nd ed.). Pacific Grove, CA: Brooks/Cole.

Foshee, V., & Bauman, K. E. (1994). Parental attachment and adolescent cigarette smoking initiation. *Journal of Adolescent Research, 9,* 88–104.

Fossati, A., Feeney, J. A., Carretta, I., Grazioli, F., Milesi, R., Leonardi, B., & Maffei, C. (2005). Modeling the relationships between adult attachment patterns and borderline personality disorder: The role of impulsivity and aggressiveness. *Journal of Social and Clinical Psychology, 24,* 520–537.

Fossati, A., Feeney, J. A., Donati, D., Donini, M., Novella, L., Bagnato, M., et al. (2003a). On the dimensionality of the Attachment Style Questionnaire in Italian clinical and nonclinical participants. *Journal of Social and Personal Relationships, 20,* 55–79.

Fossati, A., Feeney, J. A., Donati, D., Donini, M., Novella, L., Bagnato, M., et al. (2003b). Personality disorders and adult attachment dimensions in a mixed psychiatric sample: A multivariate study. *Journal of Nervous and Mental Disease, 191,* 30–37.

Fox, N. A., Kimmerly, N. L., & Schafer, W. D. (1991). Attachment to mother/attachment to father: A meta-analysis. *Child Development, 62,* 210–225.

Fraley, R. C. (2002). Attachment stability from infancy to adulthood: Meta-analysis and dynamic modeling of developmental mechanisms. *Personality and Social Psychology Review, 6,* 123–151.

Fraley, R. C., & Bonanno, G. A. (2004). Attachment and loss: A test of three competing models on the association between attachment-related avoidance and adaptation to bereavement. *Personality and Social Psychology Bulletin, 30,* 878–890.

Fraley, R. C., & Brumbaugh, C. C. (2004). A dynamical systems approach to conceptualizing and studying stability and change in attachment security. In W. S. Rholes & J. A. Simpson (Eds.), *Adult attachment: Theory, research, and clinical implications* (pp. 86–132). New York: Guilford Press.

Fraley, R. C., & Davis, K. E. (1997). Attachment formation and transfer in young adults' close friendships and romantic relationships. *Personal Relationships, 4,* 131–144.

Fraley, R. C., Fazzari, D. A., Bonanno, G. A., & Dekel, S. (2006). Attachment and psychological adaptation in high exposure survivors of the September 11th attack on the World Trade Center. *Personality and Social Psychology Bulletin, 32,* 538–551.

Fraley, R. C., Garner, J. P., & Shaver, P. R. (2000). Adult attachment and the defensive regulation of attention and memory: Examining the role of preemptive and postemptive defensive processes. *Journal of Personality and Social Psychology, 79,* 816–826.

Fraley, R. C., Niedenthal, P. M., Marks, M., Brumbaugh, C., & Vicary, A. (2006). Adult attachment and the perception of emotional expressions: Probing the hyperactivating strategies underlying anxious attachment. *Journal of Personality, 74,* 1163–1190.

Fraley, R. C., & Shaver, P. R. (1997). Adult attachment and the suppression of unwanted thoughts. *Journal of Personality and Social Psychology, 73,* 1080–1091.

Fraley, R. C., & Shaver, P. R. (1998). Airport separations: A naturalistic study of adult attachment dynamics in separating couples. *Journal of Personality and Social Psychology, 75,* 1198–1212.

Fraley, R. C., & Shaver, P. R. (1999). Loss and bereavement: Attachment theory and recent controversies concerning grief work and the nature of detachment. In J. Cassidy & P. R. Shaver (Eds.), *Handbook of attachment: Theory, research, and clinical applications* (pp. 735–759). New York: Guilford Press.

Fraley, R. C., & Shaver, P. R. (2000). Adult romantic attachment: Theoretical developments, emerging controversies, and unanswered questions. *Review of General Psychology, 4,* 132–154.

Fraley, R. C., & Spieker, S. J. (2003a). Are infant attachment patterns continuously or categorically distributed?: A taxometric analysis of strange situation behavior. *Developmental Psychology, 39,* 387–404.

Fraley, R. C., & Spieker, S. J. (2003b). What are the differences between dimensional and categorical models of individual differences in attachment?: Reply to Cassidy (2003), Cummings (2003), Sroufe (2003), and Waters and Beauchaine (2003). *Developmental Psychology, 39,* 423–429.

Fraley, R. C., & Waller, N. G. (1998). Adult attachment patterns: A test of the typological model. In J. A. Simpson & W. S. Rholes (Eds.), *Attachment theory and close relationships* (pp. 77–114). New York: Guilford Press.

Fraley, R. C., Waller, N. G., & Brennan, K. A. (2000). An item response theory analysis of self-report measures of adult attachment. *Journal of Personality and Social Psychology, 78,* 350–365.

Frazier, P. A., Byer, A. L., Fischer, A. R., Wright, D. M., & DeBord, K. A. (1996). Adult attachment style and partner choice: Correlational and experimental findings. *Personal Relationships, 3,* 117–136.

Frazier, P. A., & Cook, S. W. (1993). Correlates of distress following heterosexual relationship dissolution. *Journal of Social and Personal Relationships, 10,* 55–67.

Fredrickson, B. L. (2001). The role of positive emotions in positive psychology: The broaden-and-build theory of positive emotions. *American Psychologist, 56,* 218–226.

Freeman, H., & Brown, B. (2001). Primary attachment to parents and peers during adolescence: Differences by attachment style. *Journal of Youth and Adolescence, 30,* 653–674.

Frei, J. R., & Shaver, P. R. (2002). Respect in close relationships: Prototype definition, self-report assessment, and initial correlates. *Personal Relationships, 9,* 121–139.

Freud, S. (1953). Fragment of an analysis of a case of hysteria, In J. Strachey (Ed., & Trans.), *The standard edition of the complete psychological works of Sigmund Freud* (Vol. 7, pp. 15–122). London: Hogarth Press. (Original work published 1905)

Freud, S. (1955). *Totem and taboo.* In J. Strachey (Ed. & Trans.), *The standard edition of the complete psychological works of Sigmund Freud* (Vol. 13). London: Hogarth Press. (Original work published 1913)

Freud, S. (1957). Instincts and their vicissitudes. In J. Strachey (Ed. & Trans.), *The standard edition of the complete psychological works of Sigmund Freud* (Vol. 3, pp. 157–186). London: Hogarth Press. (Original work published 1915)

Freud, S. (1959). The future prospects of psychoanalytic counseling. In J. Reviere (Ed. & Trans.), *Sigmund Freud: Collected papers II* (pp. 285–296).

New York: Basic Books. (Original work published 1910)

Freud, S. (1961). Address delivered at the Goethe House at Frankfurt. In J. Strachey (Ed. & Trans.), *The standard edition of the complete psychological works of Sigmund Freud* (Vol. 22, pp. 208–212). London: Hogarth Press. (Original work published 1930)

Freud, S. (1963). Introductory lectures on psychoanalysis. In J. Strachey (Ed. & Trans.), *The standard edition of the complete psychological works of Sigmund Freud* (Vols. 15 & 16). London: Hogarth Press. (Original work published 1917)

Freud, S. (1975). *The future of an Illusion* (J. Strachey, Trans.). New York: Random House. (Original work published 1927)

Freud, S. (1994). *The interpretation of dreams.* (A. A. Brill, Trans.). New York: Barnes & Noble. (Original work published 1911)

Fricker, J., & Moore, S. (2002). Relationship satisfaction: The role of love styles and attachment styles. *Current Research in Social Psychology, 7,* 182–204.

Friedberg, N. L., & Lyddon, W. J. (1996). Self–other working models and eating disorders. *Journal of Cognitive Psychotherapy, 10,* 193–203.

Frijda, N. H. (1986). *The emotions.* New York: Cambridge University Press.

Fritsch, R. C., & Goodrich, W. (1990). Adolescent inpatient attachment as treatment process. In S. C. Feinstein (Ed.), *Adolescent psychiatry: Developmental and clinical studies* (Vol. 17, pp. 246–263). Chicago: University of Chicago Press.

Fritz, H., & Helgeson, V. S. (1998). Distinctions of unmitigated communion from communion: Self-neglect and over-involvement with others. *Journal of Personality and Social Psychology, 75,* 121–140.

Frodi, A., Dernevik, M., Sepa, A., Philipson, J., & Bragesjo, M. (2001). Current attachment representations of incarcerated offenders varying in degree of psychopathy. *Attachment and Human Development, 3,* 269–283.

Fuller, T. L., & Fincham, F. D. (1995). Attachment style in married couples: Relation to current marital functioning, stability over time, and method of assessment. *Personal Relationships, 2,* 17–34.

Funder, D. C., & Colvin, C. R. (1988). Friends and strangers: Acquaintanceship, agreement, and the accuracy of personality judgment. *Journal of Personality and Social Psychology, 55,* 149–158.

Furman, W., Simon, V. A., Shaffer, L., & Bouchey, H. A. (2002). Adolescents' working models and styles for relationships with parents, friends, and romantic partners. *Child Development, 73,* 241–255.

Futterman, A., Gallagher, D., Thompson, L. W., & Lovett, S. (1990). Retrospective assessment of marital adjustment and depression during the first 2 years of spousal bereavement. *Psychology and Aging, 5,* 273–280.

Fyffe, C., & Waters, E. (1997, March). *Empirical classification of adult attachment status: Predicting group membership.* Poster presented at the biennial meeting of the Society for Research in Child Development, Washington, DC.

Gabbard, G. O. (1998). Transference and countertransference in the treatment of narcissistic patients. In E. F. Ronningstam (Ed.), *Disorders of narcissism: Diagnostic, clinical, and empirical implications* (pp. 125–145). Washington, DC: American Psychiatric Association.

Gabbard, G. O. (2001). A contemporary psychoanalytic model of countertransference. *Journal of Clinical Psychology, 57*, 983–992.

Gable, S. L., & Haidt, J. (2005). What (and why) is positive psychology? *Review of General Psychology, 9*, 103–110.

Gabriel, S., Carvallo, M., Dean, K. K., Tippin, B., & Renaud, J. (2005). How I see me depends on how I see we: The role of attachment style in social comparison. *Personality and Social Psychology Bulletin, 31*, 1561–1572.

Gaines, S. O., Jr., Granrose, C. S., Rios, D. I., Garcia, B. F., Youn, M. S., Farris, K. R., & Bledsoe, K. L. (1999). Patterns of attachment and responses to accommodative dilemmas among interethnic/interracial couples. *Journal of Social and Personal Relationships, 16*, 275–285.

Gaines, S. O., Jr., & Henderson, M. C. (2002). Impact of attachment style on responses to accommodative dilemmas among same-sex couples. *Personal Relationships, 9*, 89–93.

Gaines, S. O., Jr., Reis, H. T., Summers, S., Rusbult, C. E., Cox, C. L., Wexler, M. O., et al. (1997). Impact of attachment style on reactions to accommodative dilemmas in close relationships. *Personal Relationships, 4*, 93–113.

Gaines, S. O., Jr., Work, C., Johnson, H., Youn, M. S. P., & Lai, K. (2000). Impact of attachment style and self-monitoring on individuals' responses to accommodative dilemmas across relationship types. *Journal of Social and Personal Relationships, 17*, 767–789.

Gallo, L. C., & Matthews, K. A. (2006). Adolescents' attachment orientation influences ambulatory blood pressure responses to everyday social interactions. *Psychosomatic Medicine, 68*, 253–261.

Gallo, L. C., & Smith, T. W. (2001). Attachment style in marriage: Adjustment and responses to interaction. *Journal of Social and Personal Relationships, 18*, 263–289.

Gallo, L. C., Smith, T. W., & Ruiz, J. M. (2003). An interpersonal analysis of adult attachment style: Circumplex descriptions, recalled developmental experiences, self-representations, and interpersonal functioning in adulthood. *Journal of Personality, 71*, 141–181.

Gamble, S. A., & Roberts, J. E. (2005). Adolescents' perceptions of primary caregivers and cognitive style: The roles of attachment security and gender. *Cognitive Therapy and Research, 29*, 123–141.

Gangestad, S. W., Simpson, J. A., Cousins, A. J., Garver-Apgar, C. E., & Christensen, P. N. (2004). Women's preferences for male behavioral displays. *Psychological Science, 15*, 203–206.

Gangestad, S. W., & Thornhill, R. (1997). The evolutionary psychology of extra-pair sex: The role of fluctuating asymmetry. *Evolution and Human Behavior, 18*, 69–88.

Gaston, L., Marmar, C. R., Thompson, L. W., & Gallagher, D. (1988). Relation of patient pretreat-

ment characteristics to the therapeutic alliance in diverse psychotherapies. *Journal of Consulting and Clinical Psychology, 56*, 483–489.

Geller, J. D., & Farber, B. A. (1993). Factors influencing the process of internalization in psychotherapy. *Psychotherapy Research, 3*, 166–180.

Gelso, C. J., & Carter, J. A. (1985). The relationship in counseling and psychotherapy: Components, consequences, and theoretical antecedents. *Counseling Psychologist, 13*, 155–243.

Gentzler, A. L., & Kerns, K. A. (2004). Associations between insecure attachment and sexual experiences. *Personal Relationships, 11*, 249–265.

Gentzler, A. L., & Kerns, K. A. (2006). Adult attachment and memory of emotional reactions to negative and positive events. *Cognition and Emotion, 20*, 20–42.

George, C., Kaplan, N., & Main, M. (1985). *The Adult Attachment Interview*. Unpublished protocol, Department of Psychology, University of California, Berkeley.

George, C., & Solomon, J. (1999). Attachment and caregiving: The caregiving behavioral system. In J. Cassidy & P. R. Shaver (Eds.), *Handbook of attachment: Theory, research, and clinical applications* (pp. 649–670). New York: Guilford Press.

George, C., & West, M. (2001). The development and preliminary validation of a new measure of adult attachment: The Adult Attachment Projective. *Attachment and Human Development, 3*, 30–61.

Gerlsma, C., Buunk, B. P., & Mutsaers, W. C. M. (1996). Correlates of self-reported adult attachment styles in a Dutch sample of married men and women. *Journal of Social and Personal Relationships, 13*, 313–320.

Gerlsma, C., & Luteijn, F. (2000). Attachment style in the context of clinical and health psychology: A proposal for the assessment of valence, incongruence, and accessibility of attachment representations in various working models. *British Journal of Medical Psychology, 73*, 15–34.

Germer, C. K., Siegel, R. D., & Fulton, P. R. (Eds.). (2005). *Mindfulness and psychotherapy*. New York: Guilford Press.

Gerstel, N., & Gross, H. (1984). *Commuter marriage*. New York: Guilford Press.

Gilad, G. (2002). *The integration of object relations theory and attachment theory: Object representations in the Thematic Apperception Test*. Unpublished master's thesis, Bar-Ilan University, Ramat Gan, Israel.

Gillath, O. (2003). *An analysis of the sub-goals of the sexual behavioral system*. Unpublished PhD dissertation, Bar-Ilan University, Ramat Gan, Israel.

Gillath, O., Bunge, S. A., Shaver, P. R., Wendelken, C., & Mikulincer, M. (2005). Attachment-style differences in the ability to suppress negative thoughts: Exploring the neural correlates. *NeuroImage, 28*, 835–847.

Gillath, O., & Schachner, D. A. (2006). How do sexuality and attachment interact?: Goals, motives, and strategies. In M. Mikulincer & G. S. Goodman (Eds.), *Dynamics of love: Attachment, caregiving, and sex* (pp. 337–355). New York: Guilford Press.

Gillath, O., Shaver, P. R., Mendoza, S. P., Maninger, N., & Ferrer, E. (2006, January). *Changes in salivary cortisol concentration as a function of attachment style and attachment-related emotional states.* Paper presented at the annual meeting of the Society for Personality and Social Psychology, Palm Springs, CA.

Gillath, O., Shaver, P. R., & Mikulincer, M. (2005). An attachment-theoretical approach to compassion and altruism. In P. Gilbert (Ed.), *Compassion: Conceptualizations, research, and use in psychotherapy* (pp. 121–147). London: Brunner-Routledge.

Gillath, O., Shaver, P. R., Mikulincer, M., Nitzberg, R. A., Erez, A., & van IJzendoorn, M. H. (2005). Attachment, caregiving, and volunteering: Placing volunteerism in an attachment-theoretical framework. *Personal Relationships, 12,* 425–446.

Gittleman, M. G., Klein, M. H., Smider, N. A., & Essex, M. J. (1998). Recollections of parental behavior, adult attachment, and mental health: Mediating and moderating effects. *Psychological Medicine, 28,* 1443–1455.

Gjerde, P. F., Onishi, M., & Carlson, K. S. (2004). Personality characteristics associated with romantic attachment: A comparison of interview and self-report methodologies. *Personality and Social Psychology Bulletin, 30,* 1402–1415.

Glachan, M. D., & Ney, J. (1995). First time mothers' attachment styles and their experience and management of emotional distress in themselves and their infant. *Early Child Development and Care, 105,* 21–32.

Gleason, T. R. (2002). Social provisions of real and imaginary relationships in early childhood. *Developmental Psychology, 38,* 979–992.

Gloger-Tippelt, G., Gomille, B., Koenig, L., & Vetter, J. (2002). Attachment representations in 6-year-olds: Related longitudinally to the quality of attachment in infancy and mothers' attachment representations. *Attachment and Human Development, 4,* 318–339.

Goldberg, S., Benoit, D., Blockland, K., & Madigan, S. (2003). Atypical maternal behavior, maternal representations, and infant disorganized attachment. *Development and Psychopathology, 15,* 239–257.

Goldsmith, H. H., & Alansky, J. A. (1987). Maternal and infant temperamental predictors of attachment: A meta-analytic review. *Journal of Consulting and Clinical Psychology, 55,* 805–816.

Goldwyn, R., Stanley, C., Smith, V., & Green, J. (2000). The Manchester Child Attachment Story Task: Relationship with parental AAI, SAT, and child behavior. *Attachment and Human Development, 2,* 71–84.

Goodman, G. S., Quas, J. A., Batterman-Faunce, J. M., Riddlesberger, M. M., & Kuhn, J. (1997). Children's reactions to and memory for a stressful event: Influences of age, anatomical dolls, knowledge, and parental attachment. *Applied Developmental Science, 1,* 54–75.

Goodwin, I., Holmes, G., Cochrane, R., & Mason, O. (2003). The ability of adult mental health services to meet clients' attachment needs: The development and implementation of the Service Attachment Questionnaire. *Psychology and Psychotherapy, 76,* 145–161.

Goosens, L., Marcoen, A., van Hees, S., & van de Woestijne, O. (1998). Attachment style and loneliness in adolescence. *European Journal of Psychology of Education, 13,* 529–542.

Gore, J. S., Cross, S. E., & Morris, M. L. (2006). Let's be friends: Relational self-construal and the development of intimacy. *Personal Relationships, 13,* 83–102.

Gotlib, I. H., & Hammen, C. L. (1992). *Psychological aspects of depression: Toward a cognitive-interpersonal integration.* New York: Wiley.

Gotlib, I. H., Mount, J. H., Cordy, N. I., & Whiffen, V. E. (1988). Depression and perceptions of early parenting: A longitudinal investigation. *British Journal of Psychiatry, 152,* 24–27.

Gottman, J. M. (1994). *What predicts divorce?: The relationship between marital processes and marital outcomes.* Hillsdale, NJ: Erlbaum.

Gottman, J. M., & Declaire, J. (1998). *Raising an emotionally intelligent child.* New York: Simon & Schuster.

Grabill, C. M., & Kerns, K. A. (2000). Attachment style and intimacy in friendship. *Personal Relationships, 7,* 363–378.

Granqvist, P. (1998). Religiousness and perceived childhood attachment: On the question of compensation or correspondence. *Journal for the Scientific Study of Religion, 37,* 350–367.

Granqvist, P. (2002). Attachment and religiosity in adolescence: Cross-sectional and longitudinal evaluations. *Personality and Social Psychology Bulletin, 28,* 260–270.

Granqvist, P. (2005). Building a bridge between attachment and religious coping: Tests of moderators and mediators. *Mental Health, Religion, and Culture, 8,* 35–47.

Granqvist, P., & Hagekull, B. (1999). Religiousness and perceived childhood attachment: Profiling socialized correspondence and emotional compensation. *Journal for the Scientific Study of Religion, 38,* 254–273.

Granqvist, P., & Hagekull, B. (2000). Religiosity, adult attachment, and why "singles" are more religious. *International Journal for the Psychology of Religion, 10,* 111–123.

Granqvist, P., & Hagekull, B. (2001). Seeking security in the new age: On attachment and emotional compensation. *Journal for the Scientific Study of Religion, 40,* 529–547.

Granqvist, P., & Hagekull, B. (2003). Longitudinal predictions of religious change in adolescence: Contributions from the interaction of attachment and relationship status. *Journal of Social and Personal Relationships, 20,* 793–817.

Granqvist, P., & Hagekull, B. (2005). *Religiosity and the Adult Attachment Interview: Probable experiences, state of mind, and two religious profiles.* Unpublished manuscript, Uppsala University, Sweden.

Granqvist, P., & Kirkpatrick, L. A. (2004). Religious conversion and perceived childhood attachment: A meta-analysis. *International Journal for the Psychology of Religion, 14,* 223–250.

Granqvist, P., Lantto, S., Ortiz, L., & Andersson, G. (2001). Adult attachment, perceived family support, and problems experienced by tinnitus patients. *Psychology and Health, 16,* 357–366.

Grau, I., & Doll, J. (2003). Effects of attachment styles on the experience of equity in heterosexual couples relationships. *Experimental Psychology, 50,* 298–310.

Gray, J. A. (1982). *The neuropsychology of anxiety: An enquiry into the functions of the septo-hippocampal system.* New York: Oxford University Press

Gray, J. A. (1987). *The psychology of fear and stress* (2nd ed.). Cambridge, UK: Cambridge University Press.

Gray, J. D., & Silver, R. C. (1990). Opposite sides of the same coin: Former spouses' divergent perspectives in coping with their divorce. *Journal of Personality and Social Psychology, 59,* 1180–1191.

Graziano, W. G., & Tobin, R. M. (2002). Agreeableness: Dimension of personality or social desirability artifact? *Journal of Personality, 70,* 695–727.

Green, A. (1986). *On private madness.* New York: International Universities Press.

Green, J. D., & Campbell, W. (2000). Attachment and exploration in adults: Chronic and contextual accessibility. *Personality and Social Psychology Bulletin, 26,* 452–461.

Green-Hennessy, S., & Reis, H. T. (1998). Openness in processing social information among attachment types. *Personal Relationships, 5,* 449–466.

Greenberg, J., Koole, S. L., & Pyszczynski, T. (Eds.). (2004). *Handbook of experimental existential psychology.* New York: Guilford Press.

Greenberg, J., Pyszczynski, T., & Solomon, S. (1997). Terror management theory of self-esteem and cultural worldviews: Empirical assessments and conceptual refinements. In M. P. Zanna (Ed.), *Advances in experimental social psychology* (Vol. 29, pp. 61–141). San Diego: Academic Press.

Greenberg, J., Pyszczynski, T., Solomon, S., Simon, L., & Breus, M. (1994). The role of consciousness and accessibility of death related thoughts in mortality salience effects. *Journal of Personality and Social Psychology, 67,* 627–637.

Greenberg, J. R., & Mitchell, S. A. (1983). *Object relations in psychoanalytic theory.* Cambridge, MA: Harvard University Press.

Greenberg, M. T., & Speltz, M. L. (1988). Contributions of attachment theory to the understanding of conduct problems during the preschool years. In J. Belsky & T. Nezworski (Eds.), *Clinical implications of attachment* (pp. 177–218). Hillsdale, NJ: Erlbaum.

Greenberger, E., & McLaughlin, C. S. (1998). Attachment, coping, and explanatory style in late adolescence. *Journal of Youth and Adolescence, 27,* 121–139.

Greenfield, S., & Thelen, M. (1997). Validation of the fear of intimacy scale with a lesbian and gay male population. *Journal of Social and Personal Relationships, 14,* 707–716.

Greenson, R. R. (1967). *The technique and practice of psychoanalysis* (Vol. 1). Madison, CT: International Universities Press.

Greenwald, A. G., McGhee, D. E., & Schwartz, J. L. K. (1998). Measuring individual differences in implicit cognition: The Implicit Association Test. *Journal of Personality and Social Psychology, 74,* 1464–1480.

Griffin, D. W., & Bartholomew, K. (1994a). The metaphysics of measurement: The case of adult attachment. In K. Bartholomew & D. Perlman (Eds.), *Advances in personal relationships: Attachment processes in adulthood* (Vol. 5, pp. 17–52). London: Jessica Kingsley.

Griffin, D. W., & Bartholomew, K. (1994b). Models of the self and other: Fundamental dimensions underlying measures of adult attachment. *Journal of Personality and Social Psychology, 67,* 430–445.

Gross, C. A., & Hansen, N. E. (2000). Clarifying the experience of shame: The role of attachment style, gender, and investment in relatedness. *Personality and Individual Differences, 28,* 897–907.

Gross, J. J. (1999). Emotion and emotion regulation. In O. P. John & L. A. Pervin (Eds.), *Handbook of personality: Theory and research* (2nd ed., pp. 525–552). New York: Guilford Press.

Gross J. J. (Ed.). (2007). *Handbook of emotion regulation.* New York: Guilford Press.

Grossmann, K., Fremmer-Bombik, E., Rudolph, J., & Grossmann, K. E. (1988). Maternal attachment representations as related to patterns of infant–mother attachment and maternal care during the first year. In R. A. Hinde & J. Stevenson-Hinde (Eds.), *Relationships within families* (pp. 241–260). Oxford, UK: Oxford Science Publications.

Grossmann, K., & Grossmann, K. E. (1991). Newborn behavior, early parenting quality, and later toddler–parent relationships in a group of German infants. In J. K. Nugent, B. M. Lester, & T. B. Brazelton (Eds.), *The cultural context of infancy* (pp. 3–38). Norwood, NJ: Ablex.

Grossmann, K., Grossmann, K. E., & Kindler, H. (2005). Early care and the roots of attachment and partnership representations: The Bielefeld and Regensburg longitudinal studies. In K. E. Grossmann, K. Grossmann, & E. Waters (Eds.), *Attachment from infancy to adulthood: The major longitudinal studies* (pp. 98–136). New York: Guilford Press.

Grossmann, K., Grossmann, K. E., & Zimmermann, P. (1999). A wider view of attachment and exploration: Stability and change during the years of immaturity. In J. Cassidy & P. R. Shaver (Eds.), *Handbook of attachment: Theory, research, and clinical applications* (pp. 760–786). New York: Guilford Press.

Grossmann, K. E., Grossmann, K., & Waters, E. (Eds.). (2005). *Attachment from infancy to adulthood: The major longitudinal studies.* New York: Guilford Press.

Guerrero, L. K. (1996). Attachment-style differences in intimacy and involvement: A test of the four-category model. *Communication Monographs, 63,* 269–292.

Guerrero, L. K. (1998). Attachment-style differences in the experience and expression of romantic jealousy. *Personal Relationships, 5,* 273–291.

Guerrero, L. K., & Burgoon, J. K. (1996). Attachment styles and reactions to nonverbal involvement change in romantic dyads: Patterns of reciprocity and compensation. *Human Communication Research, 22,* 335–370.

Guerrero, L. K., & Jones, S. M. (2003). Differences in one's own and one's partner's perceptions of social skills as a function of attachment style. *Communication Quarterly, 51,* 277–295.

Guidano, V. F. (1987). *Complexity of the self: A developmental approach to psychopathology and therapy.* New York: Guilford Press.

Gump, B. B., Polk, D. E., Kamarck, T. W., & Shiffman, S. M. (2001). Partner interactions are associated with reduced blood pressure in the natural environment: Ambulatory monitoring evidence from a healthy, multiethnic adult sample. *Psychosomatic Medicine, 63,* 423–433.

Gunnar, M. R. (2005). Attachment and stress in early development: Does attachment add to the potency of social regulators of infant stress? In C. S. Carter, L. Ahnert, K. E. Grossmann, S. B. Hrdy, M. E. Lamb, S. W. Porges, et al. (Eds.), *Attachment and bonding: A new synthesis* (pp. 245–256). Cambridge, MA: MIT Press.

Gur, O. (2006). *Changes in adjustment and attachment-related representations among high-risk adolescents during residential treatment: The transformational impact of the functioning of caregiving figures as a secure base.* Unpublished doctoral dissertation, Bar-Ilan University, Ramat Gan, Israel.

Gurwitz, V. (2004). *Working models of God and their accessibility in times of stress.* Unpublished doctoral dissertation, Bar-Ilan University, Ramat Gan, Israel.

Guterman, O. (2006). *Adult attachment style and sensitivity to non-verbal expressions of emotions: The facilitating role of attachment security.* Unpublished doctoral dissertation, Bar-Ilan University, Ramat Gan, Israel.

Gutzwiller, J., Oliver, J. M., & Katz, B. M. (2003). Eating dysfunctions in college women: The roles of depression and attachment to fathers. *Journal of American College Health, 52,* 27–32.

Gwadz, M. V., Clatts, M. C., Leonard, N. R., & Goldsamt, L. (2004). Attachment style, childhood adversity, and behavioral risk among young men who have sex with men. *Journal of Adolescent Health, 34,* 402–413.

Haaga, D. F., Yarmus, M., Hubbard, S., Brody, C., Solomon, A., Kirk, L., & Chamberlain, J. (2002). Mood dependency of self-rated attachment style. *Cognitive Therapy and Research, 26,* 57–71.

Haft, W. L., & Slade, A. (1989). Affect attunement and maternal attachment: A pilot study. *Infant Mental Health Journal, 10,* 157–172.

Haigler, V. F., Day, H. D., & Marshall, D. D. (1995). Parental attachment and gender-role identity. *Sex Roles, 33,* 203–220.

Hamilton, C. E. (2000). Continuity and discontinuity of attachment from infancy through adolescence. *Child Development, 71,* 690–694.

Hamilton, W. D. (1964). The genetic evolution of social behavior. *Journal of Theoretical Biology, 7,* 1–52.

Hammen, C. L. (1991). *Depression runs in families: The social context of risk and resilience in children of depressed mothers.* New York: Springer.

Hammen, C. L., Burge, D., Daley, S. E., Davila, J., Parley, B., & Rudolph, K. D. (1995). Interpersonal attachment cognitions and prediction of symptomatic responses to interpersonal stress. *Journal of Abnormal Psychology, 104,* 436–443.

Hammond, J. R., & Fletcher, G. J. (1991). Attachment styles and relationship satisfaction in the development of close relationships. *New Zealand Journal of Psychology, 20,* 56–62.

Hankin, B. L., Kassel, J. D., & Abela, J. R. Z. (2005). Adult attachment dimensions and specificity of emotional distress symptoms: Prospective investigations of cognitive risk and interpersonal stress generation as mediating mechanisms. *Personality and Social Psychology Bulletin, 31,* 136–151.

Harari, D., Furst, M., Kiryati, N., Caspi, A., & Davidson, M. (2001). A computer-based method for the assessment of body image distortions in anorexia-nervosa patients. *IEEE Transactions on Information Technology in Biomedicine, 5,* 311–319.

Hardy, G. E., Aldridge, J., Davidson, C., Rowe, C., Reilly, S., & Shapiro, D. A. (1999). Therapist responsiveness to client attachment styles and issues observed in client-identified significant events in psychodynamic-interpersonal psychotherapy. *Psychotherapy Research, 9,* 36–53.

Hardy, G. E., & Barkham, M. (1994). The relationship between interpersonal attachment styles and work difficulties. *Human Relations, 47,* 263–281.

Hardy, G. E., Cahill, J., Shapiro, D. A., Barkham, M., Rees, A., & Macaskill, N. (2001). Client interpersonal and cognitive styles as predictors of response to time-limited cognitive therapy for depression. *Journal of Clinical and Consulting Psychology, 69,* 841–845.

Harlow, H. F. (1959). Love in infant monkeys. *Scientific American, 200,* 68–86.

Harpaz-Rotem, I., & Blatt, S. J. (2005). Changes in representations of a self-designated significant other in long-term intensive inpatient treatment of seriously disturbed adolescents and young adults. *Psychiatry, 68,* 266–282.

Harris, T. O., Brown, G. W., & Bifulco, A. (1986). Loss of parent in childhood and adult psychiatric disorder: The Walthamstow study: 1. The role of lack of adequate parental care. *Psychological Medicine, 16,* 641–659.

Harris, T. O., Brown, G. W., & Bifulco, A. (1990). Depression and situational helplessness/mastery in a sample selected to study childhood parental loss. *Journal of Affective Disorders, 20,* 27–41.

Hart, J. J., Shaver, P. R., & Goldenberg, J. L. (2005). Attachment, self-esteem, worldviews, and terror management: Evidence for a tripartite security system. *Journal of Personality and Social Psychology, 88,* 999–1013.

Harvey, M., & Byrd, M. (2000). Relationships between adolescents' attachment styles and family functioning. *Adolescence, 35,* 345–356.

Harwood, I. (2003). Distinguishing between the facilitating and the self-serving charismatic group leader. *Group, 27,* 121–129.

Hayashi, G. M., & Strickland, B. R. (1998). Long-term effects of parental divorce on love relationships: Divorce as attachment disruption. *Journal of Social and Personal Relationships, 15,* 23–38.

Hazan, C., & Shaver, P. R. (1987). Romantic love conceptualized as an attachment process. *Journal of Personality and Social Psychology, 52,* 511–524.

Hazan, C., & Shaver, P. R. (1990). Love and work: An attachment-theoretical perspective. *Journal of Personality and Social Psychology, 59,* 270–280.

Hazan, C., & Shaver, P. R. (1994). Attachment as an organizational framework for research on close relationships. *Psychological Inquiry, 5,* 1–22.

Hazan, C., & Zeifman, D. (1994). Sex and the psychological tether. In K. Bartholomew & D. Perlman (Eds.), *Advances in personal relationships: Attachment processes in adulthood* (Vol. 5, pp. 151–177). London: Jessica Kingsley.

Hazan, C., & Zeifman, D. (1999). Pair-bonds as attachments: Evaluating the evidence. In J. Cassidy & P. R. Shaver (Eds.), *Handbook of attachment: Theory, research, and clinical applications* (pp. 336–354). New York: Guilford Press.

Hazan, C., Zeifman, D., & Middleton, K. (1994, July). *Adult romantic attachment, affection, and sex.* Paper presented at the 7th International Conference on Personal Relationships, Groninger, The Netherlands.

Hazen, N. L., & Durrett, M. E. (1982). Relationship of security of attachment and cognitive mapping abilities in 2-year-olds. *Development Psychology, 18,* 751–759.

Heaven, P. C. L., Da Silva, T., Carey, C., & Holen, J. (2004). Loving styles: Relationships with personality and attachment styles. *European Journal of Personality, 18,* 103–113.

Heaven, P. C. L., Mak, A., Barry, J., & Ciarrochi, J. (2002). Personality and family influences on adolescent attitudes to school and self-rated academic performance. *Personality and Individual Differences, 32,* 453–462.

Heene, E. L. D., Buysse, A., & Van Oost, P. (2005). Indirect pathways between depressive symptoms and marital distress: The role of conflict communication, attributions, and attachment style. *Family Process, 44,* 413–440.

Heider, F. (1958). *The psychology of interpersonal relations.* New York: Wiley.

Heinicke, C., & Westheimer, I. (1966). *Brief separations.* New York: International Universities Press.

Heinonen, K., Raikkonen, K., Keltikangas-Jarvinen, L., & Strandberg, T. (2004). Adult attachment dimensions and recollections of childhood family context: Associations with dispositional optimism and pessimism. *European Journal of Personality, 18,* 193–207.

Henderson, A. J. Z., Bartholomew, K., & Dutton, D. G. (1997). He loves me; he loves me not: Attachment and separation resolution of abused women. *Journal of Family Violence, 12,* 169–191.

Henderson, A. J. Z., Bartholomew, K., Trinke, S., & Kwong, M. J. (2005). When loving means hurting: An exploration of attachment and intimate abuse in a community sample. *Journal of Family Violence, 20,* 219–230.

Hendin, H. M., & Cheek, J. M. (1997). Assessing hypersensitive narcissism: A reexamination of Murray's Narcissism Scale. *Journal of Personality and Social Psychology, 31,* 588–599.

Hendrick, C., & Hendrick, S. S. (1986). A theory and method of love. *Journal of Personality and Social Psychology, 50,* 392–402.

Hendrick, C., & Hendrick, S. S. (1989). Research on love: Does it measure up? *Journal of Personality and Social Psychology, 56,* 784–794.

Hennighausen, K. H., & Lyons-Ruth, K. (2005). Disorganization of behavioral and attentional strategies toward primary attachment figures: From biologic to dialogic processes. In C. S. Carter et al. (Eds.), *Attachment and bonding: A new synthesis* (pp. 269–299). Cambridge, MA: MIT Press.

Henry, K., & Holmes, J. G. (1998). Childhood revisited: The intimate relationships of individuals from divorced and conflict-ridden families. In J.A. Simpson & W. S. Rholes (Eds.), *Attachment theory and close relationships* (pp. 280–316). New York: Guilford Press.

Henry, W. P., Schacht, T. E., & Strupp, H. H. (1990). Patient and therapist introject, interpersonal process, and differential psychotherapy outcome. *Journal of Consulting and Clinical Psychology, 58,* 768–774.

Henry, W. P., & Strupp, H. H. (1994). The therapeutic alliance as interpersonal process. In A. O. Horvath & L. S. Greenberg (Eds.), *The working alliance: Theory, research, and practice* (pp. 51–84). New York: Wiley.

Herzberg, D. S., Hammen, C., Burge, D., Daley, S. E., Davila, J., & Lindberg, N. (1999). Attachment cognitions predict perceived and enacted social support during late adolescence. *Journal of Adolescent Research, 14,* 387–404.

Hess, A. K. (1987). Psychotherapy supervision: Stages, Buber, and theory of relationship. *Professional Psychology: Research and Practice, 18,* 251–259.

Hesse, E. (1999). The Adult Attachment Interview: Historical and current perspectives. In J. Cassidy & P. R. Shaver (Eds.), *Handbook of attachment: Theory, research, and clinical applications* (pp. 395–433). New York: Guilford Press.

Hexel, M. (2003). Alexithymia and attachment style in relation to locus of control. *Personality and Individual Differences, 35,* 1261–1270.

Higgins, E. T. (1987). Self-discrepancy: A theory relating self and affect. *Psychological Review, 94,* 319–340.

Higgins, E. T. (1998). Promotion and prevention: Regulatory focus as a motivational principle. In M. P. Zanna (Ed.), *Advances in experimental social psychology* (Vol. 30, pp. 1–46). New York: Academic Press.

Higgins, E. T., Bond, R. N., Klein, R., & Strauman, T. J. (1986). Self discrepancies and emotional vulnerability: How magnitude, accessibility, and type of discrepancy influence affect. *Journal of Personality and Social Psychology, 51,* 5–15.

Hill, C. E. (1992). Research on therapist techniques in

brief individual therapy: Implications for practitioners. *Counseling Psychologist, 20,* 689–711.

Hill, E. M., Young, J. P., & Nord, J. L. (1994). Childhood adversity, attachment security, and adult relationships: A preliminary study. *Ethology and Sociobiology, 15,* 323–338.

Hill, M. A. (1984). The law of the father: Leadership and symbolic authority in psychoanalysis. In B. Kellerman (Ed.), *Leadership: A multidisciplinary perspective* (pp. 23–37). Englewood Cliffs, NJ: Prentice-Hall.

Himovitch, O. (2003). *The experience of commitment in couple relationships: An attachment theoretical perspective.* Unpublished doctoral dissertation, Bar-Ilan University, Ramat Gan, Israel.

Hinde, R. (1966). *Animal behavior: A synthesis of ethology and comparative psychology.* New York: McGraw-Hill.

Hinkley, K., & Andersen, S. M. (1996). The working self-concept in transference: Significant-other activation and self-change. *Journal of Personality and Social Psychology, 71,* 1279–1295.

Hirschberger, G., Florian, V., & Mikulincer, M. (2003). Strivings for romantic intimacy following partner complaint or partner criticism: A terror management perspective. *Journal of Social and Personal Relationships, 20,* 675–687.

Hirschi, T. (1969). *Causes of delinquency.* Berkeley: University of California Press.

Hochdorf, Z., Latzer, Y., Canetti, L., & Bachar, E. (2005). Attachment styles and attraction to death: Diversities among eating disorder patients. *American Journal of Family Therapy, 33,* 237–252.

Hoegh, D. G., & Burgeois, M. J. (2002). Prelude and postlude to the self: Correlates of achieved identity. *Youth and Society, 33,* 573–594.

Hoermann, S., Clarkin, J. F., Hull, J. W., & Fertuck, E. A. (2004). Attachment dimensions as predictors of medical hospitalizations in individuals with DSM IV Cluster B personality disorders. *Journal of Personality Disorders, 18,* 595–603.

Hofstra, J., van Oudenhoven, J. P., & Buunk, B. P. (2005). Attachment styles and majority members' attitudes towards adaptation strategies of immigrants. *International Journal of Intercultural Relations, 29,* 601–619.

Hogg, M. A. (1992). *The social psychology of group cohesiveness: From attraction to social identity.* New York: Harvester Wheatsheaf.

Hollis, J. (1998). *The Eden Project: In search of the magical other.* Toronto: Inner City Books.

Hollist, C. S., & Miller, R. B. (2005). Perceptions of attachment style and marital quality in midlife marriage. *Family Relations, 54,* 46–57.

Holloway, E. L. (1994). A bridge of knowing: The scholar–practitioner of supervision. *Counseling Psychology Quarterly, 7,* 3–15.

Holmes, J. G. (1991). Trust and the appraisal process in close relationships. In W. H. Jones & D. Perlman (Ed.), *Advances in personal relationships: A research annual* (Vol. 2, pp. 57–104). Oxford, UK: Kingsley.

Holmes, J. G., & Cameron, J. (2005). An integrative review of theories of interpersonal cognition: An interdependence theory perspective. In M. W. Baldwin (Ed.), *Interpersonal cognition* (pp. 415–447). New York: Guilford Press.

Holtzworth-Munroe, A., Stuart, G. L., & Hutchinson, G. (1997). Violent versus nonviolent husbands: Differences in attachment patterns, dependency, and jealousy. *Journal of Family Psychology, 11,* 314–331.

Honig, M. S., Farber, B. A., & Geller, J. D. (1997). The relationship of patients' pretreatment representations of mother to early treatment representations of their therapist. *Journal of the American Academy of Psychoanalysis and Dynamic Psychiatry, 25,* 357–372.

Horowitz, L. M., Rosenberg, S. E., Baer, B. A., Ureno, G., & Villasenor, L. (1988). Inventory of Interpersonal Problems: Psychometric properties and clinical applications. *Journal of Consulting and Clinical Psychology, 56,* 885–892.

Horowitz, M. J. (1982). Psychological processes induced by illness, injury, and loss. In T. Millon, C. Green, & R. Meagher (Eds.), *Handbook of clinical health psychology* (pp. 53–68). New York: Plenum Press.

Horppu, R., & Ikonen-Varila, M. (2001). Are attachment styles general interpersonal orientations? Applicants' perceptions and emotions in interaction with evaluators in a college entrance examination. *Journal of Social and Personal Relationships, 18,* 131–148.

Horppu, R., & Ikonen-Varila, M. (2004). Mental models of attachment as a part of kindergarten student teachers' practical knowledge about caregiving. *International Journal of Early Years Education, 12,* 231–243.

Horvath, A. O., & Greenberg, L. (1989). Development and validation of the Working Alliance Inventory. *Journal of Counseling Psychology, 36,* 223–232.

Horvath, A. O., & Greenberg, L. (Eds.). (1994). *The working alliance: Theory, research, and practice.* New York: Wiley.

Horvath, A. O., & Luborsky, L. (1993). The role of the therapeutic alliance in psychotherapy. *Journal of Consulting and Clinical Psychology, 61,* 561–573.

Horvath, A. O., & Symonds, D. B. (1991). Relation between working alliance and outcome in psychotherapy: A meta-analysis. *Journal of Counseling Psychology, 38,* 139–149.

House, R. J., & Howell, J. M. (1992). Personality and charismatic leadership. *Leadership Quarterly, 3,* 81–108.

Howard, M. S., & Medway, F. J. (2004). Adolescents' attachment and coping with stress. *Psychology in the Schools, 41,* 391–402.

Howell, J. M. (1988). Two faces of charisma: Socialized and personalized leadership in organizations. In J. A. Conger & R. N. Kanungo (Eds.), *Charismatic leadership: The elusive factor in organizational effectiveness* (pp. 213–236). San Francisco: Jossey-Bass.

Howes, C., & Hamilton, C. E. (1992). Children's relationships with child care teachers: Stability and concordance with parental attachments. *Child Development, 63,* 867–878.

Hrdy, S. B. (2005). Evolutionary context of human development: The cooperative breeding model. In C. S. Carter et al. (Eds.), *Attachment and bonding: A new synthesis* (pp. 9–32). Cambridge, MA: MIT Press.

Hudson, S. M., & Ward, T. (1997). Intimacy, loneliness, and attachment style in sexual offenders. *Journal of Interpersonal Violence, 12,* 323–339.

Hull, J. G., Young, R. D., & Jouriles, E. (1986). Applications of the self-awareness model of alcohol consumption: Predicting patterns of use and abuse. *Journal of Personality and Social Psychology, 51,* 790–796.

Huntsinger, E. T., & Luecken, L. J. (2004). Attachment relationships and health behavior: The mediational role of self-esteem. *Psychology and Health, 19,* 515–526.

Impett, E. A., & Peplau, L.A. (2002). Why some women consent to unwanted sex with a dating partner: Insights from attachment theory. *Psychology of Women Quarterly, 26,* 360–370.

Ireland, J. L., & Power, C. L. (2004). Attachment, emotional loneliness, and bullying behavior: A study of adult and young offenders. *Aggressive Behavior, 30,* 298–312.

Irons, C., & Gilbert, P. (2005). Evolved mechanisms in adolescent anxiety and depression symptoms: The role of the attachment and social rank systems. *Journal of Adolescence, 28,* 325–341.

Irons, C., Gilbert, P., Baldwin, M. W., Baccus, J., & Palmer, M. (2006). Parental recall, attachment relating, and self-attacking/self-reassurance: Their relationship with depression. *British Journal of Clinical Psychology, 45,* 1–12.

Isaacson, K. L. (2006). *Mary Ainsworth: A psychobiography.* Unpublished doctoral dissertation, University of California, Davis.

Iwaniec, D., & Sneddon, H. (2001). Attachment style in adults who failed to thrive as children: Outcomes of a 20-year follow-up study of factors influencing maintenance or change in attachment style. *British Journal of Social Work, 31,* 179–195.

Jacobsen, T., Edelstein, W., & Hofmann, V. (1994). A longitudinal study of the relation between representations of attachment in childhood and cognitive functioning in childhood and adolescence. *Developmental Psychology, 30,* 112–124.

Jacobsen, T., & Hofmann, V. (1997). Children's attachment representations: Longitudinal relations to school behavior and academic competency in middle childhood and adolescence. *Developmental Psychology, 33,* 703–710.

Jacobvitz, D., Curran, M., & Moller, N. (2002). Measurement of adult attachment: The place of self-report and interview methodologies. *Attachment and Human Development, 4,* 207–215.

Jaeger, E., Hahn, N.-B., & Weinraub, M. (2000). Attachment in adult daughters of alcoholic fathers. *Addiction, 95,* 267–276.

James, B. (1994). *Handbook for the treatment of attachment-trauma problems in children.* New York: Lexington Books.

James, W. (1890). *The principles of psychology.* New York: Holt.

Jang, S. A., Smith, S. W., & Levine, T. R. (2002). To stay or to leave?: The role of attachment styles in communication patterns and potential termination of romantic relationships following discovery of deception. *Communication Monographs, 69,* 236–252.

Janoff-Bulman, R. (1979). Characterological versus behavioral self-blame: Inquiries into depression and rape. *Journal of Personality and Social Psychology, 37,* 1798–1809.

Jayson, Y. (2004). *An attachment perspective on escalation of commitment.* Unpublished doctoral dissertation, Bar-Ilan University, Ramat Gan, Israel.

Jellison, W. A., & McConnell, A. R. (2003). The mediating effects of attitudes toward homosexuality between secure attachment and disclosure outcomes among gay men. *Journal of Homosexuality, 46,* 159–177.

Jerome, E. M., & Liss, M. (2005). Relationships between sensory processing style, adult attachment, and coping. *Personality and Individual Differences, 38,* 1341–1352.

Johnson, L. N., Ketring, S. A., & Abshire, C. (2003). The Revised Inventory of Parent Attachment: Measuring attachment in families. *Contemporary Family Therapy, 25,* 333–349.

Johnson, S. M. (1996). *The practice of emotionally focused marital therapy: Creating connections.* New York: Brunner/Mazel.

Johnson, S. M. (2003). Attachment theory: A guide for couple therapy. In S. M. Johnson & V. E. Whiffen (Eds.), *Attachment processes in couple and family therapy* (pp. 103–123). New York: Guilford Press.

Johnson, S. M., & Greenberg, L. S. (1985). The differential effects of experiential and problem solving interventions in resolving marital conflicts. *Journal of Consulting and Counseling Psychology, 53,* 175–184.

Johnson, S. M., Hunsley, J., Greenberg, L. S., & Schindler (1999). Emotionally focused couples therapy: Status and challenges. *Clinical Psychology: Science and Practice, 6,* 67–79.

Johnson, S. M., Makinen, J. A., & Millikin, J. W. (2001). Attachment injuries in couple relationships: A new perspective on impasses in couples therapy. *Journal of Marital and Family Therapy, 27,* 145–155.

Johnson, S. M., & Whiffen, V. E. (Eds.). (2003). *Attachment processes in couple and family therapy.* New York: Guilford Press.

Johnston, M. A. (1999). Influences of adult attachment in exploration. *Psychological Reports, 84,* 31–34.

Johnston, M. A. (2000). Delegation and organizational structure in small businesses: Influences of manager's attachment patterns. *Group and Organization Management, 25,* 4–21.

Joiner, T. E., & Coyne, J. C. (Eds.). (1999). *The interactional nature of depression: Advances in interpersonal approaches.* Washington, DC: American Psychological Association.

Joiner, T. E., Metalsky, G. I., Katz, J., & Beach, S. R. H. (1999). Depression and excessive reassurance seeking. *Psychological Inquiry, 10,* 269–278.

Joireman, J. A., Needham, T. L., & Cummings, A. L.

(2002). Relationships between dimensions of attachment and empathy. *North American Journal of Psychology, 4,* 63–80.

Jones, J. T., & Cunningham, J. D. (1996). Attachment styles and other predictors of relationship satisfaction in dating couples. *Personal Relationships, 3,* 387–399.

Joseph, B. (1989). *Psychic equilibrium and psychic change.* London: Tavistock.

Josselson, R. (1987). *Finding herself: Pathways to identity development in women.* San Francisco: Jossey-Bass.

Judge, T. A., Thoresen, C. J., Pucik, V., & Welbourne, T. M. (1999). Managerial coping with organizational change: A dispositional perspective. *Journal of Applied Psychology, 84,* 107–122.

Julian of Norwich. (2003). *Showing of love.* Collegeville, MN: Liturgical Press (Michael Glazier Books). (Handwritten in the 14th century; original work published 1670)

Julien, D., & Markman, H. J. (1991). Social support and social networks as determinants of individual and marital outcomes. *Journal of Social and Personal Relationships, 8,* 549–568.

Jung, C. G. (1958). *Psychology and religion.* Princeton, NJ: Princeton University Press.

Kachadourian, L. K., Fincham, F., & Davila, J. (2004). The tendency to forgive in dating and married couples: The role of attachment and relationship satisfaction. *Personal Relationships, 11,* 373–393.

Kafetsios, K. (2004). Attachment and emotional intelligence abilities across the life course. *Personality and Individual Differences, 37,* 129–145.

Kafetsios, K., & Nezlek, J. B. (2002). Attachment styles in everyday social interaction. *European Journal of Social Psychology, 32,* 719–735.

Kaiser, S., Kirtzeck, M., Hornschuh, G., & Sachser, N. (2003). Sex-specific difference in social support—a study in female guinea pigs. *Physiology and Behavior, 79,* 297–303.

Kaitz, M., Bar-Haim, Y., Lehrer, M., & Grossman, E. (2004). Adult attachment style and interpersonal distance. *Attachment and Human Development, 6,* 285–304.

Kalish, R. A. (1985). *Death, grief, and caring relationships.* New York: Cole.

Kamarck, T. W., Manuck, S. B., & Jennings, J. R. (1990). Social support reduces cardiovascular reactivity to psychological challenge: A laboratory model. *Psychosomatic Medicine, 52,* 42–58.

Kandel, E. R. (2006). *In search of memory: The emergence of a new science of mind.* New York: Norton.

Kanninen, K., Punamaki, R. L., & Qouta, S. (2003). Personality and trauma: Adult attachment and posttraumatic distress among former political prisoners. *Peace and Conflict: Journal of Peace Psychology, 9,* 97–126.

Kanninen, K., Salo, J., & Punamaki, R. L. (2000). Attachment patterns and working alliance in trauma therapy for victims of political violence. *Psychotherapy Research, 10,* 435–449.

Kaplan, H. S. (1974). *The new sex therapy.* New York: Brunner/Mazel.

Karen, R. (1994). *Becoming attached: Unfolding the mystery of the infant–mother bond and its impact on later life.* New York: Warner Books.

Kazarian, S. S., & Martin, R. A. (2004). Humor styles, personality, and well-being among Lebanese university students. *European Journal of Personality, 18,* 209–219.

Keelan, J. R., Dion, K. K., & Dion, K. L. (1998). Attachment style and relationship satisfaction: Test of a self-disclosure explanation. *Canadian Journal of Behavioral Science, 30,* 24–35.

Keelan, J. R., Dion, K. L., & Dion, K. K. (1994). Attachment style and heterosexual relationships among young adults: A short-term panel study. *Journal of Social and Personal Relationships, 11,* 201–214.

Keller, T. (2003). Parental images as a guide to leadership sensemaking: An attachment perspective on implicit leadership theories. *Leadership Quarterly, 14,* 141–160.

Kelley, M. L., Cash, T. F., Grant, A. R., Miles, D. L., & Santos, M. T. (2004). Parental alcoholism: Relationships to adult attachment in college women and men. *Addictive Behaviors, 29,* 1633–1636.

Kelley, M. L., Nair, V., Rawlings, T., Cash, T. F., Steer, K., & Fals Stewart, W. (2005). Retrospective reports of parenting received in their families of origin: Relationships to adult attachment in adult children of alcoholics. *Addictive Behaviors, 30,* 1479–1495.

Kemp, M. A., & Neimeyer, G. J. (1999). Interpersonal attachment: Experiencing, expressing, and coping with stress. *Journal of Counseling Psychology, 46,* 388–394.

Kennedy, J. H. (1999). Romantic attachment style and ego identity, attributional style, and family of origin in first-year college students. *College Student Journal, 33,* 171–180.

Kenny, M. E. (1987a). The extent and function of parental attachment among first-year college students. *Journal of Youth and Adolescence, 16,* 17–29.

Kenny, M. E. (1987b). Family ties and leaving home for college: Recent findings and implications. *Journal of College Student Personnel, 28,* 438–442.

Kenny, M. E. (1990). College seniors' perceptions of parental attachments: The value and stability of family ties. *Journal of College Student Development, 31,* 39–46.

Kenny, M. E. (1994). Quality and correlates of parental attachment among late adolescents. *Journal of Counseling and Development, 72,* 399–403.

Kenny, M. E., & Donaldson, G. A. (1991). Contributions of parental attachment and family structure to the social and psychological functioning of first-year college students. *Journal of Counseling Psychology, 38,* 479–486.

Kenny, M. E., & Donaldson, G. A. (1992). The relationship of parental attachment and psychological separation to the adjustment of first-year college women. *Journal of College Student Development, 33,* 431–438.

Kenny, M. E., & Gallagher, L. A. (2002). Instrumental and social/relational correlates of perceived maternal and paternal attachment in adolescence. *Journal of Adolescence, 25,* 203–219.

Kenny, M. E., Griffiths, J., & Grossman, J. (2005). Self-image and parental attachment among late adolescents in Belize. *Journal of Adolescence, 28,* 649–664.

Kenny, M. E., & Hart, K. (1992). Relationship between parental attachment and eating disorders in an inpatient and a college sample. *Journal of Counseling Psychology, 39,* 521–526.

Kenny, M. E., Lomax, R., Brabeck, M., & Fife, J. (1998). Longitudinal pathways linking adolescent reports of maternal and paternal attachments to psychological well-being. *Journal of Early Adolescence, 18,* 221–243.

Kenny, M. E., Moilanen, D. L., Lomax, R., & Brabeck, M. M. (1993). Contributions of parental attachments to view of self and depressive symptoms among early adolescents. *Journal of Early Adolescence, 13,* 408–430.

Kenny, M. E., & Perez, V. (1996). Attachment and psychological well-being among racially and ethnically diverse first-year college students. *Journal of College Student Development, 37,* 527–535.

Kerns, K. A. (1994). A longitudinal examination of links between mother–child attachment and children's friendships in early childhood. *Journal of Social and Personal Relationships, 11,* 379–381.

Kerns, K. A., Schlegelmilch, A., Morgan, T. A., & Abraham, M. M. (2005). Assessing attachment in middle childhood. In K. A. Kerns & R. A. Richardson (Eds.), *Attachment in middle childhood* (pp. 46–70). New York: Guilford Press.

Kerns, K. A., & Stevens, A. C. (1996). Parent–child attachment in late adolescence: Links to social relations and personality. *Journal of Youth and Adolescence, 25,* 323–342.

Kerr, S. L., Melley, A. M., Travea, L., & Pole, M. (2003). The relationship of emotional expression and experience to adult attachment style. *Individual Differences Research, 1,* 108–123.

Kesner, J. E., & McKenry, P. C. (1998). The role of childhood attachment factors in predicting male violence toward female intimates. *Journal of Family Violence, 13,* 417–432.

Kestenbaum, R., Farber, E. A., & Sroufe, L. A. (1989). Individual differences in empathy among preschoolers: Relation to attachment history. In N. Eisenberg (Ed.), *Empathy and related emotional competence: New directions for child development* (Vol. 44, pp. 51–64). San Francisco, CA: Jossey-Bass.

Ketterson, T. U., & Blustein, D. L. (1997). Attachment relationships and the career exploration process. *Career Development Quarterly, 46,* 167–178.

Kidd, T., & Sheffield, D. (2005). Attachment style and symptom reporting: Examining the mediating effects of anger and social support. *British Journal of Health Psychology, 10,* 531–541.

Kierkegaard, S. (1992). *Concluding unscientific postscript to philosophical fragments.* (H. V. Hong & E. H. Hong, Eds. & Trans.). Princeton, NJ: Princeton University Press. (Original work published 1846)

Kiesler, D. J. (1996). *Contemporary interpersonal theory and research: Personality, psychopathology, and psychotherapy.* New York: Wiley.

Kiesler, D. J. (2001). Therapist countertransference: In search of common themes and empirical referents. *Journal of Clinical Psychology, 57,* 1053–1063.

Kim, Y. (2005). Emotional and cognitive consequences of adult attachment: The mediating effect of the self. *Personality and Individual Differences, 39,* 913–923.

Kim, Y. (2006). Gender, attachment, and relationship duration on cardiovascular reactivity to stress in a laboratory study of dating couples. *Personal Relationships, 13,* 103–114.

King, E. B., George, J. M., & Hebl, M. R. (2005). Linking personality to helping behaviors at work: An interactional perspective. *Journal of Personality, 73,* 585–607.

Kirkpatrick, L. A. (1997). A longitudinal study of changes in religious belief and behavior as a function of individual differences in adult attachment style. *Journal for the Scientific Study of Religion, 36,* 207–217.

Kirkpatrick, L. A. (1998a). Evolution, pair-bonding, and reproductive strategies: A reconceptualization of adult attachment. In J. A. Simpson & W. S. Rholes (Eds.), *Attachment theory and close relationships* (pp. 353–393). New York: Guilford Press.

Kirkpatrick, L. A. (1998b). God as a substitute attachment figure: A longitudinal study of adult attachment style and religious change in college students. *Personality and Social Psychology Bulletin, 24,* 961–973.

Kirkpatrick, L. A. (2005). *Attachment, evolution, and the psychology of religion.* New York: Guilford Press.

Kirkpatrick, L. A., & Davis, K. E. (1994). Attachment style, gender, and relationship stability: A longitudinal analysis. *Journal of Personality and Social Psychology, 66,* 502–512.

Kirkpatrick, L. A., & Hazan, C. (1994). Attachment styles and close relationships: A four-year prospective study. *Personal Relationships, 1,* 123–142.

Kirkpatrick, L. A., & Shaver, P. R. (1988). Fear and affiliation reconsidered from a stress and coping perspective. *Journal of Social and Clinical Psychology, 7,* 214–233.

Kirkpatrick, L. A., & Shaver, P. R. (1990). Attachment theory and religion: Childhood attachments, religious beliefs, and conversion. *Journal for the Scientific Study of Religion, 29,* 315–334.

Kirkpatrick, L. A., & Shaver, P. R. (1992). An attachment-theoretical approach to romantic love and religious belief. *Personality and Social Psychology Bulletin, 18,* 266–275.

Kirsh, S. J. (1996). Attachment style and recognition of emotionally-laden drawings. *Perceptual and Motor Skills, 83,* 607–610.

Kivlighan, D. M., Jr., Patton, M. J., & Foote, D. (1998). Moderating effects of client attachment on the counselor experience-working alliance relationship. *Journal of Counseling Psychology, 45,* 274–278.

Klass, D., Silverman, P. R., & Nickman, S. L. (Eds.). (1996). *Continuing bonds: New understandings of grief.* Washington, DC: Taylor & Francis.

Klein, M. (1940). Mourning and its relationship with

manic–depressive states. *International Journal of Psychoanalysis, 12,* 47–82.

Klein, M. (1989). The Oedipus complex in the light of early anxieties. In R. Britton, M. Feldman, & E. O'Shaughnessy (Eds.), *The Oedipus complex today: Clinical implications.* London: Karnac Books. (Original work published 1945)

Klohnen, E. C., & Bera, S. (1998). Behavioral and experiential patterns of avoidantly and securely attached women across adulthood: A 31-year longitudinal perspective. *Journal of Personality and Social Psychology, 74,* 211–223.

Klohnen, E. C., & John, O. P. (1998). Working models of attachment: A theory-based prototype approach. In J. A. Simpson & W. S. Rholes (Eds.), *Attachment theory and close relationships* (pp. 115–140). New York: Guilford Press.

Klohnen, E. C., & Luo, S. (2003). Interpersonal attraction and personality: What is attractive—self similarity, ideal similarity, complementarity or attachment security? *Journal of Personality and Social Psychology, 85,* 709–722.

Klohnen, E. C., Weller, J. A., Luo, S., & Choe, M. (2005). Organization and predictive power of general and relationship-specific attachment models: One for all, and all for one? *Personality and Social Psychology Bulletin, 31*(12), 1665–1682.

Klopfer, B., Ainsworth, M. D. S., Klopfer, W., & Holt, R. (1954). *Developments in the Rorschach technique: I. Technique and theory.* New York: World Book Company.

Knafo, A., & Plomin, R. (2006). Parental discipline and affection and children's prosocial behavior: Genetic and environmental links. *Journal of Personality and Social Psychology, 90,* 147–164.

Knobloch, L. K., Solomon, D.-H., & Cruz, M. G. (2001). The role of relationship development and attachment in the experience of romantic jealousy. *Personal Relationships, 8,* 205–224.

Kobak, R. (1993). *The adult attachment Q-sort.* Unpublished manuscript, University of Delaware, Newark.

Kobak, R., Cole, H. E., Ferenz-Gillies, R., Fleming, W. S., & Gamble, S. (1993). Attachment and emotion regulation during mother–teen problem solving: A control theory analysis. *Child Development, 64,* 231–245.

Kobak, R., & Ferenz-Gillies, R. (1995). Emotion regulation and depressive symptoms during adolescence: A functionalist perspective. *Development and Psychopathology, 7,* 183–192.

Kobak, R., Ferenz-Gillies, R., Everhart, E., & Seabrook, L. (1994). Maternal attachment strategies and emotion regulation with adolescent offspring. *Journal of Research on Adolescence, 4,* 553–566.

Kobak, R., & Hazan, C. (1991). Attachment in marriage: Effects of security and accuracy of working models. *Journal of Personality and Social Psychology, 60,* 861–869.

Kobak, R., Ruckdeschel, K., & Hazan, C. (1994). From symptom to signal: An attachment view of emotion in marital therapy. In S. M. Johnson & L. S. Greenberg (Eds.), *The heart of the matter: Perspectives on emotion in marital therapy* (pp. 46–71). New York: Brunner/Mazel.

Kobak, R., & Sceery, A. (1988). Attachment in late adolescence: Working models, affect regulation, and representations of self and others. *Child Development, 59,* 135–146.

Kobak, R., Sudler, N., & Gamble, W. (1991). Attachment and depressive symptoms during adolescence: A developmental pathways analysis. *Development and Psychopathology, 3,* 461–474.

Kobasa, S. C. (1982). The hardy personality. In G. Sanders & J. Suls (Eds.), *Social psychology of health and illness* (pp. 126–151). Hillsdale, NJ: Erlbaum.

Kogot, E. (2004). *The contribution of attachment style to cognitions, affect, and behavior in achievement settings* Unpublished doctoral dissertation, Bar-Ilan University, Ramat Gan, Israel.

Kohut, H. (1971). *The analysis of the self.* New York: International Universities Press.

Kohut, H. (1977). *The restoration of the self.* New York: International Universities Press.

Kohut, H. (1984). *How does analysis cure?* Chicago: University of Chicago Press.

Kohut, H., & Wolf, E. (1978). The disorders of the self and their treatment: An outline. *International Journal of Psycho-Analysis, 59,* 413–425.

Kokotovic, A. M., & Tracey, T. J. (1990). Working alliance in the early phase of counseling. *Journal of Counseling Psychology, 37,* 16–21.

Koopman, C., Gore-Felton, C., Marouf, F., Butler, L. D., Field, N., Gill, M., et al. (2000). Relationships of perceived stress to coping, attachment, and social support among HIV-positive persons. *AIDS Care, 12,* 663–672.

Korfmacher, J., Adam, E., Ogawa, J., & Egeland, B. (1997). Adult attachment: Implications for the therapeutic process in a home visitation intervention. *Applied Developmental Science, 1,* 43–52.

Koski, L. R., & Shaver, P. R. (1997). Attachment and relationship satisfaction across the lifespan. In R. J. Sternberg & M. Hojjat (Eds.), *Satisfaction in close relationships* (pp. 26–55). New York: Guilford Press.

Kotler, T., Buzwell, S., Romeo, Y., & Bowland, J. (1994). Avoidant attachment as a risk factor for health. *British Journal of Medical Psychology, 67,* 237–245.

Kramer, P. D. (2005). *Against depression.* New York: Viking.

Krausz, M., Bizman, A., & Braslavsky, D. (2001). Effects of attachment style on preferences for and satisfaction with different employment contracts: An exploratory study. *Journal of Business and Psychology, 16,* 299–316.

Kruglanski, A. W. (1989). *Lay epistemology and human knowledge: Cognitive and motivational bases.* New York: Plenum Press.

Kumashiro, M., & Sedikides, C. (2005). Taking on board liability-focused information: Close positive relationships as a self-bolstering resource. *Psychological Science, 16,* 732–739.

Kunce, L. J., & Shaver, P. R. (1994). An attachment-theoretical approach to caregiving in romantic relationships. In K. Bartholomew & D. Perlman (Eds.), *Advances in personal relationships: Attachment processes in adulthood* (Vol. 5, pp. 205–237). London: Kingsley.

Kunda, Z. (1999). *Social cognition: Making sense of people*. Cambridge, MA: MIT Press.

Kurdek, L. A. (2002). On being insecure about the assessment of attachment styles. *Journal of Social and Personal Relationships, 19,* 811–834.

Kurtz, A. (2005). The needs of staff who care for people with a diagnosis of personality disorder who are considered a risk to others. *Journal of Forensic Psychiatry and Psychology, 16,* 399–422.

Kuschner, H. S. (1981). *When bad things happen to good people*. New York: HarperCollins.

La Guardia, J. G., Ryan, R. M., Couchman, C. E., & Deci, E. L. (2000). Within-person variation in security of attachment: A self-determination theory perspective on attachment, need fulfillment, and well-being. *Journal of Personality and Social Psychology, 79,* 367–384.

Laible, D. J., Carlo, G., & Raffaelli, M. (2000). The differential relations of parent and peer attachment to adolescent adjustment. *Journal of Youth and Adolescence, 29,* 45–59.

Lakatos, K., Toth, I., Nemoda, Z., Ney, K., Sasvari-Szekely, M., & Gervai, J. (2000). Dopamine D4 receptor (DRD4) gene polymorphism is associated with attachment disorganization in infants. *Molecular Psychiatry, 5,* 633–637.

Lakatos, K., Nemoda, Z., Toth, I., Ronai, Z., Ney, K., Sasvari-Szekely, M., & Gervai, J. (2002). Further evidence for the role of the dopamine D4 receptor (DRD4) gene in attachment disorganization: Interaction of the exon III 48–bp repeat and the -521 C/T promoter polymorphisms. *Molecular Psychiatry, 7,* 27–31.

Lalumiere, M. L., Harris, G. T., Quinsey, V. L., & Rice, M. E. (2005). *The causes of rape*. Washington, DC: American Psychological Association.

Lamb, M. (1976). Effects of stress and cohort on mother–infant and father–infant interaction. *Developmental Psychology, 12,* 435–443.

Landolt, M. A., Bartholomew, K., Saffrey, C., Oram, D., & Perlman, D. (2004). Gender nonconformity, childhood rejection, and adult attachment: A study of gay men. *Archives of Sexual Behavior, 33,* 117–128.

Landolt, M. A., & Dutton, D. G. (1997). Power and personality: An analysis of gay male intimate abuse. *Sex Roles, 37,* 335–359.

Lapsley, D. K., & Edgerton, J. (2002). Separation-individuation, adult attachment style, and college adjustment. *Journal of Counseling and Development, 80,* 484–492.

Lapsley, D. K., Rice, K. G., & Fitzgerald, D. P. (1990). Adolescent attachment, identity, and adjustment to college: Implications for the continuity of adaptation hypothesis. *Journal of Counseling and Development, 68,* 561–565.

Larose, S., & Bernier, A. (2001). Social support processes: Mediators of attachment state of mind and adjustment in late adolescence. *Attachment and Human Development, 3,* 96–120.

Larose, S., Bernier, A., Soucy, N., & Duchesne, S. (1999). Attachment style dimensions, network orientation, and the process of seeking help from college teachers. *Journal of Social and Personal Relationships, 16,* 225–247.

Larose, S., Bernier, A., & Tarabulsy, G. M. (2005). Attachment state of mind, learning dispositions, and academic performance during the college transition. *Developmental Psychology, 41,* 281–289.

Larose, S., & Boivin, M. (1997). Structural relations among attachment working models of parents, general and specific support expectations, and personal adjustment in late adolescence. *Journal of Social and Personal Relationships, 14,* 579–601.

Larose, S., & Boivin, M. (1998). Attachment to parents, social support expectations, and socioemotional adjustment during the high school-college transition. *Journal of Research on Adolescence, 8,* 1–27.

Larose, S., Boivin, M., & Doyle, A. B. (2001). Parental representations and attachment style as predictors of support-seeking behaviors and perceptions of support in an academic counseling relationship. *Personal Relationships, 8,* 93–113.

Larose, S., Guay, F., & Boivin, M. (2002). Attachment, social support, and loneliness in young adulthood: A test of two models. *Personality and Social Psychology Bulletin, 28,* 684–693.

Laschinger, B., Purnell, C., Schwartz, J., White, K., & Wingfield, R. (2004). Sexuality and attachment from a clinical point of view. *Attachment and Human Development, 6,* 151–164.

Latty-Mann, H., & Davis, K. E. (1996). Attachment theory and partner choice: Preference and actuality. *Journal of Social and Personal Relationships, 13,* 5–23.

Latzer, Y., Hochdorf, Z., Bachar, E., & Canetti, L. (2002). Attachment style and family functioning as discriminating factors in eating disorders. *Contemporary Family Therapy: An International Journal, 24,* 581–599.

Laurenceau, J. P., Barrett, L. F., & Pietromonaco, P. R. (1998). Intimacy as an interpersonal process: The importance of self-disclosure and perceived partner responsiveness in interpersonal exchanges. *Journal of Personality and Social Psychology, 74,* 1238–1251.

Laurenceau, J. P., Barrett, L. F., & Rovine, M. J. (2005). The interpersonal process model of intimacy in marriage: A daily-diary and multilevel modeling approach. *Journal of Family Psychology, 19,* 314–323.

Lavy, S. (2006). *Expressions and consequences of intrusiveness in adult romantic relationships: An attachment theory perspective*. Unpublished doctoral dissertation, Bar-Ilan University, Ramat Gan, Israel.

Lay, C. (1988). The relationship of procrastination and optimism to judgments of time to complete an essay and anticipation of setbacks. *Journal of Social Behavior and Personality, 3,* 201–204.

Lazarus, R. S. (1991). *Emotion and adaptation*. New York: Oxford University Press.

Lazarus, R. S., & Folkman, S. (1984). *Stress, appraisal, and coping*. New York: Springer.

Leak, G. K., & Cooney, R. R. (2001). Self-determination, attachment styles, and well-being in adult romantic relationships. *Representative Research in Social Psychology, 25,* 55–62.

Leak, G. K., Gardner, L. E., & Parsons, C. J. (1998).

Jealousy and romantic attachment: A replication and extension. *Representative Research in Social Psychology, 22,* 21–27.

Learner, D. G., & Kruger, L. J. (1997). Attachment, self-concept, and academic motivation in high-school students. *American Journal of Orthopsychiatry, 67,* 485–492.

Leary, M. R. (1999). Making sense of self-esteem. *Current Directions in Psychological Science, 8,* 32–35.

Leary, M. R., & Baumeister, R. F. (2000). The nature and function of self-esteem: Sociometer theory. In M. P. Zanna (Ed.), *Advances in experimental social psychology* (Vol. 32, pp. 2–51). San Diego: Academic Press.

Leary, M. R., Cottrell, C. A., & Phillips, M. (2001). Deconfounding the effects of dominance and social acceptance on self-esteem. *Journal of Personality and Social Psychology, 81,* 898–909.

Leary, M. R., Tambor, E. S., Terdal, S. K., & Downs, D. L. (1995). Self-esteem as an interpersonal monitor: The sociometer hypothesis. *Journal of Personality and Social Psychology, 68,* 518–530.

Leary, T. (1957). *Interpersonal diagnosis of personality.* New York: Ronald.

LeDoux, J. E. (1996). *The emotional brain: The mysterious underpinnings of emotional life.* New York: Simon & Schuster.

Lee, H. Y., & Hughey, K. F. (2001). The relationship of psychological separation and parental attachment to the career maturity of college freshmen from intact families. *Journal of Career Development, 27,* 279–293.

Lee, J. A. (1977). A typology of styles of loving. *Personality and Social Psychology Bulletin, 3,* 173–182.

Lee, J. M., & Bell, N. J. (2003). Individual differences in attachment–autonomy configurations: Linkages with substance use and youth competencies. *Journal of Adolescence, 26,* 347–361.

Lehman, D. R., Ellard, J. H., & Wortman, C. B. (1986). Social support for the bereaved: Recipients' and providers' perspectives of what is helpful. *Journal of Consulting and Clinical Psychology, 54,* 438–446.

Leon, K., & Jacobvitz, D. B. (2003). Relationships between adult attachment representations and family ritual quality: A prospective longitudinal study. *Family Process, 42,* 419–432.

Leondari, A., & Kiosseoglou, G. (2000). The relationship of parental attachment and psychological separation to the psychological functioning of young adults. *Journal of Social Psychology, 140,* 451–464.

LePine, J. A., Erez, A., & Johnson, D. (2002). The nature and dimensionality of organizational citizenship behavior: A critical review and meta-analysis. *Journal of Applied Psychology, 87,* 52–65.

Le Poire, B. A., Shepard, C., & Duggan, A. (1999). Nonverbal involvement, expressiveness, and pleasantness as predicted by parental and partner attachment style. *Communication Monographs, 66,* 293–311.

Lepore, S. J., Silver, R. C., Wortman, C. B., & Wayment, H. A. (1996). Social constraints, intrusive thoughts, and depressive symptoms among bereaved mothers. *Journal of Personality and Social Psychology, 70,* 271–282.

Lessard, J. C., & Moretti, M. M. (1998). Suicidal ideation in an adolescent clinical sample: Attachment patterns and clinical implications. *Journal of Adolescence, 21,* 383–395.

Levine, J. M., & Moreland, R. L. (1990). Progress in small group research. *Annual Review of Psychology, 41,* 585–634.

Levinson, A., & Fonagy, P. (2004). Offending and attachment: The relationship between interpersonal awareness and offending in a prison population with psychiatric disorder. *Canadian Journal of Psychoanalysis, 12,* 225–251.

Levy, K. N., Blatt, S. J., & Shaver, P. R. (1998). Attachment styles and parental representations. *Journal of Personality and Social Psychology, 74,* 407–419.

Levy, K. N., & Clarkin, J. F. (2002). *Change in social cognition and behavior in borderline personality disorder: A preliminary report.* Minneapolis, MN: National Institute of Mental Health.

Levy, K. N., Kelly, K. M., & Jack, E. L. (2006). Sex differences in jealousy: A matter of evolution or attachment history? In M. Mikulincer & G. S. Goodman (Eds.), *Dynamics of romantic love* (pp. 128–145). New York: Guilford Press.

Levy, K. N., Meehan, K. B., Weber, M., Reynoso, J., & Clarkin, J. F. (2005). Attachment and borderline personality disorder: Implications for psychotherapy. *Psychopathology, 38,* 64–74.

Levy, M. B., & Davis, K. E. (1988). Love styles and attachment styles compared: Their relations to each other and to various relationship characteristics. *Journal of Social and Personal Relationships, 5,* 439–471.

Levy, T. M., & Orlans, M. (1998). *Attachment, trauma, and healing: Understanding and treating attachment disorder in children and families.* Washington, DC: Child Welfare League of America Press.

Lewis, M. (2000). Self-conscious emotions: Embarrassment, pride, shame, and guilt. In M. Lewis & J. M. Haviland-Jones (Eds.), *Handbook of emotions* (pp. 623–636). New York: Guilford Press.

Lewis, M., Feiring, C., & Rosenthal, S. (2000). Attachment over time. *Child Development, 71,* 707–720.

Lifton, R. J. (1979). *The broken connection.* New York: Simon & Schuster.

Lifton, R. J., & Olson, E. (1974). *Living and dying.* New York: Praeger.

Ligiero, D. P., & Gelso, C. J. (2002). Countertransference, attachment, and the working alliance: The therapist's contribution. *Psychotherapy, 39,* 3–11.

Lin, Y. C. (1992). *The construction of the sense of intimacy from everyday social interaction.* Unpublished doctoral dissertation, University of Rochester, New York.

Liotti, G. (1992). Disorganized/disoriented attachment in the etiology of the dissociative disorders. *Dissociation: Progress in the Dissociative Disorders, 5,* 196–204.

Litman-Ovadia, H. (2004). *An attachment perspective on the career counseling process and career exploration.* Unpublished doctoral dissertation, Bar-Ilan University, Ramat Gan, Israel.

Little, B. R. (1989). Personal project analysis: Trivial pursuits, magnificent obsessions, and the search for coherence. In D. M. Buss & N. Cantor (Eds.), *Personality psychology: Recent trends and emerging directions* (pp. 15–31). New York: Springer-Verlag.

Livesley, W. J. (1991). Classifying personality disorders: Ideal types, prototypes, or dimensions? *Journal of Personality Disorders, 5,* 52–59.

Long, M. V., & Martin, P. (2000). Personality, relationship closeness, and loneliness of oldest old adults and their children. *Journals of Gerontology: Series B, Psychological Sciences and Social Sciences, 55,* 311–319.

Lopez, F. G. (1996). Attachment-related predictors of constructive thinking among college students. *Journal of Counseling and Development, 75,* 58–63.

Lopez, F. G. (1997). Student–professor relationship styles, childhood attachment bonds, and current academic orientations. *Journal of Social and Personal Relationships, 14,* 271–282.

Lopez, F. G. (2001). Adult attachment orientations, self-other boundary regulation, and splitting tendencies in a college sample. *Journal of Counseling Psychology, 48,* 440–446.

Lopez, F. G., Fuendeling, J., Thomas, K., & Sagula, D. (1997). An attachment-theoretical perspective on the use of splitting defenses. *Counseling Psychology Quarterly, 10,* 461–472.

Lopez, F. G., & Gormley, B. (2002). Stability and change in adult attachment style over the first-year college transition: Relations to self-confidence, coping, and distress patterns. *Journal of Counseling Psychology, 49,* 355–364.

Lopez, F. G., Gover, M. R., Leskela, J., Sauer, E. M., Schirmer, L., & Wyssmann, J. (1997). Attachment styles, shame, guilt, and collaborative problem-solving orientations. *Personal Relationships, 4,* 187–199.

Lopez, F. G., Mauricio, A. M., Gormley, B., Simko, T., & Berger, E. (2001). Adult attachment orientations and college student distress: The mediating role of problem coping styles. *Journal of Counseling and Development, 79,* 459–464.

Lopez, F. G., Melendez, M. C., & Rice, K. G. (2000). Parental divorce, parent–child bonds, and adult attachment orientations among college students: A comparison of three racial/ethnic groups. *Journal of Counseling Psychology, 47,* 177–186.

Lopez, F. G., Melendez, M. C., Sauer, E. M., Berger, E., & Wyssmann, J. (1998). Internal working models, self-reported problems, and help-seeking attitudes among college students. *Journal of Counseling Psychology, 45,* 79–83.

Lopez, F. G., Mitchell, P., & Gormley, B. (2002). Adult attachment orientations and college student distress: Test of a mediational model. *Journal of Counseling Psychology, 49,* 460–467.

Lorenz, K. Z. (1952). *King Solomon's ring.* New York: Crowell.

Luborsky, L., & Crits-Christoph, P. (1998). *Understanding transference: The core conflictual relationship theme method.* Washington, DC: American Psychological Association.

Luke, M. A., Maio, G. R., & Carnelley, K. B. (2004). Attachment models of the self and others: Relations with self-esteem, humanity-esteem, and parental treatment. *Personal Relationships, 11,* 281–303.

Lupinacci, M. A. (1998). Reflections on the early stage of the Oedipus complex: The parental couple in relation to psychoanalytic work. *Journal of Child Psychotherapy, 24,* 409–421.

Lussier, Y., Sabourin, S., & Turgeon, C. (1997). Coping strategies as moderators of the relationship between attachment and marital adjustment. *Journal of Social and Personal Relationships, 14,* 777–791.

Lutz, W. J., & Hock, E. (1995). Maternal separation anxiety: Relations to adult attachment representations in mothers of infants. *Journal of Genetic Psychology, 156,* 57–72.

Lyddon, W. J., & Satterfield, W. A. (1994). Relation of client attachment to therapist first- and second-order assessments. *Journal of Cognitive Psychotherapy, 8,* 233–242.

Lyddon, W. J., & Sherry, A. (2001). Developmental personality styles: An attachment theory conceptualization of personality disorders. *Journal of Counseling and Development, 79,* 405–414.

Lyn, T. S., & Burton, D. L. (2004). Adult attachment and sexual offender status. *American Journal of Orthopsychiatry, 74,* 150–159.

Lynch, P. D., Eisenberger, R., & Armeli, S. (1999). Perceived organizational support: Inferior-versus-superior performance by wary employees. *Journal of Applied Psychology, 84,* 467–483.

Lyons-Ruth, K., Bronfman, E., & Parsons, E. (1999). Maternal frightened, frightening, or atypical behavior and disorganized infant attachment patterns. *Monographs of the Society for Research in Child Development, 64,* 67–96.

Lyons-Ruth, K., & Jacobvitz, D. (1999). Attachment disorganization: Unresolved loss, relational violence, and lapses in behavioral and attentional strategies. In J. Cassidy & P. R. Shaver (Eds.), *Handbook of attachment: Theory, research, and clinical applications* (pp. 520–554). New York: Guilford Press.

Lyons-Ruth, K., Yellin, C., Melnick, S., & Atwood, G. (2005). Expanding the concept of unresolved mental states: Hostile/helpless states of mind on the Adult Attachment Interview are associated with disrupted mother–infant communication and infant disorganization. *Development and Psychopathology, 17,* 1–23.

MacDonald, G., & Kingsbury, R. (2006). Does physical pain augment anxious attachment? *Journal of Social and Personal Relationships, 23,* 291–304.

MacDonald, G., & Leary, M. R. (2005). Why does social exclusion hurt?: The relationship between social and physical pain. *Psychological Bulletin, 131,* 202–223.

MacKinnon, J. L., & Marcia, J. E. (2002). Concurring patterns of women's identity status, styles, and understanding of children's development. *International Journal of Behavioral Development, 26,* 70–80.

Magai, C. (1999). Affect, imagery, and attachment: Working models of interpersonal affect and the socialization of emotion. In J. Cassidy & P. R. Shaver (Eds.), *Handbook of attachment: Theory, research, and clinical applications* (pp. 787–802). New York: Guilford Press.

Magai, C., & Cohen, C. I. (1998). Attachment style and emotion regulation in dementia patients and their relation to caregiver burden. *Journals of Gerontology: Series B, Psychological Sciences and Social Sciences, 53,* P147–P154.

Magai, C., Cohen, C. I., Culver, C., Gomberg, D., & Malatesta, C. (1997). Relation between premorbid personality and patterns of emotion expression in mid- to late-stage dementia. *International Journal of Geriatric Psychiatry, 12,* 1092–1099.

Magai, C., Consedine, N. S., Gillespie, M., O'Neal, C., & Vilker, R. (2004). The differential roles of early emotion socialization and adult attachment in adult emotional experience: Testing a mediator hypothesis. *Attachment and Human Development, 6,* 389–417.

Magai, C., Distel, N., & Liker, R. (1995). Emotion socialization, attachment, and patterns of adult emotional traits. *Cognition and Emotion, 9,* 461–481.

Magai, C., Hunziker, J., Mesias, W., & Culver, L. (2000). Adult attachment styles and emotional biases. *International Journal of Behavioral Development, 24,* 301–309.

Mahalik, J. R., Aldarondo, E., Gilbert-Gokhale, S., & Shore, E. (2005). The role of insecure attachment and gender role stress in predicting controlling behaviors in men who batter. *Journal of Interpersonal Violence, 20,* 617–631.

Maier, H. W. (1987). Children and youth grow and develop in group care. *Child and Youth Services, 9,* 9–33.

Maier, M. A., Bernier, A., Pekrun, R., Zimmermann, P., Strasser, K., & Grossmann, K. E. (2005). Attachment state of mind and perceptual processing of emotional stimuli. *Attachment and Human Development, 7,* 67–81.

Maier, M. A., Bernier, A., Pekrun, R., Zimmermann, P., & Grossmann, K. E. (2004). Attachment working models as unconscious structures: An experimental test. *International Journal of Behavioral Development, 28,* 180–189.

Main, M. (1990). Cross-cultural studies of attachment organization: Recent studies, changing methodologies, and the concept of conditional strategies. *Human Development, 33,* 48–61.

Main, M. (1991). Metacognitive knowledge, metacognitive monitoring, and singular (coherent) vs. multiple (incoherent) models of attachment: Findings and directions for future research. In C. M. Parkes, J. Stevenson-Hinde, & P. Marris (Eds.), *Attachment across the life cycle* (pp. 127–159). London: Tavistock/Routledge.

Main, M. (1995). Attachment: Overview with implications for clinical work. In S. Goldberg, R. Muir, & J. Kerr (Eds.), *Attachment theory: Social, devel-* *opmental, and clinical perspectives* (pp. 407–474). Hillsdale, NJ: Erlbaum.

Main, M. (1999). Epilogue: Attachment theory: Eighteen points with suggestions for future studies. In J. Cassidy & P. R. Shaver (Eds.), *Handbook of attachment: Theory, research, and clinical applications* (pp. 845–888). New York: Guilford Press.

Main, M. (2001, March). *Attachment to mother and father in infancy, as related to the Adult Attachment Interview and a self-visualization task at age 19.* Poster presented at the biennial meeting of the Society for Research in Child Development, Minneapolis, MN.

Main, M., & Goldwyn, R. (1988). *Adult attachment scoring and classification system.* Unpublished manuscript, University of California, Berkeley.

Main, M., & Hesse, E. (1990). Parents' unresolved traumatic experiences are related to infant disorganized attachment status: Is frightened and/or frightening parental behavior the linking mechanism? In M. T. Greenberg, D. Cicchetti, & E. M. Cummings (Eds.), *Attachment in the preschool years: Theory, research, and intervention* (pp. 161–182). Chicago: University of Chicago Press.

Main, M., Kaplan, N., & Cassidy, J. (1985). Security in infancy, childhood, and adulthood: A move to the level of representation. *Monographs of the Society for Research in Child Development, 50,* 66–104.

Main, M., & Solomon, J. (1990). Procedures for identifying infants as disorganized/disoriented during the Ainsworth Strange Situation. In M. T. Greenberg, D. Cicchetti, & M. Cummings (Eds.), *Attachment in the preschool years: Theory, research, and intervention* (pp. 121–160). Chicago: University of Chicago Press.

Main, M., & Weston, D. R. (1981). The quality of the toddler's relationship to mother and father: Related to conflict behavior and the readiness to establish new relationships. *Child Development, 52,* 932–940.

Main, M., & Weston, D. R. (1982). Avoidance of the attachment figure in infancy: Descriptions and interpretations. In C. Parkes & J. Stevenson-Hinde (Eds.), *The place of attachment in human behavior* (pp. 31–59). New York: Basic Books.

Maio, G. R., Fincham, F. D., & Lycett, E. J. (2000). Attitudinal ambivalence toward parents and attachment style. *Personality and Social Psychology Bulletin, 26,* 1451–1464.

Malley-Morrison, K., You, H. S., & Mills, R. B. (2000). Young adult attachment styles and perceptions of elder abuse: A cross-cultural study. *Journal of Cross Cultural Gerontology, 15,* 163–184.

Mallinckrodt, B. (1991). Clients' representations of childhood emotional bonds with parents, social support, and formation of the working alliance. *Journal of Counseling Psychology, 38,* 401–409.

Mallinckrodt, B. (2000). Attachment, social competencies, social support, and interpersonal process in psychotherapy. *Psychotherapy Research, 10,* 239–266.

Mallinckrodt, B. (2001). Interpersonal processes, attachment, and development of social competencies in individual and group psychotherapy. In B.

R. Sarason & S. Duck (Eds.), *Personal relationships: Implications for clinical and community psychology* (pp. 89–117). New York: Wiley.

Mallinckrodt, B., & Chen, E. C. (2004). Attachment and interpersonal impact perceptions of group members: A social relations model analysis of transference. *Psychotherapy Research, 14,* 210–230.

Mallinckrodt, B., Coble, H. M., & Gantt, D. L. (1995). Working alliance, attachment memories, and social competencies of women in brief therapy. *Journal of Counseling Psychology, 42,* 79–84.

Mallinckrodt, B., Gantt, D. L., & Coble, H. M. (1995). Attachment patterns in the psychotherapy relationship: Development of the Client Attachment to Therapist Scale. *Journal of Counseling Psychology, 42,* 307–317.

Mallinckrodt, B., King, J. L., & Coble, H. M. (1998). Family dysfunction, alexithymia, and client attachment to therapist. *Journal of Counseling Psychology, 45,* 497–504.

Mallinckrodt, B., McCreary, B. A., & Robertson, A. K. (1995). Co-occurrence of eating disorders and incest: The role of attachment, family environment, and social competencies. *Journal of Counseling Psychology, 42,* 178–186.

Mallinckrodt, B., Porter, M. J., & Kivlighan, D. M., Jr. (2005). Client attachment to therapist, depth of in-session exploration, and object relations in brief psychotherapy. *Psychotherapy, 42,* 85–100.

Mallinckrodt, B., & Wei, M. (2005). Attachment, social competencies, social support, and psychological distress. *Journal of Counseling Psychology, 52,* 358–367.

Man, K. O., & Hamid, P. (1998). The relationship between attachment prototypes, self-esteem, loneliness, and causal attributions in Chinese trainee teachers. *Personality and Individual Differences, 24,* 357–371.

Manassis, K., Bradley, S., Goldberg, S., Hood, J., & Swinson, R. P. (1994). Attachment in mothers with anxiety disorders and their children. *Journal of the American Academy of Child and Adolescent Psychiatry, 33,* 1106–1113.

Manassis, K., Owens, M., Adam, K. S., West, M., & Sheldon-Keller, A. E. (1999). Assessing attachment: Convergent validity of the Adult Attachment Interview and the Parental Bonding Instrument. *Australian and New Zealand Journal of Psychiatry, 33,* 559–567.

Marchand, J. F. (2004). Husbands' and wives' marital quality: The role of adult attachment orientations, depressive symptoms, and conflict resolution behaviors. *Attachment and Human Development, 6,* 99–112.

Marchand, J. F., Schedler, S., & Wagstaff, D. A. (2004). The role of parents' attachment orientations, depressive symptoms, and conflict behaviors in children's externalizing and internalizing behavior problems. *Early Childhood Research Quarterly, 19,* 449–462.

Marcia, J. E. (1980). Identity in adolescence. In J. Adelson (Ed.), *Handbook of adolescent psychology* (pp. 154–187). New York: Wiley.

Markiewicz, D., Doyle, A. B., & Brendgen, M. (2001). The quality of adolescents' friendships: Associations with mothers' interpersonal relationships, attachments to parents and friends, and prosocial behaviors. *Journal of Adolescence, 24,* 429–445.

Markiewicz, D., Reis, M., & Gold, D. P. (1997). An exploration of attachment styles and personality traits in caregiving for dementia patients. *International Journal of Aging and Human Development, 45,* 111–132.

Markman, H. J., Stanley, S., & Blumberg, S. L. (1994). *Fighting for your marriage: Positive steps for preventing divorce and preserving a lasting love.* San Francisco: Jossey-Bass.

Marmarosh, C. L., Franz, V. A., Koloi, M., Majors, R. C., Rahimi, A. M., Ronquillo, J. G., et al. (2006). Therapists' group attachments and their expectations of patients' attitudes about group therapy. *International Journal of Group Psychotherapy, 56,* 325–338.

Marsa, F., O'Reilly, G., Carr, A., Murphy, P., O'Sullivan, M., Cotter, A., & Hevey, D. (2004). Attachment styles and psychological profiles of child sex offenders in Ireland. *Journal of Interpersonal Violence, 19,* 228–251.

Marsh, P., McFarland, F., Allen, J. P., McElhaney, K. B., & Land, D. (2003). Attachment, autonomy, and multifinality in adolescent internalizing and risky behavioral symptoms. *Development and Psychopathology, 15,* 451–467.

Marshall, W. L., Serran, G. A., & Cortoni, F. A. (2000). Childhood attachments, sexual abuse, and their relationship to adult coping in child molesters. *Sexual Abuse: Journal of Research and Treatment, 12,* 17–26.

Maslow, A. H. (1954). *Motivation and personality.* New York: Harper & Row.

Maslow, A. H. (1968). *Toward a psychology of being* (2nd ed.). New York: Van Nostrand.

Maslow, A. H. (1971). *The farther reaches of human nature.* New York: Viking.

Masterson, J. F. (1977). Primary anorexia nervosa. In P. Hartocollis (Ed.), *Borderline personality disorders* (pp. 475–494). New York: International Universities Press.

Matas, L., Arend, R., & Sroufe, L. A. (1978). Continuity of adaptation in the second year: The relationship between quality of attachment and later competence. *Child Development, 49,* 547–556.

Mathews, A., & MacLeod, C. (1985). Selective processing of threat cues in anxiety states. *Behaviour Research and Therapy, 23,* 563–569.

Maunder, R. G., & Hunter, J. J. (2001). Attachment and psychosomatic medicine: Developmental contributions to stress and disease. *Psychosomatic Medicine, 63,* 556–567.

Maunder R. G., Lancee, W. J., Greenberg, G., Hunter, J. J., & Fernandes, B. (2000). Insecure attachment in a subgroup of ulcerative colitis defined by ANCA status. *Digestive Diseases Science, 45,* 2127–2132.

Maunder, R. G., Lancee, W. J., Nolan, R. P., Hunter, J. J., & Grerenberg, G. R. (2005). Attachment insecurity moderates the relationship between disease activity and depressive symptoms in ulcerative colitis. *Inflammatory Bowel Disease, 11,* 919–926.

Maunder, R. G., Lancee, W. J., Nolan, R. P., Hunter, J. J., & Tannenbaum, D. W. (2006). The relationship of attachment insecurity to subjective stress and autonomic function during standardized acute stress in healthy adults. *Journal of Psychosomatic Research, 60,* 283–290.

Maunder, R. G., Panzer, A., Viljoen, M., Owen, J., Human, S., & Hunter, J. J. (2006). Physicians' difficulty with emergency department patients is related to patients' attachment style. *Social Science and Medicine, 63,* 552–562.

Mauricio, A. M., & Gormley, B. (2001). Male perpetration of physical violence against female partners. *Journal of Interpersonal Violence, 16,* 1066–1081.

Mawson, A. R. (1980). Aggression, attachment behavior, and crimes of violence. In T. Hirschi & M. Gottfredson (Eds.), *Understanding crime: Current theory and research* (pp. 103–116). Beverly Hills, CA: Sage.

Mayer, J. (2004, February 16). Contract sport: What did the Vice President do for Halliburton? *New Yorker,* pp. 80–91.

Mayseless, O. (1991). Adult attachment patterns and courtship violence. *Family Relations: Interdisciplinary Journal of Applied Family Studies, 40,* 21–28.

Mayseless, O. (1993). Gifted adolescents and intimacy in close same-sex friendships. *Journal of Youth and Adolescence, 22,* 135–146.

Mayseless, O. (2004). Home leaving to military service: Attachment concerns, transfer of attachment functions from parents to peers, and adjustment. *Journal of Adolescent Research, 19,* 533–558.

Mayseless, O., Danieli, R., & Sharabany, R. (1996). Adults' attachment patterns: Coping with separations. *Journal of Youth and Adolescence, 25,* 667–690.

Mayseless, O., & Popper, M. (in press). Reliance on leaders and social institutions: An attachment perspective. *Attachment and Human Development.*

Mayseless, O., & Scharf, M. (in press). Adolescents' attachment representations and their capacity for intimacy in close relationships. *Journal of Research on Adolescence.*

Mayseless, O., & Scher, A. (2000). Mother's attachment concerns regarding spouse and infant's temperament as modulators of maternal separation anxiety. *Journal of Child Psychology and Psychiatry, 41,* 917–925.

Mayseless, O., Sharabany, R., & Sagi, A. (1997). Attachment concerns of mothers as manifested in parental, spousal, and friendship relationships. *Personal Relationships, 4,* 255–269.

McCarthy, G. (1999). Attachment style and adult love relationships and friendships: A study of a group of women at risk of experiencing relationship difficulties. *British Journal of Medical Psychology, 72,* 305–321.

McCarthy, G., & Taylor, A. (1999). Avoidant/ambivalent attachment style as a mediator between abusive childhood experiences and adult relationship difficulties. *Journal of Child Psychology and Psychiatry, 40,* 465–477.

McCluskey, U. (2002). The dynamics of attachment and systems-centered group psychotherapy. *Group Dynamics, 6,* 131–142.

McCormick, C. B., & Kennedy, J. H. (1994). Parent–child attachment working models and self-esteem in adolescence. *Journal of Youth and Adolescence, 23,* 1–18.

McCrae, R. R., & Costa, P. T. (1989). The structure of interpersonal traits: Wiggins's circumplex and the five-factor model. *Journal of Personality and Social Psychology, 56,* 586–595.

McCrae, R. R., & Costa, P. T. (1990). *Personality in adulthood.* New York: Guilford Press.

McCullough, M. E. (2000). Forgiveness as human strength: Theory, measurement, and links to well-being. *Journal of Social and Clinical Psychology, 19,* 43–55.

McCullough, M. E., Emmons, R. A., & Tsang, J. (2002). The grateful disposition: A conceptual and empirical topography. *Journal of Personality and Social Psychology, 82,* 112–127.

McCullough, M. E., Rachal, K. C., Sandage, S. J., Worthington, E. L., Brown, S. W., & Hight, T. L. (1998). Interpersonal forgiving in close relationships: II. Theoretical elaboration and measurement. *Journal of Personality and Social Psychology, 75,* 1586–1603.

McCullough, M. E., Worthington, E. L., & Rachal, K. C. (1997). Interpersonal forgiving in close relationships. *Journal of Personality and Social Psychology, 73,* 321–336.

McCurdy, S. J., & Scherman, A. (1996). Effects of family structure on the adolescent separation–individuation process. *Adolescence, 31,* 307–319.

McDonald, A., Beck, R., Allison, S., & Norsworthy, L. (2005). Attachment to God and parents: Testing the correspondence vs. compensation hypotheses. *Journal of Psychology and Christianity, 24,* 21–28.

McElhaney, K. B., Immele, A., Smith, F. D., & Allen, J. P. (2006). Attachment organization as a moderator of the link between friendship quality and adolescent delinquency. *Attachment and Human Development, 8,* 33–46.

McGowan, S. (2002). Mental representations in stressful situations: The calming and distressing effects of significant others. *Journal of Experimental Social Psychology, 38,* 152–161.

McKinney, K. G. (2002). Engagement in community service among college students: Is it affected by significant attachment relationships? *Journal of Adolescence, 25,* 139–154.

McMahon, C., Barnett, B., Kowalenko, N., & Tennant, C. (2005). Psychological factors associated with persistent postnatal depression: Past and current relationships, defense styles, and the mediating role of insecure attachment style. *Journal of Affective Disorders, 84,* 15–24.

McNally, A. M., Palfai, T. P., Levine, R. V., & Moore, B. M. (2003). Attachment dimensions and drinking-related problems among young adults the mediational role of coping motives. *Addictive Behaviors, 28,* 1115–1127.

McNally, R. J. (1998). Experimental approaches to cognitive abnormality in posttraumatic stress disorder. *Clinical Psychology Review, 18,* 971–982.

McNamara, P., Andresen, J., Clark, J., Zborowski,

M., & Duffy, C. A. (2001). Impact of attachment styles on dream recall and dream content: A test of the attachment hypothesis of REM sleep. *Journal of Sleep Research, 10*, 117–127.

Meaney, M. J. (2004). The nature of nurture: Maternal effects and chromatin remodeling. In J. T. Cacioppo (Ed.), *Essays in social neuroscience* (pp. 1–14). Cambridge, MA: MIT Press.

Mearns, J. (1991). Coping with a breakup: Negative mood regulation expectancies and depression following the end of a romantic relationship. *Journal of Personality and Social Psychology, 60*, 327–334.

Medway, F. J., Davis, K. E., Cafferty, T. P., Chappell, K. D., & O'Hearn, R. E. (1995). Family disruption and adult attachment correlates of spouse and child reactions to separation and reunion due to Operation Desert Storm. *Journal of Social and Clinical Psychology, 14*, 97–118.

Meesters, C., & Muris, P. (2002). Attachment style and self-reported aggression. *Psychological Reports, 90*, 231–235.

Meeus, W., Oosterwegel, A., & Vollebergh, W. (2002). Parental and peer attachment and identity development in adolescence. *Journal of Adolescence, 25*, 93–106.

Meredith, P. J., & Noller, P. (2003). Attachment and infant difficultness in postnatal depression. *Journal of Family Issues, 24*, 668–686.

Meredith, P. J., Strong, J., & Feeney, J. A. (2005). Evidence of a relationship between adult attachment variables and appraisals of chronic pain. *Pain Research and Management, 10*, 191–200.

Meredith, P. J., Strong, J., & Feeney, J. A. (2006a). The relationship of adult attachment to emotion, catastrophizing, control, threshold and tolerance, in experimentally-induced pain. *Pain, 120*, 44–52.

Meredith, P. J., Strong, J., & Feeney, J. A. (2006b). Adult attachment, anxiety, and pain self-efficacy as predictors of pain intensity and disability. *Pain, 123*, 146–154.

Merrill, L. L., Thomsen, C. J., Crouch, J. L., May, P., Gold, S. R., & Milner, J. S. (2005). Predicting adult risk of child physical abuse from childhood exposure to violence: Can interpersonal schemata explain the association? *Journal of Social and Clinical Psychology, 24*, 981–1002.

Metz, M. E., & Epstein, N. (2002). Assessing the role of relationship conflict in sexual dysfunction. *Journal of Sex and Marital Therapy, 28*, 139–164.

Meyer, B., Olivier, L., & Roth, D. A. (2005). Please don't leave me!: BIS/BAS, attachment styles, and responses to a relationship threat. *Personality and Individual Differences, 38*, 151–162.

Meyer, B., & Pilkonis, P. A. (2001). Attachment style. *Psychotherapy, 38*, 466–472.

Meyer, B., & Pilkonis, P. A. (2005). An attachment model of personality disorders. In M. F. Lenzenweger & J. F. Clarkin (Eds.), *Major theories of personality disorder* (2nd ed., pp. 231–281). New York: Guilford Press.

Meyer, B., Pilkonis, P. A., & Beevers, C. G. (2004). What's in a (neutral) face?: Personality disorders, attachment styles, and the appraisal of ambiguous social cues. *Journal of Personality Disorders, 18*, 320–336.

Meyer, B., Pilkonis, P. A., Proietti, J. M., Heape, C. L., & Egan, M. (2001). Attachment styles and personality disorders as predictors of symptom course. *Journal of Personality Disorders, 15*, 371–389.

Meyer, D. E., & Schvaneveldt, R. W. (1971). Facilitation in recognizing pairs of words: Evidence of dependence between retrieval operations. *Journal of Experimental Psychology, 90*, 227–234.

Meyer, J. P., Allen, N. J., & Smith, C. A. (1993). Commitment to organizations and occupations: Extension and test of a three-component conceptualization. *Journal of Applied Psychology, 78*, 538–551.

Meyers, S. A. (1998). Personality correlates of adult attachment style. *Journal of Social Psychology, 138*, 407–409.

Meyers, S. A., & Landsberger, S. A. (2002). Direct and indirect pathways between adult attachment style and marital satisfaction. *Personal Relationships, 9*, 159–172.

Mickelson, K. D., Kessler, R. C., & Shaver, P. R. (1997). Adult attachment in a nationally representative sample. *Journal of Personality and Social Psychology, 73*, 1092–1106.

Mikail, S. F., Henderson, P. R., & Tasca, G. A. (1994). An interpersonally based model of chronic pain: An application of attachment theory. *Clinical Psychology Review, 14*, 1–16.

Mikulincer, M. (1994). *Human learned helplessness.* New York: Plenum Press.

Mikulincer, M. (1995). Attachment style and the mental representation of the self. *Journal of Personality and Social Psychology, 69*, 1203–1215.

Mikulincer, M. (1997). Adult attachment style and information processing: Individual differences in curiosity and cognitive closure. *Journal of Personality and Social Psychology, 72*, 1217–1230.

Mikulincer, M. (1998a). Adult attachment style and affect regulation: Strategic variations in self-appraisals. *Journal of Personality and Social Psychology, 75*, 420–435.

Mikulincer, M. (1998b). Adult attachment style and individual differences in functional versus dysfunctional experiences of anger. *Journal of Personality and Social Psychology, 74*, 513–524.

Mikulincer, M. (1998c). Attachment working models and the sense of trust: An exploration of interaction goals and affect regulation. *Journal of Personality and Social Psychology, 74*, 1209–1224.

Mikulincer, M., & Arad, D. (1999). Attachment working models and cognitive openness in close relationships: A test of chronic and temporary accessibility effects. *Journal of Personality and Social Psychology, 77*, 710–725.

Mikulincer, M., Birnbaum, G., Woddis, D., & Nachmias, O. (2000). Stress and accessibility of proximity-related thoughts: Exploring the normative and intraindividual components of attachment theory. *Journal of Personality and Social Psychology, 78*, 509–523.

Mikulincer, M., Dolev, T., & Shaver, P. R. (2004). Attachment-related strategies during thought suppression: Ironic rebounds and vulnerable self-representations. *Journal of Personality and Social Psychology, 87*, 940–956.

Mikulincer, M., & Erev, I. (1991). Attachment style and the structure of romantic love. *British Journal of Social Psychology, 30*, 273–291.

Mikulincer, M., & Florian, V. (1995). Appraisal of and coping with a real-life stressful situation: The contribution of attachment styles. *Personality and Social Psychology Bulletin, 21*, 406–414.

Mikulincer, M., & Florian, V. (1997). Are emotional and instrumental supportive interactions beneficial in times of stress?: The impact of attachment style. *Anxiety, Stress and Coping: An International Journal, 10*, 109–127.

Mikulincer, M., & Florian, V. (1998). The relationship between adult attachment styles and emotional and cognitive reactions to stressful events. In J. A. Simpson & W. S. Rholes (Eds.), *Attachment theory and close relationships* (pp. 143–165). New York: Guilford Press.

Mikulincer, M., & Florian, V. (1999a). The association between parental reports of attachment style and family dynamics, and offspring's reports of adult attachment style. *Family Process, 38*, 243–257.

Mikulincer, M., & Florian, V. (1999b). The association between spouses' self-reports of attachment styles and representations of family dynamics. *Family Process, 38*, 69–83.

Mikulincer, M., & Florian, V. (1999c). Maternal–fetal bonding, coping strategies, and mental health during pregnancy: The contribution of attachment style. *Journal of Social and Clinical Psychology, 18*, 255–276.

Mikulincer, M., & Florian, V. (2000). Exploring individual differences in reactions to mortality salience: Does attachment style regulate terror management mechanisms? *Journal of Personality and Social Psychology, 79*, 260–273.

Mikulincer, M., Florian, V., Birnbaum, G., & Malishkevich, S. (2002). The death-anxiety buffering function of close relationships: Exploring the effects of separation reminders on death-thought accessibility. *Personality and Social Psychology Bulletin, 28*, 287–299.

Mikulincer, M., Florian, V., Cowan, P. A., & Cowan, C. P. (2002). Attachment security in couple relationships: A systemic model and its implications for family dynamics. *Family Process, 41*, 405–434.

Mikulincer, M., Florian, V., & Hirschberger, G. (2003). The existential function of close relationships: Introducing death into the science of love. *Personality and Social Psychology Review, 7*, 20–40.

Mikulincer, M., Florian, V., & Tolmacz, R. (1990). Attachment styles and fear of personal death: A case study of affect regulation. *Journal of Personality and Social Psychology, 58*, 273–280.

Mikulincer, M., Florian, V., & Weller, A. (1993). Attachment styles, coping strategies, and posttraumatic psychological distress: The impact of the Gulf War in Israel. *Journal of Personality and Social Psychology, 64*, 817–826.

Mikulincer, M., Gillath, O., Halevy, V., Avihou, N., Avidan, S., & Eshkoli, N. (2001). Attachment theory and reactions to others' needs: Evidence that activation of the sense of attachment security promotes empathic responses. *Journal of Personality and Social Psychology, 81*, 1205–1224.

Mikulincer, M., Gillath, O., Sapir-Lavid, Y., Yaakobi, E., Arias, K., Tal-Aloni, L., & Bor, G. (2003). Attachment theory and concern for others' welfare: Evidence that activation of the sense of secure base promotes endorsement of self-transcendence values. *Basic and Applied Social Psychology, 25*, 299–312.

Mikulincer, M., Gillath, O., & Shaver, P. R. (2002). Activation of the attachment system in adulthood: Threat-related primes increase the accessibility of mental representations of attachment figures. *Journal of Personality and Social Psychology, 83*, 881–895.

Mikulincer, M., & Goodman, G. S. (Eds.). (2006). *Dynamics of romantic love: Attachment, caregiving, and sex.* New York: Guilford Press.

Mikulincer, M., Hirschberger, G., Nachmias, O., & Gillath, O. (2001). The affective component of the secure base schema: Affective priming with representations of attachment security. *Journal of Personality and Social Psychology, 81*, 305–321.

Mikulincer, M., & Horesh, N. (1999). Adult attachment style and the perception of others: The role of projective mechanisms. *Journal of Personality and Social Psychology, 76*, 1022–1034.

Mikulincer, M., Horesh, N., Eilati, I., & Kotler, M. (1999). The association between adult attachment style and mental health in extreme life-endangering conditions. *Personality and Individual Differences, 27*, 831–842.

Mikulincer, M., Horesh, N., Levy-Shiff, R., Manovich, R., & Shalev, J. (1998). The contribution of adult attachment style to the adjustment to infertility. *British Journal of Medical Psychology, 71*, 265–280.

Mikulincer, M., & Nachshon, O. (1991). Attachment styles and patterns of self-disclosure. *Journal of Personality and Social Psychology, 61*, 321–331.

Mikulincer, M., & Orbach, I. (1995). Attachment styles and repressive defensiveness: The accessibility and architecture of affective memories. *Journal of Personality and Social Psychology, 68*, 917–925.

Mikulincer, M., Orbach, I., & Iavnieli, D. (1998). Adult attachment style and affect regulation: Strategic variations in subjective self–other similarity. *Journal of Personality and Social Psychology, 75*, 436–448.

Mikulincer, M., & Selinger, M. (2001). The interplay between attachment and affiliation systems in adolescents' same-sex friendships: The role of attachment style. *Journal of Social and Personal Relationships, 18*, 81–106.

Mikulincer, M., & Shaver, P. R. (2001). Attachment theory and intergroup bias: Evidence that priming the secure base schema attenuates negative reactions to out-groups. *Journal of Personality and Social Psychology, 81*, 97–115.

Mikulincer, M., & Shaver, P. R. (2003). The attachment behavioral system in adulthood: Activation, psychodynamics, and interpersonal processes. In M. P. Zanna (Ed.), *Advances in experimental social psychology* (Vol. 35, pp. 53–152). New York: Academic Press.

Mikulincer, M., & Shaver, P. R. (2004). Security-based self-representations in adulthood: Contents and processes. In W. S. Rholes & J. A. Simpson (Eds.), *Adult attachment: Theory, research, and clinical implications* (pp. 159–195). New York: Guilford Press.

Mikulincer, M., & Shaver, P. R. (2005a). Mental representations of attachment security: Theoretical foundation for a positive social psychology. In M. W. Baldwin (Ed.), *Interpersonal cognition* (pp. 233–266). New York: Guilford Press.

Mikulincer, M., & Shaver, P. R. (2005b). Attachment theory and emotions in close relationships: Exploring the attachment-related dynamics of emotional reactions to relational events. *Personal Relationships, 12,* 149–168.

Mikulincer, M., & Shaver, P. R. (in press). An attachment perspective on bereavement. In M. Stroebe, R. O. Hansson, H. A. W. Schut, & W. Stroebe (Eds.), *Handbook of bereavement research and practice: 21st century perspectives.* Washington, DC: American Psychological Association.

Mikulincer, M., & Shaver, P. R. (2007). Contributions of attachment theory and research to motivation science. In J. Shah & W. Gardner (Eds.), *Handbook of motivation science.* New York: Guilford Press.

Mikulincer, M., Shaver, P. R., Gillath, O., & Nitzberg, R. A. (2005). Attachment, caregiving, and altruism: Boosting attachment security increases compassion and helping. *Journal of Personality and Social Psychology, 89,* 817–839.

Mikulincer, M., Shaver, P. R., & Horesh, N. (2006). Attachment bases of emotion regulation and posttraumatic adjustment. In D. K. Snyder, J. A. Simpson, & J. N. Hughes (Eds.), *Emotion regulation in families: Pathways to dysfunction and health* (pp. 77–99). Washington, DC: American Psychological Association.

Mikulincer, M., Shaver, P. R., & Pereg, D. (2003). Attachment theory and affect regulation: The dynamics, development, and cognitive consequences of attachment-related strategies. *Motivation and Emotion, 27,* 77–102.

Mikulincer, M., Shaver, P. R., & Slav, K. (2006). Attachment, mental representations of others, and gratitude and forgiveness in romantic relationships. In M. Mikulincer & G. S. Goodman (Eds.), *Dynamics of romantic love: Attachment, caregiving, and sex* (pp. 190–215). New York: Guilford Press.

Mikulincer, M., & Sheffi, E. (2000). Adult attachment style and cognitive reactions to positive affect: A test of mental categorization and creative problem solving. *Motivation and Emotion, 24,* 149–174.

Miljkovitch, R., Pierrehumbert, B., Bretherton, I., & Halfon, O. (2004). Associations between parental and child attachment representations. *Attachment and Human Development, 6,* 305–325.

Miljkovitch, R., Pierrehumbert, B., Karmaniola, A., Bader, M., & Halfon, O. (2005). Assessing attachment cognitions and their associations with depression in youth with eating or drug misuse disorders. *Substance Use and Misuse, 40,* 605–623.

Miller, A. L., Notaro, P. C., & Zimmerman, M. A. (2002). Stability and change in internal working models of friendship: Associations with multiple domains of urban adolescent functioning. *Journal of Social and Personal Relationships, 19,* 233–259.

Miller, G. A., Galanter, E., & Pribram, K. H. (1960). *Plans and the structure of behavior.* New York: Holt, Rinehart & Winston.

Miller, G. A., & Rice, K.G. (1993). A factor analysis of a university counseling center problem checklist. *Journal of College Student Development, 34,* 98–102.

Miller, L. C., Berg, J. H., & Archer, R. L. (1983). Openers: Individuals who elicit intimate self-disclosure. *Journal of Personality and Social Psychology, 44,* 1234–1244.

Milligan, K., Atkinson, L., Trehub, S. E., Benoit, D., & Poulton, L. (2003). Maternal attachment and the communication of emotion through song. *Infant Behavior and Development, 26,* 1–13.

Millon, T., & Davis, R. D. (1996). *Disorders of personality: DSM-IV and beyond.* New York: Wiley.

Minuchin, P. (1985). Families and individual development: Provocations from the field of family therapy. *Child Development, 56,* 289–302.

Mirels, H. L., Greblo, P., & Dean, J. B. (2002). Judgmental self-doubt: Beliefs about one's judgmental prowess. *Personality and Individual Differences, 33,* 741–758.

Mitchell, S. (1998). *The essence of wisdom.* New York: Broadway Books.

Mohr, J. J. (1999). Same-sex romantic attachment. In J. Cassidy & P. R. Shaver (Eds.), *Handbook of attachment: Theory, research, and clinical applications* (pp. 378–394). New York: Guilford Press.

Mohr, J. J., & Fassinger, R. E. (2003). Self-acceptance and self-disclosure of sexual orientation in lesbian, gay and bisexual adults: An attachment perspective. *Journal of Counseling Psychology, 50,* 482–495.

Mohr, J. J., Gelso, C. J., & Hill, C. E. (2005). Client and counselor trainee attachment as predictors of session evaluation and countertransference behavior in first counseling sessions. *Journal of Counseling Psychology, 52,* 298–309.

Moller, N. P., Fouladi, R. T., McCarthy, C. J., & Hatch, K. D. (2003). Relationship of attachment and social support to college students' adjustment following a relationship breakup. *Journal of Counseling and Development, 81,* 354–369.

Moller, N. P., McCarthy, C. J., & Fouladi, R. T. (2002). Earned attachment security: Its relationship to coping resources and stress symptoms among college students following relationship breakup. *Journal of College Student Development, 43,* 213–230.

Moncher, F. J. (1996). The relationship of maternal adult attachment style and risk of physical child abuse. *Journal of Interpersonal Violence, 11,* 335–350.

Montebarocci, O., Codispoti, M., Baldaro, B., & Rossi, N. (2004). Adult attachment style and alexithymia. *Personality and Individual Differences, 36,* 499–507.

Moore, K., Moretti, M. M., & Holland, R. (1998). A new perspective on youth care programs: Using attachment theory to guide interventions for troubled youth. *Residential Treatment for Children and Youth, 15,* 1–24.

Moras, K., & Strupp, H. H. (1982). Pretherapy interpersonal relations, patients' alliance, and outcome in brief therapy. *Archives of General Psychiatry, 39,* 405–409.

Moreira, J. M., Bernardes, S., Andrez, M., Aguiar, P., Moleiro, C., & de Fatima Silva, M. (1998). Social competence, personality and adult attachment style in a Portuguese sample. *Personality and Individual Differences, 24,* 565–570.

Moreira, J. M., de Fatima Silva, M., Moleiro, C., Aguiar, P., Andrez, M., Bernardes, S., & Afonso, H. (2003). Social support as an offshoot of attachment style. *Personality and Individual Differences, 34,* 485–501.

Moretti, M. M., Holland, R., & Peterson, S. (1994). Long term outcome of an attachment-based program for conduct disorder. *Canadian Journal of Psychiatry, 39,* 360–370.

Morf, C. C., & Rhodewalt, F. (2001). Unraveling the paradoxes of narcissism: A dynamic self-regulatory processing model. *Psychological Inquiry, 12,* 177–196.

Morgan, H. J., & Shaver, P. R. (1999). Attachment processes and commitment to romantic relationships. In J. M. Adams & W. H. Jones (Eds.), *Handbook of interpersonal commitment and relationship stability* (pp. 109–124). New York: Plenum Press.

Morrison, T. L., Goodlin-Jones, B. L., & Urquiza, A. J. (1997). Attachment and the representation of intimate relationships in adulthood. *Journal of Psychology: Interdisciplinary and Applied, 131,* 57–71.

Morrison, T. L., Urquiza, A. J., & Goodlin-Jones, B. L. (1997). Attachment, perceptions of interaction, and relationship adjustment. *Journal of Social and Personal Relationships, 14,* 627–642.

Mosheim, R., Zachhuber, U., Scharf, L., Hofmann, A., Kemmler, G., Danzl, C., et al. (2000). Quality of attachment and interpersonal problems as possible predictors of inpatient therapy outcome. *Psychotherapeut, 45,* 223–229.

Moss, E., & St.-Laurent, D. (2001). Attachment at school age and academic performance. *Developmental Psychology, 37,* 863–874.

Mothersead, P. K., Kivlighan, D. M., Jr., & Wynkoop, T. F. (1998). Attachment, family dysfunction, parental alcoholism, and interpersonal distress in late adolescence: A structural model. *Journal of Counseling Psychology, 45,* 196–203.

MoveOn Bulletin. (July 10, 2002). Who is Dick Cheney? (*www.moveon.org*).

Mullen, B., & Cooper, C. (1994). The relationship between group cohesiveness and performance: An integration. *Psychological Bulletin, 115,* 210–227.

Muller, R. T., & Lemieux, K. E. (2000). Social support, attachment, and psychopathology in high risk formerly maltreated adults. *Child Abuse and Neglect, 24,* 883–900.

Muller, R. T., Sicoli, L. A., & Lemieux, K. E. (2000). Relationship between attachment style and posttraumatic stress symptomatology among adults who report the experience of childhood abuse. *Journal of Traumatic Stress, 13,* 321–332.

Mullis, R. L., Hill, E., & Readdick, C. A. (1999). Attachment and social support among adolescents. *Journal of Genetic Psychology, 160,* 500–502.

Muran, J. C., Segal, Z. V., Samstag, L. W., & Crawford, C. E. (1994). Patient pretreatment interpersonal problems and therapeutic alliance in short-term cognitive therapy. *Journal of Consulting and Clinical Psychology, 62,* 185–190.

Muris, P., & Meesters, C. (2002). Attachment, behavioral inhibition, and anxiety disorders symptoms in normal adolescents. *Journal of Psychopathology and Behavioral Assessment, 24,* 97–106.

Muris, P., Meesters, C., Morren, M., & Moorman, L. (2004). Anger and hostility in adolescents: Relationships with self-reported attachment style and perceived parental rearing styles. *Journal of Psychosomatic Research, 57,* 257–264.

Muris, P., Meesters, C., & van den Berg, S. (2003). Internalizing and externalizing problems as correlates of self-reported attachment style and perceived parental rearing in normal adolescents. *Journal of Child and Family Studies, 12,* 171–183.

Muris, P., Meesters, C., van Melick, M., & Zwambag, L. (2001). Self-reported attachment style, attachment quality, and symptoms of anxiety and depression in young adolescents. *Personality and Individual Differences, 30,* 809–818.

Murphy, B., & Bates, G. W. (1997). Adult attachment style and vulnerability to depression. *Personality and Individual Differences, 22,* 835–844.

Murphy, S. A. Braun, T., Tillery, L., Cain, K. C., Johnson, L. C., & Beaton, R. B. (1999). PTSD among bereaved parents following the violent deaths of their 12– to 28-year-old children: A longitudinal prospective analysis. *Journal of Traumatic Stress, 12,* 273–291.

Murray, S. L., Holmes, J. G., & Collins, N. L. (2006). The relational signature of felt security. *Psychological Bulletin, 132,* 641–666.

Myers, L. B., & Vetere, A. (2002). Adult romantic attachment styles and health-related measures. *Psychology, Health, and Medicine, 7,* 175–180.

Myhr, G., Sookman, D., & Pinard, G. (2004). Attachment security and parental bonding in adults with obsessive–compulsive disorder: A comparison with depressed out-patients and healthy controls. *Acta Psychiatrica Scandinavica, 109,* 447–456.

Nachmias, M., Gunnar, M., Mangelsdorf, S., Parritz, R. H., & Buss, K. (1996). Behavioral inhibition and stress reactivity: The moderating role of attachment security. *Child Development, 67,* 508–522.

Nada-Raja, S., McGee, R., & Stanton, W. R. (1992). Perceived attachments to parents and peers and psychological well-being in adolescence. *Journal of Youth and Adolescence, 21,* 471–485.

Nager, E. A., & de Vries, B. (2004). Memorializing on the World Wide Web: Patterns of grief and attachment in adult daughters of deceased mothers. *Omega, 49,* 43–56.

Nakash-Eisikovits, O., Dutra, L., & Westen, D. (2002). Relationship between attachment patterns and personality pathology in adolescents. *Journal of the American Academy of Child and Adolescent Psychiatry, 41,* 1111–1123.

National Center for Health Statistics. (1995). *Health, United States, 1994.* Hyattsville, MD: U.S. Public Health Service.

Neff, K. D. (2003). Self-compassion: An alternative conceptualization of a healthy attitude toward oneself. *Self and Identity, 2,* 85–102.

Neria, Y., Guttmann-Steinmetz, S., Koenen, K., Levinovsky, L., Zakin, G., & Dekel, R. (2001). Do attachment and hardiness relate to each other and to mental health in real-life stress? *Journal of Social and Personal Relationships, 18,* 844–858.

Neswald-McCalip, R. (2001). Development of the secure counselor: Case examples supporting Pistole & Watkins's (1995) discussion of attachment theory in counseling supervision. *Counselor Education and Supervision, 41,* 18–27.

Neyer, F. J., & Voigt, D. (2004). Personality and social network effects on romantic relationships: A dyadic approach. *European Journal of Personality, 18,* 279–299.

NICHD Early Child Care Research Network. (1994). Child care and child development: The NICHD Study of Early Child Care. In S. Friedman & H. Haywood (Eds.), *Developmental follow-up: Concepts, domains, and methods* (pp. 377–396). New York: Academic Press.

NICHD Early Child Care Research Network. (2001). Child care and family predictors of MacArthur preschool attachment and stability from infancy. *Developmental Psychology, 37,* 847–862.

Nickell, A. D., Waudby, C. J., & Trull, T. J. (2002). Attachment, parental bonding, and borderline personality disorder features in young adults. *Journal of Personality Disorders, 16,* 148–159.

Niedenthal, P. M., Brauer, M., Robin, L., & Innes-Ker, A. H. (2002). Adult attachment and the perception of facial expression of emotion. *Journal of Personality and Social Psychology, 82,* 419–433.

Nitzberg, R. E., Shaver, P. R., & Conger, R. D. (2007). *Romantic attachment style in the age period from 18 to 20: Stability and connections with parental and partner social interactions.* Manuscript under review.

Noftle, E. E., & Shaver, P. R. (2006). Attachment dimensions and the Big Five personality traits: Associations and comparative ability to predict relationship quality. *Journal of Research in Personality, 40,* 179–208.

Noller, P. (2005). Attachment insecurity as a filter in the decoding and encoding of nonverbal behavior in close relationships. *Journal of Nonverbal Behavior, 29,* 171–176.

Noller, P., & Feeney, J. A. (1994). Relationship satisfaction, attachment, and nonverbal accuracy in early marriage. *Journal of Nonverbal Behavior, 18,* 199–221.

Noller, P., & Feeney, J. A. (2002). *Understanding marriage: Developments in the study of couple interaction.* New York: Cambridge University Press.

Noom, M. J., Dekovic, M., & Meeus, W. H. J. (1999). Autonomy, attachment, and psychosocial adjustment during adolescence: A double-edged sword? *Journal of Adolescence, 22,* 771–783.

Noyes, R., Jr., Stuart, S. P., Langbehn, D. R., Happel, R. L., Longley, S. L., Muller, B. A., & Yagla. S. J. (2003). Test of an interpersonal model of hypochondriasis. *Psychosomatic Medicine, 65,* 292–300.

Oatley, K., & Jenkins, J. M. (1996). *Understanding emotions.* Cambridge, MA: Blackwell.

Obegi, J. H., & Berant, E. (Eds.). (in press). *Clinical applications of adult attachment.* New York: Guilford Press.

Obegi, J. H., Morrison, T. L., & Shaver, P. R. (2004). Exploring intergenerational transmission of attachment style in young female adults and their mothers. *Journal of Social and Personal Relationships, 21,* 625–638.

O'Brien, K. M. (1996). The influence of psychological separation and parental attachment on the career development of adolescent women. *Journal of Vocational Behavior, 48,* 257–274.

O'Brien, K. M., & Fassinger, R. E. (1993). A causal model of the career orientation and career choice of adolescent women. *Journal of Counseling Psychology, 40,* 456–469.

O'Brien, K. M., Friedman, S.-M., Tipton, L. C., & Linn, S. G. (2000). Attachment, separation, and women's vocational development: A longitudinal analysis. *Journal of Counseling Psychology, 47,* 301–315.

O'Connor, T. G. (2005). Attachment disturbances associated with early severe deprivation. In C. S. Carter et al. (Eds.), *Attachment and bonding: A new synthesis* (pp. 257–268). Cambridge, MA: MIT Press.

O'Connor, T. G., & Croft, C. M. (2001). A twin study of attachment in preschool children. *Child Development, 72,* 1501–1511.

Ogawa, J. R., Sroufe, L. A., Weinfield, N. S., Carlson, E. A., & Egeland, B. (1997). Development and the fragmented self: Longitudinal study of dissociative symptomatology in a nonclinical sample. *Development and Psychopathology, 9,* 855–879.

Ognibene, T. C., & Collins, N. L. (1998). Adult attachment styles, perceived social support, and coping strategies. *Journal of Social and Personal Relationships, 15,* 323–345.

O'Hearn, R. E., & Davis, K. E. (1997). Women's experience of giving and receiving emotional abuse. *Journal of Interpersonal Violence, 12,* 375–391.

O'Kearney, R. (1996). Attachment disruption in anorexia nervosa and bulimia nervosa: A review of theory and empirical research. *International Journal of Eating Disorders, 20,* 115–127.

O'Koon, J. (1997). Attachment to parents and peers in late adolescence and their relationship with self-image. *Adolescence, 32,* 471–482.

Oliver, L. E., & Whiffen, V. E. (2003). Perceptions of parents and partners and men's depressive symptoms. *Journal of Social and Personal Relationships, 20,* 621–635.

Oman, D., & Thoresen, C. E. (2003). Spiritual modeling: A key to spiritual and religious growth? *International Journal for the Psychology of Religion, 13,* 149–165.

Onishi, M., Gjerde, P. F., & Block, J. (2001). Personality implications of romantic attachment patterns in young adults: A multi-method, multi-informant study. *Personality and Social Psychology Bulletin, 27*, 1097–1110.

Orbach, I. (1997). A taxonomy of factors related to suicidal behavior. *Clinical Psychology: Science and Practice, 4*, 208–224.

Organ, D. W. (1997). Organizational citizenship behavior: It's construct clean-up time. *Human Performance, 10*, 85–97.

Orzolek-Kronner, C. (2002). The effect of attachment theory in the development of eating disorders: Can symptoms be proximity-seeking? *Child and Adolescent Social Work Journal, 19*, 421–435.

Osterweis, M., Solomon, F., & Green, M. (Eds.). (1984). *Bereavement: Reactions, consequences, and care.* Washington, DC: National Academy Press.

Otway, L. J., & Vignoles, V. L. (2006). Narcissism and childhood recollections: A quantitative test of psychoanalytic predictions. *Personality and Social Psychology Bulletin, 32*, 104–116.

Overall, N. C., Fletcher, G. J. O., & Friesen, M. D. (2003). Mapping the intimate relationship mind: Comparisons between three models of attachment representations. *Personality and Social Psychology Bulletin, 29*, 1479–1493.

Owen, M. T., Easterbrooks, M. A., Chase-Lansdale, L., & Goldberg, W. A. (1984). The relation between maternal employment status and the stability of attachments to mother and to father. *Child Development, 55*, 1894–1901.

Owens, G., Crowell, J. A., Pan, H., Treboux, D., O'Connor, E., & Waters, E. (1995). The prototype hypothesis and the origins of attachment working models: Adult relationships with parents and romantic partners. *Monographs of the Society for Research in Child Development, 60*, 216–233.

Oyen, A. S., Landy, S., & Hilburn-Cobb, C. (2000). Maternal attachment and sensitivity in an at-risk sample. *Attachment and Human Development, 2*, 203–217.

Palazzoli, M. (1978). *Self-starvation.* New York: Aronson.

Paley, B., Cox, M. J., Burchinal, M. R., & Payne, C. (1999). Attachment and marital functioning: Comparison of spouses with continuous-secure, earned-secure, dismissing, and preoccupied attachment stances. *Journal of Family Psychology, 13*, 580–597.

Paley, B., Cox, M. J., Harter, K. S. M., & Margand, N. A. (2002). Adult attachment stance and spouses' marital perceptions during the transition to parenthood. *Attachment and Human Development, 4*, 340–360.

Paley, B., Cox, M. J., Kanoy, K. W., Harter, K. S. M., Burchinal, M., & Margand, N. A. (2005). Adult attachment and marital interaction as predictors of whole family interactions during the transition to parenthood. *Journal of Family Psychology, 19*, 420–429.

Papini, D. R., & Roggman, L. A. (1992). Adolescent perceived attachment to parents in relation to competence, depression, and anxiety: A longitudinal study. *Journal of Early Adolescence, 12*, 420–440.

Papini, D. R., & Roggman, L. A. (1993). Parental attachment to early adolescents and parents' emotional and marital adjustment: A longitudinal study. *Journal of Early Adolescence, 13*, 311–328.

Papini, D. R., Roggman, L. A., & Anderson, J. (1991). Early-adolescent perceptions of attachment to mother and father: A test of emotional-distancing and buffering hypotheses. *Journal of Early Adolescence, 11*, 258–275.

Parish, M., & Eagle, M. N. (2003). Attachment to the therapist. *Psychoanalytic Psychology, 20*, 271–286.

Park, K. A., & Waters, E. (1989). Security of attachment and preschool friendships. *Child Development, 60*, 1076–1081.

Park, L. E., Crocker, J., & Mickelson, K. D. (2004). Attachment styles and contingencies of self-worth. *Personality and Social Psychology Bulletin, 30*, 1243–1254.

Parkes, C. M. (1985). Bereavement. *British Journal of Psychiatry, 146*, 11–17.

Parkes, C. M. (2001). A historical overview of the scientific study of bereavement. In M. S. Stroebe, W. Stroebe, R. O. Hansson, & H. Schut (Eds.), *Handbook of bereavement research: Consequences, coping, and care* (pp. 25–45). Washington, DC: American Psychological Association.

Parkes, C. M. (2003). *Attachment patterns in childhood: Relationships, coping, and psychological state in adults seeking psychiatric help after bereavement.* Unpublished manuscript, St. Christopher's Hospice, London.

Parkes, C. M., & Weiss, R. S. (1983) *Recovery from bereavement.* New York: Basic Books.

Paterson, J. E., Field, J., & Pryor, J. (1994). Adolescents' perceptions of their attachment relationships with their mothers, fathers, and friends. *Journal of Youth and Adolescence, 23*, 579–600.

Paterson, J. E., Pryor, J., & Field, J. (1995). Adolescent attachment to parents and friends in relation to aspects of self-esteem. *Journal of Youth and Adolescence, 24*, 365–376.

Patrick, M., Hobson, R., Castle, D., Howard, R., & Maughan, B (1994). Personality disorder and the mental representation of early social experience. *Development and Psychopathology, 6*, 375–388.

Paul, E. L., McManus, B., & Hayes, A. (2000). "Hookups": Characteristics and correlates of college students' spontaneous and anonymous sexual experiences. *Journal of Sex Research, 37*, 76–88.

Pearson, J. L., Cohn, D. A., Cowan, P. A., & Cowan, C. P. (1994). Earned- and continuous-security in adult attachment: Relation to depressive symptomatology and parenting style. *Development and Psychopathology, 6*, 359–373.

Pearson, J. L., Cowan, P. A., Cowan, C. P., & Cohn, D. A. (1993). Adult attachment and adult child–older parent relationships. *American Journal of Orthopsychiatry, 63*, 606–613.

Pederson, D. R., Gleason, K. E., Moran, G., & Bento, S. (1998). Maternal attachment representations, maternal sensitivity, and the infant–mother attachment relationship. *Developmental Psychology, 34*, 925–933.

Pelham, B. W., & Swann, W. B. (1989). From self-conceptions to self-worth: On the sources and structure of global self-esteem. *Journal of Personality and Social Psychology, 57,* 672–680.

Pelham, B. W., & Swann, W. B. (1994). The juncture of intrapersonal and interpersonal knowledge: Self-certainty and interpersonal congruence. *Personality and Social Psychology Bulletin, 20,* 349–357.

Peplau, L. A., & Perlman, D. (Eds.). (1982). *Loneliness: A sourcebook of current theory, research, and therapy.* New York: Wiley.

Pereg, D., & Mikulincer, M. (2004). Attachment style and the regulation of negative affect: Exploring individual differences in mood congruency effects on memory and judgment. *Personality and Social Psychology Bulletin, 30,* 67–80.

Perris, C., & Andersson, P. (2000). Experiences of parental rearing and patterns of attachment in adulthood. *Clinical Psychology and Psychotherapy, 7,* 279–288.

Pesonen, A. K., Raikkonen, K., Keltikangas-Jarvinen, L., Strandberg, T., & Jarvenpaa, A. L. (2003). Parental perception of infant temperament: Does parents' joint attachment matter? *Infant Behavior and Development, 26,* 167–182.

Pesonen, A. K., Raikkonen, K., Strandberg, T., Kelitikangas-Jarvinen, L., & Jarvenpaa, A. L. (2004). Insecure adult attachment style and depressive symptoms: Implications for parental perceptions of infant temperament. *Infant Mental Health Journal, 25,* 99–116.

Pettem, O., West, M., Mahoney, A., & Keller, A. (1993). Depression and attachment problems. *Journal of Psychiatry and Neuroscience, 18,* 78–81.

Pfaller, J., Kiselica, M., & Gerstein, L. (1998). Attachment style and family dynamics in young adults. *Journal of Counseling Psychology, 45,* 353–357.

Phelps, J. L., Belsky, J., & Crnic, K. (1998). Earned security, daily stress, and parenting: A comparison of five alternative models. *Development and Psychopathology, 10,* 21–38.

Piaget, J. (1953). *Origins of intelligence in the child.* London: Routledge.

Picardi, A., Mazzotti, E., Gaetano, P., Cattaruzza, M. S., Baliva, G., Melchi, C. F., et al. (2005). Stress, social support, emotional regulation, and exacerbation of diffuse plaque psoriasis. *Psychosomatics: Journal of Consultation Liaison Psychiatry, 46,* 556–564.

Picardi, A., Pasquini, P., Cattaruzza, M. S., Gaetano, P., Melchi, C. F., Baliva, G., et al. (2003). Stressful life events, social support, attachment security and alexithymia in vitiligo: A case–control study. *Psychotherapy and Psychosomatics, 72,* 150–158.

Picardi, A., Toni, A., & Caroppo, E. (2005). Stability of alexithymia and its relationships with the "Big Five" factors, temperament, character, and attachment style. *Psychotherapy and Psychosomatics, 74,* 371–378.

Pielage, S., Gerlsma, C., & Schaap, C. (2000). Insecure attachment as a risk factor for psychopathology: The role of stressful events. *Clinical Psychology and Psychotherapy, 7,* 296–302.

Pierce, T., & Lydon, J. (1998). Priming relational schemas: Effects of contextually activated and chronically accessible interpersonal expectations on responses to a stressful event. *Journal of Personality and Social Psychology, 75,* 1441–1448.

Pierce, T., & Lydon, J. (2001). Global and specific relational models in the experience of social interactions. *Journal of Personality and Social Psychology, 80,* 613–631.

Pietromonaco, P. R., & Barrett, L. F. (1997). Working models of attachment and daily social interactions. *Journal of Personality and Social Psychology, 73,* 1409–1423.

Pietromonaco, P. R., & Barrett, L. F. (2000). The internal working models concept: What do we really know about the self in relation to others? *Review of General Psychology, 4,* 155–175.

Pietromonaco, P. R., & Carnelley, K. B. (1994). Gender and working models of attachment: Consequences for perceptions of self and romantic relationships. *Personal Relationships, 1,* 63–82.

Pincus, A. L., Dickinson, K. A., Schut, A. J., Castonguay, L. G., & Bedics, J. (1999). Integrating interpersonal assessment and adult attachment using SASB. *European Journal of Psychological Assessment, 15,* 206–220.

Pincus, A. L., & Gurtman, M. B. (1995). The three faces of interpersonal dependency: Structural analyses of self-report dependency measures. *Journal of Personality and Social Psychology, 69,* 744–758.

Pincus, A. L., & Wilson, K. R. (2001). Interpersonal variability in dependent personality. *Journal of Personality, 69,* 223–251.

Pines, A. M. (2004). Adult attachment styles and their relationship to burnout: A preliminary cross-cultural investigation. *Work and Stress, 18,* 66–80.

Piotrkowski, C. S., & Gornick, L. K. (1987). Effects of work-related separations on children and families. In J. Bloom-Feshbach & S. Feshbach (Eds.), *The psychology of separation and loss* (pp. 267–299). San Francisco: Jossey-Bass.

Pistole, M. C. (1989). Attachment in adult romantic relationships: Style of conflict resolution and relationship satisfaction. *Journal of Social and Personal Relationships, 6,* 505–512.

Pistole, M. C. (1993). Attachment relationships: Self-disclosure and trust. *Journal of Mental Health Counseling, 15,* 94–106.

Pistole, M. C. (1994). Adult attachment styles: Some thoughts on closeness–distance struggles. *Family Process, 33,* 147–159.

Pistole, M. C. (1995a). Adult attachment style and narcissistic vulnerability. *Psychoanalytic Psychology, 12,* 115–126.

Pistole, M. C. (1995b). College students' ended love relationships: Attachment style and emotion. *Journal of College Student Development, 36,* 53–60.

Pistole, M. C., & Arricale, F. (2003). Understanding attachment: Beliefs about conflict. *Journal of Counseling and Development, 81,* 318–328.

Pistole, M., Clark, E. M., & Tubbs, A. L. (1995). Love relationships: Attachment style and the investment model. *Journal of Mental Health Counseling, 17,* 199–209.

Pistole, M. C., & Tarrant, N. (1993). Attachment style and aggression in male batterers. *Family Therapy, 20,* 165–173.

Pistole, M. C., & Vocaturo, L. C. (1999). Attachment and commitment in college students' romantic relationships. *Journal of College Student Development, 40,* 710–720.

Pistole, M. C., & Watkins, C. (1995). Attachment theory, counseling process, and supervision. *Counseling Psychologist, 23,* 457–478.

Pope, K. S. (1994). *Sexual involvement with therapists: Patient assessment, subsequent therapy, forensics.* Washington, DC: American Psychological Association.

Popper, M. (2001). *Hypnotic leadership.* Westport, CT: Praeger

Popper, M. (2002). Narcissism and attachment patterns of personalized and socialized charismatic leaders. *Journal of Social and Personal Relationships, 19,* 797–809.

Popper, M., Amit, K., Gal, R., Mishkal-Sinai, M., & Lisak, A. (2004). The capacity to lead: Major psychological differences between leaders and nonleaders. *Military Psychology, 16,* 245–263.

Popper, M., & Mayseless, O. (2003). Back to basics: Applying a parenting perspective to transformational leadership. *Leadership Quarterly, 14,* 41–65.

Popper, M., Mayseless, O., & Castelnovo, O. (2000). Transformational leadership and attachment. *Leadership Quarterly, 11,* 267–289.

Pottharst, K. (Ed.). (1990a). *Explorations in adult attachment.* New York: Peter Lang.

Pottharst, K. (1990b). The search for methods and measures. In K. Pottharst (Ed.), *Explorations in adult attachment* (pp. 9–37). New York: Peter Lang.

Powers, S. I., Pietromonaco, P. R., Gunlicks, M., & Sayer, A. (2006). Dating couples' attachment styles and patterns of cortisol reactivity and recovery in response to a relationship conflict. *Journal of Personality and Social Psychology, 90,* 613–628.

Powers, W. T. (1973). *Behavior: The control of perception.* Chicago: Aldine.

Priel, B., & Besser, A. (2000). Adult attachment styles, early relationships, antenatal attachment, and perceptions of infant temperament: A study of first-time mothers. *Personal Relationships, 7,* 291–310.

Priel, B., & Besser, A. (2001). Bridging the gap between attachment and object relations theories: A study of the transition to motherhood. *British Journal of Medical Psychology, 74,* 85–100.

Priel, B., Mitrany, D., & Shahar, G. (1998). Closeness, support, and reciprocity: A study of attachment styles in adolescence. *Personality and Individual Differences, 25,* 1183–1197.

Priel, B., & Shamai, D. (1995). Attachment style and perceived social support: Effects on affect regulation. *Personality and Individual Differences, 19,* 235–241.

Pyszczynski, T., Greenberg, J., & Koole, S. L. (2004). Experimental existential psychology: Exploring the human confrontation with reality. In J. Greenberg, S. L Koole, & T. Pyszczynski (Eds.), *Handbook of experimental existential psychology* (pp. 3–9). New York: Guilford Press.

Pyszczynski, T., Greenberg, J., & LaPrelle, J. (1985). Social comparison after success and failure: Biased search for information consistent with a self-serving conclusion. *Journal of Experimental Social Psychology, 21,* 195–211.

Racanelli, C. (2005). Attachment and compassion fatigue among American and Israeli mental health clinicians working with traumatized victims of terrorism. *International Journal of Emergency Mental Health, 7,* 115–124.

Radecki-Bush, C., Farrell, A. D., & Bush, J. P. (1993). Predicting jealous responses: The influence of adult attachment and depression on threat appraisal. *Journal of Social and Personal Relationships, 10,* 569–588.

Rainer, J. P. (2000). Compassion fatigue: When caregiving begins to hurt. In L. Vandecreek & T. L. Jackson (Eds.), *Innovations in clinical practice: A source book* (Vol. 18, pp. 441–453). Sarasota, FL: Professional Resource Exchange.

Rainey, L. M., & Borders, L. D. (1997). Influential factors in career orientation and career aspiration of early adolescent girls. *Journal of Counseling Psychology, 44,* 160–172.

Ramacciotti, A., Sorbello, M., Pazzagli, A., Vismara, L., Mancone, & Pallanti, S. (2001). Attachment processes in eating disorders. *Eating and Weight Disorders, 6,* 166–170.

Rando, T. A. (1992). The increased prevalence of complicated mourning: The onslaught is just beginning. *Omega, 26,* 43–60.

Rank, O. (1945). *Will therapy and truth and reality.* New York: Knopf.

Rankin, L. B., Saunders, D. G., & Williams, R. A. (2000). Mediators of attachment style, social support, and sense of belonging in predicting woman abuse by African American men. *Journal of Interpersonal Violence, 15,* 1060–1080.

Raskin, P. M., Kummel, P., & Bannister, T. (1998). The relationship between coping styles, attachment, and career salience in partnered working women with children. *Journal of Career Assessment, 6,* 403–416.

Rauh, H., Ziegenhain, U., Muller, B., & Wijnroks, L. (2000). Stability and change in infant–mother attachment in the second year of life: Relations to parenting quality and varying degrees of day-care experience. In P. M. Crittenden & A. H. Claussen (Eds.), *The organization of attachment relationships: Maturation, culture, and context* (pp. 251–276). New York: Cambridge University Press.

Raval, V., Goldberg, S., Atkinson, L., Benoit, D., Myhal, N., Poulton, L., & Zwiers, M. (2001). Maternal attachment, maternal responsiveness, and infant attachment. *Infant Behavior and Development, 24,* 281–304.

Raz, A. (2002). *Personality, core relationship themes, and interpersonal competence among young adults experiencing difficulties in establishing long-term relationships.* Unpublished doctoral dissertation, Haifa University, Haifa, Israel.

Reese-Weber, M., & Marchand, J. F. (2002). Family and individual predictors of late adolescents' romantic relationships. *Journal of Youth and Adolescence, 31,* 197–206.

Reich, W. A., & Siegel, H. I. (2002). Attachment, ego-identity development, and exploratory interest in university students. *Asian Journal of Social Psychology, 5,* 125–134.

Reinecke, M. A., & Rogers, G. M. (2001). Dysfunctional attitudes and attachment style among clinically depressed adults. *Behavioural and Cognitive Psychotherapy, 29,* 129–141.

Reis, H. T. (in press). Steps toward the ripening of relationship science. *Personal Relationships.*

Reis, H. T., Clark, M. S., & Holmes, J. G. (2004). Perceived partner responsiveness as an organizing construct in the study of intimacy and closeness. In D. J. Mashek & A. Aron (Eds.), *Handbook of closeness and intimacy* (pp. 201–225). Mahwah, NJ: Erlbaum.

Reis, H. T., & Shaver, P. R. (1988). Intimacy as an interpersonal process. In S. Duck (Ed.), *Handbook of research in personal relationships* (pp. 367–389). London: Wiley.

Reis, H.T., & Wheeler, L. (1991). Studying social interaction with the Rochester Interaction Record. In M. P. Zanna (Ed.), *Advances in experimental social psychology* (Vol. 24, pp. 270–318). San Diego: Academic Press.

Reis, S., & Grenyer, B. F. S. (2004). Fear of intimacy in women: Relationship between attachment styles and depressive symptoms. *Psychopathology, 37,* 299–303.

Resnick, S. (1997). *The pleasure zone.* Berkeley, CA: Conari Press.

Rholes, W. S., & Simpson, J. A. (Eds.). (2004). *Adult attachment: Theory, research, and clinical implications.* New York: Guilford Press.

Rholes, W. S., Simpson, J. A., & Blakely, B. S. (1995). Adult attachment styles and mothers' relationships with their young children. *Personal Relationships, 2,* 35–54.

Rholes, W. S., Simpson, J. A., Blakely, B. S., Lanigan, L., & Allen, E. A. (1997). Adult attachment styles, the desire to have children, and working models of parenthood. *Journal of Personality, 65,* 357–385.

Rholes, W. S., Simpson, J. A., Campbell, L., & Grich, J. (2001). Adult attachment and the transition to parenthood. *Journal of Personality and Social Psychology, 81,* 421–435.

Rholes, W. S., Simpson, J. A., & Friedman, M. (2006). Avoidant attachment and the experience of parenting. *Personality and Social Psychology Bulletin, 32,* 275–285.

Rholes, W. S., Simpson, J. A., & Orina, M. (1999). Attachment and anger in an anxiety-provoking situation. *Journal of Personality and Social Psychology, 76,* 940–957.

Ricciuti, H. N. (1974). Fear and the development of social attachments in the first year of life. In M. Lewis & L. Rosenblum (Eds.), *Origins of fear* (pp. 73–106). New York: Wiley.

Rice, K. G., Fitzgerald, D. P., Whaley, T. J., & Gibbs, C. L. (1995). Cross-sectional and longitudinal examination of attachment, separation–individuation, and college student adjustment. *Journal of Counseling and Development, 73,* 463–474.

Rice, K. G., & Lopez, F. G. (2004). Maladaptive perfectionism, adult attachment, and self-esteem in college students. *Journal of College Counseling, 7,* 118–128.

Rice, K. G., Lopez, F. G., & Vergara, D. (2005). Parental/social influences on perfectionism and adult attachment orientations. *Journal of Social and Clinical Psychology, 24,* 580–605.

Rice, K. G., & Mirzadeh, S.-A. (2000). Perfectionism, attachment, and adjustment. *Journal of Counseling Psychology, 47,* 238–250.

Rice, K. G., & Whaley, T. J. (1994). A short-term longitudinal study of within-semester stability and change in attachment and college student adjustment. *Journal of College Student Development, 35,* 324–330.

Ricks, M. H. (1985). The social transmission of parental behavior: Attachment across generations. In I. Bretherton & E. Waters (Eds.), *Growing points in attachment theory and research. Monographs of the Society for Research in Child Development, 50* (1–2, Serial No. 209), 211–227.

Ridge, S. R., & Feeney, J. A. (1998). Relationship history and relationship attitudes in gay males and lesbians: Attachment style and gender differences. *Australian and New Zealand Journal of Psychiatry, 32,* 848–859.

Riggio, R. E. (1986). Assessment of basic social skills. *Journal of Personality and Social Psychology, 51,* 649–660.

Riggio, R. E. (1993). Social interaction skills and nonverbal behavior. In R. S. Feldman (Ed.), *Applications of nonverbal behavioral theories and research* (pp. 3–30). Hillsdale, NJ: Erlbaum.

Riggs, S. A., & Jacobvitz, D. (2002). Expectant parents' representations of early attachment relationships: Associations with mental health and family history. *Journal of Consulting and Clinical Psychology, 70,* 195–204.

Riggs, S. A., Jacobvitz, D., & Hazen, N. (2002). Adult attachment and history of psychotherapy in a normative sample. *Psychotherapy: Theory, Research, Practice, Training, 39,* 344–353.

Robbins, S. B. (1995). Attachment perspectives on the counseling relationship: Comment on Mallinckrodt, Gantt, and Coble (1995). *Journal of Counseling Psychology, 42,* 318–319.

Roberto, K. A., & Stanis, P. I. (1994). Reactions of older women to the death of their close friends. *Omega, 29,* 17–28.

Roberts, J. E., Gotlib, I. H., & Kassel, J. D. (1996). Adult attachment security and symptoms of depression: The mediating roles of dysfunctional attitudes and low self-esteem. *Journal of Personality and Social Psychology, 70,* 310–320.

Roberts, L. J., & Greenberg, D. R. (2002). Observational "windows" to intimacy processes in marriage. In P. Noller & J. A. Feeney (Eds.), *Understanding marriage: Developments in the study of couple interaction* (pp. 118–149). New York: Cambridge University Press.

Roberts, N., & Noller, P. (1998). The associations between adult attachment and couple violence: The role of communication patterns and relationship satisfaction. In J. A. Simpson & W. S. Rholes (Eds.), *Attachment theory and close relationships* (pp. 317–350). New York: Guilford Press.

Robertson, J., & Bowlby, J. (1952). Responses of young children to separation from their mothers.

Courier of the International Children's Center, Paris, 2, 131–140.

Robins, R. W., Caspi, A., & Moffitt, T. E. (2002). It's not just who you're with, it's who you are: Personality and relationship experiences across multiple relationships. *Journal of Personality, 70,* 925–964.

Roche, D. N., Runtz, M. G., & Hunter, M. A. (1999). Adult attachment: A mediator between child sexual abuse and later psychological adjustment. *Journal of Interpersonal Violence, 14,* 184–207.

Rogers, C. R. (1961). *On becoming a person.* Boston: Houghton Mifflin.

Rogers, W. S., Bidwell, J., & Wilson, L. (2005). Perception of and satisfaction with relationship power, sex, and attachment styles: A couple level analysis. *Journal of Family Violence, 20,* 241–251.

Roisman, G. I., Bahadur, M. A., & Oster, H. (2000). Infant attachment security as a discriminant predictor of career development in late adolescence. *Journal of Adolescent Research, 15,* 531–545.

Roisman, G. I., Collins, W. A., Sroufe, L. A., & Egeland, B. (2005). Predictors of young adults' representations of and behavior in their current romantic relationship: Prospective tests of the prototype hypothesis. *Attachment and Human Development, 7,* 105–121.

Roisman, G. I., Fortuna, K., & Holland, A. (2006). An experimental manipulation of retrospectively defined earned and continuous attachment security. *Child Development, 77,* 59–71.

Roisman, G. I., Madsen, S. D., Hennighausen, K. H., Sroufe, L. A., & Collins, W. A. (2001). The coherence of dyadic behavior across parent–child and romantic relationships as mediated by the internalized representation of experience. *Attachment and Human Development, 3,* 156–172.

Roisman, G. I., Padron, E., Sroufe, L. A., & Egeland, B. (2002). Earned-secure attachment status in retrospect and prospect. *Child Development, 73,* 1204–1219.

Roisman, G. I., Tsai, J. L., & Chiang, K. H. S. (2004). The emotional integration of childhood experience: Physiological, facial expressions, and self-reported emotional response during the Adult Attachment Interview. *Developmental Psychology, 40,* 776–789.

Rom, E., & Mikulincer, M. (2003). Attachment theory and group processes: The association between attachment style and group-related representations, goals, memories, and functioning. *Journal of Personality and Social Psychology, 84,* 1220–1235.

Roney, A., Meredith, P., & Strong, J. (2004). Attachment styles and factors affecting career choice of occupational therapy students. *British Journal of Occupational Therapy, 67,* 133–141.

Rook, K. S. (1998). Investigating the positive and negative sides of personal relationships: Through a lens darkly? In B. H. Spitzberg & W. R. Cupach (Eds.), *The dark side of close relationships* (pp. 369–393). Mahwah, NJ: Erlbaum.

Rorschach, H. (1942). *Psychodiagnostics: A diagnostic test based on perception* (P. Lenkau & B. Kroneberg, Trans.). New York: Grune & Stratton.

Roseman, I. J., & Evdokas, A. (2004). Appraisals cause experienced emotions: Experimental evidence. *Cognition and Emotion, 18,* 1–28.

Rosenblatt, A., Greenberg, J., Solomon, S., Pyszczynski, T., & Lyon, D. (1989). Evidence for terror management theory I: The effects of mortality salience on reactions to those who violate or uphold cultural values. *Journal of Personality and Social Psychology, 57,* 681–690.

Rosenfarb, I. S., Becker, J., & Khan, A. (1994). Perceptions of parental and peer attachments by women with mood disorders. *Journal of Abnormal Psychology, 103,* 637–644.

Rosenstein, D. S., & Horowitz, H. A. (1996). Adolescent attachment and psychopathology. *Journal of Consulting and Clinical Psychology, 64,* 244–253.

Rosenthal, R., & Jacobson, L. (1968). *Pygmalion in the classroom.* New York: Holt, Rinehart & Winston.

Rosenzweig, D. L., Farber, B. A., & Geller, J. D. (1996). Clients' representations of their therapists over the course of psychotherapy. *Journal of Clinical Psychology, 52,* 197–207.

Rothbart, M. K., & Ahadi, S. A. (1994). Temperament and the development of personality. *Journal of Abnormal Psychology, 103,* 55–66.

Rothbart, M. K., & Derryberry, D. (1981). Development of individual differences in temperament. In M. E. Lamb & A. L. Brown (Eds.), *Advances in developmental psychology* (Vol. 1, pp. 37–86). Hillsdale, NJ: Erlbaum.

Rowatt, W. C., & Kirkpatrick, L. A. (2002). Two dimensions of attachment to God and their relation to affect, religiosity, and personality constructs. *Journal for the Scientific Study of Religion, 41,* 637–651.

Rowe, A., & Carnelley, K. B. (2003). Attachment style differences in the processing of attachment-relevant information: Primed-style effects on recall, interpersonal expectations, and affect. *Personal Relationships, 10,* 59–75.

Rowe, A. C., & Carnelley, K. B. (2005). Preliminary support for the use of a hierarchical mapping technique to examine attachment networks. *Personal Relationships, 12,* 499–519.

Rowe, A. C., & Carnelley, K. B. (2006). *Long lasting effects of repeated priming of attachment security on views of self and relationships.* Paper presented at the 13th European Conference on Personality, Athens, Greece.

Rozov, E. J. (2002). Therapist attachment style and emotional trait biases: A study of therapist contribution to the working alliance. *Dissertation Abstracts International: Section B: Sciences and Engineering, 62*(9), 4235.

Rubenstein, C., & Shaver, P. R. (1982). The experience of loneliness. In L. A. Peplau & D. Perlman (Eds.), *Loneliness: A sourcebook of current theory, research, and therapy* (pp. 206–223). New York: Wiley.

Rubin, K. H., Bukowski, W., & Parker, J. G. (1998). Peer interactions, relationships, and groups. In W. Damon (Series Ed.) & N. Eisenberg (Vol. Ed.), *Handbook of child psychology* (5th ed., Vol. 3, pp. 619–700). New York: Wiley.

Rubin, S. S. (1991). Adult child loss and the two-track model of bereavement. *Omega, 24,* 183–202.

Rubino, G., Barker, C., Roth, T., & Fearon, P. (2000). Therapist empathy and depth of interpretation in response to potential alliance ruptures: The role of therapist and patient attachment styles. *Psychotherapy Research, 10,* 408–420.

Rusbult, C. E. (1983). A longitudinal test of the investment model: The development (and deterioration) of satisfaction and commitment in heterosexual involvements. *Journal of Personality and Social Psychology, 45,* 101–117.

Rusbult, C. E., Verette, J., Whitney, G. A., Slovik, L. F., & Lipkus, I. (1991). Accommodation processes in close relationships: Theory and preliminary empirical evidence. *Journal of Personality and Social Psychology, 60,* 53–78.

Rutter, M. (1981). *Maternal deprivation reassessed* (2nd ed.). New York: Penguin.

Ruvolo, A. P., Fabin, L. A., & Ruvolo, C. M. (2001). Relationship experiences and change in attachment characteristics of young adults: The role of relationship breakups and conflict avoidance. *Personal Relationships, 8,* 265–281.

Ryan, E. R., & Cicchetti, D. V. (1985). Predicting quality of alliance in the initial psychotherapy interview. *Journal of Nervous and Mental Disease, 173,* 717–725.

Ryan, N. E., Solberg, V., & Brown, S. D. (1996). Family dysfunction, parental attachment, and career search self-efficacy among community college students. *Journal of Counseling Psychology, 43,* 84–89.

Sachser, N. (2005). Adult social bonding: Insights from studies in nonhuman mammals. In C. S. Carter et al. (Eds.), *Attachment and bonding: A new synthesis* (pp. 119–135). Cambridge, MA: MIT Press.

Sachser, N., Durschlag, M., & Hirzel, D. (1998). Social relationships and the management of stress. *Psychoneuroendocrinology, 23,* 891–904.

Sack, A., Sperling, M. B., Fagen, G., & Foelsch, P. (1996). Attachment style, history, and behavioral contrasts for a borderline and normal sample. *Journal of Personality Disorders, 10,* 88–102.

Safford, S. M., Alloy, L. B., Crossfield, A. G., Morocco, A. M., & Wang, J. C. (2004). The relationship of cognitive style and attachment style to depression and anxiety in young adults. *Journal of Cognitive Psychotherapy, 18,* 25–41.

Safran, J. D. (1993). Breaches in the therapeutic alliance: An arena for negotiating authentic relatedness. *Psychotherapy: Theory, Research, Practice, Training, 30,* 11–24.

Safran, J. D., & Muran, J. C. (1996). The resolution of ruptures in the therapeutic alliance. *Journal of Clinical and Consulting Psychology, 64,* 447–458.

Sagi, A., Lamb, M. E., Lewkowicz, K. S., Shoham, R., Dvir, R., & Estes, D. (1985). Security of infant–mother, –father, and –metapelet attachment among kibbutz-reared Israeli children. *Monographs of the Society for Research in Child Development, 50*(1–2, Serial No. 209), 257–275.

Sagi, A., van IJzendoorn, M. H., Aviezer, O., Donnell, F., Koren-Karie, N., Joels, T., & Harel, Y. (1995). Attachments in a multiple-caregiver and multiple-infant environment: The case of the Israeli kibbut-

zim. *Monographs of the Society for Research in Child Development, 60,* 71–91.

Sagi, A., van IJzendoorn, M. H., Aviezer, O., Donnell, F., & Mayseless, O. (1994). Sleeping out of home in a kibbutz communal arrangement: It makes a difference for infant–mother attachment. *Child Development, 65,* 992–1004.

Sagi, A., van IJzendoorn, M. H., Scharf, M., Joels, T., Koren-Karie, N., Mayseless, O., et al. (1997). Ecological constraints for intergenerational transmission of attachment. *International Journal of Behavioral Development, 20,* 287–299.

Sagi-Schwartz, A., & Aviezer, O. (2005). Correlates of attachment to multiple caregivers in kibbutz children from birth to emerging adulthood: The Haifa longitudinal study. In K. E. Grossmann, K. Grossmann, & E. Waters (Eds.), *Attachment from infancy to adulthood: The major longitudinal studies* (pp. 165–197). New York: Guilford Press.

Salzman, J. P. (1996). Primary attachment in female adolescents: Association with depression, self-esteem, and maternal identification. *Psychiatry: Interpersonal and Biological Processes, 59,* 20–33.

Salzman, J. P. (1997). Ambivalent attachment in female adolescents: Association with affective instability and eating disorders. *International Journal of Eating Disorders, 21,* 251–259.

Samuolis, J., Layburn, K., & Schiaffino, K. M. (2001). Identity development and attachment to parents in college students. *Journal of Youth and Adolescence, 30,* 373–384.

Sampson, M. C. (2003, March). *Examining early correlates of self-report measures of adult attachment: A prospective longitudinal view.* Poster presented at the biennial meeting of the Society for Research in Child Development, Tampa, FL.

Sanford, K. (1997). Two dimensions of adult attachment: Further validation. *Journal of Social and Personal Relationships, 14,* 133–143.

Sarason, B. R., Pierce, G. R., & Sarason, I. G. (1990). Social support: The sense of acceptance and the role of relationships. In B. R. Sarason, G. R. Pierce, & I. G. Sarason (Eds.), *Social support: An interactional view* (pp. 97–128). New York: Wiley.

Saroglou, V., Kempeneers, A., & Seynhaeve, I. (2003). Need for closure and adult attachment dimensions as predictors of religion and reading interests. In P. Roelofsma, J. Corveleyn, & J. van Saane (Eds.), *One hundred years of psychology and religion* (pp. 139–154). Amsterdam: Vrije University Press.

Saroglou, V., Pichon, I., Trompette, L., Verschueren, M., & Dernelle, R. (2005). Prosocial behavior and religion: New evidence based on projective measures and peer ratings. *Journal for the Scientific Study of Religion, 44,* 323–348.

Saroglou, V., & Scariot, C. (2002). Humor Styles Questionnaire: Personality and educational correlates in Belgian high school and college students. *European Journal of Personality, 16,* 43–54.

Satterfield, W. A., & Lyddon, W. J. (1995). Client attachment and perceptions of the working alliance with counselor trainees. *Journal of Counseling Psychology, 42,* 187–189.

Satterfield, W. A., & Lyddon, W. J. (1998). Client

attachment and the working alliance. *Counseling Psychology Quarterly, 11,* 407–415.

Sauer, E. M., Lopez, F. G., & Gormley, B. (2003). Respective contributions of therapist and client adult attachment orientations to the development of the early working alliance: A preliminary growth modeling study. *Psychotherapy Research, 13,* 371–382.

Sawle, G. A., & Kear-Colwell, J. (2001). Adult attachment style and pedophilia: A developmental perspective. *International Journal of Offender Therapy and Comparative Criminology, 45,* 32–50.

Sbarra, D. A. (2006). Predicting the onset of emotional recovery following nonmarital relationship dissolution: Survival analyses of sadness and anger. *Personality and Social Psychology Bulletin, 32,* 298–312.

Sbarra, D. A., & Emery, R. E. (2005). The emotional sequelae of nonmarital relationship dissolution: Analysis of change and intraindividual variability over time. *Personal Relationships, 12,* 213–232.

Schachner, D. A. (2006). *Attachment and long-term singlehood.* Unpublished doctoral dissertation, University of California, Davis.

Schachner, D. A., & Shaver, P. R. (2002). Attachment style and human mate poaching. *New Review of Social Psychology, 1,* 122–129.

Schachner, D. A., & Shaver, P. R. (2004). Attachment dimensions and sexual motives. *Personal Relationships, 11,* 179–195.

Schachner, D. A., Shaver, P. R., & Mikulincer, M. (2005). Patterns of nonverbal behavior and sensitivity in the context of attachment relationships. *Journal of Nonverbal Behavior, 29,* 141–169.

Schachter, S. (1959). *The psychology of affiliation.* Stanford, CA: Stanford University Press.

Schafer, R. (1968). *Aspects of internalization.* New York: International Universities Press.

Schaller, M., & Cialdini, R. B. (1988). The economics of empathic helping: Support for a mood management motive. *Journal of Experimental Social Psychology, 24,* 163–181.

Scharf, M. (2001). A "natural experiment" in childrearing ecologies and adolescents' attachment and separation representations. *Child Development, 72,* 236–251.

Scharf, M., Mayseless, O., & Kivenson-Baron, I. (2004). Adolescents' attachment representations and developmental tasks in emerging adulthood. *Developmental Psychology, 40,* 430–444.

Scharfe, E. (2003). Stability and change of attachment representations from cradle to grave. In S. M. Johnson & V. E. Whiffen (Eds.), *Attachment processes in couple and family therapy* (pp. 64–84). New York: Guilford Press.

Scharfe, E., & Bartholomew, K. (1994). Reliability and stability of adult attachment patterns. *Personal Relationships, 1,* 23–43.

Scharfe, E., & Bartholomew, K. (1995). Accommodation and attachment representations in young couples. *Journal of Social and Personal Relationships, 12,* 389–401.

Scharfe, E., & Eldredge, D. (2001). Associations between attachment representations and health behaviors in late adolescence. *Journal of Health Psychology, 6,* 295–307.

Scher, A., & Dror, E. (2003). Attachment, caregiving, and sleep: The tie that keeps infants and mothers awake. *Sleep and Hypnosis, 5,* 27–37.

Scher, A., & Mayseless, O. (1994). Mothers' attachment with spouse and parenting in the first year. *Journal of Social and Personal Relationships, 11,* 601–609.

Schimel, J., Arndt, J., Pyszczynski, T., & Greenberg, J. (2001). Being accepted for who we are: Evidence that social validation of the intrinsic self reduces general defensiveness. *Journal of Personality and Social Psychology, 80,* 35–52.

Schindler, A., Thomasius, R., Sack, P. M., Gemeinhardt, B., Kustner, U., & Eckert, J. (2005). Attachment and substance use disorders: A review of the literature and a study in drug dependent adolescents. *Attachment and Human Development, 7,* 207–228.

Schirmer, L. L., & Lopez, F. G. (2001). Probing the social support and work strain relationship among adult workers: Contributions of adult attachment orientations. *Journal of Vocational Behavior, 59,* 17–33.

Schlenker, B. R. (1980). *Impression management: The self-concept, social identity, and interpersonal relations.* Monterey, CA: Brooks/Cole.

Schmidt, S., Nachtigall, C., Wuethrich-Martone, O., & Strauss, B. (2002). Attachment and coping with chronic disease. *Journal of Psychosomatic Research, 53,* 763–773.

Schmitt, D. P. (2002). Personality, attachment, and sexuality related to dating relationship outcomes: Constrasting three perspectives on personal attribute interaction. *British Journal of Social Psychology, 41,* 589–610.

Schmitt, D. P. (2005). Is short-term mating the maladaptive result of insecure attachment?: A test of competing evolutionary perspectives. *Personality and Social Psychology Bulletin, 31,* 747–768.

Schmitt, D. P., & Allik, J. (2005). Simultaneous administration of the Rosenberg Self-Esteem Scale in 53 nations: Exploring the universal and culture-specific features of global self-esteem. *Journal of Personality and Social Psychology, 89,* 623–642.

Schneider, B. H., Atkinson, L., & Tardif, C. (2001). Child–parent attachment and children's peer relations: A quantitative review. *Developmental Psychology, 37,* 86–100.

Schneider, B. H., & Younger, A. J. (1996). Adolescent–parent attachment and adolescents' relations with their peers: A closer look. *Youth and Society, 28,* 95–108.

Schuengel, C., Bakermans-Kranenburg, M. J., & van IJzendoorn, M. H. (1999). Frightening maternal behavior linking unresolved loss and disorganized infant attachment. *Journal of Consulting and Clinical Psychology, 67,* 54–63.

Schuengel, C., & van IJzendoorn, M. H. (2001). Attachment in mental health institutions: A critical review of assumptions, clinical implications, and research strategies. *Attachment and Human Development, 3,* 304–323.

Schuengel, C., van IJzendoorn, M. H., Bakermans-

Kranenburg, M. J., & Blom, M. (1998). Frightening maternal behavior, unresolved loss, and disorganized infant attachment: A pilot study. *Journal of Reproductive and Infant Psychology, 16,* 277–283.

Schultheiss, D. E. P., & Blustein, D. L. (1994). Contributions of family relationship factors to the identity formation process. *Journal of Counseling and Development, 73,* 159–166.

Schultheiss, D. E. P., Kress, H. M., Manzi, A. J., & Glasscock, J. M. J. (2001). Relational influences in career development: A qualitative inquiry. *Counseling Psychologist, 29,* 214–239.

Schut, H. A. W., Stroebe, M., de Keijser, J., & van den Bout, J. (1997). Intervention for the bereaved: Gender differences in the efficacy of grief counseling. *British Journal of Clinical Psychology, 36,* 63–72.

Schwartz, J. P., Waldo, M., & Higgins, A. J. (2004). Attachment styles: Relationship to masculine gender role conflict in college men. *Psychology of Men and Masculinity, 5,* 143–146.

Schwarzer, R., & Leppin, A. (1989). Social support and health: A meta-analysis. *Psychology and Health, 3,* 1–15.

Schwarzer, R., & Schwarzer, C. (1996). A critical survey of coping instruments. In M. Zeidner & N. S. Endler (Eds.), *Handbook of coping: Theory, research, and applications* (pp. 107–132). Oxford, UK: Wiley.

Scinta, A., & Gable, S. L. (2005). Performance comparisons and attachment: An investigation of competitive responses in close relationships. *Personal Relationships, 12,* 357–372.

Scott, D. J., & Church, A. (2001). Separation/attachment theory and career decidedness and commitment: Effects of parental divorce. *Journal of Vocational Behavior, 58,* 328–347.

Scott, R. L., & Cordova, J. V. (2002). The influence of adult attachment styles on the association between marital adjustment and depressive symptoms. *Journal of Family Psychology, 16,* 199–208.

Searle, B., & Meara, N. M. (1999). Affective dimensions of attachment styles: Exploring self-reported attachment style, gender, and emotional experience among college students. *Journal of Counseling Psychology, 46,* 147–158.

Segrin, C. (1998). Disrupted interpersonal relationships and mental health problems. In W. R. Cupach & B. H. Spitzberg (Eds.), *The dark side of close relationships* (pp. 327–365). Mahwah, NJ: Erlbaum.

Seiffge-Krenke, I., & Beyers, W. (2005). Coping trajectories from adolescence to young adulthood: Links to attachment state of mind. *Journal of Research on Adolescence, 15,* 561–582.

Seligman, M. E. P. (2002). *Authentic happiness: Using the new positive psychology to realize your potential for lasting fulfillment.* New York: Free Press.

Senchak, M., & Leonard, K. E. (1992). Attachment styles and marital adjustment among newlywed couples. *Journal of Social and Personal Relationships, 9,* 51–64.

Shafer, A. B. (2001). The Big Five and sexuality trait terms as predictors of relationships and sex. *Journal of Research in Personality, 35,* 313–338.

Shamir, B. (1999). Taming charisma for better understanding and greater usefulness: A response to Beyer. *Leadership Quarterly, 10,* 555–562.

Shamir, B., House, R. J., & Arthur, M. B. (1993). The motivational effects of charismatic leadership: A self-concept based theory. *Organizational Science, 4,* 577–593.

Shapiro, D. L., & Levendosky, A. A. (1999). Adolescent survivors of childhood sexual abuse: The mediating role of attachment style and coping in psychological and interpersonal functioning. *Child Abuse and Neglect, 23,* 1175–1191.

Sharabany, R., Mayseless, O., Edri, G., & Lulav, D. (2001). Ecology, childhood experiences, and adult attachment styles of women in the kibbutz. *International Journal of Behavioral Development, 25,* 214–225.

Sharpe, T. M., Killen, J. D., Bryson, S. W., Shisslak, C. M., Estes, L. S., Gray, N., et al. (1998). Attachment style and weight concerns in preadolescent and adolescent girls. *International Journal of Eating Disorders, 23,* 39–44.

Sharpsteen, D. J., & Kirkpatrick, L. A. (1997). Romantic jealousy and adult romantic attachment. *Journal of Personality and Social Psychology, 72,* 627–640.

Shaver, P. R. (1980). The public mistrust. *Psychology Today, 14,* 44–49, 102.

Shaver, P. R., Belsky, J., & Brennan, K. A. (2000). The Adult Attachment Interview and self-reports of romantic attachment: Associations across domains and methods. *Personal Relationships, 7,* 25–43.

Shaver, P. R., & Brennan, K. A. (1992). Attachment styles and the "Big Five" personality traits: Their connections with each other and with romantic relationship outcomes. *Personality and Social Psychology Bulletin, 18,* 536–545.

Shaver, P. R., & Clark, C. L. (1994). The psychodynamics of adult romantic attachment. In J. M. Masling & R. F. Bornstein (Eds.), *Empirical perspectives on object relations theories* (pp. 105–156). Washington, DC: American Psychological Association.

Shaver, P. R., Collins, N. L., & Clark, C. L. (1996). Attachment styles and internal working models of self and relationship partners. In G. J. O. Fletcher & J. Fitness (Eds.), *Knowledge structures in close relationships: A social psychological approach* (pp. 25–61). Mahwah, NJ: Erlbaum.

Shaver, P. R., & Hazan, C. (1984). Incompatibility, loneliness, and limerence. In W. Ickes (Ed.), *Compatible and incompatible relationships* (pp. 163–184). New York: Springer-Verlag.

Shaver, P. R., & Hazan, C. (1987). Being lonely, falling in love: Perspectives from attachment theory. *Journal of Social Behavior and Personality, 2,* 105–124.

Shaver, P. R., & Hazan, C. (1988). A biased overview of the study of love. *Journal of Social and Personal Relationships, 5,* 473–501.

Shaver, P. R., & Hazan, C. (1993). Adult romantic attachment: Theory and evidence. In D. Perlman & W. Jones (Eds.), *Advances in personal relationships* (Vol. 4, pp. 29–70). London: Jessica Kingsley.

Shaver, P. R., Hazan, C., & Bradshaw, D. (1988). Love as attachment: The integration of three behavioral systems. In R. J. Sternberg & M. Barnes (Eds.), *The psychology of love* (pp. 68–99). New Haven, CT: Yale University Press.

Shaver, P. R., & Klinnert, M. (1982). Schachter's theories of affiliation and emotions: Implications of developmental research. In L. Wheeler (Ed.), *Review of personality and social psychology* (Vol. 3, pp. 37–71). Beverly Hills, CA: Sage.

Shaver, P. R., & Mikulincer, M. (2002a). Attachment-related psychodynamics. *Attachment and Human Development, 4*, 133–161.

Shaver, P. R., & Mikulincer, M. (2002b). Dialogue on adult attachment: Diversity and integration. *Attachment and Human Development, 4*, 243–257.

Shaver, P. R., & Mikulincer, M. (2004). What do self-report attachment measures assess? In W. S. Rholes & J. A. Simpson (Eds.), *Adult attachment: Theory, research, and clinical implications* (pp. 17–54). New York: Guilford Press.

Shaver, P. R., & Mikulincer, M. (2005). Attachment theory and research: Resurrection of the psychodynamic approach to personality. *Journal of Research in Personality, 39*, 22–45.

Shaver, P. R., & Mikulincer, M. (2006). A behavioral systems approach to romantic love relationships: Attachment, caregiving, and sex. In R. J. Sternberg & K. Weis (Eds.), *The new psychology of love* (pp. 35–64). New Haven, CT: Yale University Press.

Shaver, P. R., & Mikulincer, M. (2007). Adult attachment theory and the regulation of emotion. In J. J. Gross (Ed.), *Handbook of emotion regulation* (pp. 446–465). New York: Guilford Press.

Shaver, P. R., & Norman, A. J. (1995). Attachment theory and counseling psychology: A commentary. *Counseling Psychologist, 23*, 491–500.

Shaver, P. R., Papalia, D., Clark, C. L., Koski, L. R., Tidwell, M., & Nalbone, D. (1996). Androgyny and attachment security: Two related models of optimal personality. *Personality and Social Psychology Bulletin, 22*, 582–597.

Shaver, P. R., Schachner, D. A., & Mikulincer, M. (2005). Attachment style, excessive reassurance seeking, relationship processes, and depression. *Personality and Social Psychology Bulletin, 31*, 343–359.

Shaver, P. R., Schwartz, J., Kirson, D., & O'Connor, C. (1987). Emotion knowledge: Further exploration of a prototype approach. *Journal of Personality and Social Psychology, 52*, 1061–1086.

Shaver, P. R., & Tancredy, C. M. (2001). Emotion, attachment, and bereavement: A conceptual commentary. In M. S. Stroebe, W. Stroebe, R. O. Hansson, & H. Schut (Eds.), *Handbook of bereavement research: Consequences, coping, and care* (pp. 63–88). Washington, DC: American Psychological Association.

Shealy, C. N. (1995). From Boys Town to *Oliver Twist*: Separating fact from fiction in welfare reform and out-of-home placement of children and youth. *American Psychologist, 50*, 565–580.

Shechtman, Z., & Rybko, J. (2004). Attachment style and observed initial self-disclosure as explanatory variables of group functioning. *Group Dynamics, 8*, 207–220.

Sheehan, G., & Noller, P. (2002). Adolescents' percep-tions of differential parenting: Links with attachment style and adolescent adjustment. *Personal Relationships, 9*, 173–190.

Shedler, J., Mayman, M., & Manis, M. (1993). The illusion of mental health. *American Psychologist, 48*, 1117–1131.

Sheldon, A. E., & West, M. (1990). Attachment pathology and low social skills in avoidant personality disorder: An exploratory study. *Canadian Journal of Psychiatry, 35*, 596–599.

Shi, L. (2003). The association between adult attachment styles and conflict resolution in romantic relationships. *American Journal of Family Therapy, 31*, 143–157.

Shields, C. G., Travis, L. A., & Rousseau, S. L. (2000). Marital attachment and adjustment in older couples coping with cancer. *Aging and Mental Health, 4*, 223–233.

Shorey, H. S., Snyder, C. R., Yang, X., & Lewin, M. R. (2003). The role of hope as a mediator in recollected parenting, adult attachment, and mental health. *Journal of Social and Clinical Psychology, 22*, 685–715.

Shuchter, S. R., & Zisook, S. (1993). The course of normal grief. In M. Stroebe, W. Stroebe, & R. O. Hansson (Eds.), *Handbook of bereavement* (pp. 23–43). New York: Cambridge University Press.

Sibley, C. G., Fischer, R., & Liu, J. H. (2005). Reliability and validity of the revised Experiences in Close Relationships (ECR-R) self-report measure of adult romantic attachment. *Personality and Social Psychology Bulletin, 31*, 1524–1536.

Sibley, C. G., & Liu, J. H. (2004). Short-term temporal stability and factor structure of the revised experiences in close relationships (ECR-R) measure of adult attachment. *Personality and Individual Differences, 36*, 969–975.

Silverberg, S. B., Vazsonyi, A. T., Schlegel, A. E., & Schmidt, S. (1998). Adolescent apprentices in Germany: Adult attachment, job expectations, and delinquency attitudes. *Journal of Adolescent Research, 13*, 254–271.

Simpson, J. A. (1990). Influence of attachment styles on romantic relationships. *Journal of Personality and Social Psychology, 59*, 971–980.

Simpson, J. A., & Gangestad, S. W. (1991). Individual differences in sociosexuality: Evidence for convergent and discriminant validity. *Journal of Personality and Social Psychology, 60*, 870–883.

Simpson, J. A., Ickes, W., & Blackstone, T. (1995). When the head protects the heart: Empathic accuracy in dating relationships. *Journal of Personality and Social Psychology, 69*, 629–641.

Simpson, J. A., Ickes, W., & Grich, J. (1999). When accuracy hurts: Reactions of anxious–ambivalent dating partners to a relationship-threatening situation. *Journal of Personality and Social Psychology, 76*, 754–769.

Simpson, J. A., & Rholes, W. S. (Eds.). (1998). *Attachment theory and close relationships*. New York: Guilford Press.

Simpson, J. A., & Rholes, W. S. (2002a). Attachment orientations, marriage, and the transition to parenthood. *Journal of Research in Personality, 36*, 622–628.

Simpson, J. A., & Rholes, W. S. (2002b). Fearful-avoidance, disorganization, and multiple working models: Some directions for future theory and research. *Attachment and Human Development, 4,* 223–229.

Simpson, J. A., & Rholes, W. S. (2004). Anxious attachment and depressive symptoms: An interpersonal perspective. In W. S. Rholes & J. A. Simpson (Eds.), *Adult attachment: Theory, research, and clinical implications* (pp. 408–437). New York: Guilford Press.

Simpson, J. A., Rholes, W. S., Campbell, L., Tran, S., & Wilson, C. L. (2003). Adult attachment, the transition to parenthood, and depressive symptoms. *Journal of Personality and Social Psychology, 84,* 1172–1187.

Simpson, J. A., Rholes, W. S., Campbell, L., & Wilson, C. L. (2003). Changes in attachment orientations across the transitions to parenthood. *Journal of Experimental Social Psychology, 39,* 317–331.

Simpson, J. A., Rholes, W. S., & Nelligan, J. S. (1992). Support seeking and support giving within couples in an anxiety-provoking situation: The role of attachment styles. *Journal of Personality and Social Psychology, 62,* 434–446.

Simpson, J. A., Rholes, W. S., Orina, M., & Grich, J. (2002). Working models of attachment, support giving, and support seeking in a stressful situation. *Personality and Social Psychology Bulletin, 28,* 598–608.

Simpson, J. A., Rholes, W. S., & Phillips, D. (1996). Conflict in close relationships: An attachment perspective. *Journal of Personality and Social Psychology, 71,* 899–914.

Skinner, B. F. (1953). *Science and human behavior.* New York: Macmillan.

Skovholt, T. M., Grier, T. L., & Hanson, M. R. (2001). Career counseling for longevity: Self-care and burnout prevention strategies for counselor resilience. *Journal of Career Development, 27,* 167–176.

Slade, A. (1999). Attachment theory and research: Implications for the theory and practice of individual psychotherapy with adults. In J. Cassidy & P. R. Shaver (Eds.), *Handbook of attachment: Theory, research, and clinical applications* (pp. 575–594). New York: Guilford Press.

Slade, A., Belsky, J., Aber, J., & Phelps, J. L. (1999). Mothers' representations of their relationships with their toddlers: Links to adult attachment and observed mothering. *Developmental Psychology, 35,* 611–619.

Slade, A., & Cohen, L. J. (1996). The process of parenting and the remembrance of things past. *Infant Mental Health Journal, 17,* 217–238.

Slade, A., Grienenberger, J., Bernbach, E., Levy, D., & Locker, A. (2005). Maternal reflective functioning, attachment, and the transmission gap: A preliminary study. *Attachment and Human Development, 7,* 283–298.

Smallbone, S. W., & Dadds, M. R. (1998). Childhood attachment and adult attachment in incarcerated adult male sex offenders. *Journal of Interpersonal Violence, 13,* 555–573.

Smallbone, S. W., & Dadds, M. R. (2000). Attach-ment and coercive sexual behavior. *Sexual Abuse: Journal of Research and Treatment, 12,* 3–15.

Smallbone, S. W., & Dadds, M. R. (2001). Further evidence for a relationship between attachment insecurity and coercive sexual behavior in nonoffenders. *Journal of Interpersonal Violence, 16,* 22–35.

Smith, C. A., & Ellsworth, P. C. (1987). Patterns of appraisal and emotion related to taking an exam. *Journal of Personality and Social Psychology, 52,* 475–488.

Smith, E. R., Murphy, J., & Coats, S. (1999). Attachment to groups: Theory and management. *Journal of Personality and Social Psychology, 77,* 94–110.

Smith, K. D., Keating, J. P., & Stotland, E. (1989). Altruism revisited: The effect of denying feedback on a victim's status to an empathic witness. *Journal of Personality and Social Psychology, 57,* 641–650.

Smolewska, K., & Dion, K. L. (2005). Narcissism and adult attachment: A multivariate approach. *Self and Identity, 4,* 59–68.

Snapp, C. M., & Leary, M. R. (2001). Hurt feelings among new acquaintances: Moderating effects of interpersonal familiarity. *Journal of Social and Personal Relationships, 18,* 315–326.

Snell, W. E. Jr., Overbey, G. A., & Brewer, A. L. (2005). Parenting perfectionism and the parenting role. *Personality and Individual Differences, 39,* 613–624.

Soares, I., Lemos, M. S., & Almeida, C. (2005). Attachment and motivational strategies in adolescence: Exploring links. *Adolescence, 40,* 129–154.

Solomon, J., & George, C. (1999). The measurement of attachment security in infancy and childhood. In J. Cassidy & P. R. Shaver (Eds.), *Handbook of attachment: Theory, research, and clinical applications* (pp. 287–316). New York: Guilford Press.

Solomon, Z., Ginzburg, K., Mikulincer, M., Neria, Y., & Ohry, A. (1998). Coping with war captivity: The role of attachment style. *European Journal of Personality, 12,* 271–285.

Sonnby-Borgstrom, M., & Jonsson, P. (2003). Models-of-self and models-of-others as related to facial muscle reactions at different levels of cognitive control. *Scandinavian Journal of Psychology, 44,* 141–151.

Sonnby-Borgstrom, M., & Jonsson, P. (2004). Dismissing-avoidant pattern of attachment and mimicry reactions at different levels of information processing. *Scandinavian Journal of Psychology, 45,* 103–113.

Sörensen, S., Webster, J. D., & Roggman, L. A. (2002). Adult attachment and preparing to provide care for older relatives. *Attachment and Human Development, 4,* 84–106.

Spangler, G., & Zimmermann, P. (1999). Attachment representation and emotion regulation in adolescents: A psychobiological perspective on internal working models. *Attachment and Human Development, 1,* 270–290.

Sperling, M. B., & Berman, W. H. (1991). An attachment classification of desperate love. *Journal of Personality Assessment, 56,* 45–55.

Sperling, M. B., & Berman, W. H. (Eds.). (1994). *Attachment in adults: Clinical and developmental perspectives.* New York: Guilford Press.

Sperling, M. B., & Berman, W. H., & Fagen, G. (1992). Classification of adult attachment: An integrative taxonomy from attachment and psychoanalytic theories. *Journal of Personality Assessment, 59,* 239–247.

Sperling, M. B., Sharp, J. L., & Fishler, P. H. (1991). On the nature of attachment in a borderline population: A preliminary investigation. *Psychological Reports, 68,* 543–546.

Sprecher, S., & Cate, R. M. (2004). Sexual satisfaction and sexual expression as predictors of relationship satisfaction and stability. In J. H. Harvey, A. Wenzel, & S. Sprecher (Eds.), *Handbook of sexuality in close relationships* (pp. 235–256). Mahwah, NJ: Erlbaum.

Sprecher, S., Felmlee, D., Metts, S., Fehr, B., & Vanni, D. (1998). Factors associated with distress following the breakup of a close relationship. *Journal of Social and Personal Relationships, 15,* 791–809.

Sprecher, S., & Regan, P. C. (1998). Passionate and companionate love in courting and young married couples. *Sociological Inquiry, 68,* 163–185.

Srivastava, S., & Beer, J. S. (2005). How self-evaluations relate to being liked by others: Integrating sociometer and attachment perspectives. *Journal of Personality and Social Psychology, 89,* 966–977.

Sroufe, L. A. (1978). Attachment and the roots of competence. *Human Nature, 1,* 50–57.

Sroufe, L. A. (1979). Socioemotional development. In J. Osofsky (Ed.), *Handbook of infant development* (pp. 462–516). New York: Wiley.

Sroufe, L. A. (1983). Infant–caregiver attachment and patterns of adaptation in preschool: The roots of maladaptation and competence. In M. Perlmutter (Ed.), *Minnesota Symposia on Child Psychology* (Vol. 16, pp. 16, 41–81). Minneapolis: University of Minnesota Press.

Sroufe, L. A., Egeland, B., Carlson, E., & Collins, W. A. (2005). *The development of the person: The Minnesota study of risk and adaptation from birth to adulthood.* New York: Guilford Press.

Sroufe, L. A., Egeland, B., & Kreutzer, T. (1990). The fate of early experience following developmental change: Longitudinal approaches to individual adaptation in childhood. *Child Development, 61,* 1363–1373.

Sroufe, L. A., Fox, N., & Pancake, V. (1983). Attachment and dependency in developmental perspective. *Child Development, 54,* 1615–1627.

Sroufe, L. A., & Waters, E. (1977a). Heart rate as a convergent measure in clinical and developmental research. *Merrill–Palmer Quarterly, 23,* 3–27.

Sroufe, L. A., & Waters, E. (1977b). Attachment as an organizational construct. *Child Development, 48,* 1184–1199.

Stackert, R. A., & Bursik, K. (2003). Why am I unsatisfied?: Adult attachment style, gendered irrational relationship beliefs, and young adult romantic relationship satisfaction. *Personality and Individual Differences, 34,* 1419–1429.

Stalker, C. A., & Davies, F. (1995). Attachment organization and adaptation in sexually abused women. *Canadian Journal of Psychiatry, 40,* 234–240.

Stalker, C. A., & Davies, F. (1998). Working models of attachment and representations of the object in a clinical sample of sexually abused women. *Bulletin of the Menninger Clinic, 62,* 334–335.

Stanojević, T.S. (2004). Adult attachment and prediction of close relationships. *Facta Universitatis, 3,* 67–81.

Steele, H., Phibbs, E., & Woods, R. T. (2004). Coherence of mind in daughter caregivers of mothers with dementia: Links with their mothers' joy and relatedness on reunion in a Strange Situation. *Attachment and Human Development, 6,* 439–450.

Steele, H., & Steele, M. (2005). Understanding and resolving emotional conflict: The London Parent–Child Project. In K. E. Grossmann, K. Grossmann, & E. Waters (Eds.), *Attachment from infancy to adulthood: The major longitudinal studies* (pp. 137–164). New York: Guilford Press.

Steele, H., Steele, M., & Fonagy, P. (1996). Associations among attachment classifications of mothers, fathers, and their infants. *Child Development, 67,* 541–555.

Stein, H., Koontz, A., Fonagy, P., Allen, J. G., Fultz, J., Brethour, J. R., et al. (2002). Adult attachment: What are the underlying dimensions? *Psychology and Psychotherapy, 75,* 77–91.

Steiner-Pappalardo, N. L., & Gurung, R. A. R. (2002). The femininity effect: Relationship quality, sex, gender, attachment, and significant-other concepts. *Personal Relationships, 9,* 313–325.

Stephan, C. W., & Bachman, G. F. (1999). What's sex got to do with it?: Attachment, love schemas, and sexuality. *Personal Relationships, 6,* 111–123.

Stern, J. (2003). *Terror in the name of God: Why religious militants kill.* New York: HarperCollins.

Sternberg, K. J., Lamb, M. E., Guterman, E., Abbott, C. B., & Dawud Noursi, S. (2005). Adolescents' perceptions of attachments to their mothers and fathers in families with histories of domestic violence: A longitudinal perspective. *Child Abuse and Neglect, 29,* 853–869.

Stober, J. (2003). Self-pity: Exploring the links to personality, control beliefs, and anger. *Journal of Personality, 71,* 183–220.

Strodl, E., & Noller, P. (2003). The relationship of adult attachment dimensions to depression and agoraphobia. *Personal Relationships, 10,* 171–185.

Stroebe, M., Hansson, R. O., Stroebe, W., & Schut, H. A. W. (Eds.). (2001). *Handbook of bereavement research: Consequences, coping, and care.* Washington, DC: American Psychological Association.

Stroebe, M., & Schut, H. A. W. (1999). The dual process model of coping with bereavement: Rationale and description. *Death Studies, 23,* 1–28.

Stroebe, M., Schut, H., & Stroebe, W. (2005). Attachment in coping with bereavement: A theoretical integration. *Review of General Psychology, 9,* 48–66.

Stroebe, W., & Stroebe, M. (1987). *Bereavement and health: The psychological and physical consequences of partner loss.* New York: Cambridge University Press.

Stroop, J. R. (1938). Factors affecting speed in serial verbal reactions. *Psychological Monographs, 50,* 38–48.

Styron, T., & Janoff-Bulman, R. (1997). Childhood attachment and abuse: Long-term effects on adult attachment, depression, and conflict resolution. *Child Abuse and Neglect, 21,* 1015–1023.

Sullivan, H. S. (1953). *The interpersonal theory of psychiatry.* New York: Norton.

Sumer, H., & Knight, P. A. (2001). How do people with different attachment styles balance work and family?: A personality perspective on work–family linkage. *Journal of Applied Psychology, 86,* 653–663.

Sumer, N., & Cozzarelli, C. (2004). The impact of adult attachment on partner and self-attributions and relationship quality. *Personal Relationships, 11,* 355–371.

Super, D. E., Savickas, M. L., & Super, C. M. (1996). The life-span, life-space approach to careers. In D. Brown & L. Brooks (Eds.), *Career choice and development: Applying contemporary theories to practice* (pp. 121–178). San Francisco: Jossey-Bass.

Susman-Stillman, A., Kalkose, M., Egeland, B., & Waldman, I. (1996). Infant temperament and maternal sensitivity as predictors of attachment security. *Infant Behavior and Development, 19,* 33–47.

Suomi, S. J. (1999). Attachment in rhesus monkeys. In J. Cassidy & P. R. Shaver (Eds.), *Handbook of attachment: Theory, research, and clinical applications* (pp. 181–197). New York: Guilford Press.

Swann, W. B., Jr. (1990). To be adored or to be known: The interplay of self-enhancement and self-verification. In R. M. Sorrentino & E. T. Higgins (Eds.), *Motivation and cognition* (Vol. 2, pp. 33–66). New York: Guilford Press.

Swanson, B., & Mallinckrodt, B. (2001). Family environment, love withdrawal, childhood sexual abuse, adult attachment. *Psychotherapy Research, 11,* 455–472.

Tacon, A. M., Caldera, Y. M., & Bell, N. J. (2001). Attachment style, emotional control, and breast cancer. *Families, Systems and Health, 19,* 319–326.

Tait, L., Birchwood, M., & Trower, P. (2004). Adapting to the challenge of psychosis: Personal resilience and the use of sealing-over (avoidant) coping strategies. *British Journal of Psychiatry, 185,* 410–415.

Tajfel, H. (1982). Social psychology and intergroup relations. *Annual Review of Psychology, 33,* 1–39.

Tajfel, H., & Turner, J. C. (1986). The social identity theory of intergroup behavior. In S. Worchel & W. Austin (Eds.), *Psychology of intergroup relations* (pp. 7–24). Chicago: Nelson.

Tangney, J. P. (1992). Situational determinants of shame and guilt in young adulthood. *Personality and Social Psychology Bulletin, 18,* 199–206.

Tangney, J. P., Baumeister, R. F., Boone, A. L. (2004). High self-control predicts good adjustment, less pathology, better grades, and interpersonal success. *Journal of Personality, 72,* 271–322.

Tangney, J. P., Hill-Barlow, D., Wagner, P. E., Marschall, D. E., Borenstein, J. K., Sanftner, J., et al. (1996). Assessing individual differences in constructive versus destructive responses to anger across the lifespan. *Journal of Personality and Social Psychology, 70,* 780–796.

Tarabulsy, G. M., Bernier, A., Provost, M. A., Maranda, J., Larose, S., Moss, E., et al. (2005). Another look inside the gap: Ecological contributions to the transmission of attachment in a sample of adolescent mother–infant dyads. *Developmental Psychology, 41,* 212–224.

Tasca, G. A., Ritchie, K., Conrad, G., Balfour, L., Gayton, J., Lybanon, V., & Bissada, H. (2006). Attachment scales predict outcome in a randomized controlled trial of two group therapies for binge eating disorder: An aptitude by treatment interaction. *Psychotherapy Research, 16,* 106–121.

Taubman-Ben-Ari, O., Findler, L., & Mikulincer, M. (2002). The effects of mortality salience on relationship strivings and beliefs: The moderating role of attachment style. *British Journal of Social Psychology, 41,* 419–441.

Tavecchio, L. W. C., & Thomeer, M. A. E. (1999). Attachment, social network, and homelessness in young people. *Social Behavior and Personality, 27,* 247–262.

Tayler, L., Parker, G., & Roy, K. (1995). Parental divorce and its effects on the quality of intimate relationships in adulthood. *Journal of Divorce and Remarriage, 24,* 181–202.

Taylor, R. E., Mann, A. H., White, N. J., & Goldberg, D. P. (2000). Attachment style in patients with unexplained physical complaints. *Psychological Medicine, 30,* 931–941.

Taylor, S. E., & Brown, J. D. (1988). Illusion and well-being: A social psychological perspective on mental health. *Psychology Bulletin, 103,* 193–210.

Tedeschi, R. G., & Calhoun, L. G. (2004). Posttraumatic growth: Conceptual foundations and empirical evidence. *Psychological Inquiry, 15,* 1–18.

TenElshof, J. K., & Furrow, J. L. (2000). The role of secure attachment in predicting spiritual maturity of students at a conservative seminary. *Journal of Psychology and Theology, 28,* 99–108.

Tennov, D. (1979). *Love and limerence: The experience of being in love.* New York: Stein & Day.

Teti, D. M., Sakin, J. W., Kucera, E., Corns, K. M., & Eiden, R. D. (1996). And baby makes four: Predictors of attachment security among preschool-age firstborns during the transition to siblinghood. *Child Development, 67,* 579–596.

Thelen, M. H., Sherman, M. D., & Borst, T. S. (1998). Fear of intimacy and attachment among rape survivors. *Behavior Modification, 22,* 108–116.

Thibault, J. W., & Kelley, H. H. (1959). *The social psychology of groups.* New York: Wiley.

Thoits, P. A. (1986). Social support as coping assistance. *Journal of Consulting and Clinical Psychology, 54,* 416–423.

Thomas, A., & Chess, S. (1977). *Temperament and development.* New York: Brunner/Mazel.

Thompson, R., & Zuroff, D. C. (1999). Development of self-criticism in adolescent girls: Roles of maternal dissatisfaction, maternal coldness, and insecure attachment. *Journal of Youth and Adolescence, 28,* 197–210.

Thompson, R., & Zuroff, D. C. (2004). The levels of self-criticism scale: Comparative self-criticism and internalized self-criticism. *Personality and Individual Differences, 36*, 419–430.

Thompson, R. A. (1999). Early attachment and later development. In J. Cassidy & P. R. Shaver (Eds.), *Handbook of attachment: Theory, research, and clinical applications* (pp. 265–286). New York: Guilford Press.

Thornhill, R., & Palmer, C. T. (2000). *A natural history of rape: Biological bases of sexual coercion.* Cambridge, MA: MIT Press.

Thorpe, S. J., & Salkovskis, P. M. (1995). Phobia beliefs: Do cognitive factors play a role in specific phobias? *Behaviour Research and Therapy, 33*, 805–816.

Tidwell, M. C. O., Reis, H. T., & Shaver, P. R. (1996). Attachment, attractiveness, and social interaction: A diary study. *Journal of Personality and Social Psychology, 71*, 729–745.

Tognoli, P. L. (1987). Reflection on Oedipus in Sophocles' tragedy and in clinical practice. *International Review of Psychoanalysis, 14*, 475–482.

Tokar, D. M., Withrow, J. R., Hall, R. J., & Moradi, B. (2003). Psychological separation, attachment security, vocational self-concept crystallization, and career indecision: A structural equation analysis. *Journal of Counseling Psychology, 50*, 3–19.

Tolmacz, R. (2001). The secure-base function in a therapeutic community for adolescents. *Therapeutic Communities: International Journal for Therapeutic and Supportive Organizations, 22*, 115–130.

Torquati, J. C., & Raffaelli, M. (2004). Daily experiences of emotions and social contexts of securely and insecurely attached young adults. *Journal of Adolescent Research, 19*, 740–758.

Torquati, J. C., & Vazsonyi, A. T. (1999). Attachment as an organizational construct for affect, appraisals, and coping of late adolescent females. *Journal of Youth and Adolescence, 28*, 545–562.

Touris, M., Kromelow, S., & Harding, C. (1995). Mother–firstborn attachment and the birth of a sibling. *American Journal of Orthopsychiatry, 65*, 293–297.

Townsend, A. L., & Franks, M. M. (1995). Binding ties: Closeness and conflict in adult children's caregiving relationships. *Psychology and Aging, 10*, 343–351.

Tracy, J. L., Shaver, P. R., Albino, A. W., & Cooper, M. L. (2003). Attachment styles and adolescent sexuality. In P. Florsheim (Ed.), *Adolescent romance and sexual behavior: Theory, research, and practical implications* (pp. 137–159). Mahwah, NJ: Erlbaum.

Travis, L. A., Bliwise, N. G., Binder, J. L., & Horne-Moyer, H. (2001). Changes in clients' attachment styles over the course of time-limited dynamic psychotherapy. *Psychotherapy, 38*, 149–159.

Treboux, D., Crowell, J. A., & Waters, E. (2004). When "new" meets "old": Configurations of adult attachment representations and their implications for marital functioning. *Developmental Psychology, 40*, 295–314.

Trinke, S. J., & Bartholomew, K. (1997). Hierarchies of attachment relationships in young adulthood. *Journal of Social and Personal Relationships, 14*, 603–625.

Troisi, A., & D'Argenio, A. (2004). The relationship between anger and depression in a clinical sample of young men: The role of insecure attachment. *Journal of Affective Disorders, 79*, 269–272.

Troisi, A., D'Argenio, A., Peracchio, F., & Petti, P. (2001). Insecure attachment and alexithymia in young men with mood symptoms. *Journal of Nervous and Mental Disease, 189*, 311–316.

Troisi, A., Massaroni, P., & Cuzzolaro, M. (2005). Early separation anxiety and adult attachment style in women with eating disorders. *British Journal of Clinical Psychology, 44*, 89–97.

Trull, T. J., Widiger, T. A., & Frances, A. J. (1987). Covariation of avoidant, schizoid, and dependent personality disorder criteria sets. *American Journal of Psychiatry, 144*, 767–771.

Trusty, J., Ng, K. M., & Watts, R. E. (2005). Model of effects of adult attachment on emotional empathy of counseling students. *Journal of Counseling and Development, 83*, 66–77.

Tucker, J. S., & Anders, S. L. (1998). Adult attachment style and nonverbal closeness in dating couples. *Journal of Nonverbal Behavior, 22*, 109–124.

Tucker, J. S., & Anders, S. L. (1999). Attachment style, interpersonal perception accuracy, and relationship satisfaction in dating couples. *Personality and Social Psychology Bulletin, 25*, 403–412.

Turan, B., Osar, Z., Turan, J. M., Ilkova, H., & Damci, T. (2003). Dismissing attachment and outcome in diabetes: The mediating role of coping. *Journal of Social and Clinical Psychology, 22*, 607–626.

Twaite, J. A., & Rodriguez-Srednicki, O. (2004). Childhood sexual and physical abuse and adult vulnerability to PTSD: The mediating effects of attachment and dissociation. *Journal of Child Sexual Abuse, 13*, 17–38.

Tweed, R. G., & Dutton, D. G. (1998). A comparison of impulsive and instrumental subgroups of batterers. *Violence and Victims, 13*, 217–230.

Tyrrell, C. L., & Dozier, M. (1997, March). *The role of attachment in therapeutic process and outcome for adults with serious psychiatric disorders.* Paper presented at the biennial meeting of Society for Research in Child Development, Washington, DC.

Tyrrell, C. L., Dozier, M., Teague, G. B., & Fallot, R. D. (1999). Effective treatment relationships for persons with serious psychiatric disorders: The importance of attachment states of mind. *Journal of Consulting and Clinical Psychology, 67*, 725–733.

van den Boom, D. C. (1994). The influence of temperament and mothering on attachment and exploration: An experimental manipulation of sensitive responsiveness among lower-class mothers with irritable infants. *Child Development, 65*, 1457–1477.

Van der Mark, I. L., van IJzendoorn, M. H., & Bakermans-Kranenburg, M. J. (2002). Development of empathy in girls during the second year of life: Associations with parenting, attachment, and temperament. *Social Development, 11*, 451–468.

Van Doorn, C., Kasl, S. V., Beery, L. C., Jacobs, S. C., & Prigerson, H. G. (1998). The influence of marital quality and attachment styles on traumatic grief and depressive symptoms. *Journal of Nervous and Mental Disease, 186,* 566–573.

van Ecke, Y., Chope, R. C., & Emmelkamp, P. M. G. (2005). Immigrants and attachment status: Research findings with Dutch and Belgian immigrants in California. *Social Behavior and Personality, 33,* 657–673.

Van Emmichoven, I. A., van IJzendoorn, M. H., de Ruiter, C., & Brosschot, J. F. (2003). Selective processing of threatening information: Effects of attachment representation and anxiety disorder on attention and memory. *Development and Psychopathology, 15,* 219–237.

van IJzendoorn, M. (1995). Adult attachment representations, parental responsiveness, and infant attachment: A meta-analysis on the predictive validity of the Adult Attachment Interview. *Psychological Bulletin, 117,* 387–403.

van IJzendoorn, M. (1996). Commentary. *Human Development, 39,* 224–231.

van IJzendoorn, M. H., & Bakermans-Kranenburg, M. J. (1997). Intergenerational transmission of attachment: A move to the contextual level. In L. Atkinson & J. K. Zucker (Eds.), *Attachment and psychopathology* (pp. 135–170). New York: Guilford Press.

van IJzendoorn, M. H., & Bakermans-Kranenburg, M. J. (2004). Maternal sensitivity and infant temperament in the formation of attachment. In G. Bremner & A. Slater (Eds.), *Theories of infant development* (pp. 233–257). Malden, MA: Blackwell.

van IJzendoorn, M. H., Feldbrugge, J., Derks, F. C. H., de Ruiter, C., Verhagen M. F., Philipse, M. W., et al. (1997). Attachment representations of personality-disordered criminal offenders. *American Journal of Orthopsychiatry, 67,* 449–459.

van IJzendoorn, M. H., Kranenburg, M. J., Zwart-Woudstra, H. A., Van Busschbach, A. M., & Lambermon, M. W. E. (1991). Parental attachment and children's socio-emotional development: Some findings on the validity of the Adult Attachment Interview in the Netherlands. *International Journal of Behavioral Development, 14,* 375–394.

van IJzendoorn, M. H., & Sagi, A. (1999). Cross-cultural patterns of attachment: Universal and contextual dimensions. In J. Cassidy & P. R. Shaver (Eds.), *Handbook of attachment: Theory, research, and clinical applications* (pp. 713–734). New York: Guilford Press.

van IJzendoorn, M. H., & Zwart-Woudstra, H. A. (1995). Adolescents' attachment representations and moral reasoning. *Journal of Genetic Psychology, 156,* 359–372.

Van Lange, P. A. M., DeBruin, E. M. N., Otten, W., & Joireman, J. A. (1997). Development of prosocial, individualistic, and competitive orientations: Theory and preliminary evidence. *Journal of Personality and Social Psychology, 73,* 733–746.

Van Overwalle, F., Mervielde, I., & De Schuyter, J. (1995). Structural modeling of the relationships between attributional dimensions, emotions, and performance of college freshmen. *Cognition and Emotion, 9,* 59–85.

Vasquez, K., Durik, A. M., & Hyde, J. S. (2002).

Family and work: Implications of adult attachment styles. *Personality and Social Psychology Bulletin, 28,* 874–886.

Vaughn, B. E., & Bost, K. K. (1999). Attachment and temperament: Redundant, independent, or interacting influences on interpersonal adaptation and personality development? In J. Cassidy & P. R. Shaver (Eds.), *Handbook of attachment: Theory, research, and clinical applications* (pp. 198–225). New York: Guilford Press.

Vaughn, B. E., Egeland, B. R., Sroufe, L. A., & Waters, E. (1979). Individual differences in infant–mother attachment at 12 and 18 months: Stability and change in families under stress. *Child Development, 50,* 971–975.

Versace, R., & Nevers, B. (2003). Word frequency effect on repetition priming as a function of prime duration and delay between the prime and the target. *British Journal of Psychology, 94,* 389–408.

Verschueren, K., & Marcoen, A. (1999). Representation of self and socioemotional competence in kindergartners: Differential and combined effects of attachment to mother and father. *Child Development, 70,* 183–201.

Vetere, A., & Myers, L. B. (2002). Repressive coping style and adult romantic attachment style: Is there a relationship? *Personality and Individual Differences, 32,* 799–807.

Vignoli, E., Croity Belz, S., Chapeland, V., de Fillipis, A., & Garcia, M. (2005). Career exploration in adolescents: The role of anxiety, attachment, and parenting style. *Journal of Vocational Behavior, 67,* 153–168.

Vivona, J. M. (2000). Parental attachment styles of late adolescents: Qualities of attachment relationships and consequences for adjustment. *Journal of Counseling Psychology, 47,* 316–329.

Vogel, D. L., & Wei, M. (2005). Adult attachment and help-seeking intent: The mediating roles of psychological distress and perceived social support. *Journal of Counseling Psychology, 52,* 347–357.

Volling, B. L., Notaro, P. C., & Larsen, J. J. (1998). Adult attachment styles: Relations with emotional well-being, marriage, and parenting. *Family Relations, 47,* 355–367.

Vondra, J. I., Hommerding, K. D., & Shaw, D. S. (1999). Stability and change in infant attachment style in a low-income sample. *Monographs of the Society for Research in Child Development, 64,* 119–144.

Vorauer, J. D., Cameron, J. J., Holmes, J. G., & Pearce, D. G. (2003). Invisible overtures: Fears of rejection and the signal amplification bias. *Journal of Personality and Social Psychology, 84,* 793–812.

Vormbrock, J. K. (1993). Attachment theory as applied to wartime and job-related marital separation. *Psychological Bulletin, 114,* 122–144.

Vrij, A., Paterson, B., Nunkoosing, K., Soukara, S., & Oosterwegel, A. (2003). Perceived advantages and disadvantages of secrets disclosure. *Personality and Individual Differences, 35,* 593–602.

Vungkhanching, M., Sher, K. J., Jackson, K. M., & Parra, G. R. (2004). Relation of attachment style to family history of alcoholism and alcohol use disorders in early adulthood. *Drug and Alcohol Dependence, 75,* 47–53.

Waddington, C. H. (1957). *The strategy of the genes.* London: Allen & Unwin.

Wade, T. J., & Brannigan, A. (1998). The genesis of adolescent risk-taking: Pathways through family, school, and peers. *Canadian Journal of Sociology, 23,* 1–19.

Waite, L. J., & Joyner, K. (2001). Emotional satisfaction and physical pleasure in sexual unions: Time horizon, sexual behavior, and sexual exclusivity. *Journal of Marriage and the Family, 63,* 247–264.

Waldinger, R. J., Seidman, E. L., Gerber, A. J., Liem, J. H., Allen, J. P., & Hauser, S. T. (2003). Attachment and core relationship themes: Wishes for autonomy and closeness in the narratives of securely and insecurely attached adults. *Psychotherapy Research, 13,* 77–98.

Walker, L. J., & Pitts, R. C. (1998). Naturalistic conceptions of moral maturity. *Developmental Psychology, 34,* 403–419.

Wallace, B. A. (2006). *The attention revolution: Unlocking the powers of the focused mind.* Boston: Wisdom.

Wallace, J. L., & Vaux, A. (1993). Social support network orientation: The role of adult attachment style. *Journal of Social and Clinical Psychology, 12,* 354–365.

Waller, E., Scheidt, C. E., & Hartmann, A. (2004). Attachment representation and illness behavior in somatoform disorders. *Journal of Nervous and Mental Disease, 192,* 200–209.

Walsh, A. (1992). Drug use and sexual behavior: Users, experimenters, and abstainers. *Journal of Social Psychology, 132,* 691–693.

Wampler, K. S., Shi, L., Nelson, B. S., & Kimball, T. G. (2003). The Adult Attachment Interview and observed couple interaction: Implications for an intergenerational perspective on couple therapy. *Family Process, 42,* 497–515.

Ward, A., Ramsay, R., & Treasure, J. (2000). Attachment research in eating disorders. *British Journal of Medical Psychology, 73,* 35–51.

Ward, A., Ramsay, R., Turnbull, S., Benedettini, M., & Treasure, J. (2000). Attachment patterns in eating disorders: Past in the present. *International Journal of Eating Disorders, 28,* 370–376.

Ward, A., Ramsay, R., Turnbull, S., Steele, M., Steele, H., & Treasure, J. (2001). Attachment in anorexia nervosa: A transgenerational perspective. *British Journal of Medical Psychology, 74,* 497–505.

Ward, M. J., & Carlson, E. A. (1995). Associations among adult attachment representations, maternal sensitivity, and infant–mother attachment in a sample of adolescent mothers. *Child Development, 66,* 69–79.

Ward, T., Hudson, S. M., & Marshall, W. L. (1996). Attachment style in sex offenders: A preliminary study. *Journal of Sex Research, 33,* 17–26.

Waskowic, T. D., & Chartier, B. M. (2003). Attachment and the experience of grief following the loss of a spouse. *Omega, 47,* 77–91.

Waters, E. (1978). The reliability and stability of individual differences in infant–mother attachment. *Child Development, 49,* 483–494.

Waters, E. (1994). *Attachment Behavior Q-set (Version 3).* Unpublished manuscript, State University of New York, Stony Brook.

Waters, E., Crowell, J., Elliott, M., Corcoran, D., & Treboux, D. (2002). Bowlby's secure base theory and the social/personality psychology of attachment styles: Work(s) in progress. *Attachment and Human Development, 4,* 230–242.

Waters, E., Merrick, S., Treboux, D., Crowell, J., & Albersheim, L. (2000). Attachment security in infancy and early adulthood: A twenty-year longitudinal study. *Child Development, 71,* 684–689.

Waters, H. S., Rodrigues, L. M., & Ridgeway, D. (1998). Cognitive underpinnings of narrative attachment assessment. *Journal of Experimental Child Psychology, 71,* 211–234.

Watt, M. C., McWilliams, L. A., & Campbell, A. G. (2005). Relations between anxiety sensitivity and attachment style dimensions. *Journal of Psychopathology and Behavioral Assessment, 27,* 191–200.

Watts, F. N., & Sharrock, R. (1984). Questionnaire dimensions of spider phobia. *Behaviour Research and Therapy, 22,* 575–580.

Wautier, G., & Blume, L. B. (2004). The effects of ego identity, gender role, and attachment on depression and anxiety in young adults. *Identity, 4,* 59–76.

Wayment, H. A. (2006). Attachment style, empathy, and helping following a collective loss: Evidence from the September 11 terrorist attack. *Attachment and Human Development, 8,* 1–9.

Wayment, H. A., & Vierthaler, J. (2002). Attachment style and bereavement reactions. *Journal of Loss and Trauma, 7,* 129–149.

Wearden, A. J., Cook, L., & Vaughan-Jones, J. (2003). Adult attachment, alexithymia, symptom reporting, and health-related coping. *Journal of Psychosomatic Research, 55,* 341–347.

Wearden, A. J., Lamberton, N., Crook, L., & Walsh, V. (2005). Adult attachment, alexithymia, and symptom reporting: An extension to the four category model of attachment. *Journal of Psychosomatic Research, 58,* 279–288.

Weems, C. F., Berman, S. L., Silverman, W. K., & Rodriguez, E. T. (2002). The relation between anxiety sensitivity and attachment style in adolescence and early adulthood. *Journal of Psychopathology and Behavioral Assessment, 24,* 159–168.

Weger, H., Jr., & Polcar, L. E. (2002). Attachment style and person-centered comforting. *Western Journal of Communication, 66,* 84–103.

Wegner, D. M. (1994). Ironic processes of mental control. *Psychological Review, 101,* 34–52.

Wegner, D. M., Erber, R., & Zanakos, S. (1993). Ironic processes in the mental control of mood and mood-related thoughts. *Journal of Personality and Social Psychology, 65,* 1093–1104.

Wegner, D. M., & Smart, L. (1997). Deep cognitive activation: A new approach to the unconscious. *Journal of Consulting and Clinical Psychology, 65,* 984–995.

Wei, M., Heppner, P., & Mallinckrodt, B. (2003). Perceived coping as a mediator between attachment and psychological distress: A structural equation modeling approach. *Journal of Counseling Psychology, 50,* 438–447.

Wei, M., Heppner, P. P., Russell, D. W., & Young, S. K. (2006). Maladaptive perfectionism and ineffective coping as mediators between attachment and future depression: A prospective analysis. *Journal of Counseling Psychology, 53,* 67–79.

Wei, M., Mallinckrodt, B., Larson, L. M., & Zakalik, R. A. (2005). Adult attachment, depressive symptoms, and validation from self versus others. *Journal of Counseling Psychology, 52,* 368–377.

Wei, M., Mallinckrodt, B., Russell, D. W., & Abraham, W. (2004). Maladaptive perfectionism as a mediator and moderator between adult attachment and depressive mood. *Journal of Counseling Psychology, 51,* 201–212.

Wei, M., Russell, D. W., Mallinckrodt, B., & Zakalik, R. A. (2004). Cultural equivalence of adult attachment across four ethnic groups: Factor structure, structured means, and associations with negative mood. *Journal of Counseling Psychology, 51,* 408–417.

Wei, M., Russell, D. W., & Zakalik, R. A. (2005). Adult attachment, social self-efficacy, self-disclosure, loneliness, and subsequent depression for freshman college students: A longitudinal study. *Journal of Counseling Psychology, 52,* 602–614.

Wei, M., Shaffer, P. A., Young, S. K., & Zakalik, R. A. (2005). Adult attachment, shame, depression, and loneliness: The mediating role of basic psychological needs satisfaction. *Journal of Counseling Psychology, 52,* 591–601.

Wei, M., Vogel, D. L., Ku, T. Y., & Zakalik, R. A. (2005). Adult attachment, affect regulation, negative mood, and interpersonal problems: The mediating roles of emotional reactivity and emotional cutoff. *Journal of Counseling Psychology, 52,* 14–24.

Weimer, B. L., Kerns, K. A., & Oldenburg, C. M. (2004). Adolescents' interactions with a best friend: Associations with attachment style. *Journal of Experimental Child Psychology, 88,* 102–120.

Weiner, B. (1985). An attributional theory of achievement motivation and emotion. *Psychological Review, 92,* 548–573.

Weinfield, N. S., Sroufe, L., & Egeland, B. (2000). Attachment from infancy to early adulthood in a high-risk sample: Continuity, discontinuity, and their correlates. *Child Development, 71,* 695–702.

Weinfield, N. S., Sroufe, L. A., Egeland, B., & Carlson, E. A. (1999). The nature of individual differences in infant–caregiver attachment. In J. Cassidy & P. R. Shaver (Eds.), *Handbook of attachment: Theory, research, and clinical applications* (pp. 68–88). New York: Guilford Press.

Weiss, R. S. (1973). *Loneliness: The experience of emotional and social isolation.* Cambridge, MA: MIT Press.

Weiss, R. S. (1975). *Marital separation.* New York: Basic Books.

Weiss, R. S. (1976). The emotional impact of marital separation. *Journal of Social Issues, 32,* 135–145.

Weiss, R. S. (1982). Attachment in adult life. In C. M. Parkes & J. Stevenson-Hinde (Eds.), *The place of attachment in human behavior* (pp. 171–184). New York: Basic Books.

Weiss, R. S. (1993). Loss and recovery. In M. S. Stroebe, W. Stroebe, & R. O. Hansson (Eds.), *Handbook of bereavement* (pp. 271–284). New York: Cambridge University Press.

Weiss, R. S. (1998). A taxonomy of relationships. *Journal of Social and Personal Relationships, 15,* 671–683.

Wekerle, C., & Wolfe, D. A. (1998). The role of child maltreatment and attachment style in adolescent relationship violence. *Development and Psychopathology, 10,* 571–586.

Wells, G. (2003). Lesbians in psychotherapy: Relationship of shame and attachment style. *Journal of Psychology and Human Sexuality, 15,* 101–116.

Wells, G., & Hansen, N. D. (2003). Lesbian shame: Its relationship to identity integration and attachment. *Journal of Homosexuality, 45,* 93–110.

West, M., & George, C. (2002). Attachment and dysthymia: The contributions of preoccupied attachment and agency of self to depression in women. *Attachment and Human Development, 4,* 278–293.

West, M., Keller, A., Links, P. S., & Patrick, J. (1993). Borderline disorder and attachment pathology. *Canadian Journal of Psychiatry, 38,* 16–22.

West, M., Rose, S. M., & Brewis, C. S. (1995). Anxious attachment and psychological distress in cardiac rehabilitation patients. *Journal of Clinical Psychology in Medical Settings, 2,* 167–178.

West, M., Rose, S. M., & Sheldon, A. (1993). Anxious attachment as a determinant of adult psychopathology. *Journal of Nervous and Mental Disease, 181,* 422–427.

West, M., Rose, S. M., & Sheldon-Keller, A. E. (1994). Assessment of patterns of insecure attachment in adults and application to dependent and schizoid personality disorders. *Journal of Personality Disorders, 8,* 249–256.

West, M., Rose, S. M., Verhoef, M. J., Spreng, S., & Bobey, M. (1998). Anxious attachment and self-reported depressive symptomatology in women. *Canadian Journal of Psychiatry, 43,* 294–297.

West, M., & Sheldon, A. E. (1988). The classification of pathological attachment patterns in adults. *Journal of Personality Disorders, 2,* 153–160.

West, M., & Sheldon-Keller, A. E. (1992). The assessment of dimensions relevant to adult reciprocal attachment. *Canadian Journal of Psychiatry, 37,* 600–606.

West, M., & Sheldon-Keller, A. E. (1994). *Patterns of relating: An adult attachment perspective.* New York: Guilford Press.

West, M., Spreng, S. W., Rose, S. M., & Adam, K. S. (1999). Relationship between attachment–felt security and history of suicidal behaviors in clinical adolescents. *Canadian Journal of Psychiatry, 44,* 578–582.

Westen, D. (1991). Clinical assessment of object relations using the TAT. *Journal of Personality Assessment, 56,* 56–74.

Westen, D. (1998). The scientific legacy of Sigmund Freud: Toward a psychodynamically informed psychological science. *Psychological Bulletin, 124,* 252–283.

Westmaas, J., & Silver, R. C. (2001). The role of

attachment in responses to victims of life crises. *Journal of Personality and Social Psychology, 80*, 425–438.

Whiffen, V. E. (2005). The role of partner characteristics in attachment insecurity and depressive symptoms. *Personal Relationships, 12*, 407–423.

Whiffen, V. E., Aube, J. A., Thompson, J. M., & Campbell, T. (2000). Attachment beliefs and interpersonal contexts associated with dependency and self-criticism. *Journal of Social and Clinical Psychology, 19*, 184–205.

Whiffen, V. E., Judd, M. E., & Aube, J. A. (1999). Intimate relationships moderate the association between childhood sexual abuse and depression. *Journal of Interpersonal Violence, 14*, 940–954.

Whiffen, V. E., Kallos-Lilly, A., & MacDonald, B. J. (2001). Depression and attachment in couples. *Cognitive Therapy and Research, 25*, 577–590.

Whiffen, V. E., Kerr, M. A., & Kallos-Lilly, V. (2005). Maternal depression, adult attachment, and children's emotional distress. *Family Process, 44*, 93–103.

Whisman, M. A., & Allan, L. E. (1996). Attachment and social cognition theories of romantic relationships: Convergent or complementary perspectives? *Journal of Social and Personal Relationships, 13*, 263–278.

Whisman, M. A., & McGarvey, A. L. (1995). Attachment, depressotypic cognitions, and dysphoria. *Cognitive Therapy and Research, 19*, 633–650.

Whitaker, D. J., Beach, S. R. H., Etherton, J., Wakefield, R., & Anderson, P. L. (1999). Attachment and expectations about future relationships: Moderation by accessibility. *Personal Relationships, 6*, 41–56.

White, R. W. (1965). The experience of schizophrenia. *Psychiatry, 28*, 199–211.

Whiters, L. A., & Vernon, L. L. (2006). To err is human: Embarrassment, attachment, and communication apprehension. *Personality and Individual Differences, 40*, 99–110.

Widiger, T. A., & Frances, A. (1985). The DSM-III personality disorders: Perspectives from psychology. *Archives of General Psychiatry, 42*, 615–623.

Wieselquist, J., Rusbult, C. E., Foster, C. A., & Agnew, C. R. (1999). Commitment, pro-relationship behavior, and trust in close relationships. *Journal of Personality and Social Psychology, 77*, 942–966.

Wiggins, J. S. (1979). A psychological taxonomy of trait descriptive terms: The interpersonal domain. *Journal of Personality and Social Psychology, 37*, 395–412.

Wiggins, J. S. (1991). Agency and communion as conceptual coordinates for the understanding and measurement of interpersonal behavior. In W. Grove & D. Cicchetti (Eds.), *Thinking clearly about psychology: Essays in honor of Paul E. Meehl* (Vol. 2, pp. 89–113). Minneapolis: University of Minnesota Press.

Wilkinson, R. B., & Walford, W. A. (2001). Attachment and personality in the psychological health of adolescents. *Personality and Individual Differences, 31*, 473–484.

Williams, N. L., & Riskind, J. H. (2004). Adult romantic attachment and cognitive vulnerabilities to anxiety and depression: Examining the interpersonal basis of vulnerability models. *Journal of Cognitive Psychotherapy, 18*, 7–24.

Williamson, G. M., Walters, A. S., & Shaffer, D. R. (2002). Caregiver models of self and others, coping, and depression: Predictors of depression in children with chronic pain. *Health Psychology, 21*, 405–410.

Wilson, J. S., & Costanzo, P. R. (1996). A preliminary study of attachment, attention, and schizotypy in early adulthood. *Journal of Social and Clinical Psychology, 15*, 231–260.

Wink, P. (1991). Two faces of narcissism. *Journal of Personality and Social Psychology, 61*, 590–597.

Winnicott, D. (1953). Transitional objects and transitional phenomena. *International Journal of Psycho-Analysis, 34*, 89–97.

Winnicott, D. W. (1965). *The maturational process and the facilitating environment*. London: Hogarth Press.

Wiseman, H., Mayseless, O., & Sharabany, R. (2005). Why are they lonely?: Perceived quality of early relationships with parents, attachment, personality predispositions, and loneliness in first-year university students. *Personality and Individual Differences, 40*, 237–248.

Wisman, A., & Koole, S. L. (2003). Hiding in the crowd: Can mortality salience promote affiliation with others who oppose one's worldview. *Journal of Personality and Social Psychology, 84*, 511–527.

Wismer Fries, A. B., Ziegler, T. E., Kurian, J. R., Jacoris, S., & Pollak, S. D. (2005). Early experience in humans is associated with changes in neuropeptides critical for regulating social behavior. *Proceedings of the National Academy of Sciences USA, 102*, 17237–17240.

Woike, B. A., Osier, T. J., & Candela, K. (1996). Attachment styles and violent imagery in thematic stories about relationships. *Personality and Social Psychology Bulletin, 22*, 1030–1034.

Wolpe, J. (1969). *The practice of behavior therapy*. New York: Pergamon Press.

Wolszon, L. R. (1998). Women's body image theory and research: A hermeneutic critique. *American Behavioral Scientist, 41*, 542–557.

Woodhouse, S. S., Schlosser, L. Z., Crook, R. E., Ligiero, D. P., & Gelso, C. J. (2003). Client attachment to therapist: Relations to transference and client recollections of parental caregiving. *Journal of Counseling Psychology, 50*, 395–408.

Wrosch, C., Scheier, M. F., Miller, G. E., Schultz, R., & Carver, C. S. (2003). Adaptive self-regulation of unattainable goals: Goal disengagement, goal reengagement, and subjective well-being. *Personality and Social Psychology Bulletin, 29*, 1494–1508.

Yalom, I. (1980). *Existential psychotherapy*. New York: Basic Books.

You, H. S., & Malley-Morrison, K. (2000). Young adult attachment styles and intimate relationships with close friends: A cross-cultural study of Koreans and Caucasian Americans. *Journal of Cross-Cultural Psychology, 31*, 528–534.

Young, A. M., & Acitelli, L. K. (1998). The role of attachment style and relationship status of the perceiver in the perceptions of romantic partner.

Journal of Social and Personal Relationships, 15, 161–173.

Young, J. Z. (1964). *A model for the brain.* London: Oxford University Press.

Zaleznik, A. (1992). Managers and leaders: Are they different? *Harvard Business Review,* 126–133.

Zakin, G., Solomon, Z., & Neria, Y. (2003). Hardiness, attachment style, and long-term psychological distress among Israeli POWs and combat veterans. *Personality and Individual Differences, 34,* 819–829.

Zayas, V., & Shoda, Y. (2005). Do automatic reactions elicited by thoughts of romantic partner, mother, and self relate to adult romantic attachment? *Personality and Social Psychology Bulletin, 31,* 1011–1025.

Zautra, A., Smith, B., Affleck, G., & Tennen, H. (2001). Examinations of chronic pain and affect relationships: Applications of a dynamic model of affect. *Journal of Consulting and Clinical Psychology, 69,* 786–795.

Zeanah, C. H., Benoit, D., Barton, M., Regan, C., Hirshberg, L. M., & Lipsitt, L. P. (1993). Representations of attachment in mothers and their one-year-old infants. *Journal of the American Academy of Child and Adolescent Psychiatry, 32,* 278–286.

Zeanah, C. H., Smyke, A. T., Koga, S. F., & Carlson, E. (2005). Attachment in institutionalized and community children in Romania. *Child Development, 76,* 1015–1028.

Zedeck, S. (1992). Introduction: Exploring the domain of work and family concerns. In S. Zedeck (Ed.), *Work, families, and organizations* (pp. 1–32). San Francisco: Jossey-Bass.

Zeidner, M., & Endler, N. S. (Eds.). (1996). *Handbook of coping: Theory, research, and applications.* Oxford, UK: Wiley.

Zeifman, D., & Hazan, C. (1997). A process model of adult attachment formation. In S. Duck (Ed.), *Handbook of personal relationships* (pp. 179–195). Chichester, UK: Wiley.

Zelenko, M., Kraemer, H., Huffman, L., Gschwendt, M., Pageler, N., & Steiner, H. (2005). Heart rate correlates of attachment status in young mothers and their infants. *Journal of the American Academy of Child and Adolescent Psychiatry, 44,* 470–476.

Zerbe, K. (1993). *The body betrayed: A deeper understanding of women, eating disorders, and treatment.* Carlsbad, CA: Gurze Books.

Zhang, F., & Hazan, C. (2002). Working models of attachment and person perception processes. *Personal Relationships, 9,* 225–235.

Zhang, F., & Labouvie-Vief, G. (2004). Stability and fluctuation in adult attachment style over a 6-year period. *Attachment and Human Development, 6,* 419–437.

Zimmermann, P. (2004). Attachment representations and characteristics of friendship relations during adolescence. *Journal of Experimental Child Psychology, 88,* 83–101.

Zimmermann, P., & Becker-Stoll, F. (2002). Stability of attachment representations during adolescence: The influence of ego-identity status. *Journal of Adolescence, 25,* 107–124.

Zimmermann, P., Fremmer-Bombik, E., Spangler, G., & Grossmann, K. E. (1997). Attachment in adolescence: A longitudinal perspective. In W. Koops, J. B. Hoeksma, & D. C. Van den Boom (Eds.), *Development of interaction and attachment: Traditional and non-traditional approaches* (pp. 281–292). Amsterdam: North-Holland.

Zimmermann, P., Maier, M. A., Winter, M., & Grossmann, K. E. (2001). Attachment and adolescents' emotion regulation during a joint problem-solving task with a friend. *International Journal of Behavioral Development, 25,* 331–343.

Zimmermann, P., Wulf, K., & Grossmann, K. E. (1997, July). *Attachment representation: You can see it in the face.* Poster presented at the biennial meeting of the International Society for the Study of Behavioral Development, Quebec, Canada.

Zisook, S., Schuchter, S. R., Sledge, P. A., Paulus, M. P., & Judd, L. W. (1994). The spectrum of depressive phenomena after spousal bereavement. *Journal of Clinical Psychiatry, 55,* 29–36.

Zuroff, D. C., & Blatt, S. J. (2006). The therapeutic relationship in the brief treatment of depression: Contributions to clinical improvement and enhanced adaptive capacities. *Journal of Consulting and Clinical Psychology, 74,* 199–206.

Zuroff, D. C., & Fitzpatrick, D. K. (1995). Depressive personality styles: Implications for adult attachment. *Personality and Individual Differences, 18,* 253–365.

Zuroff, D. C., Moskowitz, D. S., & Cote, S. (1999). Dependency, self-criticism, interpersonal behavior and affect: Evolutionary perspectives. *British Journal of Clinical Psychology, 38,* 231–250.

Index